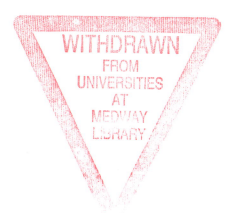

Handbook of Iron Overload Disorders

Handbook of Iron Overload Disorders

Edited by

James C. Barton
Medical Director, Southern Iron Disorders Center and Clinical Professor, Department of Medicine,
University of Alabama at Birmingham, Birmingham, Alabama, USA.

Corwin Q. Edwards
Director of Graduate Medical Education, Intermountain Medical Center and LDS Hospital, Professor of Medicine, Associate Director,
Internal Medicine Training Program, University of Utah School of Medicine, Salt Lake City, Utah, USA.

Pradyumna D. Phatak
Head, Hematology/Medical Oncology Unit, Rochester General Hospital, Rochester and Clinical Professor of Oncology,
Roswell Park Cancer Institute, Buffalo, New York, USA.

Robert S. Britton
Associate Research Professor, Department of Internal Medicine,
Saint Louis University School of Medicine, St. Louis, Missouri, USA.

Bruce R. Bacon
Director, Division of Gastroenterology and Hepatology,
Saint Louis University School of Medicine, St. Louis, Missouri, USA.

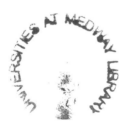

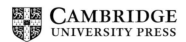

CAMBRIDGE
UNIVERSITY PRESS

CAMBRIDGE UNIVERSITY PRESS
Cambridge, New York, Melbourne, Madrid, Cape Town, Singapore,
São Paulo, Delhi, Dubai, Tokyo

Cambridge University Press
The Edinburgh Building, Cambridge CB2 8RU, UK

Published in the United States of America by
Cambridge University Press, New York

www.cambridge.org
Information on this title: www.cambridge.org/9780521873437

First published 2010

Printed in the United Kingdom at the University Press, Cambridge

A catalog record for this publication is available from the British Library

Library of Congress Cataloging-in-Publication Data
Handbook of iron overload disorders / James C. Barton ... [et al.].
     p. ; cm.
   Includes bibliographical references and index.
   ISBN 978-0-521-87343-7 (hardback)
1. Iron–Metabolism–Disorders–Handbooks, manuals, etc.   I. Barton,
James C.   II. Title.
   [DNLM: 1. Iron overload–physiopathology.   2. Iron–metabolism.
3. Iron overload–diagnosis.   4. Iron overload–therapy.
WD 200.5.I7 H236 2010]
   RC632.I7H36 2010
   616.1′52–dc22
                                                                          2010008738

ISBN 978-0-521-87343-7 Hardback

Contents

The color plates are to be found between 214 and 215.

Foreword

When Jim Barton and Corwin Edwards edited their multi-authored text *Hemochromatosis: Genetics, Pathophysiology, Diagnosis, and Treatment* published in 2000 by Cambridge University Press, it filled a void in learning resources for iron overload disorders, in particular those related to the then-recently discovered *HFE* gene and its common deleterious mutations. I commented in my Foreword to that text that "phenotypic expression ... was virtually invariable in individuals possessing the abnormal allele on both chromosomes 6." That statement has proved to be incorrect in the light of subsequent research demonstrating that phenotypic expression of *HFE* C282Y homozygous mutation is both unpredictable and variable in its manifestations. This reversal of previous dogma in genetic hemochromatosis and other important new data illustrate the need for an update on iron overload disorders in general.

In the 10 years since the publication of that text, much information has been discovered that provides new insights into the regulation of iron metabolism, and the causation and cosmopolitan distribution of diverse iron overload disorders. These discoveries have come about through the combined research efforts of many investigators, including biochemists, molecular biologists, experimental and clinical pathologists, geneticists, epidemiologists, clinical and research hematologists, and hepatologists. New iron-regulatory proteins and their genes have been discovered that provide an emerging awareness of the complexity of the integration and interactions of all genes, proteins, and tissues that participate in iron homeostasis in humans and other vertebrates.

It is not surprising that this awareness has brought confusion to the practicing clinician, who is often faced with the interpretation of an array of clinical data, laboratory tests, mutation analyses, and histopathological, epidemiological, and public health observations. Add to this confusion, patient questions regarding genetic guidance and one can understand the need for a succinct *Handbook of Iron Overload Disorders*.

Therefore, the decision to change from a multi-authored, highly detailed, large textbook to a smaller, more succinct, practical handbook may well have been prompted by these perceived needs of practicing clinicians. It is a tribute to the earlier editors and to Cambridge University Press that this has been achieved by condensing the author/editor team to just five experts, all recognized, authoritative "ferrophiles" (or "ferrophobes" – depending on their particular vantage points in the spectrum of iron-related disorders). They are, respectively, two hematologists, an internist/epidemiologist, a research experimental pathologist, and a clinical investigator/hepatologist. It is admirable that this combined endeavor has avoided compartmentation of their efforts by assuring that, while each of the five has taken primary responsibility for individual chapters, they have come together as a team to produce a cohesive product. Because each of them has contributed to every topic, one finds no identification of individual authorship for each chapter. In this way, the reader is offered the combined wisdom of some very wise, highly experienced experts.

The overall product of these efforts is unique in my experience, namely, a comprehensible handbook of practical information written with the authoritative imprimatur of recognized experts, while retaining a most accessible, succinct style worthy of the best monographs so respected by those of us who grew up in the era of the revered, professorial authority. In the relatively short space of 368 pages, readers will find valuable information and guidance on a myriad of iron overload disorders relevant to their respective practices. In addition to those disorders primarily related to dysregulation of iron absorption and metabolism, the reader will find new information about conditions, both genetic and acquired, in which iron is emerging as a significant contributor to progression or complications. Newer diagnostic tests are described and practical information is offered for the availability and interpretation of molecular genetic tests. Finally, innovative pharmacologic approaches to iron removal are described that offer renewed hope among those afflicted with iron overload disorders that are not amenable to phlebotomy management.

It remains a privilege for me to be able to write a Foreword to this most worthy handbook, with the knowledge that all who access the information and guidance contained within it will come away enthused by the topic of iron metabolism and iron overload disorders, and be far better equipped to handle the challenges of iron overload disorders in their daily practice.

Anthony S. Tavill MD, FACP, FRCP (London)
Professor Emeritus of Medicine, Case Western
Reserve University, Cleveland, Ohio, USA

Consultant Hepatologist and Morton Stone
Professor of Digestive and Liver Diseases,
Cleveland Clinic, Cleveland, Ohio, USA

Preface

Hemochromatosis and iron overload comprise a group of common disorders. Their ascent from curiosities at necropsy in the nineteenth century to clinically important conditions in the twenty-first century has been a long and difficult one. Eighty years passed from Trousseau's description of hemochromatosis in 1855 to Sheldon's suggestion in 1935 that this disorder was possibly heritable. Thirty-nine years later, Saddi and Feingold reported that the common type of hemochromatosis was inherited as an autosomal recessive trait. In 1975, Simon and colleagues demonstrated linkage of hemochromatosis to the human leukocyte antigen (HLA) complex on the short arm of chromosome 6, especially HLA-A*03. In 1988, Edwards and colleagues reported their observations of 11 065 Utah blood donors and their families who were evaluated with iron phenotyping, liver biopsies, and HLA typing. This landmark study demonstrated that hemochromatosis in western European whites is common, heritable, and often undetected. In 1996, Feder and colleagues discovered a HLA-linked hemochromatosis gene, now known as *HFE*. Subsequent important discoveries include those of non-*HFE* types of hemochromatosis, and the central role of hepcidin in controlling iron absorption.

The discovery of *HFE* stimulated a renaissance of learning about iron biology and disease. Using diverse plant and animal models and in vitro systems, basic scientists have explored the genetics, molecular biology, and toxicology of iron absorption and metabolism. Clinician scientists have sought unusual cases in their clinical rosters, study of which has permitted greater understanding of the genetics and pathophysiology of iron overload. Cooperative investigator groups have performed large screening studies to identify population and individual characteristics associated with hemochromatosis, iron overload, and deleterious iron-related mutations, and their respective implications for personal and public health.

Biochemists have designed new drugs to diminish morbidity and mortality among persons with heritable and acquired iron overload disorders. After almost 150 years, hemochromatosis and iron overload are recognized as common, treatable, and cosmopolitan disorders. The present authors contributed to a Cambridge University Press monograph entitled *"Hemochromatosis: Genetics, Pathophysiology, Diagnosis and Treatment"* published in 2000. Today, its applicability to diagnosis and treatment is limited, consistent with advances of the last decade.

Many patients with hemochromatosis or iron overload remain undiagnosed or untreated. Until now, there were few practical yet comprehensive learning resources for clinicians and other experts about these disorders. The Cambridge University Press *Handbook of Iron Overload Disorders* fulfills a need for a handy and affordable text on this topic. This up-to-date volume describes the signs and symptoms, laboratory and pathology testing, imaging procedures, genetics, differential diagnosis, and management of iron overload disorders in a convenient format supplemented with informative tables and figures. This handbook was designed to be used by primary care and internal medicine physicians, gastroenterologists, hepatologists, hematologists, endocrinologists, oncologists, cardiologists, rheumatologists, geneticists, genetic counselors, translational research investigators, and public health scientists. The ascent of hemochromatosis and iron overload to importance in daily office and hospital practice in 2010 inspired us to write the present handbook, and we hope that you will enjoy it.

James C. Barton, MD,
Corwin Q. Edwards, MD,
Pradyumna D. Phatak, MD,
Robert S. Britton, PhD, and
Bruce R. Bacon, MD.

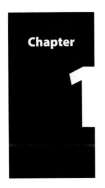

History of iron overload disorders

In 1704 in Berlin, Heinrich Diesbach and Johann Konrad Dippel attempted to manufacture a synthetic red pigment. By accident, Dippel mixed potash, animal oil derived from blood, and iron sulfate. Thereafter, he discovered that he had produced an insoluble, light-fast, dark blue pigment. This color was first used extensively to dye the uniforms of the Prussian army, and became known as "Prussian blue." Almost 150 years later, physicians and scientists recognized the feasibility of visualizing iron in tissue using a similar staining sequence. After more than 250 years, it became practical to quantify iron in blood and tissue, permitting case finding and screening for hemochromatosis and iron overload. Maneuvers to treat iron overload began in the same era. In the interval 1994–1996, the genetic bases of four different iron disorders (X-linked sideroblastic anemia, aceruloplasminemia, hereditary hyperferritinemia-cataract syndrome, and *HFE* hemochromatosis) were elucidated. The pace of basic science, clinical, and sociological revelations pertinent to hemochromatosis and iron overload disorders continues to accelerate. This chapter provides an abbreviated chronology of these discoveries.

Iron in tissue

In 1847, Rudolph Virchow reported the occurrence of golden brown granular pigment at sites of hemorrhage and congestion in tissue examined by microscopy. The pigment was soluble in sulfuric acid, yielded a red ash on ignition, and produced a positive Prussian blue reaction.[1] In 1867, Max Perls formulated the first practical acidified ferrocyanide reaction for histologic analysis of iron, and applied the staining reaction to a variety of tissues.[2] In 1962, Scheuer and colleagues reported a method of grading iron stained using Perls' technique in hepatic biopsy specimens in patients with hemochromatosis and their relatives, and described the characteristic gradient of iron distribution in hepatocytes in hemochromatosis.[3] The method is widely used today.

Iron overload disorders

Armand Trousseau described the syndrome of hepatic cirrhosis, pancreatic fibrosis, and cutaneous hyperpigmentation in 1865, but he did not recognize the involvement of iron in its pathogenesis (Table 1.1).[4] Troisier's account of *diabète bronzé et cirrhose pigmentaire* in 1871 confirmed and extended that of Trousseau, and described in detail the iron-reactive pigment in various tissues.[5] Troisier's syndromic triad became the *sine qua non* of hemochromatosis diagnosis for decades. In 1889, von Recklinghausen reported the use of the methods of Virchow and Perls to identify excess iron in tissues obtained at autopsy of persons who had *hämochromatose*.[6] Following the theories of Virchow, von Recklinghausen believed that the iron-containing pigment was derived from blood (due to hemorrhage or hemolysis), rather than from the primary deposition of iron. The syndrome of "juvenile hemochromatosis" was first recognized and described by French authors in the early 1930s who called it *le syndrome endocrine-hepato-cardiaque*.[7,8] Early cases were summarized by Royer de Vericourt in his 1935 thesis (Table 1.1).[9]

The first substantive characterization of iron overload in non-European peoples was published in 1929 by Scottish medical student A.S. Strachan.[10] He was appointed as the first Professor of Pathology in 1926 at the newly created Medical School of the University of the Witwatersrand in Johannesburg.[11] His 1929 thesis was based on a necropsy study of 876 individuals from several parts of southern and central Africa who died in Johannesburg from 1925 to 1928. Strachan concluded that

> haemochromatosis is a not uncommon disease in the South African native; the chief factor in its production

Table 1.1. An abbreviated chronology of major heritable primary iron overload disorders[a]

Disorder	Date, author of first clinical report	Gene (protein)	Date, author of first genetic definition	Reference(s)
HFE hemochromatosis	1871, Troisier	*HFE* (HFE)	1996, Feder	5,43
Early age-of-onset ("juvenile") hemochromatosis	1932, Bezançon	*TFR2* (transferrin receptor-2)	2000, Camaschella	65
		HAMP (hepcidin)	2003, Merryweather-Clarke; Roetto	66,67
		HJV (hemojuvelin)	2004, Papanikolaou	68
		SLC40A1 (ferroportin)[c]	2005, Sham	69
X-linked sideroblastic anemia	1945, Cooley	*ALAS2* (δ-aminolevulinate synthase)	1994, Cotter	70,71
Atransferrinemia	1961, Heilmeyer	*TF* (transferrin)	2000, Beutler	72,73
Aceruloplasminemia	1987, Miyajima	*CP* (ceruloplasmin)	1995, Harris; Yoshida	74–76
Hereditary hyperferritinemia-cataract syndrome[b]	1995, Beaumont; Girelli	*FTL* (ferritin light chain)	1995, Beaumont; Girelli	77–79
Autosomal dominant iron overload with predominance of macrophage iron deposition	1999, Pietrangelo	*SLC40A1* (ferroportin)[d]	2001, Montosi	80,81
Autosomal dominant iron overload	2001, Kato	*FTH1* (ferritin heavy chain)	2001, Kato	82
DMT1 hemochromatosis	2004, Priwitzerova	*DMT1* (divalent metal transporter-1)	2005, Mims	83,84
Anemia and iron overload due to glutaredoxin-5 deficiency	2007, Camaschella	*GLRX5* (glutaredoxin-5)	2007, Camaschella	85

Notes: [a]The clinical descriptions of the disorder and the genetic definitions were not necessarily made from the same subjects or kinships. There may be a heritable component of African iron overload, although a putative African iron overload gene[86] remains unidentified.
[b]Hereditary hyperferritinemia-cataract syndrome is not associated with iron overload, but is included here because it mimics autosomal iron overload in many kinships.
[c]"Gain-of function" *SLC40A1* mutations are typically associated with this phenotype.
[d]"Loss-of function" *SLC40A1* mutations are typically associated with this phenotype.

appears to be the diet. The development of the complete picture of bronzed diabetes depends on the degree of deposition of the pigment and the rate of its deposition.[10,11]

Possible causes of iron overload

In 1935, the English gerontologist Joseph H. Sheldon[12] (Fig. 1.1) summarized 311 carefully selected "haemochromatosis" cases from the literature.[13] He concluded that the absorption of iron (and possibly that of other metals) is increased in hemochromatosis, and suggested that the disorder is an inborn error of metabolism that primarily affects men. Sheldon rejected hypotheses that diabetes, infections, intoxication, alcoholism, and other conditions cause hemochromatosis, and he viewed Strachan's findings with skepticism.[11] In the 1960s, Richard A. MacDonald opined that iron overload and tissue and organ injury in whites with hemochromatosis are typical consequences of alcoholism and other nutritional factors, and not the result of an inborn error that enhances intestinal absorption of iron.[14] MacDonald

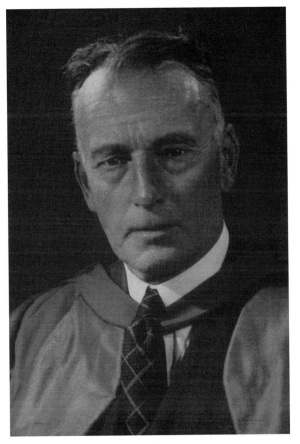

Fig. 1.1. Dr. Joseph H. Sheldon, an English gerontologist, was the author of the first monograph on hemochromatosis; his text was published in 1935.[12,13] Sheldon's observations on 311 cases carefully selected from the literature led him to conclude that iron absorption is increased in persons with hemochromatosis, and to suggest that the hemochromatosis is an inborn error of metabolism that primarily affects men.[13]

derived support of his opinion from Strachan's report of alcohol consumption and nutritional deficits in Native Africans with iron overload.

Many investigators subsequently published evidence of the central role of a heritable factor that increased iron absorption in whites with hemochromatosis, and recognized that the clinical phenotype of hemochromatosis was influenced by age, sex, and other attributes. In contrast, it was apparent in 1964 that the severity of iron overload in sub-Saharan Native Africans was directly related to their rate of consumption of iron contained in traditional beer.[15] In this disorder, hepatic iron concentrations usually exceeded those typical of alcoholism, and most Native Africans with iron overload

did not have histologic abnormalities of the liver typical of alcoholism.[11]

Diagnosis of hemochromatosis and iron overload

The 1962 histologic grading method of Scheuer and colleagues, and the availability of reliable clinical measurements of serum iron, total serum iron-binding capacity, and serum ferritin provided the standard basis for ascertaining the iron phenotype of hemochromatosis for more than 30 years. Phenotype variability among probands and the respective family members with hemochromatosis could be demonstrated using these techniques.[16,17] The hepatic iron index helped to distinguish presumed hemochromatosis homozygotes from heterozygotes and persons with alcoholism and other conditions,[18] although validity of the index in evaluating persons with non-*HFE* hemochromatosis or iron overload has not been established. SQUID (superconducting quantum interference device) and magnetic resonance imaging have been used as non-invasive techniques to estimate organ iron content since 1982 and 1983, respectively.[19,20]

Complications of iron overload

Since Troisier's account,[5] it has been generally acknowledged that the liver is the major target organ of iron overload in hemochromatosis (and many other iron overload disorders).[21] Bassett and co-workers demonstrated that the hepatic iron concentrations in hemochromatosis are directly related to the occurrence of cirrhosis.[18] This argues strongly for early diagnosis and treatment of iron overload, although some reports suggest that phlebotomy therapy may reverse cirrhosis in some patients.[22] Diabetes mellitus, once attributed only to iron overload of the pancreatic islets, is now associated primarily with insulin resistance, coincidental inheritance of other diabetogenic genes, and other factors. Accordingly, iron depletion changes diabetes control very little in most patients. Cardiac siderosis with cardiomyopathy and arrhythmias were first described in the 1930s,[9] and occur almost exclusively in persons with early age-of-onset ("juvenile") hemochromatosis due to mutations in the genes that encode transferrin receptor-2, hemojuvelin, hepcidin, or ferroportin. Hypogonadotrophic hypogonadism is widely recognized as the cause of *infantilisme* in children and young adults with early age-of-onset hemochromatosis, but also explains loss of libido and muscle mass and the development of osteoporosis in some men with *HFE* hemochromatosis. In 1964, Schumacher described a distinctive type of arthropathy that affects some persons with hemochromatosis.[23] Factor(s) other than hemochromatosis alleles or iron overload may cause this condition. The cutaneous abnormalities of hemochromatosis are more diverse than the hyperpigmentation described by Trousseau and Troisier.[24]

Iron overload injures the liver and other organs by causing discrete biochemical and microanatomical lesions.[25] Two major (but not mutually exclusive) mechanisms have been proposed to describe the toxicity induced by iron overload at the cellular and subcellular levels.[25] The oxidative injury hypothesis postulates that iron overload in vivo results in the formation of oxyradicals, with resultant damage to cellular constituents and impairment of cellular function. The lysosomal injury hypothesis proposes that excessive accumulation of iron within lysosomes can lead to lysosomal fragility, impaired lysosomal function, and eventual cellular injury through the release of hydrolytic enzymes and stored iron into the cytoplasm. In addition to lysosomes, iron-induced oxyradicals may damage hepatic mitochondria, endoplasmic reticulum, plasma membranes, and DNA.[25]

Iron is carcinogenic in humans and in laboratory animals.[26] The incidence rate of primary liver cancer in persons with hemochromatosis is high, especially in those with cirrhosis, as reported by Deugnier and colleagues in 1993.[27,28] African iron overload may be a risk factor for esophageal carcinoma. Mechanisms whereby iron may be involved in carcinogenesis include induction of oxidative damage of DNA, facilitation of tumor proliferation, and modifications of the immune system.[26] Common hepatic disorders such as alcoholism, steatosis, and viral hepatitis may augment liver injury and dysfunction in persons with hemochromatosis, and may also enhance liver iron deposition in persons with hemochromatosis or African iron overload.

Iron and immunity

Iron is essential to the normal function of neutrophils, macrophages, and lymphocytes, but iron overload impairs many functions of these cells.[29] Over several decades, there have been case reports of fulminant infections by unusual siderophilic bacteria, fungi, or trypanosomes in persons with hemochromatosis, iron overload, or chronic liver disease.[29,30] Infections are not generally reported as major causes of morbidity or mortality in persons with hemochromatosis, although a re-evaluation of the 1929 work of Strachan revealed that tuberculosis was a significant cause of death in black South Africans with iron overload.[10,11] In 1978, de Sousa and co-workers reported fundamental relationships of hemochromatosis, iron overload, and numbers of CD8+ lymphocytes.[31] In 2003, it was reported that approximately 30% of hemochromatosis probands have a form of heritable antibody deficiency linked to chromosome 6p.[32] In 2005, a significant inverse relationship of total blood lymphocyte counts and severity of iron overload in hemochromatosis probands was described,[33] extending the previous conclusions of de Sousa and co-workers. Altogether, immunity in patients with iron overload encompasses functions of infection resistance, modulation of iron overload, and tumor surveillance, and these may be decreased in some respects in many patients.

Treatment and outcomes

In 1952, Davis and Arrowsmith reported treating three persons with hemochromatosis with repeated phlebotomy.[34] A long-term study published in 1988 demonstrated that the longevity of hemochromatosis patients treated with phlebotomy was greater than that of untreated subjects.[35] Phlebotomy also permits an accurate (although retrospective) quantification of total body iron burdens in patients with hemochromatosis. In a prospective trial, Niederau and colleagues published in 1996 that hemochromatosis patients without hepatic cirrhosis or diabetes mellitus who undergo iron depletion have normal actuarial survival.[36]

In 1962, Sephton-Smith reported the use of the parenteral iron chelator deferoxamine to manage iron overload associated with severe thalassemia.[37] By 1994, it was demonstrated that the early use of deferoxamine in an amount proportional to the transfusion iron load reduces the body iron burden and helps protect against diabetes mellitus, cardiac disease, and early death in patients with thalassemia major.[38] In 1983, Kontoghiorghes and colleagues first reported the treatment of iron overload in thalassemia with the oral iron chelator deferiprone ("L1").[39] In 2003, Galanello and colleagues first reported the treatment of iron overload in thalassemia with the oral iron chelator deferasirox.[40]

Genetic basis of iron overload syndromes

In 1975, Simon and colleagues reported in a letter that the genetic factor associated with hemochromatosis was closely linked to the human leukocyte antigen (HLA)-A*03 locus on chromosome 6p.[41] By the late 1970s, HLA immunophenotyping was used to identify relatives of probands who also inherited two HLA-linked hemochromatosis alleles, sometimes before iron overload occurred. In 1977, Utah investigators reported the utility of various iron measures as diagnostic criteria for stages of hemochromatosis in patients and relatives.[16] In 1988, Edwards and colleagues used iron phenotyping and HLA typing to screen more than 11 000 white Utah blood donors for hemochromatosis, demonstrating clearly that hemochromatosis is a common heritable disorder expressed more prominently and frequently in men than women.[42]

In the half-century between 1945 and 1995, X-linked sideroblastic anemia, aceruloplasminemia, hereditary hyperferritinemia-cataract syndrome, and ferroportin hemochromatosis were described, and the heritable nature of each condition was proven or strongly suspected at first publication (Table 1.1).

In 1996, Feder and colleagues discovered a previously undocumented atypical major histocompatibility (MHC) class I gene on chromosome 6p by analyzing whites with hemochromatosis. In almost every case, the gene (later named *HFE*) contained the missense mutations C282Y or H63D (Table 1.1).[43] *HFE*, expressed only by certain tissues, encodes a protein that binds transferrin receptor and participates in controlling iron absorption. The C282Y mutation causes a significant disruption in the tertiary structure of HFE protein, and thereby a consequential loss of function. Homozygosity for *HFE* C282Y mutation occurs in approximately 90% of persons with hemochromatosis phenotypes, and this genotype defines "classical" hemochromatosis. As expected, C282Y occurs almost exclusively in whites of European descent. In contrast, the *HFE* H63D mutation occurs in almost all population groups worldwide, although it causes little change in HFE protein structure and thus is infrequently associated with increased iron absorption.

Today, *HFE* genotyping facilitates routine clinical evaluation and population screening for hemochromatosis, especially in European white populations. The discovery of *HFE* also kindled renewed enthusiasm for the study of iron among scientists and clinicians, leading to a "golden age" of discovery of many previously unknown proteins and control mechanisms germane to iron absorption and homeostasis, and to the clinical and genetic characterization of iron overload syndromes less common but no less informative than *HFE* hemochromatosis (Table 1.1).[44]

Population screening for hemochromatosis and iron overload

Severe iron overload is common in series of patients diagnosed to have hemochromatosis in medical care, and thus it was generally presumed for many years that most hemochromatosis (or C282Y) homozygotes would eventually develop injurious iron overload. Accordingly, population screening using iron phenotyping of white populations was promoted to achieve early diagnosis and permit timely treatment to alleviate iron overload.[45] In 2000, Beutler and colleagues reported the results of screening a large multiracial adult population in southern California using iron phenotyping and *HFE* genotyping. They revealed, to the surprise of many, that most C282Y homozygotes do not have symptoms or signs attributable to iron overload, that few have evidence of consequential liver disease, and that life expectancy for most is normal.[46,47] Other large screening studies in Norway, Australia, and North America confirmed the essence of these outcomes.[48–50] Each of two large screening studies in North America, including one that oversampled African Americans, Hispanics, and Asians, demonstrated that few non-whites had evidence of *HFE* hemochromatosis or non-transfusion iron overload.[46,50] In 2006, the US Preventive Services Task Force concluded that "Research addressing genetic screening for hereditary hemochromatosis remains insufficient to confidently project the impact of, or estimate the benefit from, widespread or high-risk genetic screening for hereditary hemochromatosis."[51,52] Regardless, there is substantial and rational support for hemochromatosis screening in certain subpopulations of whites, including selected family members of probands,[16,53,54] men,[42,55] persons with undiagnosed liver disease,[56] and those with serum ferritin >1000 μg/L.[57]

Social issues

After the discovery of *HFE* in 1996, there was heightened concern about the potentially negative social implications of phenotype or genotype diagnoses of heritable disorders, especially one as common as hemochromatosis. In 2003, Shaheen and colleagues reported that insurance denial and increased premium rates were reported commonly by hemochromatosis patients without end organ damage diagnosed in medical care, but the overall proportions with active insurance, good quality of life, and psychological well-being were similar to those of siblings without hemochromatosis.[58] In the HEIRS Study, there were only minor negative emotional responses to the genetic testing.[59,60] The risk of insurance or employment problems 1 year after phenotype and genotype screening for hemochromatosis and iron overload was also very low.[61] In the last decade, there has been much interest in utilizing hemochromatosis patients as blood donors. Altogether, many hemochromatosis patients and their donated units meet current blood bank criteria for acceptability, and policy changes to permit treatment-related blood donations without "labeling" the harvested blood units have been enacted.[62–64]

Conclusions

Pursuit of the etiology and treatment of hemochromatosis first described in western Europeans in the nineteenth century has led to a plethora of basic science discoveries and clinical revelations since 1996, the magnitude of which is unparalleled in the history of iron studies in living organisms. Many other important basic science and clinical truths about hemochromatosis and other iron overload disorders probably remain to be discovered and published. Future directions for clinical and basic science research in hemochromatosis and iron overload are discussed in Chapter 39.

References

1. Virchow R. *Die pathologischen Pigmente.* Arch Pathol Anat 1847; **1**: 379–486.

2. Perls M. *Nachweis von Eisenoxyd in gewissen Pigmenten. Virchow Arch Pathol Anat* 1867; **39**: 42–8.

3. Scheuer PJ, Williams R, Muir AR. Hepatic pathology in relatives of patients with haemochromatosis. *J Pathol Bacteriol* 1962; **84**: 53–64.

4. Trousseau A. *Glycosurie, diabète sucré.* Paris, J.-B. Baillière. 1865; 663–98.

5. Troisier M. *Diabète sucré. Bull Soc Anat Paris* 1871; **16**: 231–5.

6. von Recklinghausen FD. *Über hämochromatose. Tagebl Versamml Natur Ärtze Heidelberg* 1889; **62**: 324–5.

7. Bezançon F, de Gennes L, Delarue J, Oumensky V. *Cirrhose pigmentaire avec infantilisme et insuffisance cardiaque et aplasie endocriniennes multiples. Bull Mém Soc Med Hôp Paris* 1932; **48**: 967–74.

8. de Gennes L, Delarue J, de Vericourt R. *Sur un nouveau cas de cirrhose pigmentaire avec infantilisme et myocarde. Le syndrome endocrine-hepato-cardiaque. Bull Mem Soc Méd Hôp Paris* 1935; **51**: 1228.

9. de Vericourt R. *Le syndrome endocrino-hepato-myocardique (sur un aspect des cirrhoses pigmentaires).* Paris, 1935.

10. Strachan AS. Haemosiderosis and haemochromatosis in South African natives with a comment on the eiology of haemochromatosis. MD Thesis. University of Glasgow, 1929.

11. Gordeuk VR, McLaren CE, MacPhail AP, Deichsel G, Bothwell TH. Associations of iron overload in Africa with hepatocellular carcinoma and tuberculosis: Strachan's 1929 thesis revisited. *Blood* 1996; **87**: 3470–6.

12. Bacon BR. Joseph H. Sheldon and hereditary hemochromatosis: historical highlights. *J Lab Clin Med* 1989; **113**: 761–2.

13. Sheldon JH. *Haemochromatosis.* London, Oxford University Press, 1935.

14. MacDonald RA. *Hemochromatosis and Hemosiderosis.* Springfield, Charles C. Thomas, 1964.

15. Bothwell TH, Seftel H, Jacobs P, Torrance JD, Baumslag M. Iron overload in Bantu subjects. Studies on the availability of iron in Bantu beer. *Am J Clin Nutr* 1964; **14**: 47–51.

16. Edwards CQ, Carroll M, Bray P, Cartwright GE. Hereditary hemochromatosis. Diagnosis in siblings and children. *N Engl J Med* 1977; **297**: 7–13.

17. Cartwright GE, Edwards CQ, Kravitz K, *et al.* Hereditary hemochromatosis. Phenotypic expression of the disease. *N Engl J Med* 1979; **301**: 175–9.

18. Bassett ML, Halliday JW, Powell LW. Value of hepatic iron measurements in early hemochromatosis and determination of the critical iron level associated with fibrosis. *Hepatology* 1986; **6**: 24–9.

19. Brittenham GM, Farrell DE, Harris JW, *et al.* Magnetic-susceptibility measurement of human iron stores. *N Engl J Med* 1982; **307**: 1671–5.

20. Runge VM, Clanton JA, Smith FW, *et al.* Nuclear magnetic resonance of iron and copper disease states. *Am J Roentgenol* 1983; **141**: 943–8.

21. Brown KE, Bacon BR. Hepatic iron metabolism in hemochromatosis. In: Barton JC, Edwards CQ, eds. *Hemochromatosis. Genetics, Pathophysiology, Diagnosis and Treatment.* Cambridge, Cambridge University Press. 2000; 157–62.

22. Adams PC, Barton JC. Haemochromatosis. *Lancet* 2007; **370**: 1855–60.

23. Schumacher HRJ. Hemochromatosis and arthritis. *Arth Rheum* 1964; 7: 50.

24. Chevrant-Breton J. Cutaneous manifestations of hemochromatosis. In: Barton JC, Edwards CQ, eds. *Hemochromatosis. Genetics, Pathophysiology, Diagnosis and Treatment.* Cambridge, Cambridge University Press. 2000; 290–6.

25. Britton RS. Mechanisms of iron toxicity. In: Barton JC, Edwards CQ, eds. *Hemochromatosis. Genetics, Pathophysiology, Diagnosis and Treatment.* Cambridge, Cambridge University Press. 2000; 229–38.

26. Deugnier Y, Loréal O. Iron as a carcinogen. In: Barton JC, Edwards CQ, eds. *Hemochromatosis. Genetics, Pathophysiology, Diagnosis and Treatment.* Cambridge, Cambridge University Press. 2000; 239–49.

27. Deugnier YM, Charalambous P, le Quilleuc D, *et al.* Preneoplastic significance of hepatic iron-free foci in genetic hemochromatosis: a study of 185 patients. *Hepatology* 1993; **18**: 1363–9.

28. Deugnier YM, Guyader D, Crantock L, *et al.* Primary liver cancer in genetic hemochromatosis: a clinical, pathological, and pathogenetic study of 54 cases. *Gastroenterology* 1993; **104**: 228–34.

29. Brock JH. Role of iron in infections and immunity. In: Barton JC, Edwards CQ, eds. *Hemochromatosis. Genetics, Pathophysiology, Diagnosis and Treatment.* Cambridge, Cambridge University Press. 2000; 371–80.

30. Bullen JJ. Bacterial infections in hemochromatosis. In: Barton JC, Edwards CQ, eds. *Hemochromatosis. Genetics, Pathophysiology, Diagnosis and Treatment.* Cambridge, Cambridge University Press. 2000; 381–6.

31. de Sousa M, Porto G, Arosa FA, *et al.* T-lymphocyte expression and function in hemochromatosis. In: Barton JC, Edwards CQ, eds. *Hemochromatosis. Genetics, Pathophysiology, Diagnosis and Treatment.* Cambridge, Cambridge University Press. 2000; 396–410.

32. Barton JC, Bertoli LF, Acton RT. Common variable immunodeficiency and IgG subclass deficiency in central Alabama hemochromatosis probands homozygous for *HFE* C282Y. *Blood Cells Mol Dis* 2003; **31**: 102–11.

33. Barton JC, Wiener HW, Acton RT, Go RC. Total blood lymphocyte counts in hemochromatosis probands with *HFE* C282Y homozygosity: relationship to severity of iron overload and HLA-A and -B alleles and haplotypes. *BMC Blood Disord* 2005; **5**: 5.

34. Davis WD Jr, Arrowsmith WR. The effect of repeated phlebotomies in hemochromatosis; report of three cases. *J Lab Clin Med* 1952; **39**: 526–32.

35. Niederau C, Fischer R, Sonnenberg A, Stremmel W, Trampisch HJ, Strohmeyer G. Survival and causes of death in cirrhotic and in noncirrhotic patients with primary hemochromatosis. *N Engl J Med* 1985; **313**: 1256–62.

36. Niederau C, Fischer R, Purschel A, Stremmel W, Haussinger D, Strohmeyer G. Long-term survival in patients with hereditary hemochromatosis. *Gastroenterology* 1996; **110**: 1107–19.

37. Sephton-Smith R. Iron excretion in thalassemia major after administration of chelating agents. *Br Med J* 1962; **2**: 1577.

38. Brittenham GM, Griffith PM, Nienhuis AW, *et al.* Efficacy of deferoxamine in preventing complications of iron overload in patients with thalassemia major. *N Engl J Med* 1994; **331**: 567–73.

39. Kontoghiorghes GJ, Aldouri MA, Sheppard L, Hoffbrand AV. 1,2-Dimethyl-3-hydroxypyrid-4-one, an orally active chelator for treatment of iron overload. *Lancet* 1987; **1**: 1294–5.

40. Galanello R, Piga A, Alberti D, Rouan MC, Bigler H, Sechaud R. Safety, tolerability, and pharmacokinetics of ICL670, a new orally active iron-chelating agent in patients with transfusion-dependent iron overload due to beta-thalassemia. *J Clin Pharmacol* 2003; **43**: 565–72.

41. Simon M, Pawlotsky Y, Bourel M, Fauchet R, Genetet B. Hémochromatose idiopathique: maladie associée a l'antigéne tissulaire HLA 3? *Nouv Presse Méd* 1975; **19**: 1432.

42. Edwards CQ, Griffen LM, Goldgar D, Drummond C, Skolnick MH, Kushner JP. Prevalence of hemochromatosis among 11 065 presumably healthy blood donors. *N Engl J Med* 1988; **318**: 1355–62.

43. Feder JN, Gnirke A, Thomas W, *et al.* A novel MHC class I-like gene is mutated in patients with hereditary haemochromatosis. *Nat Genet* 1996; **13**: 399–408.

44. Andrews NC. Forging a field: the golden age of iron biology. *Blood* 2008; **112**: 219–30.

45. Phatak PD, Sham RL, Raubertas RF, *et al.* Prevalence of hereditary hemochromatosis in 16031 primary care patients. *Ann Intern Med* 1998; **129**: 954–61.

46. Beutler E, Felitti V, Gelbart T, Ho N. The effect of *HFE* genotypes on measurements of iron overload in

patients attending a health appraisal clinic. *Ann Intern Med* 2000; **133**: 329–37.

47. Beutler E, Felitti VJ. The C282Y mutation does not shorten life span. *Arch Intern Med* 2002; **162**: 1196–7.

48. Asberg A, Hveem K, Thorstensen K, *et al.* Screening for hemochromatosis: high prevalence and low morbidity in an unselected population of 65 238 persons. *Scand J Gastroenterol* 2001; **36**: 1108–15.

49. Olynyk JK, Cullen DJ, Aquilia S, Rossi E, Summerville L, Powell LW. A population-based study of the clinical expression of the hemochromatosis gene. *N Engl J Med* 1999; **341**: 718–24.

50. Adams PC, Reboussin DM, Barton JC, *et al.* Hemochromatosis and iron overload screening in a racially diverse population. *N Engl J Med* 2005; **352**: 1769–78.

51. Whitlock EP, Garlitz BA, Harris EL, Beil TL, Smith PR. Screening for hereditary hemochromatosis: a systematic review for the U.S. Preventive Services Task Force. *Ann Intern Med* 2006; **145**: 209–23.

52. Screening for hemochromatosis: recommendation statement. *Ann Intern Med* 2006; **145**: 204–8.

53. Barton JC, Rothenberg BE, Bertoli LF, Acton RT. Diagnosis of hemochromatosis in family members of probands: a comparison of phenotyping and *HFE* genotyping. *Genet Med* 1999; **1**: 89–93.

54. Acton RT, Barton JC, Passmore LV, *et al.* Accuracy of family history of hemochromatosis or iron overload: the hemochromatosis and iron overload screening study. *Clin Gastroenterol Hepatol* 2008.

55. Barton JC, Acton RT. Population screening for hemochromatosis: has the time finally come? *Curr Gastroenterol Rep* 2000; **2**: 18–26.

56. Bacon BR, Olynyk JK, Brunt EM, Britton RS, Wolff RK. *HFE* genotype in patients with hemochromatosis and other liver diseases. *Ann Intern Med* 1999; **130**: 953–62.

57. Waalen J, Felitti VJ, Gelbart T, Beutler E. Screening for hemochromatosis by measuring ferritin levels: a more effective approach. *Blood* 2008; **111**: 3373–6.

58. Shaheen NJ, Lawrence LB, Bacon BR, *et al.* Insurance, employment, and psychosocial consequences of a diagnosis of hereditary hemochromatosis in subjects without end organ damage. *Am J Gastroenterol* 2003; **98**: 1175–80.

59. Hicken BL, Calhoun DA, Barton JC, Tucker DC. Attitudes about and psychosocial outcomes of *HFE* genotyping for hemochromatosis. *Genet Test* 2004; **8**: 90–7.

60. Power TE, Adams PC, Barton JC, *et al.* Psychosocial impact of genetic testing for hemochromatosis in the HEIRS Study: a comparison of participants recruited in Canada and in the United States. *Genet Test* 2007; **11**: 55–64.

61. Hall MA, Barton JC, Adams PC, *et al.* Genetic screening for iron overload: No evidence of discrimination at 1 year. *J Fam Pract* 2007; **56**: 829–34.

62. Barton JC, Grindon AJ, Barton NH, Bertoli LF. Hemochromatosis probands as blood donors. *Transfusion* 1999; **39**: 578–85.

63. Brittenham GM, Klein HG, Kushner JP, Ajioka RS. Preserving the national blood supply. *Hematology Am Soc Hematol Educ Program* 2001; 422–32.

64. Power TE, Adams PC. Hemochromatosis patients as voluntary blood donors. *Can J Gastroenterol* 2004; **18**: 393–6.

65. Camaschella C, Roetto A, Cali A, *et al.* The gene *TFR2* is mutated in a new type of haemochromatosis mapping to 7q22. *Nat Genet* 2000; **25**: 14–15.

66. Merryweather-Clarke AT, Cadet E, Bomford A, *et al.* Digenic inheritance of mutations in *HAMP* and *HFE* results in different types of haemochromatosis. *Hum Mol Genet* 2003; **12**: 2241–7.

67. Roetto A, Papanikolaou G, Politou M, *et al.* Mutant antimicrobial peptide hepcidin is associated with severe juvenile hemochromatosis. *Nat Genet* 2003; **33**: 21–2.

68. Papanikolaou G, Samuels ME, Ludwig EH, *et al.* Mutations in *HFE2* cause iron overload in chromosome 1q-linked juvenile hemochromatosis. *Nat Genet* 2004; **36**: 77–82.

69. Sham RL, Phatak PD, West C, Lee P, Andrews C, Beutler E. Autosomal dominant hereditary hemochromatosis associated with a novel ferroportin mutation and unique clinical features. *Blood Cells Mol Dis* 2005; **34**: 157–61.

70. Cooley TB. A severe type of hereditary anemia with elliptocytosis: interesting sequence of splenectomy. *Am J Med Sci* 1945; **209**: 561–8.

71. Cotter PD, Rucknagel DL, Bishop DF. X-linked sideroblastic anemia: identification of the mutation in the erythroid-specific delta-aminolevulinate synthase gene (*ALAS2*) in the original family described by Cooley. *Blood* 1994; **84**: 3915–24.

72. Heilmeyer L, Keller W, Vivell O, *et al.* [Congenital atransferrinemia in a 7-year-old girl.] *Dtsch Med Wochenschr* 1961; **86**: 1745–51.

73. Beutler E, Gelbart T, Lee P, Trevino R, Fernandez MA, Fairbanks VF. Molecular characterization of a case of atransferrinemia. *Blood* 2000; **96**: 4071–4.

74. Miyajima H, Nishimura Y, Mizoguchi K, Sakamoto M, Shimizu T, Honda N. Familial apoceruloplasmin deficiency associated with blepharospasm and retinal degeneration. *Neurology* 1987; **37**: 761–7.

75. Harris ZL, Takahashi Y, Miyajima H, Serizawa M, MacGillivray RT, Gitlin JD. Aceruloplasminemia:

molecular characterization of this disorder of iron metabolism. *Proc Natl Acad Sci USA* 1995; **92**: 2539–43.

76. Yoshida K, Furihata K, Takeda S, *et al.* A mutation in the ceruloplasmin gene is associated with systemic hemosiderosis in humans. *Nat Genet* 1995; **9**: 267–72.

77. Beaumont C, Leneuve P, Devaux I, *et al.* Mutation in the iron responsive element of the L ferritin mRNA in a family with dominant hyperferritinaemia and cataract. *Nat Genet* 1995; **11**: 444–6.

78. Girelli D, Corrocher R, Bisceglia L, *et al.* Molecular basis for the recently described hereditary hyperferritinemia-cataract syndrome: a mutation in the iron-responsive element of ferritin L-subunit gene (the "Verona mutation"). *Blood* 1995; **86**: 4050–3.

79. Girelli D, Olivieri O, De Franceschi L, Corrocher R, Bergamaschi G, Cazzola M. A linkage between hereditary hyperferritinaemia not related to iron overload and autosomal dominant congenital cataract. *Br J Haematol* 1995; **90**: 931–4.

80. Pietrangelo A, Montosi G, Totaro A, *et al.* Hereditary hemochromatosis in adults without pathogenic mutations in the hemochromatosis gene. *N Engl J Med* 1999; **341**: 725–32.

81. Montosi G, Donovan A, Totaro A, *et al.* Autosomal-dominant hemochromatosis is associated with a mutation in the ferroportin (*SLC11A3*) gene. *J Clin Invest* 2001; **108**: 619–23.

82. Kato J. [Mutation of H-ferritin gene in a family associated with hereditary iron overload: a new iron overload-related gene?] *Rinsho Ketsueki* 2001; **42**: 403–7.

83. Priwitzerova M, Pospisilova D, Prchal JT, *et al.* Severe hypochromic microcytic anemia caused by a congenital defect of the iron transport pathway in erythroid cells. *Blood* 2004; **103**: 3991–2.

84. Mims MP, Guan Y, Pospisilova D, *et al.* Identification of a human mutation of *DMT1* in a patient with microcytic anemia and iron overload. *Blood* 2005; **105**: 1337–42.

85. Camaschella C, Campanella A, De Falco L, *et al.* The human counterpart of zebrafish *shiraz* shows sideroblastic-like microcytic anemia and iron overload. *Blood* 2007; **110**: 1353–8.

86. Gordeuk V, Mukiibi J, Hasstedt SJ, *et al.* Iron overload in Africa. Interaction between a gene and dietary iron content. *N Engl J Med* 1992; **326**: 95–100.

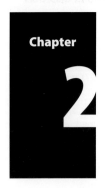

Chapter

2

Normal iron absorption and metabolism

Iron is essential to life because it is the central oxygen ligand in the heme proteins hemoglobin and myoglobin. Accordingly, there are many interactions between iron homeostasis and oxygen regulation and delivery. Iron is also required for cytochrome P-450 enzyme oxidative metabolism and DNA synthesis. In health, body iron content is controlled by absorption that responds to iron losses and the rate of erythropoiesis. Multiple mechanisms provide functional feedback control of iron homeostasis, tissue oxygen sensing and delivery, and the tempo of red blood cell production. The physiologic capacity to excrete iron is very limited. Thus, body iron content is regulated almost entirely by controlled absorption.[1,2] This chapter reviews the basic physiologic and molecular characteristics of iron metabolism and homeostasis, and their pertinence to iron overload disorders.

Iron physiology

Normal iron homeostasis is maintained by absorption of iron from the diet that precisely balances iron loss, and by controlled iron distribution in the body.[1,3] Normal healthy adults have 4000–5000 mg of iron (Table 2.1). Daily iron loss occurs due to perspiration, desquamation from skin, and minor injuries, and from the gastrointestinal tract. The rate of this unavoidable iron loss is proportional to body iron stores. Women lose additional iron due to menstruation, pregnancy and childbirth, and lactation. Overall, daily iron losses in adult men and post-menopausal women are approximately 1.0 mg and in menstruating women approximately 1.5 mg. The median iron loss ascribable to pregnancy is 500 mg.[4] Iron requirements of growth and development in infants or adolescents may exceed those of normal adults severalfold.

Hemoglobin in erythrocytes constitutes the largest normal body iron pool. Developing erythroid cells in the bone marrow highly express surface transferrin receptors to obtain iron for hemoglobin synthesis. In healthy adults, red blood cell production is ∼2 million cells/second. Normal erythropoiesis requires the delivery of ∼25 mg Fe daily to erythroid cells via transferrin. This amount far exceeds the amount of iron needed to replenish stores. The quantity of iron in the circulating erythrocyte mass is usually stable, although this may change as an adaptation to altitude, lung disease, cigarette smoking, or other conditions that affect oxygen availability. Erythropoiesis stimulated by blood loss, hemolysis, erythropoietin, or hypoxemia requires an additional 10–40 mg Fe daily. Mature erythrocytes filled with hemoglobin circulate in the blood. Many physiology experiments of past decades sought to identify the "erythropoiesis regulator," a substance now generally acknowledged to be erythropoietin.

Hepatocytes and macrophages (including Kupffer cells) contain storage iron, and represent the second largest normal iron pool. In health, the quantity of iron present in hepatocytes and macrophages is nonetheless relatively small in comparison with the erythroid compartment, especially in women of reproductive age. Amounts of stored iron in these sites sometimes increases with age. Many physiology experiments of past decades also sought to identify the "stores regulator," now acknowledged to be hepcidin.

Myoglobin, the third largest iron pool, contains heme moieties in myoglobin that are necessary for normal muscle and cardiac function. The quantity of iron in myoglobin iron is relatively stable, although it increases with growth and development and decreases with age or catabolism. At high altitude, iron needed for erythropoiesis may be donated by myoglobin.

Typical daily western diets contain 10–20 mg of iron. Many vegetarian diets contain less iron, but the quantity is nonetheless sufficient to replace daily iron losses. There are two major forms of intrinsic food

Table 2.1. Iron in healthy adults[a]

Location	Primary function(s)	Amount, mg
Erythrocytes	O_2 transport via hemoglobin	1800
Liver	Storage as ferritin, hemosiderin	1000
Muscle (including heart, smooth muscle)	Energy storage, transfer by myoglobin	300
Marrow	Hemoglobin in erythroblasts; macrophage stores as ferritin, hemosiderin after phagocytosis of senescent erythrocytes	300
Multiple tissues	Energy storage, transfer as cytochromes, catalase, peroxidase; iron sensing as iron-responsive proteins	8
Plasma	Transport by transferrin[b]	3
Skin, gastrointestinal tract, uterus, other sites	Unavoidable losses due to desquamation, minor trauma, menstruation, pregnancy, lactation	1–3[c]
Small intestine	Absorption[d]	1–3

Notes: [a]Most normal body cells contain iron. Iron quantities in most sites is typically greater in men than in women. Body iron increases with age. Normal brain and heart function depend critically on iron, although absolute levels of iron in these organs are difficult to measure directly, except at necropsy. Relative quantities can be estimated using magnetic resonance imaging techniques or a superconducting quantum interference device (SQUID) (Chapter 4).
[b]Average daily iron transport is ~24 mg.
[c]Average cumulative daily iron losses.
[d]Equals cumulative unavoidable daily iron losses.

iron: (1) non-heme iron compounds inherent to many animal and plant foodstuffs; and (2) heme iron in hemoglobin, myoglobin, and other heme compounds.[2] Extrinsic inorganic iron is sometimes used to fortify foodstuffs, and may be inadvertently imparted to foods from soil or iron cooking vessels, or ingested as dietary, or medicinal supplements. In general, dietary inorganic iron occurs in a greater proportion but is less readily absorbed than heme iron. Dietary and intraluminal factors in the gastrointestinal tract also alter the suitability of iron for absorption, largely by affecting secretion of gastric acid, promoting or inhibiting the release of iron compounds from foodstuffs, or altering the solubility of iron moieties.[2]

Iron homeostasis
Iron storage

Ferritin is an intracellular storage molecule that sequesters iron (Table 2.2). This prevents or reduces intracellular damage due to the formation of oxyradicals. Apoferritin, a heteropolymer of 24 subunits, forms a hollow nanocage that can store as many as 4500 ferric ions (Fe^{3+}) per molecule.[5] Ferritin is composed of L (light or liver) and H (heavy or heart) chains or subunits. L-subunits have ferroxidase activity that is necessary for entry of iron into the ferritin shell.[6–8] H-subunits facilitate formation of the iron core of ferritin.[6–8] Most ferritin is intracellular. Hepatocytes and reticuloendothelial macrophages contain relatively large amounts of ferritin; smaller quantities occur in early erythroid precursors, myocardial fibers, and a variety of other cells.

A small proportion of ferritin undergoes glycosylation and is secreted into the plasma, although the function of this ferritin is unknown. Injury of cells that normally contain large quantities of ferritin, e.g. hepatocytes, may increase serum ferritin levels. Certain types of neoplastic cells autonomously produce large quantities of apoferritin without regard to body iron quantities. Chronic ethanol ingestion stimulates hepatic synthesis or secretion of ferritin in some subjects. Accordingly, levels of ferritin in plasma or serum are indicators not only of the degree of iron repletion, but elevated levels are also markers of liver injury, myocardial infarction, inflammation, or malignancy. Ferritin is the primary component of hemosiderin, an aggregate of partially degraded ferritin, lysosomes, and other material.[9] Ferritin depleted of iron undergoes ubiquitination and destruction in proteasomes.[10]

Iron procurement

Transferrin is a glycoprotein that binds and transports iron (Table 2.3). Most transferrin in the plasma is produced by hepatocytes; smaller quantities are

Table 2.2. Some proteins that alter the chemical form of iron or heme

Protein	Location	Function, properties	Gene; chromosome	OMIM designation[a]
Ferritin L-subunit	Hepatocytes, macrophages, most other cells	Forms 24-mer nanocage with H-subunits for iron storage as ferrihydrite; promotes iron entry into nanocage	*FTL*; 9q13.3–q13.4	*134790
Ferritin H-subunit	Hepatocytes, macrophages, most other cells	Forms 24-mer nanocage with L-subunits for iron storage as ferrihydrite; facilitates formation of iron core	*FTH1*; 11q12–q13	*134770
Cytochrome b reductase 1 (duodenal cytochrome b; DCYTB)	Duodenal microvilli	Reduces Fe^{3+} to Fe^{2+}, promotes iron entry into luminal surfaces of enterocytes	*CYBRD1* (*DCYTB*); 2	*605745
Ceruloplasmin	Synthesized by liver; found in brain, lung, other tissues, plasma; not in intestine	Multicopper oxidase, oxidizes Fe^{2+} to Fe^{3+}, promotes iron-binding to transferrin; homologue of hephaestin	*CP*; 3q23–q24	*117700
Hephaestin	Basolateral surfaces of villus tip enterocytes, central nervous system, retina	Multicopper oxidase, oxidizes Fe^{2+} to Fe^{3+}, promotes iron egress from enterocytes; homologue of ceruloplasmin	*HEPH*; Xq11–q12	*300167
Heme oxygenase 1	Enterocytes, macrophages, lung, many other cell types	Cleaves heme to form biliverdin; essential for heme catabolism; inducible	*HMOX1*; 22q12	+141250
Heme oxygenase 2	Endothelial cells, adventitial nerves of blood vessels, neurons in autonomic ganglia, lung	Cleaves heme to form biliverdin; enzyme is constitutive	*HMOX2*; 16q13.3	*141251

Note: [a]Online Mendelian Inheritance in Man database. (http://www.ncbi.nlm.nih.gov/sites/entrez?db=omim).

produced by other cell types. In mammals, transferrin without bound iron (apotransferrin) contains two iron-binding lobes that probably arose due to duplication of a primitive transferrin gene that encoded mono-sited transferrin. Human apotransferrin can bind two ferric (Fe^{3+}) ions per molecule in a pH-dependent manner; iron-saturated transferrin is called holotransferrin. Most iron that normally circulates in the plasma or in extracellular fluid is bound to transferrin, and this prevents cellular injury that could be caused by highly reactive, non-transferrin-bound iron (NTBI). Although transferrin-bound iron is a relatively small body compartment by static measurements, this iron pool turns over approximately

eight times daily in normal persons. In health, approximately one-third of the total iron-binding sites on transferrin molecules in the plasma are saturated with iron. The ratio of iron bound to transferrin to the total iron-binding capacity of transferrin is expressed as transferrin saturation. In certain types of hemochromatosis or iron overload of some other causes, transferrin saturation is typically elevated (Chapters 4, 8). Transferrin saturation is typically normal or low in other iron overload disorders and in iron deficiency.

Transferrin delivers iron to cells that bear the classical transferrin receptor TFR1 (Table 2.3). These cells preferentially bind diferric transferrin.

Table 2.3. Some proteins that bind or transport iron or heme

Protein	Location	Function, properties	Gene; chromosome	OMIM designation[a]
Transferrin	Plasma, bile; produced in liver	Plasma iron transport	TF; 3q21	*190000
Transferrin receptor-1 (TFR1)	Surfaces of most cells, especially erythroid cells, hepatocytes, macrophages	Binds iron-laden transferrin for cellular iron uptake	TFRC; 3q29	*190010
Transferrin receptor-2 (TFR2)	Surfaces of liver, spleen, lung, muscle, prostate, blood mononuclear cells (alpha transcript); all tissues tested (beta transcript)	Binds iron-laden transferrin; modulates hepcidin expression	TFR2; 7q22	*604720
Divalent metal transporter-1 (DMT1)	All tissues	Transports iron and other divalent metal cations not bound to transferrin	SLC11A2; 12q13	*600523
Surface receptor CD163	Macrophages	Scavenges haptoglobin-hemoglobin complex	CD163; 12q13.3	*605545
Surface receptor LRP/CD91	Macrophages	Scavenges hemopexin-heme complex	LRP1; 12q13.1–q13.3	*10770
Mitoferrin	Mitochondria	Promotes mitochondrial iron uptake	SLC25A37; 8p21	*610387
Ferroportin	Enterocytes, macrophages, hepatocytes, placental syncytiotrophoblasts	Act as hepcidin receptor; exports iron from cells	SLC40A1 (FPN1); 2q32	*604653
FLVCR (feline leukemia virus subgroup C receptor)	Erythroid cells, macrophages, liver; probably other cells	Exports heme from erythroid cells; may protect against heme toxicity; mediates heme export from macrophages that ingest senescent red cells; regulates hepatic iron	FLVCR; 1931.3	*609144
Heme receptor (HCP1)	Enterocyte microvillus surfaces	Binds heme, heme-hemopexin; transports folate	SLC46A1; 17q11.1	*611672
Lactoferrin	Neutrophils, external secretions; not expressed in intestine; modulates iron metabolism, hematopoiesis, and immunologic reactions	Promotes iron sequestration in macrophages in local areas of inflammation; homologous to transferrin	LTF; 3q21–q23	*150210
Calreticulin	Enterocyte brush borders; erythroid cells; perhaps other cells	Alternate carrier for inorganic Fe^{3+} uptake	CALR; 19p13.2	*109091

Note: [a]Online Mendelian Inheritance in Man database. (http://www.ncbi.nlm.nih.gov/sites/entrez?db=omim).

TFR1 receptors are highly expressed by bone marrow erythroid precursors, rapidly dividing cells, and activated lymphocytes. In mice, early lymphoid cells and neuroepithelial cells also require transferrin receptor for normal differentiation, although the basis of this phenomenon is incompletely understood.[11,12] Cells that express surface TFR1 internalize transferrin-iron

Table 2.4. Some proteins that regulate iron homeostasis

Protein	Location	Function, properties	Gene; chromosome	OMIM designation[a]
IRE-binding protein 1 (IRP1, aconitase)	Many cell types	Bifunctional; binds IRE or cytosolic iron-sulfur cluster	*ACO1* (*IREB1*); 9p22–p13	*1008880
IRE-binding protein 2 (IRP2)	Intestine, brain	Senses iron concentrations, modulates IRE-binding activity at physiologic oxygen tensions	*IREB2*; 15	*147582
HFE	Hepatocytes, macrophages, basolateral surfaces of enterocytes, some other cells; not expressed by erythrocytes	Co-localizes with β_2-microglobulin, binds transferrin receptor; modulates hepcidin expression	*HFE*; 6p21.3	+235200
Hepcidin	Highest in liver, moderate in heart and brain; also in lung and other tissues	Binds ferroportin in enterocytes and macrophages, decreases iron export	*HAMP*; 19q13	*606464
Hemojuvelin	Liver, heart, skeletal muscle	Increases hepatic hepcidin expression; secondarily decreases ferroportin expression in enterocytes, macrophages	*HJV* (*HFE2*); 1q21	*608374

Note: [a]Online Mendelian Inheritance in Man database. (http://www.ncbi.nlm.nih.gov/sites/entrez?db=omim).

complexes into clathrin-coated pits. These invaginate to form endosomes that become acidified due to proton influx. Acidification of the endosomes induces conformational changes in transferrin that result in the release of inorganic ferric (Fe^{3+}) iron from transferrin. The ferrireductase STEAP3 converts the iron to ferrous (Fe^{2+}) ions;[13] they are subsequently transported across the endosomal membrane by divalent metal transporter-1 (DMT1) (Table 2.3).[14,15] Transport of Fe^{2+} across membranes by DMT1 typically requires proton co-transport,[15,16] consistent with the low pH of endosomes generated during receptor-mediated transferrin uptake. DMT1 may also participate in the transport of non-transferrin-bound iron into cells.[17] HFE protein does not appear to alter the unloading of iron from transferrin in the endosome (Table 2.4).[18] Apotransferrin is recycled to and released at the cell surface. The transferrin cycle appears to have no direct role in the control of intestinal iron absorption. Persons with atransferrinemia have the paradoxical combination of microcytic anemia, a consequence of iron-restricted erythropoiesis, and iron overload (Chapter 19).

Intracellular iron homeostasis

Iron-responsive (or regulatory) elements (IREs), are highly conserved regulatory sequences that occur in the untranslated regions (UTRs) of mRNA encoded by genes of certain iron-associated proteins.[19–26] IREs assume a characteristic secondary "stem-loop" configuration.[27] Cytoplasmic iron-responsive (or regulatory) proteins (IRPs) bind the stem-loop of IREs in mRNA in a specific manner and repress corresponding protein translation or degradation (Table 2.4).[22,25,28–32] The two known IRPs share sequence homology. IRP1, also known as aconitase, is a bifunctional protein that performs mutually exclusive roles as an IRP or as the cytoplasmic isoform of aconitase, an iron–sulfur protein that requires a 4Fe 4S iron–sulfur cluster for enzymatic activity.[33–36] Extensive conformational changes related to IRE binding or presence of an iron–sulfur cluster account for the alternate functions of IRP1 as either an mRNA regulator or an enzyme.[34,36] In this manner, intracellular iron levels are communicated to IREs.[37] IRP2 dominates regulation of mammalian iron homeostasis because it alone registers iron concentrations and modulates its RNA-binding activity at physiologic oxygen tensions.[38] In conditions of low iron availability, quantities of IRP accumulate, whereas an abundance of iron promotes IRP2 degradation.[34]

Ferritin IRE occurs in the 5′ UTR proximal to the start codon for translation. IRP binding to ferritin IRE prevents translation.[39] In conditions of low iron availability, ferritin production is decreased. When iron is plentiful, IRP levels fall, permitting synthesis of ferritin H- and L-subunits for iron storage. There are multiple IREs of TFR1 situated in the 3′ UTR of its mRNA.[21] In this case, IRP binding protects TFR1 mRNA from destruction in the cytoplasm. When iron is abundant, nucleases attack sequences adjacent to the IREs and destabilize TFR1 mRNA. 5′ IREs also occur in association with mRNAs of ferroportin and aminolevulinic acid synthase, and a 3′ IRE occurs in the mRNA of DMT1, although the regulatory roles of these IREs are incompletely defined.[24,26] Mutations in the ferritin light chain IRE result in constitutive upregulation of L-ferritin subunit production, and thereby cause the syndrome of autosomal dominant hyperferritinemia (without iron overload) and cataract (Chapter 17). A mutation in the ferritin heavy chain IRE discovered in a Japanese family caused autosomal dominant iron overload (Chapter 16).

Regulation of iron availability

Hepcidin is the major, direct regulator of iron absorption from the intestine and iron release from macrophage and hepatocyte stores (Table 2.4).[40] Hepcidin is a 25-amino-acid peptide with four internal disulfide bonds that is produced predominantly in the liver. Derived from a larger precursor molecule,[41–44] hepcidin is secreted into the circulation. Because hepcidin molecules are small, hepcidin is filtered by the kidneys and is readily detected and quantified in urine. Most regulation of serum hepcidin levels probably occurs at the level of production.[45] Hepcidin mRNA and urine levels are decreased in types of hemochromatosis due to mutations in the genes HFE, HJV, and TFR2 (Chapters 8, 13, 15).[46–48] HFE C282Y homozygotes have a blunted urine hepcidin response to an oral iron challenge.[49]

Hepcidin is encoded by the HAMP gene. The proximal region of the HAMP promoter is highly conserved in mammals,[50] and includes important motifs responsive to bone morphogenetic proteins (BMPs) and STAT.[51,52] Mutations in the coding region of the hepcidin gene (HAMP) may modify hemochromatosis phenotypes in persons who also inherit common HFE mutations (Chapters 8, 14).[53,54] In a patient homozygous for a HAMP promoter mutation, there was steady-state transcription but failed upregulation of hepcidin levels by iron.[55] Inactivation of the hepcidin gene in mice causes severe iron overload,[56,57] and its transgenic overexpression causes iron deficiency.[58,59] Hepcidin transcription is responsive to diverse physiologic and pathologic needs. In mice, hepcidin mRNA is elevated in iron overload[43] and decreased in iron deficiency and tissue hypoxia.[60,61] The amount of hepcidin mRNA in hepatocytes is decreased in response to hypoxia and ineffective erythropoiesis[60,62] and induced in response to treatment with lipopolysaccharide or by other inflammatory stimuli.[43,60] Altogether, these mechanisms permit increased iron availability for erythropoiesis when hepcidin levels are low, and iron sequestration and iron withholding from pathogenic bacteria during infection.[63–65]

Hepcidin expression is induced by the BMP signaling pathway.[66,67] BMP is a powerful stimulus for hepcidin expression[67] and the BMP/Smad pathway is the most potent known activator of hepcidin transcription.[45] In mice, inactivation of Smad4 in the liver results in severe iron overload.[68] The BMP pathway involves members of the transforming growth factor beta (TGF-β) superfamily of ligands that act by binding BMP receptors. Binding induces phosphorylation of the BMP receptors that, in turn, phosphorylate a subset of Smad proteins. These form heteromeric complexes with the common mediator Smad4, and they translocate to the nucleus where they regulate the transcription of specific targets.[45,69–71] The region of the HAMP promoter between 1.6 kb and 1.8 kb upstream from the start of translation appears to be essential for the response to iron.[72] This region responds to stimulation with BMPs, but differs from an area responsive to stimulation with lipopolysaccharide and interleukin-6.[72] Hemojuvelin acts as a BMP co-receptor to stimulate hepcidin transcription.[67] Treatment of hepatocytes with BMPs stimulates hepcidin expression, in a manner dependent on the presence of Smad4, BMPs, and hemojuvelin.[66,68] Induction of hepcidin production in inflammation is upregulated by a STAT3 binding site through a signaling pathway triggered by interleukin-6.[50,73] The von Hippel-Lindau/hypoxia-inducible transcription factor (HIF)-1α acts as a repressor when it binds the *HAMP* promoter.[74] Other factors may also bind to the hepcidin promoter, but their role in physiologic regulation of hepcidin expression is not well defined.[45]

The receptor of hepcidin is ferroportin (SLC40A1), a glycoprotein iron exporter expressed by enterocytes (basolateral surfaces), macrophages, hepatocytes, and placental syncytiotrophoblasts (Table 2.3). During evolution, the ferroportin-binding site of hepcidin has been highly conserved.[75] It has been postulated that ferroportin exists as a dimer,[76] although recent evidence suggests it functions as a monomer.[77] In health, hepcidin binds to ferroportin and promotes its internalization and destruction by ubiquitination within cells, resulting in cellular retention of iron.[78,79] Relatively greater quantities of hepcidin therefore decrease internal iron availability from two major sources: absorptive enterocytes and macrophages. Conversely, inappropriately low quantities of hepcidin promote iron absorption and release of iron from macrophage stores. Mutations in the ferroportin gene *SLC40A1* induce autosomal dominant iron overload of two major types, both attributed to the "dominant negative" effects of the abnormal member of each dimer (Chapter 12).

Iron and specific cell types

Enterocytes

Inorganic iron is absorbed primarily via the apical (luminal) microvillus membranes (brush borders) of mature enterocytes on or near the tips of small intestinal villi.[2,80] Iron absorption occurs primarily in the proximal duodenum (and to a lesser extent in the jejunum and ileum).[2,80] Most dietary non-heme iron is in the ferric (Fe^{3+}) form. Transport of iron across the microvillus membranes requires that the iron be converted to a ferrous (Fe^{2+}) form, either by reducing agents in the luminal contents of the gut[2] or by duodenal cytochrome b (DCYTB = CYBRD1) (Table 2.2) (Fig. 2.1).[81] STEAP ferrireductase proteins expressed in the intestine may participate in the reduction of non-heme ferric iron and its subsequent absorption.[82]

In the intestine, DMT1 is most highly expressed in the apical microvillus membrane of duodenal enterocytes.[83] The intestinal form of this protein occurs in a splice isoform that differs from that which participates in the transferrin cycle.[24,84] DMT1 transports ferrous iron (Fe^{2+}) iron across the microvillus membranes of absorptive enterocytes (Tables 2.2, 2.3).[16,85] The action of DMT1 after the administration of oral iron may mediate the physiologic "mucosal block" phenomenon.[86] Observations in a patient with a mutation in the *SLC11A2* gene that encodes DMT1 suggests that the human intestinal absorption may compensate for deficient ferrous iron uptake by absorbing more heme iron.[87] Intestinal DMT1-mediated iron transport requires proton co-transport. The protons are presumably supplied by gastric acid that enters the duodenum (Fig. 2.1). This partly explains why achlorhydria, antacids, or gastric acid blockers can reduce inorganic iron absorption.[2] DMT1 probably transports other divalent metal cations such as Mn^{2+}, Co^{2+}, Zn^{2+}, Cu^{2+}, and Pb^{2+},[15] the absorption of which is increased in iron deficiency and in *HFE* hemochromatosis (Chapters 4, 5). Calreticulin homologues that bind iron and other transitional metals, may also function in enterocyte uptake of iron and non-ferrous metals (Table 2.2).[88,89]

Heme iron is transported from the gut lumen via a brush-border receptor/transporter.[90–93] Evidence that heme receptor (heme carrier protein-1, HCP1) is responsible for heme importation into duodenal enterocytes is conflicting (Table 2.3).[94,95] Once within enterocytes, heme oxygenase degrades heme and releases its iron for subsequent handling in a manner that is probably similar to that of non-heme inorganic iron (Tables 2.1, 2.2). Other transmembrane iron transporters may exist, but their physiologic significance is not well defined.[45]

Most iron taken up by enterocytes from the luminal contents is retained for local use or storage, and is subsequently lost into the gastrointestinal tract by exfoliation.[2] Other iron, derived both from inorganic and heme sources, enters a common "intracellular iron pool" and is transported into the blood via the basolateral membrane.[80] The basolateral iron transporter is ferroportin[22,23,96,97] that probably transports iron in its ferrous (Fe^{2+}) form.[45] Ferroportin mRNA contains a 5' UTR IRE,[22,23,25] indicating that protein translation should be enhanced when iron is plentiful. This is the case for HepG2 and Kupffer cells, but not for duodenal enterocytes.[22,25,32] Thus, IRE regulation of ferroportin production is cell-specific, suggesting the presence of other control mechanisms in enterocytes.[98]

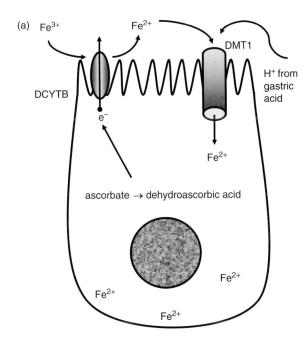

(a)

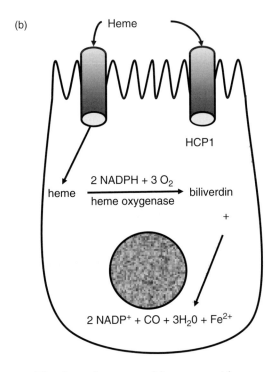

(b)

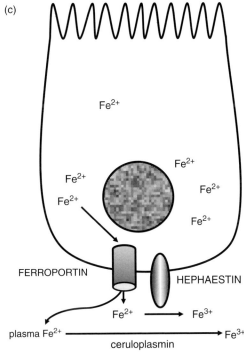

(c)

Fig. 2.1. (a) Iron transport in duodenal enterocytes. Intraluminal ferric iron (Fe^{3+}) is converted to ferrous iron (Fe^{2+}) at the brush border by acquisition of an electron donated by ascorbic acid. Divalent metal transporter-1 (DMT1) transports Fe^{2+} into the cytoplasm. This requires co-transport of protons presumably supplied by gastric acid that enters the duodenum. (b) Intraluminal heme is transported intracellularly, possibly by heme carrier protein-1 (HCP1). Fe^{2+} is released from heme by the action of heme oxygenase. (c) Under control of hepcidin, ferroportin exports Fe^{2+} that is converted to Fe^{3+} by a multicopper oxidase (hephaestin at the basolateral membrane, ceruloplasmin in the plasma).

The homologous multicopper oxidases ceruloplasmin (serum) and hephaestin (basolateral membranes of enterocytes) enhance iron export from enterocytes (Table 2.2).[86,99–102] In the small intestine, hephaestin is expressed almost entirely by enterocytes of the villus tips where iron absorption is maximal; crypt enterocytes have little or no hephaestin. Ceruloplasmin participates in the oxidation of ferrous (Fe^{2+}) iron extruded from the basolateral surfaces of enterocytes by ferroportin. Ceruloplasmin is also required to maintain ferroportin localization on cell membranes.[103] Enterocytes express transferrin and transferrin receptors only on their basolateral membranes.[104] The receptors interact with the regulatory protein HFE, although the precise interplay of transferrin, transferrin receptor, and HFE at this location is incompletely understood (Tables 2.3, 2.4).[105,106]

17

Erythroid cells

Iron exerts self-regulatory control over its uptake in erythroblasts via IRPs that bind reversibly to IRE sequences of the mRNAs of transferrin receptor, δ-aminolevulinate synthase-2, H- and L-ferritin subunits, and ferroportin.[19–26] The circulating erythrocyte mass is maintained by adjusting rate of marrow erythrocyte production from a stable compartment of stem cells that precisely replaces erythrocyte losses. Bone marrow erythroid precursors have the highest surface density of TFR1, and thus the highest rate of iron uptake from plasma transferrin. Erythroid precursors also require TFR1 for normal differentiation (Table 2.2). It is presumed that this is due predominantly to the role of TFR1 in delivering iron for hemoglobin synthesis. In normal erythroid cells, most iron that enters the cytoplasm is incorporated into heme or other compounds, or is stored in endosomes as ferritin/hemosiderin (siderosomes).

Importation of iron into mitochondria for heme synthesis is effected by mitoferrin, a highly conserved protein expressed in hematopoietic cells that supplies iron to ferrochelatase for incorporation into protoporphyrin IX (Table 2.3).[107] To date, mutations in mitoferrin are known only from the zebrafish mutant *frascati* that is characterized by profound hypochromic anemia and erythroid maturation arrest due to defective mitochondrial iron uptake.[107] The first and the rate-limiting enzyme of heme biosynthesis is δ-aminolevulinate synthase-2 (ALAS2). The enzyme requires glycine and succinyl coenzyme A as substrates, and pyridoxal 5′-phosphate as a cofactor; this condensation reaction occurs within mitochondria. Mutations in the X-linked *ALAS2* gene cause defective hemoglobinization of erythrocytes; some patients develop iron overload (Chapter 25). A heme exporter, FLVCR, permits erythroblasts to expel excessive and potentially toxic heme (Table 2.3).[108] FLVCR also mediates heme export from macrophages that ingest senescent red cells, and regulates hepatic iron.[109] Disruption of the *FLVCR* ortholog in mice demonstrates that heme export is important for normal erythropoiesis and somatic development.[109]

HIF plays a central role in regulating oxygen-associated gene expression.[110,111] There is an absolute requirement of HIF-prolyl hydroxylase (PHD) for dioxygen and iron. This suggests that HIF-PHD functions directly as a cellular oxygen sensor. Interaction of HIF-1 and von Hippel-Lindau (VHL) protein is iron-dependent, and is necessary for oxygen-dependent degradation of HIF-1α subunits. In oxygenated and iron-replete cells, HIF-1α subunits are rapidly destroyed by the ubiquitin-proteasome pathway. In conditions of hypoxia or iron chelation, the HIF-1/VHL complex is stable and thus allows transcriptional activation of erythropoietin.[112,113] The hematopoietic microenvironment required for erythropoiesis is dynamically regulated by oxygen through the functions of HIF-2α in endothelial cells.[114]

Hypoxia activates the erythropoietin gene via a 3′ enhancer sequence that responds primarily to hypoxia-induced stabilization of HIF-1. Erythropoietin synthesis occurs in renal cortical interstitial cells and is regulated at level of transcription. Erythropoietin binds, dimerizes and cross-links its receptor on erythroblasts, and functions as a differentiating stimulus, mitogen, and anti-apoptotic agent.[115] The erythropoietin receptor is a member of the cytokine receptor superfamily. In its native form, it exists as a single chain. Erythropoietin-binding induces dimerization and activation of the receptor. This initiates signaling that includes JAK2 protein activation by phosphorylation.[115] Erythropoietin does not stimulate iron absorption.

Hepcidin is suppressed by post-phlebotomy anemia or erythropoiesis. This suppression is reversed by inhibitors of erythropoiesis, but is not directly mediated by anemia, tissue hypoxia, or erythropoietin. The effect of anemia on hepcidin (and iron availability) appears to be mediated by a "regulator" released during erythropoiesis. This putative substance may use pathways to release iron preferentially from hemoglobin-recycling macrophages, and not from ferritin/hemosiderin.[110,116,117] Growth/differentiation factor 15 (GDF15), a member of the transforming growth factor-beta superfamily, may be such a "regulator." There was increased expression and secretion of GDF15 in erythroblast transcriptome profiles from healthy donors during erythroblast maturation.[118] In comparison, individuals with beta-thalassemia syndromes had elevated GDF15 serum levels that were positively correlated with the levels of soluble transferrin receptor, erythropoietin, and ferritin. Serum from thalassemia patients suppressed hepcidin mRNA expression in human hepatocytes, and depletion of GDF15 reversed hepcidin suppression.

These results suggest that GDF15 over expression arising from an expanded erythroid compartment contributes to iron overload in thalassemia syndromes (or other types of anemia associated with ineffective erythropoiesis) by inhibiting hepcidin expression.[118] In contrast, volunteer blood superdonors have markedly decreased serum hepcidin levels, but most have normal GDF15 expression. This indicates that GDF15 over expression arising from the expanded erythroid pool necessary to replace donated red cells is not the biochemical mechanism for their decreased serum hepcidin levels.[119] To date, there are no reports of GDF15 expression in hemochromatosis.

Hepatocytes

The liver plays a central role in iron metabolism in health and in iron overload.[120] Hepatocytes synthesize hepcidin and thus influence iron absorption and iron release from stores. Hepatocytes express other molecules involved in iron transport and regulation of iron homeostasis.[98] Approximately 8% of plasma iron turnover in humans is attributable to the liver, particularly hepatocytes.[121,122] The liver is also a major storage site for iron. Approximately 80% of iron in hepatocytes is contained in ferritin, and 2%–3% is present as heme. The remainder is either bound to transferrin or is present in an intracellular pool.[123] Iron within hepatocytes is either used locally or is stored in ferritin molecules. Ferroportin is the sole mediator of iron release from hepatocytes,[124] although ferroportin expression in hepatocytes is less than that in Kupffer cells.[22,125,126]

Hepatocytes express surface transferrin receptors (TFR1) that promote internalization of diferric transferrin.[127,128] In hemochromatosis, hepatic transferrin receptors are down-regulated in accordance with iron overload.[129,130] Hepatocytes also have a low-affinity, transferrin-mediated route of iron uptake.[122,131,132] This pathway accounts for most hepatocyte iron uptake.[131,133,134] because hepatocyte TFR1 would be saturated at the concentrations of transferrin present in plasma.[98] Transferrin receptor 2 (TFR2) does not appear to explain the low-affinity transferrin-mediated iron uptake mechanism (Table 2.3).[135,136] TFR2 protein is expressed on the basolateral surfaces of hepatocytes.[137] There is binding of TFR2 to membrane-anchored HFE,[138] although the physiologic significance of this interaction has not been defined. TFR2 mRNA does not

contain IREs, and cellular iron levels do not appear to change TFR2 mRNA expression.[139] Regulation of TFR2-mediated iron uptake is greater in proliferating cells than in non-dividing cells, and in the presence of dietary transferrin.[98,140,141] TFR2 protein levels are increased in genetic models of iron overload, such as hemochromatosis, but not in the atransferrinemic mouse which has impaired transferrin synthesis.[142,143] TFR2 may participate in regulating hepcidin expression.[138,144] Mutations in *TFR2* in humans cause a hemochromatosis phenotype, often severe (Chapter 15).

NTBI in plasma is bound predominantly to citrate.[145–147] The uptake of NTBI by hepatocytes is linear, concentration-dependent, and saturable.[98] NTBI uptake in vitro is increased in hepatocytes and hepatocellular carcinoma cells in which DMT1 mRNA and protein expression are up-regulated.[17,148] Diferric transferrin inhibits DMT1-mediated iron uptake by hepatocytes.[149–151] In mice, DMT1 protein staining of hepatocyte plasma membranes is greatest in iron-loaded animals, lower in control animals, and inapparent after iron depletion.[152] Altogether, these observations indicate that DMT1 is a major transporter of NTBI in hepatocytes.[98] In conditions in which available plasma iron exceeds the iron-binding capacity of plasma transferrin, NTBI may enter hepatocytes directly via a DMT1 mechanism.[17] This mechanism of hepatocyte iron uptake is also important in *HFE* hemochromatosis and other disorders in which transferrin saturation with iron is often markedly elevated.[146] Concentrations of certain non-ferrous divalent metals such as zinc and manganese are increased in the livers of patients with hemochromatosis; their transport into hepatocytes may be another consequence of transferrin or DMT1 pathways (Chapters 4, 5).

Hepatocytes clear other proteins from plasma that bind or contain iron, including ferritin, lactoferrin, and the hemoglobin-haptoglobin and heme-hemopexin complexes. Hepatocytes bear specific surface receptors for ferritin; bound ferritin enters the cells by endocytosis.[153–155] The ferritin may be catabolized in lysosomes, excreted in the bile, or retained in the ferritin pool of hepatocytes.[98] The receptor-mediated uptake of hemoglobin–haptoglobin and heme–hemopexin complexes is similar to that in other cells.[156,157] Heme and hemoglobin may be degraded by hepatocyte lysosomes.[157,158] Hemoglobin or its catabolites may also be excreted into the canaliculi and excreted into the bile.[159] Two non-specific lactoferrin-binding sites have been described on hepatocyte surfaces: a low-density lipoprotein receptor-related protein (LRP)[160] and the major subunit of the asialoglyco-protein receptor.[161] Lactoferrin is internalized via receptor-mediated endocytosis and degraded in lysosomes.[160–162]

Hepcidin is produced by hepatocytes under conditions of iron availability.[41–43] It is unknown if hepcidin acts in an autocrine manner by binding ferroportin expressed by hepatocytes.[98] Hemojuvelin is expressed at the basolateral membranes of peri-portal hepatocytes.[47,137,163] In hemojuvelin knockout mice ($Hjv^{-/-}$), hepcidin production by the liver is decreased and liver iron loading occurs.[163,164] The major function of hemojuvelin in hepatocytes appears to be regulation of hepcidin. Adult liver expresses predominantly STEAP3 but also produces small amounts of STEAP1.[13,82] These proteins co-localize partially in endosomal compartments with transferrin and TFR1. HFE expression is greatest in the liver, and it requires β_2-microglobulin for correct cell surface localization.[165] HFE protein may exert its iron-regulatory activity principally in hepatocytes by modulating the production of hepcidin.[166]

Macrophages

Macrophages, especially those in the bone marrow, spleen, lymph nodes, and liver (Kupffer cells), engulf senescent or injured erythrocytes (and other blood cells) and salvage their iron.[167] Macrophage surface CD163 scavenger receptor molecules capture hemoglobin and heme that is bound to haptoglobin, respectively (Table 2.2).[157,168,169] Surface expression of LRP/CD91 mediates hemopexin-heme internalization by a similar mechanism (Table 2.3).[157] Heme transporter heme carrier protein 1 (HCP-1) is also expressed in human macrophages. Within early endosomes, HCP-1 co-localizes with endocytosed hemoglobin-haptoglobin complexes taken up via the CD163 scavenger receptor pathway. The hemoglobin–haptoglobin complex passes the DMT1 endosomal compartment *en route* from the macrophage surface to lysosomes. Macrophage capture of heme iron by CD163 and LRP/CD91 pathways stimulates heme-oxygenase 1 mRNA transcription and cell surface expression of ferroportin.[157,169–171] Heme degradation products generated by Kupffer cells are excreted in the bile.[172] These findings highlight a dual mechanism of ferroportin regulation in macrophages, characterized by early induction of gene transcription predominantly mediated by heme, followed by iron-mediated post-transcriptional regulation of ferroportin.[173]

Macrophages, including Kupffer cells, express ferroportin transcript and protein.[126,171] Macrophages release iron into the plasma via ferroportin under the control of hepcidin. When ferroportin expression is up-regulated through iron treatment or erythrophagocytosis, ferroportin expression is strongly augmented at the plasma membrane of macrophages, and iron release is enhanced.[174,175] When hepcidin levels are relatively low, more ferroportin laden with iron is expressed at the surfaces of macrophages and hepatocytes, permitting iron export into plasma.[173,176] When hepcidin levels are increased, macrophage ferroportin protein levels are decreased[174] due to tyrosine phosphorylation of ferroportin at the plasma membrane, and subsequent ferroportin internalization, dephosphorylation, and degradation by ubiquitination.[79] Accordingly, iron efflux from macrophages is reduced significantly.[78,175] Iron released from storage cells is converted into the ferric (Fe^{3+}) state by ceruloplasmin (Table 2.2). Recycled ferric iron readily binds plasma apotransferrin. Ferritin synthesis in macrophages is increased in conditions of iron excess.[177] Thus, hepcidin participates in regulation of plasma iron levels and tissue distribution of iron by post-translational regulation of ferroportin. Likewise, either reduced synthesis of ferroportin in macrophages[178] or a "loss-of-function" *SCL40A1* mutations[179–182] increases iron retention in macrophages, including that in Kupffer cells (Chapter 12).

Lactoferrin, an iron-binding glycoprotein homologous to transferrin, is released by neutrophils in areas of inflammation or infection, binds iron at acidic values of pH (unlike transferrin), and may convey iron to macrophages or monocytes via their surface lactoferrin receptors (Table 2.3).[183,184] The iron is incorporated rapidly into ferritin.[183] This mechanism may enhance the sequestration of iron mediated by the action of hepcidin on ferroportin during infection or inflammation.[65] Monocytes and macrophages express surface transferrin receptors of relatively low affinity, but it is unlikely that they recycle stored iron through receptor-bound apotransferrin.[185] Kupffer cells also express transferrin receptors (TFR1)[186] and high levels of HFE protein.[187]

References

1. Finch CA, Deubelbeiss K, Cook JD, *et al.* Ferrokinetics in man. *Medicine (Baltimore)* 1970; **49**: 17–53.

2. Conrad ME, Barton JC. Factors affecting iron balance. *Am J Hematol* 1981; **10**: 199–225.

3. Chung J, Wessling-Resnick M. Molecular mechanisms and regulation of iron transport. *Crit Rev Clin Lab Sci* 2003; **40**: 151–82.

4. Bothwell TH, Charlton RW, Cook JD, Finch CA. Iron loss. *Iron Metabolism in Man.* Oxford, Blackwell Scientific Publications. 1979; 245–55.

5. Harrison PM, Fischbach FA, Hoy TG, Haggis GH. Ferric oxyhydroxide core of ferritin. *Nature* 1967; **216**: 1188–90.

6. Theil EC. Ferritin: structure, gene regulation, and cellular function in animals, plants, and microorganisms. *Annu Rev Biochem* 1987; **56**: 289–315.

7. Levi S, Yewdall SJ, Harrison PM, *et al.* Evidence of H-and L-chains have co-operative roles in the iron-uptake mechanism of human ferritin. *Biochem J* 1992; **288** (Pt 2): 591–6.

8. Harrison PM, Arosio P. The ferritins: molecular properties, iron storage function and cellular regulation. *Biochim Biophys Acta* 1996; **1275**: 161–203.

9. Wixom RL, Prutkin L, Munro HN. Hemosiderin: nature, formation, and significance. *Int Rev Exp Pathol* 1980; **22**: 193–225.

10. de Domenico I, Vaughn MB, Li L, *et al.* Ferroportin-mediated mobilization of ferritin iron precedes ferritin degradation by the proteasome. *EMBO J* 2006; **25**: 5396–404.

11. Levy JE, Jin O, Fujiwara Y, Kuo F, Andrews NC. Transferrin receptor is necessary for development of erythrocytes and the nervous system. *Nat Genet* 1999; **21**: 396–9.

12. Ned RM, Swat W, Andrews NC. Transferrin receptor 1 is differentially required in lymphocyte development. *Blood* 2003; **102**: 3711–18.

13. Ohgami RS, Campagna DR, Greer EL, *et al.* Identification of a ferrireductase required for efficient transferrin-dependent iron uptake in erythroid cells. *Nat Genet* 2005; **37**: 1264–9.

14. Fleming MD, Trenor CC, III, Su MA, *et al.* Microcytic anaemia mice have a mutation in *Nramp2*, a candidate iron transporter gene. *Nat Genet* 1997; **16**: 383–6.

15. Gunshin H, Mackenzie B, Berger UV, *et al.* Cloning and characterization of a mammalian proton-coupled metal-ion transporter. *Nature* 1997; **388**: 482–8.

16. Gunshin H, Fujiwara Y, Custodio AO, Direnzo C, Robine S, Andrews NC. Slc11a2 is required for intestinal iron absorption and erythropoiesis but dispensable in placenta and liver. *J Clin Invest* 2005; **115**: 1258–66.

17. Shindo M, Torimoto Y, Saito H, *et al.* Functional role of DMT1 in transferrin-independent iron uptake by human hepatocyte and hepatocellular carcinoma cell, HLF. *Hepatol Res* 2006; **35**: 152–62.

18. Davies PS, Zhang AS, Anderson EL, *et al.* Evidence for the interaction of the hereditary haemochromatosis protein, HFE, with the transferrin receptor in endocytic compartments. *Biochem J* 2003; **373**: 145–53.

19. Aziz N, Munro HN. Iron regulates ferritin mRNA translation through a segment of its 5' untranslated region. *Proc Natl Acad Sci USA* 1987; **84**: 8478–82.

20. Hentze MW, Rouault TA, Caughman SW, Dancis A, Harford JB, Klausner RD. A cis-acting element is necessary and sufficient for translational regulation of human ferritin expression in response to iron. *Proc Natl Acad Sci USA* 1987; **84**: 6730–4.

21. Casey JL, Koeller DM, Ramin VC, Klausner RD, Harford JB. Iron regulation of transferrin receptor mRNA levels requires iron-responsive elements and a rapid turnover determinant in the 3' untranslated region of the mRNA. *EMBO J* 1989; **8**: 3693–9.

22. Abboud S, Haile DJ. A novel mammalian iron-regulated protein involved in intracellular iron metabolism. *J Biol Chem* 2000; **275**: 19 906–12.

23. McKie AT, Marciani P, Rolfs A, *et al.* A novel duodenal iron-regulated transporter, IREG1, implicated in the basolateral transfer of iron to the circulation. *Mol Cell* 2000; **5**: 299–309.

24. Hubert N, Hentze MW. Previously uncharacterized isoforms of divalent metal transporter (DMT)-1: implications for regulation and cellular function. *Proc Natl Acad Sci USA* 2002; **99**: 12 345–50.

25. Lymboussaki A, Pignatti E, Montosi G, Garuti C, Haile DJ, Pietrangelo A. The role of the iron-responsive element in the control of ferroportin 1/IREG1/MTP1 gene expression. *J Hepatol* 2003; **39**: 710–15.

26. Leipuviene R, Theil EC. The family of iron-responsive RNA structures regulated by changes in cellular iron and oxygen. *Cell Mol Life Sci* 2007; **64**: 2945–55.

27. Casey JL, Hentze MW, Koeller DM, *et al.* Iron-responsive elements: regulatory RNA sequences that control mRNA levels and translation. *Science* 1988; **240**: 924–8.

28. Hentze MW, Caughman SW, Rouault TA, *et al.* Identification of the iron-responsive element for the translational regulation of human ferritin mRNA. *Science* 1987; **238**: 1570–3.

29. Caughman SW, Hentze MW, Rouault TA, Harford JB, Klausner RD. The iron-responsive element is the single

element responsible for iron-dependent translational regulation of ferritin biosynthesis. Evidence for function as the binding site for a translational repressor. *J Biol Chem* 1988; **263**: 19 048–52.

30. Leibold EA, Munro HN. Cytoplasmic protein binds in vitro to a highly conserved sequence in the 5′ untranslated region of ferritin heavy- and light-subunit mRNAs. *Proc Natl Acad Sci USA* 1988; **85**: 2171–5.

31. Rouault TA, Hentze MW, Caughman SW, Harford JB, Klausner RD. Binding of a cytosolic protein to the iron-responsive element of human ferritin messenger RNA. *Science* 1988; **241**: 1207–10.

32. Chen Y, Qian ZM, Du J, *et al.* Iron loading inhibits ferroportin 1 expression in PC12 cells. *Neurochem Int* 2005; **47**: 507–13.

33. Hentze MW, Argos P. Homology between IRE-BP, a regulatory RNA-binding protein, aconitase, and isopropylmalate isomerase. *Nucleic Acids Res* 1991; **19**: 1739–40.

34. Kaptain S, Downey WE, Tang C, *et al.* A regulated RNA-binding protein also possesses aconitase activity. *Proc Natl Acad Sci USA* 1991; **88**: 10 109–13.

35. Eisenstein RS. Iron regulatory proteins and the molecular control of mammalian iron metabolism. *Annu Rev Nutr* 2000; **20**: 627–62.

36. Walden WE, Selezneva AI, Dupuy J, *et al.* Structure of dual function iron regulatory protein 1 complexed with ferritin IRE-RNA. *Science* 2006; **314**: 1903–8.

37. Haile DJ, Hentze MW, Rouault TA, Harford JB, Klausner RD. Regulation of interaction of the iron-responsive element-binding protein with iron-responsive RNA elements. *Mol Cell Biol* 1989; **9**: 5055–61.

38. Meyron-Holtz EG, Ghosh MC, Iwai K, *et al.* Genetic ablations of iron regulatory proteins 1 and 2 reveal why iron regulatory protein 2 dominates iron homeostasis. *EMBO J* 2004; **23**: 386–95.

39. Muckenthaler M, Gray NK, Hentze MW. IRP-1 binding to ferritin mRNA prevents the recruitment of the small ribosomal subunit by the cap-binding complex eIF4F. *Mol Cell* 1998; **2**: 383–8.

40. Ganz T. Hepcidin and its role in regulating systemic iron metabolism. *Hematology Am Soc Hematol Educ Program* 2006; 29–35.

41. Krause A, Neitz S, Magert HJ, *et al.* LEAP-1, a novel highly disulfide-bonded human peptide, exhibits antimicrobial activity. *FEBS Lett* 2000; **480**: 147–50.

42. Park CH, Valore EV, Waring AJ, Ganz T. Hepcidin, a urinary antimicrobial peptide synthesized in the liver. *J Biol Chem* 2001; **276**: 7806–10.

43. Pigeon C, Ilyin G, Courselaud B, *et al.* A new mouse liver-specific gene, encoding a protein homologous to

human antimicrobial peptide hepcidin, is overexpressed during iron overload. *J Biol Chem* 2001; **276**: 7811–19.

44. Scamuffa N, Basak A, Lalou C, *et al.* Regulation of prohepcidin processing and activity by the subtilisin-like pro-protein convertases Furin, PC5, PACE4, and PC7. *Gut* 2008; **57**: 1573–82.

45. Andrews NC. Forging a field: the golden age of iron biology. *Blood* 2008; **112**: 219–30.

46. Gehrke SG, Kulaksiz H, Herrmann T, *et al.* Expression of hepcidin in hereditary hemochromatosis: evidence for a regulation in response to the serum transferrin saturation and to non-transferrin-bound iron. *Blood* 2003; **102**: 371–6.

47. Papanikolaou G, Samuels ME, Ludwig EH, *et al.* Mutations in *HFE2* cause iron overload in chromosome 1q-linked juvenile hemochromatosis. *Nat Genet* 2004; **36**: 77–82.

48. Nemeth E, Roetto A, Garozzo G, Ganz T, Camaschella C. Hepcidin is decreased in *TFR2* hemochromatosis. *Blood* 2005; **105**: 1803–6.

49. Piperno A, Girelli D, Nemeth E, *et al.* Blunted hepcidin response to oral iron challenge in *HFE*-related hemochromatosis. *Blood* 2007; **110**: 4096–100.

50. Wrighting DM, Andrews NC. Interleukin-6 induces hepcidin expression through STAT3. *Blood* 2006; **108**: 3204–9.

51. Truksa J, Lee P, Beutler E. Two BMP responsive elements, STAT, and bZIP/HNF4/COUP motifs of the hepcidin promoter are critical for BMP, SMAD1, and HJV responsiveness. *Blood* 2009; **113**: 688–95.

52. Casanovas G, Mleczko-Sanecka K, Altamura S, Hentze MW, Muckenthaler MU. Bone morphogenetic protein (BMP)-responsive elements located in the proximal and distal hepcidin promoter are critical for its response to HJV/BMP/SMAD. *J Mol Med* 2009; **87**: 471–80.

53. Merryweather-Clarke AT, Cadet E, Bomford A, *et al.* Digenic inheritance of mutations in *HAMP* and *HFE* results in different types of haemochromatosis. *Hum Mol Genet* 2003; **12**: 2241–7.

54. Jacolot S, Le Gac G, Scotet V, Quere I, Mura C, Ferec C. *HAMP* as a modifier gene that increases the phenotypic expression of the *HFE* pC282Y homozygous genotype. *Blood* 2004; **103**: 2835–40.

55. Porto G, Roetto A, Daraio F, *et al.* A Portuguese patient homozygous for the -25G>A mutation of the *HAMP* promoter shows evidence of steady-state transcription but fails to up-regulate hepcidin levels by iron. *Blood* 2005; **106**: 2922–3.

56. Nicolas G, Bennoun M, Devaux I, *et al.* Lack of hepcidin gene expression and severe tissue iron

overload in upstream stimulatory factor 2 (USF2) knockout mice. *Proc Natl Acad Sci USA* 2001; **98**: 8780–5.

57. Lesbordes-Brion JC, Viatte L, Bennoun M, *et al.* Targeted disruption of the hepcidin 1 gene results in severe hemochromatosis. *Blood* 2006; **108**: 1402–5.

58. Nicolas G, Bennoun M, Porteu A, *et al.* Severe iron deficiency anemia in transgenic mice expressing liver hepcidin. *Proc Natl Acad Sci USA* 2002; **99**: 4596–601.

59. Roy CN, Mak HH, Akpan I, Losyev G, Zurakowski D, Andrews NC. Hepcidin antimicrobial peptide transgenic mice exhibit features of the anemia of inflammation. *Blood* 2007; **109**: 4038–44.

60. Nicolas G, Chauvet C, Viatte L, *et al.* The gene encoding the iron regulatory peptide hepcidin is regulated by anemia, hypoxia, and inflammation. *J Clin Invest* 2002; **110**: 1037–44.

61. Weinstein DA, Roy CN, Fleming MD, Loda MF, Wolfsdorf JI, Andrews NC. Inappropriate expression of hepcidin is associated with iron refractory anemia: implications for the anemia of chronic disease. *Blood* 2002; **100**: 3776–81.

62. Adamsky K, Weizer O, Amariglio N, *et al.* Decreased hepcidin mRNA expression in thalassemic mice. *Br J Haematol* 2004; **124**: 123–4.

63. Ashrafian H. Hepcidin: the missing link between hemochromatosis and infections. *Infect Immun* 2003; **71**: 6693–700.

64. Ganz T. Hepcidin–a peptide hormone at the interface of innate immunity and iron metabolism. *Curr Top Microbiol Immunol* 2006; **306**: 183–98.

65. Paradkar PN, De Domenico I, Durchfort N, Zohn I, Kaplan J, Ward DM. Iron depletion limits intracellular bacterial growth in macrophages. *Blood* 2008; **112**: 866–74.

66. Babitt JL, Huang FW, Xia Y, Sidis Y, Andrews NC, Lin HY. Modulation of bone morphogenetic protein signaling in vivo regulates systemic iron balance. *J Clin Invest* 2007; **117**: 1933–9.

67. Babitt JL, Huang FW, Wrighting DM, *et al.* Bone morphogenetic protein signaling by hemojuvelin regulates hepcidin expression. *Nat Genet* 2006; **38**: 531–9.

68. Wang RH, Li C, Xu X, *et al.* A role of SMAD4 in iron metabolism through the positive regulation of hepcidin expression. *Cell Metab* 2005; **2**: 399–409.

69. Anderson GJ, Frazer DM. Iron metabolism meets signal transduction. *Nat Genet* 2006; **38**: 503–4.

70. Kautz L, Meynard D, Monnier A, *et al.* Iron regulates phosphorylation of Smad1/5/8 and gene expression of Bmp6, Smad7, Id1, and Atoh8 in the mouse liver. *Blood* 2008; **112**: 1503–9.

71. McReynolds LJ, Gupta S, Figueroa ME, Mullins MC, Evans T. Smad1 and Smad5 differentially regulate embryonic hematopoiesis. *Blood* 2007; **110**: 3881–90.

72. Truksa J, Lee P, Peng H, Flanagan J, Beutler E. The distal location of the iron-responsive region of the hepcidin promoter. *Blood* 2007; **110**: 3436–7.

73. Verga Falzacappa MV, Vujic SM, Kessler R, Stolte J, Hentze MW, Muckenthaler MU. STAT3 mediates hepatic hepcidin expression and its inflammatory stimulation. *Blood* 2007; **109**: 353–8.

74. Peyssonnaux C, Zinkernagel AS, Schuepbach RA, *et al.* Regulation of iron homeostasis by the hypoxia-inducible transcription factors (HIFs). *J Clin Invest* 2007; **117**: 1926–32.

75. de Domenico I, Nemeth E, Nelson JM, *et al.* The hepcidin-binding site on ferroportin is evolutionarily conserved. *Cell Metab* 2008; **8**: 146–56.

76. de Domenico I, Ward DM, Musci G, Kaplan J. Evidence for the multimeric structure of ferroportin. *Blood* 2007; **109**: 2205–9.

77. Schimanski LM, Drakesmith H, Talbott C, *et al.* Ferroportin: lack of evidence for multimers. *Blood Cells Mol Dis* 2008; **40**: 360–9.

78. Nemeth E, Tuttle MS, Powelson J, *et al.* Hepcidin regulates cellular iron efflux by binding to ferroportin and inducing its internalization. *Science* 2004; **306**: 2090–3.

79. de Domenico I, Ward DM, Langelier C, *et al.* The molecular mechanism of hepcidin-mediated ferroportin down-regulation. *Mol Biol Cell* 2007; **18**: 2569–78.

80. Parmley RT, Barton JC, Conrad ME, Austin RL. Ultrastructural cytochemistry of iron absorption. *Am J Pathol* 1978; **93**: 707–27.

81. McKie AT, Barrow D, Latunde-Dada GO, *et al.* An iron-regulated ferric reductase associated with the absorption of dietary iron. *Science* 2001; **291**: 1755–9.

82. Ohgami RS, Campagna DR, McDonald A, Fleming MD. The Steap proteins are metalloreductases. *Blood* 2006; **108**: 1388–94.

83. Canonne-Hergaux F, Gruenheid S, Ponka P, Gros P. Cellular and subcellular localization of the Nramp2 iron transporter in the intestinal brush border and regulation by dietary iron. *Blood* 1999; **93**: 4406–17.

84. Lam-Yuk-Tseung S, Touret N, Grinstein S, Gros P. Carboxyl-terminus determinants of the iron transporter DMT1/SLC11A2 isoform II (-IRE/1B) mediate internalization from the plasma membrane into recycling endosomes. *Biochemistry* 2005; **44**: 12 149–59.

85. Andrews NC. The iron transporter DMT1. *Int J Biochem Cell Biol* 1999; **31**: 991–4.

23

86. Frazer DM, Wilkins SJ, Becker EM, *et al.* A rapid decrease in the expression of DMT1 and Dcytb but not Ireg1 or hephaestin explains the mucosal block phenomenon of iron absorption. *Gut* 2003; **52**: 340–6.

87. Priwitzerova M, Pospisilova D, Prchal JT, *et al.* Severe hypochromic microcytic anemia caused by a congenital defect of the iron transport pathway in erythroid cells. *Blood* 2004; **103**: 3991–2.

88. Conrad ME, Umbreit JN, Moore EG. Rat duodenal iron-binding protein mobilferrin is a homologue of calreticulin. *Gastroenterology* 1993; **104**: 1700–4.

89. Conrad ME, Umbreit JN, Peterson RD, Moore EG, Harper KP. Function of integrin in duodenal mucosal uptake of iron. *Blood* 1993; **81**: 517–21.

90. Grasbeck R, Kouvonen I, Lundberg M, Tenhunen R. An intestinal receptor for heme. *Scand J Haematol* 1979; **23**: 5–9.

91. Parmley RT, Barton JC, Conrad ME, Austin RL, Holland RM. Ultrastructural cytochemistry and radioautography of hemoglobin–iron absorption. *Exp Mol Pathol* 1981; **34**: 131–44.

92. Grasbeck R, Majuri R, Kouvonen I, Tenhunen R. Spectral and other studies on the intestinal haem receptor of the pig. *Biochim Biophys Acta* 1982; **700**: 137–42.

93. Uc A, Stokes JB, Britigan BE. Heme transport exhibits polarity in Caco-2 cells: evidence for an active and membrane protein-mediated process. *Am J Physiol Gastrointest Liver Physiol* 2004; **287**: G1150–7.

94. Shayeghi M, Latunde-Dada GO, Oakhill JS, *et al.* Identification of an intestinal heme transporter. *Cell* 2005; **122**: 789–801.

95. Qiu A, Jansen M, Sakaris A, *et al.* Identification of an intestinal folate transporter and the molecular basis for hereditary folate malabsorption. *Cell* 2006; **127**: 917–28.

96. Donovan A, Brownlie A, Zhou Y, *et al.* Positional cloning of zebrafish ferroportin 1 identifies a conserved vertebrate iron exporter. *Nature* 2000; **403**: 776–81.

97. Zoller H, Theurl I, Koch R, Kaser A, Weiss G. Mechanisms of iron mediated regulation of the duodenal iron transporters divalent metal transporter 1 and ferroportin 1. *Blood Cells Mol Dis* 2002; **29**: 488–97.

98. Graham RM, Chua AC, Herbison CE, Olynyk JK, Trinder D. Liver iron transport. *World J Gastroenterol* 2007; **13**: 4725–36.

99. Osaki S, Johnson DA, Frieden E. The possible significance of the ferrous oxidase activity of ceruloplasmin in normal human serum. *J Biol Chem* 1966; **241**: 2746–51.

100. Roeser HP, Lee GR, Nacht S, Cartwright GE. The role of ceruloplasmin in iron metabolism. *J Clin Invest* 1970; **49**: 2408–17.

101. Vulpe CD, Kuo YM, Murphy TL, *et al.* Hephaestin, a ceruloplasmin homologue implicated in intestinal iron transport, is defective in the *sla* mouse. *Nat Genet* 1999; **21**: 195–99.

102. Anderson GJ, Frazer DM, Wilkins SJ, *et al.* Relationship between intestinal iron-transporter expression, hepatic hepcidin levels and the control of iron absorption. *Biochem Soc Trans* 2002; **30**: 724–6.

103. de Domenico I, Ward DM, di Patti MC, *et al.* Ferroxidase activity is required for the stability of cell surface ferroportin in cells expressing GPI-ceruloplasmin. *EMBO J* 2007; **26**: 2823–31.

104. Parmley RT, Barton JC, Conrad ME. Ultrastructural localization of transferrin, transferrin receptor, and iron-binding sites on human placental and duodenal microvilli. *Br J Haematol* 1985; **60**: 81–9.

105. Feder JN, Penny DM, Irrinki A, *et al.* The hemochromatosis gene product complexes with the transferrin receptor and lowers its affinity for ligand binding. *Proc Natl Acad Sci USA* 1998; **95**: 1472–7.

106. Lebron JA, Bennett MJ, Vaughn DE, *et al.* Crystal structure of the hemochromatosis protein HFE and characterization of its interaction with transferrin receptor. *Cell* 1998; **93**: 111–23.

107. Shaw GC, Cope JJ, Li L, *et al.* Mitoferrin is essential for erythroid iron assimilation. *Nature* 2006; **440**: 96–100.

108. Quigley JG, Yang Z, Worthington MT, *et al.* Identification of a human heme exporter that is essential for erythropoiesis. *Cell* 2004; **118**: 757–66.

109. Keel SB, Doty RT, Yang Z, *et al.* A heme export protein is required for red blood cell differentiation and iron homeostasis. *Science* 2008; **319**: 825–8.

110. Ponka P, Sheftel AD. It's hepcidin again, but is it the only master? *Blood* 2006; **108**: 3631–2.

111. Yoon D, Pastore YD, Divoky V, *et al.* Hypoxia-inducible factor-1 deficiency results in dysregulated erythropoiesis signaling and iron homeostasis in mouse development. *J Biol Chem* 2006; **281**: 25 703–11.

112. Jaakkola P, Mole DR, Tian YM, *et al.* Targeting of HIF-alpha to the von Hippel-Lindau ubiquitylation complex by O_2-regulated prolyl hydroxylation. *Science* 2001; **292**: 468–72.

113. Takeda K, Aguila HL, Parikh NS, *et al.* Regulation of adult erythropoiesis by prolyl hydroxylase domain proteins. *Blood* 2008; **111**: 3229–35.

114. Yamashita T, Ohneda O, Sakiyama A, Iwata F, Ohneda K, Fujii-Kuriyama Y. The microenvironment for erythropoiesis is regulated by HIF-2alpha through VCAM-1 in endothelial cells. *Blood* 2008; **112**: 1482–92.

115. Chong ZZ, Kang JQ, Maiese K. Hematopoietic factor erythropoietin fosters neuroprotection through novel

signal transduction cascades. *J Cereb Blood Flow Metab* 2002; **22**: 503–14.

116. Vokurka M, Krijt J, Sulc K, Necas E. Hepcidin mRNA levels in mouse liver respond to inhibition of erythropoiesis. *Physiol Res* 2006; **55**: 667–74.

117. Pak M, Lopez MA, Gabayan V, Ganz T, Rivera S. Suppression of hepcidin during anemia requires erythropoietic activity. *Blood* 2006; **108**: 3730–5.

118. Tanno T, Bhanu NV, Oneal PA, *et al.* High levels of GDF15 in thalassemia suppress expression of the iron regulatory protein hepcidin. *Nat Med* 2007; **13**: 1096–101.

119. Mast AE, Foster TM, Pinder HL, *et al.* Behavioral, biochemical, and genetic analysis of iron metabolism in high-intensity blood donors. *Transfusion* 2008; **48**: 2197–204.

120. Brown KE, Bacon BR. Hepatic iron metabolism in hemochromatosis. In: Barton JC, Edwards CQ, eds. *Hemochromatosis: Genetics, Pathophysiology, Diagnosis and Treatment*. Cambridge, Cambridge University Press. 2000; 157–62.

121. Hershko C, Cook JD, Finch DA. Storage iron kinetics, 3. Study of desferrioxamine action by selective radioiron labels of RE and parenchymal cells. *J Lab Clin Med* 1973; **81**: 876–86.

122. Morgan EH, Smith GD, Peters TJ. Uptake and subcellular processing of ^{59}Fe-^{125}I-labeled transferrin by rat liver. *Biochem J* 1986; **237**: 163–73.

123. Young SP, Roberts S, Bomford A. Intracellular processing of transferrin and iron by isolated rat hepatocytes. *Biochem J* 1985; **232**: 819–23.

124. Donovan A, Lima CA, Pinkus JL, *et al.* The iron exporter ferroportin/Slc40a1 is essential for iron homeostasis. *Cell Metab* 2005; **1**: 191–200.

125. Bastin J, Drakesmith H, Rees M, Sargent I, Townsend A. Localization of proteins of iron metabolism in the human placenta and liver. *Br J Haematol* 2006; **134**: 532–43.

126. Canonne-Hergaux F, Donovan A, Delaby C, Wang HJ, Gros P. Comparative studies of duodenal and macrophage ferroportin proteins. *Am J Physiol Gastrointest Liver Physiol* 2006; **290**: G156–63.

127. Lu JP, Hayashi K, Awai M. Transferrin receptor expression in normal, iron-deficient and iron-overloaded rats. *Acta Pathol Jpn* 1989; **39**: 759–64.

128. Trinder D, Morgan EH, Baker E. The effects of an antibody to the rat transferrin receptor and of rat serum albumin on the uptake of diferric transferrin by rat hepatocytes. *Biochim Biophys Acta* 1988; **943**: 440–6.

129. Sciot R, Paterson AC, Van den Oord JJ, Desmet VJ. Lack of hepatic transferrin receptor expression in hemochromatosis. *Hepatology* 1987; **7**: 831–7.

130. Lombard M, Bomford A, Hynes M, *et al.* Regulation of the hepatic transferrin receptor in hereditary hemochromatosis. *Hepatology* 1989; **9**: 1–5.

131. Morgan EH, Baker E. Iron uptake and metabolism by hepatocytes. *Fed Proc* 1986; **45**: 2810–16.

132. Trinder D, Zak O, Aisen P. Transferrin receptor-independent uptake of differic transferrin by human hepatoma cells with antisense inhibition of receptor expression. *Hepatology* 1996; **23**: 1512–20.

133. Thorstensen K, Romslo I. Albumin prevents non-specific transferrin-binding and iron uptake by isolated hepatocytes. *Biochim Biophys Acta* 1984; **804**: 393–7.

134. Cole ES, Glass J. Transferrin-binding and iron uptake in mouse hepatocytes. *Biochim Biophys Acta* 1983; **762**: 102–10.

135. Kawabata H, Yang R, Hirama T, *et al.* Molecular cloning of transferrin receptor 2. A new member of the transferrin receptor-like family. *J Biol Chem* 1999; **274**: 20826–32.

136. Chua AC, Delima RD, Morgan EH, *et al.* Iron uptake from plasma transferrin by a transferrin receptor 2 mutant mouse model of haemochromatosis, *J Hepatol* 2010; **52**: 425–31.

137. Merle U, Theilig F, Fein E, *et al.* Localization of the iron regulatory proteins hemojuvelin and transferrin receptor 2 to the basolateral membrane domain of hepatocytes. *Histochem Cell Biol* 2007; **127**: 221–6.

138. Goswami T, Andrews NC. Hereditary hemochromatosis protein, HFE, interaction with transferrin receptor 2 suggests a molecular mechanism for mammalian iron sensing. *J Biol Chem* 2006; **281**: 28 494–8.

139. Fleming RE, Migas MC, Holden CC, *et al.* Transferrin receptor 2: continued expression in mouse liver in the face of iron overload and in hereditary hemochromatosis. *Proc Natl Acad Sci USA* 2000; **97**: 2214–19.

140. Deaglio S, Capobianco A, Cali A, *et al.* Structural, functional, and tissue distribution analysis of human transferrin receptor 2 by murine monoclonal antibodies and a polyclonal antiserum. *Blood* 2002; **100**: 3782–9.

141. Lee AW, Oates PS, Trinder D. Effects of cell proliferation on the uptake of transferrin-bound iron by human hepatoma cells. *Hepatology* 2003; **38**: 967–77.

142. Robb A, Wessling-Resnick M. Regulation of transferrin receptor 2 protein levels by transferrin. *Blood* 2004; **104**: 4294–9.

25

143. Johnson MB, Enns CA. Diferric transferrin regulates transferrin receptor 2 protein stability. *Blood* 2004; **104**: 4287–93.

144. Camaschella C. Why do humans need two types of transferrin receptor? Lessons from a rare genetic disorder. *Haematologica* 2005; **90**: 296.

145. Sarkar B. State of iron(3) in normal human serum: low molecular weight and protein ligands besides transferrin. *Can J Biochem* 1970; **48**: 1339–50.

146. Batey RG, Lai Chung FP, Shamir S, Sherlock S. A non-transferrin-bound serum iron in idiopathic hemochromatosis. *Dig Dis Sci* 1980; **25**: 340–6.

147. Stojkovski S, Goumakos W, Sarkar B. Iron(III)-binding polypeptide in human cord and adult serum: isolation, purification and partial characterization. *Biochim Biophys Acta* 1992; **1137**: 155–61.

148. Chua AC, Olynyk JK, Leedman PJ, Trinder D. Non-transferrin-bound iron uptake by hepatocytes is increased in the Hfe knockout mouse model of hereditary hemochromatosis. *Blood* 2004; **104**: 1519–25.

149. Trinder D, Morgan E. Inhibition of uptake of transferrin-bound iron by human hepatoma cells by non-transferrin-bound iron. *Hepatology* 1997; **26**: 691–8.

150. Graham RM, Morgan EH, Baker E. Ferric citrate uptake by cultured rat hepatocytes is inhibited in the presence of transferrin. *Eur J Biochem* 1998; **253**: 139–45.

151. Scheiber-Mojdehkar B, Zimmermann I, Dresow B, Goldenberg H. Differential response of non-transferrin-bound iron uptake in rat liver cells on long-term and short-term treatment with iron. *J Hepatol* 1999; **31**: 61–70.

152. Trinder D, Oates PS, Thomas C, Sadleir J, Morgan EH. Localization of divalent metal transporter 1 (DMT1) to the microvillus membrane of rat duodenal enterocytes in iron deficiency, but to hepatocytes in iron overload. *Gut* 2000; **46**: 270–6.

153. Worwood M, Dawkins S, Wagstaff M, Jacobs A. The purification and properties of ferritin from human serum. *Biochem J* 1976; **157**: 97–103.

154. Mack U, Powell LW, Halliday JW. Detection and isolation of a hepatic membrane receptor for ferritin. *J Biol Chem* 1983; **258**: 4672–5.

155. Osterloh K, Aisen P. Pathways in the binding and uptake of ferritin by hepatocytes. *Biochim Biophys Acta* 1989; **1011**: 40–5.

156. Kristiansen M, Graversen JH, Jacobsen C, *et al.* Identification of the haemoglobin scavenger receptor. *Nature* 2001; **409**: 198–201.

157. Hvidberg V, Maniecki MB, Jacobsen C, Hojrup P, Moller HJ, Moestrup SK. Identification of the receptor scavenging hemopexin-heme complexes. *Blood* 2005; **106**: 2572–9.

158. Oshiro S, Nakajima H. Intrahepatocellular site of the catabolism of heme and globin moiety of hemoglobin-haptoglobin after intravenous administration to rats. *J Biol Chem* 1988; **263**: 16032–8.

159. Hinton RH, Dobrota M, Mullock BM. Haptoglobin-mediated transfer of haemoglobin from serum into bile. *FEBS Lett* 1980; **112**: 247–50.

160. Meilinger M, Haumer M, Szakmary KA, *et al.* Removal of lactoferrin from plasma is mediated by binding to low-density lipoprotein receptor-related protein/alpha 2-macroglobulin receptor and transport to endosomes. *FEBS Lett* 1995; **360**: 70–4.

161. Ziere GJ, van Dijk MC, Bijsterbosch MK, van Berkel TJ. Lactoferrin uptake by the rat liver. Characterization of the recognition site and effect of selective modification of arginine residues. *J Biol Chem* 1992; **267**: 11 229–35.

162. Bennatt DJ, Ling YY, McAbee DD. Isolated rat hepatocytes bind lactoferrins by the RHL-1 subunit of the asialoglycoprotein receptor in a galactose-independent manner. *Biochemistry* 1997; **36**: 8367–76.

163. Niederkofler V, Salie R, Arber S. Hemojuvelin is essential for dietary iron sensing, and its mutation leads to severe iron overload. *J Clin Invest* 2005; **115**: 2180–6.

164. Huang FW, Pinkus JL, Pinkus GS, Fleming MD, Andrews NC. A mouse model of juvenile hemochromatosis. *J Clin Invest* 2005; **115**: 2187–91.

165. Feder JN, Tsuchihashi Z, Irrinki A, *et al.* The hemochromatosis founder mutation in *HLA-H* disrupts beta2-microglobulin interaction and cell surface expression. *J Biol Chem* 1997; **272**: 14 025–8.

166. Ganz T. Iron homeostasis: fitting the puzzle pieces together. *Cell Metab* 2008; **7**: 288–90.

167. Terpstra V, van Berkel TJ. Scavenger receptors on liver Kupffer cells mediate the in vivo uptake of oxidatively damaged red blood cells in mice. *Blood* 2000; **95**: 2157–63.

168. Dennis C. Haemoglobin scavenger. *Nature* 2001; **409**: 141.

169. Schaer DJ, Schaer CA, Buehler PW, *et al.* CD163 is the macrophage scavenger receptor for native and chemically modified hemoglobins in the absence of haptoglobin. *Blood* 2006; **107**: 373–80.

170. Knutson MD, Vafa MR, Haile DJ, Wessling-Resnick M. Iron loading and erythrophagocytosis increase ferroportin 1 (FPN1) expression in J774 macrophages. *Blood* 2003; **102**: 4191–7.

171. Zhang AS, Xiong S, Tsukamoto H, Enns CA. Localization of iron metabolism-related mRNAs in rat

liver indicate that HFE is expressed predominantly in hepatocytes. *Blood* 2004; **103**: 1509–14.

172. Maines MD, Gibbs PE. Thirty some years of heme oxygenase: from a "molecular wrecking ball" to a "mesmerizing" trigger of cellular events. *Biochem Biophys Res Commun* 2005; **338**: 568–77.

173. Delaby C, Pilard N, Puy H, Canonne-Hergaux F. Sequential regulation of ferroportin expression after erythrophagocytosis in murine macrophages: early mRNA induction by heme followed by iron-dependent protein expression. *Biochem J* 2008; **411**: 123–31.

174. Delaby C, Pilard N, Goncalves AS, Beaumont C, Canonne-Hergaux F. Presence of the iron exporter ferroportin at the plasma membrane of macrophages is enhanced by iron loading and down-regulated by hepcidin. *Blood* 2005; **106**: 3979–84.

175. Knutson MD, Oukka M, Koss LM, Aydemir F, Wessling-Resnick M. Iron release from macrophages after erythrophagocytosis is up-regulated by ferroportin 1 over expression and down-regulated by hepcidin. *Proc Natl Acad Sci USA* 2005; **102**: 1324–8.

176. Kondo H, Saito K, Grasso JP, Aisen P. Iron metabolism in the erythrophagocytosing Kupffer cell. *Hepatology* 1988; **8**: 32–8.

177. Galli A, Bergamaschi G, Recalde H, *et al.* Ferroportin gene silencing induces iron retention and enhances ferritin synthesis in human macrophages. *Br J Haematol* 2004; **127**: 598–603.

178. Valenti L, Guido M, Dongiovanni P, Cremonesi L, Fracanzani AL, Fargion S. Ferroportin 1 in the recurrence of hepatic iron overload after liver transplantation. *Dig Liver Dis* 2009; **41**: e17–20.

179. Jouanolle AM, Douabin-Gicquel V, Halimi C, *et al.* Novel mutation in ferroportin 1 gene is associated with autosomal dominant iron overload. *J Hepatol* 2003; **39**: 286–9.

180. Wallace DF, Clark RM, Harley HA, Subramaniam VN. Autosomal dominant iron overload due to a novel mutation of ferroportin 1 associated with parenchymal iron loading and cirrhosis. *J Hepatol* 2004; **40**: 710–13.

181. Drakesmith H, Schimanski LM, Ormerod E, *et al.* Resistance to hepcidin is conferred by hemochromatosis-associated mutations of ferroportin. *Blood* 2005; **106**: 1092–7.

182. de Domenico I, Ward DM, Musci G, Kaplan J. Iron overload due to mutations in ferroportin. *Haematologica* 2006; **91**: 92–5.

183. Birgens HS, Kristensen LO, Borregaard N, Karle H, Hansen NE. Lactoferrin-mediated transfer of iron to intracellular ferritin in human monocytes. *Eur J Haematol* 1988; **41**: 52–7.

184. Butler TW, Heck LW, Berkow R, Barton JC. Radioimmunometric quantification of surface lactoferrin in blood mononuclear cells. *Am J Med Sci* 1994; **307**: 102–7.

185. Andreesen R, Sephton RG, Gadd S, Atkins RC, De Abrew S. Human macrophage maturation in vitro: expression of functional transferrin-binding sites of high affinity. *Blut* 1988; **57**: 77–83.

186. van Berkel TJ, Dekker CJ, Kruijt JK, van Eijk HG. The interaction in vivo of transferrin and asialotransferrin with liver cells. *Biochem J* 1987; **243**: 715–22.

187. Bastin JM, Jones M, O'Callaghan CA, Schimanski L, Mason DY, Townsend AR. Kupffer cell staining by an HFE-specific monoclonal antibody: implications for hereditary haemochromatosis. *Br J Haematol* 1998; **103**: 931–41.

Iron toxicity

Iron is an essential element, but in excess it can result in cell injury (Table 3.1).[1–5] When storage mechanisms are overwhelmed, iron in low molecular weight forms can play a catalytic role in the initiation of free radical reactions. The resulting oxyradicals have the potential to damage cellular lipids, nucleic acids, proteins, and carbohydrates, resulting in wide-ranging impairment in cellular function and integrity. The rate of free radical production must overwhelm the cytoprotective defenses of cells before injury occurs.

In *HFE* hemochromatosis, there can be a pathologic expansion of body iron stores due to an increase in the absorption of dietary iron. Transferrin saturation is increased and non-transferrin-bound iron (which is redox-active) may be present. The excess iron is preferentially deposited in the cytoplasm of parenchymal cells of various organs and tissues including the liver, pancreas, heart, endocrine glands, skin, and joints.[6,7] Damage can result in micronodular cirrhosis of the liver and atrophy of the pancreas (primarily islets). Hepatocellular carcinoma, usually in the presence of cirrhosis, is another consequence of excess iron deposition in the liver. Symptoms are related to damage of involved organs and include liver failure (from cirrhosis), diabetes mellitus, arthritis, cardiac dysfunction (arrhythmias and failure), and hypogonadotrophic hypogonadism.[6,7] Important co-factors of iron-induced liver injury include chronic hepatitis C and excess alcohol consumption.[6,7] Although cadmium and lead may also be transported by divalent metal transporter-1, the major apical iron transporter in enterocytes, excess iron is considered to be the major cause of toxicity in hemochromatosis.[1–5]

In disorders of erythropoiesis and in some forms of chronic liver disease, increased iron absorption and tissue iron deposition can occur. A common factor in the iron-loading anemias is refractory anemia with a hypercellular bone marrow and ineffective erythropoiesis.[8] These conditions include β-thalassemia and sideroblastic anemias. In these syndromes, clinical and pathologic consequences similar to those seen in *HFE* hemochromatosis can occur. In disorders of erythropoiesis in which there are concomitant blood transfusions, the iron burden can increase very rapidly through the combined impact of increased iron absorption and transfusion-derived iron (in hemoglobin). Therefore, these patients may present with the consequences of iron toxicity to the liver, heart, and pancreas many years earlier than patients with *HFE* hemochromatosis.[8]

The degree of structural and functional damage to the liver, heart, and endocrine organs generally parallels the degree of parenchymal iron overload.[6,7] Excess iron can be stored as ferritin in both the cytoplasm and lysosomes, or as hemosiderin in lysosomes. The hepatic concentration of iron is an important factor in determining hepatotoxicity, since removal of excess iron by phlebotomy or chelation results in clinical improvement.[6,7]

Two major hypotheses have been proposed to explain iron-induced toxicity: the oxidative injury hypothesis and the lysosomal injury hypothesis.[1–5] These hypotheses concerning iron-induced damage are not mutually exclusive, since there is evidence of oxidative damage to lysosomal lipids which may contribute to lysosomal injury in iron overload.

Oxidative injury hypothesis

The oxidative injury hypothesis postulates that iron overload in vivo can result in the formation of oxyradicals, with resultant damage to cellular constituents and impairment in cellular function. This section will summarize how iron catalyzes the formation of oxyradicals, the potential cellular targets of these radicals, and the evidence that iron can cause free radical production in vivo.

Table 3.1. Iron toxicity

Iron in excess can cause cell injury through the generation of oxyradicals

Oxyradicals can damage cellular lipids, nucleic acids, proteins, and carbohydrates

Mitochondrial injury, decreased cellular ATP levels, impaired cellular calcium homeostasis, and lysosomal fragility may all contribute to cellular injury in iron overload

Iron-induced damage to DNA may play a role in hepatocarcinogenesis

Hepatic iron overload can lead to fibrogenesis, and potentiating factors include chronic viral hepatitis and excess alcohol consumption

Iron potentiates the cardiotoxicity of anthracycline chemotherapeutic drugs and the pulmonary toxicity of bleomycin

Iron catalyzes the formation of oxyradicals

Abundant evidence now exists from in vitro experiments that iron can catalyze the production of oxyradicals, when iron is available in a redox-active form.[1,2] Two important radicals that can result from these reactions are lipid radicals and hydroxyl radicals. One type of reaction promoted by iron that leads to the formation of lipid radicals is the decomposition of preformed lipid hydroperoxides. Ferrous (Fe^{2+}) iron chelates and ferric (Fe^{3+}) iron chelates can react with lipid hydroperoxides to form alkoxyl and peroxyl radicals, respectively.

Iron can also catalyze the production of hydroxyl radicals through Fenton or Haber–Weiss chemistry.[1,2] These reactions require the presence of hydrogen peroxide and superoxide radical, which are often found in biological systems. The hydroxyl radical is extremely reactive and can attack many cell constituents including lipids, nucleic acids, and proteins. Since the polyunsaturated fatty acids of membrane phospholipids are particularly susceptible to oxidative attack, the process of lipid peroxidation has been widely studied after iron overload.

Iron causes lipid peroxidation and oxidant stress in vivo

After initiation of lipid peroxidation by hydroxyl radicals or another radical species, a number of products are produced including conjugated dienes, lipid hydroperoxides, and a large number of lipid breakdown products.[1–4] The latter include the reactive aldehydes malondialdehyde (MDA) and 4-hydroxynonenal (HNE). MDA and HNE can react with proteins and the resulting adducts can serve as markers of lipid peroxidation.

Substantial evidence has now accumulated that iron overload in experimental animals can result in hepatic lipid peroxidation in vivo.[1] A number of lipid peroxidation products have been detected in the liver including conjugated dienes, thiobarbituric acid-reactants (TBA-reactants), HNE, fluorescent products, and protein adducts of MDA. High concentrations of iron in the liver seem to be required to produce lipid peroxidation, suggesting that the normal storage pathways have to be overwhelmed before iron is available to catalyze oxyradical production.

Although oxyradicals have the potential to cause damage to lipids, proteins, carbohydrates, and DNA, cells contain cytoprotective mechanisms (antioxidants, scavenging enzymes, repair processes) whose action counteracts the effects of oxyradical production.[9] Thus, the net effect of oxyradicals on cellular function will depend on the balance between radical production and these cytoprotective systems. Vitamin E (α-tocopherol) is an important lipid-soluble antioxidant, which acts to quench lipid peroxidation; in doing so, vitamin E is oxidized. Although water-soluble, ascorbate also plays an important role in the defense against lipid peroxidation through the regeneration of vitamin E from oxidized vitamin E. Levels of both of these critical antioxidants can be decreased under pro-oxidant conditions. In experimental iron overload, hepatic and plasma vitamin E levels are low, and plasma ascorbate levels are also reduced.

There is substantial evidence in experimental animals that iron overload can induce oxidative stress and depletion of antioxidants, but there are fewer studies that address this issue in patients with iron overload (Table 3.2). Young et al.[10] reported that the mean plasma level of TBA-reactants was increased in a group of 15 hemochromatosis patients, compared to the level in 15 matched healthy controls. Concurrent

Table 3.2. Evidence for lipid peroxidation in patients with iron overload

Observations
TBA-reactants in plasma
MDA-protein adducts in liver
HNE-protein adducts in liver
Etheno-DNA adducts in liver
8-iso-prostaglandin F2α in urine

measurement of the plasma concentrations of vitamin E and ascorbate revealed that these were decreased in the hemochromatosis group. Direct evidence of hepatic lipid peroxidation in hemochromatosis patients has been demonstrated by increased amounts of MDA-protein adducts and HNE-protein adducts in liver biopsies.[11,12] After phlebotomy therapy, the levels of these adducts in the liver was substantially reduced, indicating that their presence was dependent on elevated hepatic iron levels.[12] In addition, hemochromatosis patients have increased levels of 8-iso-prostaglandin F2α, a marker of oxidative stress, in their urine.[13] Patients with iron overload due to beta-thalassemia also have increased plasma levels of TBA-reactants and decreased circulating concentrations of vitamin E and ascorbate.[14]

Taken together with the results in experimental animals, these studies in patients with iron overload support the concept that iron overload can induce oxidant stress when the body iron stores are substantially elevated.

Lysosomal injury hypothesis

Accumulation of intracellular iron in lysosomes is commonly seen in patients with iron overload.[15] It is generally considered that sequestration of iron within lysosomes serves a protective role by removing this redox-active metal from the cytoplasm and by providing a route for removal from the liver through lysosome-mediated biliary excretion. The lysosomal injury hypothesis[16–19] proposes that excessive accumulation of iron within lysosomes can lead to lysosomal fragility, impaired lysosomal function, and eventual cellular injury through the release of hydrolytic enzymes and stored iron into the cytoplasm. One mechanism which may contribute to the increased lysosomal fragility found in iron overload is lipid peroxidation.[18,19] While lysosomal changes have been observed in patients with iron overload and in iron-loaded animals, it remains to be determined if fragile lysosomes release their contents into the cytoplasm in vivo with resultant cellular injury.

Cellular organelle dysfunction in iron overload

In addition to lysosomes, iron-induced oxyradicals may damage hepatic mitochondria, the endoplasmic reticulum, and the plasma membrane.

Mitochondria

Mitochondrial oxidative metabolism is susceptible to iron-induced impairment. Hepatic mitochondria from iron-loaded rats show significant decreases in respiratory rate at moderate degrees of hepatic iron overload.[20] At hepatic iron concentrations at which there were decreases in oxidative metabolism, there was also evidence of mitochondrial lipid peroxidation. The effects of iron overload on hepatic mitochondrial respiration are caused primarily by a decrease in cytochrome C oxidase activity.[21] The impairment in mitochondrial oxidative capacity caused by iron overload results in a substantial decrease in hepatic ATP concentrations.[1,21] This decrease in hepatic ATP levels may disturb hepatocellular function and compromise cellular integrity.

Endoplasmic reticulum

Hepatic microsomal lipid peroxidation was found in vivo in rats with chronic dietary iron overload, when the hepatic iron content exceeded a certain threshold.[22] In addition, decreases in microsomal cytochrome P-450, aminopyrine demethylase activity, and cytochrome b_5 were associated with microsomal lipid peroxidation in this model.[22] Another microsomal function which is sensitive to the damaging effects of peroxidation is calcium sequestration. Chronic dietary iron overload in rats resulted in an impairment in hepatic microsomal calcium sequestration,[23] and this may alter hepatocellular calcium homeostasis and contribute to cell injury.

Plasma membrane

In a series of detailed studies, Hershko and co-workers have studied the toxicity of non-transferrin-bound iron

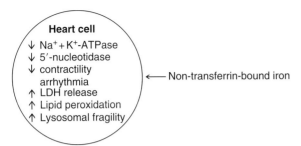

Fig. 3.1. Effects of non-transferrin-bound iron on cultured heart cells. Taken from James C. Barton and Corwin Q. Edwards (eds), Hemochromatosis: Genetics, Pathophysiology, Diagnosis, and Treatment, Cambridge University Press 2000. Reproduced with permission.

in rat myocardial cells in culture.[24] Exposure of cardiac myocytes to ferric ammonium citrate resulted in lipid peroxidation, decreased contractility and arrhythmias (Fig. 3.1). These investigators have identified thiol-rich enzymes (such as Na^+-$+K^+$-ATPase and $5'$-nucleotidase) in the plasma membrane as possible primary targets of iron toxicity, and suggested that oxidative modification of these enzymes may impair their activity. Because Na^+-$+K^+$-ATPase plays a key role in maintaining the cell membrane potential, a decrease in its activity may contribute to the functional activities observed. Most effects of non-transferrin-bound iron on myocytes can be prevented or reversed by iron chelators. Non-transferrin-bound iron also impaired mitochondrial respiration and increased lysosomal fragility in these myocardial cells, indicating that damage to mitochondria and lysosomes may also play a role in myocardial injury caused by iron overload. Interestingly, *Hfe* knockout mice (a model of *HFE* hemochromatosis) have increased susceptibility to cardiotoxicity induced by the anthracycline chemotherapeutic agent, doxorubicin.[25] The pulmonary toxicity of bleomycin is also potentiated by iron. These results suggest that genetic mutations related to abnormalities in iron metabolism may contribute to the toxicity of certain chemotherapeutic agents in humans.

Iron can cause DNA damage and carcinogenesis

Hemochromatosis patients with long-standing iron overload and cirrhosis have an increased risk for developing hepatocellular carcinoma.[26] Accordingly, it has been proposed that hepatocellular carcinoma in these patients may be a consequence of iron-induced oxidative damage to hepatic DNA, combined with the replicative stimulus provided by cirrhotic nodular regeneration. Iron salts have been shown to produce DNA strand breaks when incubated in vitro with either purified DNA or with isolated nuclei.[27] In addition to these in vitro data, it has been demonstrated that endogenous iron plays a key role in the DNA damage produced by hydrogen peroxide in mammalian cells, since pretreatment with iron-chelating agents diminishes this damage. It is thought that some iron is bound to DNA in vivo and that this iron, in the presence of superoxide and hydrogen peroxide, can catalyze the formation of "site-directed" hydroxyl radicals which cause DNA damage. Lipid peroxidation products in the presence of iron can also produce DNA damage in vitro through a mechanism that also may involve the hydroxyl radical.[28]

Chronic iron overload in vivo results in damage to hepatic DNA based on a number of measures including strand breaks, fragmentation and 8-hydroxydeoxyguanosine (a marker of oxidative DNA damage).[1,27,29] Several studies have investigated the possibility of DNA damage in patients with iron overload. Carmichael *et al.*[30] examined hepatic DNA samples from 6 hemochromatosis patients, and bulky DNA lesions were detected which contained from 2 to 50 base modifications per 100 million nucleotides. It has also been demonstrated that iron-loaded patients have increased levels of lipid peroxidation-derived etheno-DNA adducts in their livers.[31] Of interest, these DNA adducts are associated with an increased frequency of mutations in the p53 tumor suppressor gene (codon 249) in hemochromatosis liver.[32]

Therefore, evidence has accumulated indicating that iron can produce injury to DNA in patients with hemochromatosis and in experimental animals. This damage might be an important step leading to carcinogenesis, especially when coupled with a proliferative stimulus such as that provided by concomitant cirrhosis of the liver.

Summary

Figure 3.2 summarizes several proposed mechanisms of iron-induced toxicity. It has long been suspected that free radicals may play a role in iron-induced cell toxicity because of the powerful pro-oxidant action of iron salts in vitro. In the presence of available cellular reductants, iron in low-molecular-weight forms may play a catalytic role in the initiation of free radical reactions. The resulting oxyradicals have the potential

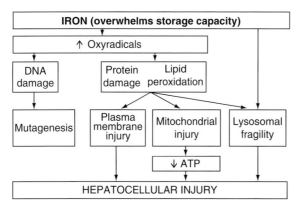

Fig. 3.2. Mechanisms of cellular toxicity induced by iron overload. Taken from James C. Barton and Corwin Q. Edwards (eds), Hemochromatosis: Genetics, Pathophysiology, Diagnosis, and Treatment, Cambridge University Press 2000. Reproduced with permission.

to damage cellular lipids, nucleic acids, proteins, and carbohydrates, resulting in wide-ranging impairment in cellular function and integrity. Nonetheless, cells are endowed with cytoprotective mechanisms (antioxidants, scavenging enzymes, repair processes) which act to counteract the effects of free radical production. Thus, the net effect of iron-induced free radicals on cellular function will depend on the balance between radical production and the cytoprotective systems. As a result, the rate of free radical production may need to overwhelm the cytoprotective defenses before cellular injury occurs.

There is substantial evidence that iron overload in experimental animals can result in oxidative damage to lipids in vivo, once the concentration of iron exceeds a threshold level. In the liver, this lipid peroxidation is associated with impairment of membrane-dependent functions of mitochondria (oxidative metabolism) and lysosomes (membrane integrity, fluidity, pH). Although these findings do not prove causality, it seems likely that lipid peroxidation is involved, since similar functional defects are produced by iron-induced lipid peroxidation in these organelles in vitro. Iron overload impairs hepatic mitochondrial respiration primarily through a decrease in cytochrome C oxidase activity. In iron overload, hepatocellular calcium homeostasis may be impaired through damage to mitochondrial and microsomal calcium sequestration. DNA has also been reported to be a target of iron-induced damage and this may have consequences as regards malignant transformation. Mitochondrial respiratory enzymes and

plasma membrane enzymes such as Na^{+}-$+K^{+}$-ATPase may be key targets of damage by non-transferrin-bound iron in cardiac myocytes. Levels of some antioxidants such as vitamin E are decreased during iron overload, which is also suggestive of ongoing oxidative stress. Reduced cellular ATP levels, lysosomal fragility, impaired cellular calcium homeostasis, and damage to DNA may all contribute to cellular injury in iron overload.

Evidence is accumulating that free radical production is increased in patients with iron overload. Iron-loaded patients have elevated plasma levels of TBA-reactants and increased hepatic levels of MDA-protein and HNE-protein adducts, indicative of lipid peroxidation. Hepatic DNA of iron-loaded patients shows evidence of damage including mutations of the tumor suppressor gene p53.

References

1. Britton RS. Mechanisms of iron toxicity. In: Barton JC, Edwards CQ, eds. *Hemochromatosis. Genetics, Pathophysiology, Diagnosis and Treatment*. Cambridge, Cambridge University Press. 2000; 229–38.

2. Pietrangelo A. Mechanism of iron toxicity. *Adv Exp Med Biol* 2002; **509**: 19–43.

3. Britton RS, Leicester KL, Bacon BR. Iron toxicity and chelation therapy. *Int J Hematol* 2002; **76**: 219–28.

4. Papanikolaou G, Pantopoulos K. Iron metabolism and toxicity. *Toxicol Appl Pharmacol* 2005; **202**: 119–211.

5. Ramm GA, Ruddell RG. Hepatotoxicity of iron overload: Mechanisms of iron-induced hepatic fibrogenesis. *Semin Liver Dis* 2005; **25**: 433–49.

6. Bacon BR. Hemochromatosis: Diagnosis and management. *Gastroenterology* 2001; **120**: 718–25.

7. Powell LW. Hereditary hemochromatosis and iron overload diseases. *J Gastroenterol Hepatol* 2002; **17** (Suppl 1): 191–5.

8. Bottomley SS. Secondary iron overload disorders. *Semin Hematol* 1998; **35**: 77–86.

9. Halliwell B, Gutteridge JMC. *Free Radicals in Biology and Medicine*. 3rd edition. Oxford, Oxford University Press, 1999.

10. Young IS, Trouton TG, Torney JJ, McMaster D, Callender ME, Trimble ER. Antioxidant status and lipid peroxidation in hereditary haemochromatosis. *Free Radic Biol Med* 1994; **16**: 393–7.

11. Niemela O, Parkkila S, Britton RS, Brunt E, Janney C, Bacon BR. Hepatic lipid peroxidation in hereditary hemochromatosis and alcoholic liver injury. *J Lab Clin Med* 1999; **133**: 451–60.

12. Houglum K, Ramm GA, Crawford DHG, Witztum JL, Powell LW, Chojkier M. Excess iron induces hepatic oxidative stress and transforming growth factor β1 in genetic hemochromatosis. *Hepatology* 1997; **26**: 605–10.

13. Kom GD, Schwedhelm E, Nielsen P, Boger RH. Increased urinary excretion of 8-iso-prostaglandin F2alpha in patients with HFE-related hemochromatosis: A case-control study. *Free Radic Biol Med* 2006; **40**: 1194–200.

14. Livrea MA, Tesoriere L, Pintaudi AM, *et al.* Oxidative stress and antioxidant status in β-thalassemia major: Iron overload and depletion of lipid-soluble antioxidants. *Blood* 1996; **88**: 3608–14.

15. Iancu TC, Shiloh H. Morphological observations in iron overload: An update. *Adv Exp Med Biol* 1994; **356**: 255–65.

16. Selden C, Owen M, Hopkins JMP, Peters TJ. Studies on the concentration and intracellular localization of iron proteins in liver biopsy specimens from patients with iron overload with special reference to their role in lysosomal disruption. *Br J Haematol* 1980; **44**: 593–603.

17. Peters TJ, O'Connell MJ, Ward RJ. Role of free-radical mediated lipid peroxidation in the pathogenesis of hepatic damage by lysosomal disruption. In: Poli G, Cheeseman KH, Dianzani MU, Slater TF, eds. *Free Radicals in Liver Injury*. Oxford, IRL Press. 1985; 107–15.

18. O'Connell M, Halliwell B, Moorhouse CP, Aruoma OI, Baum H, Peters TJ. Formation of hydroxyl radicals in the presence of ferritin and haemosiderin. Is haemosiderin formation a biological protective mechanism? *Biochem J* 1986; **234**: 727–31.

19. Myers BM, Prendergast FG, Holman R, Kuntz SM, LaRusso NF. Alterations in the structure, physicochemical properties, and pH of hepatocyte lysosomes in experimental iron overload. *J Clin Invest* 1991; **88**: 1207–15.

20. Bacon BR, Park CH, Brittenham GM, O'Neill R, Tavill AS. Hepatic mitochondrial oxidative metabolism in rats with chronic dietary iron overload. *Hepatology* 1985; **5**: 789–97.

21. Bacon BR, O'Neill R, Britton RS. Hepatic mitochondrial energy production in rats with chronic iron overload. *Gastroenterology* 1993; **105**: 1134–40.

22. Bacon BR, Healey JF, Brittenham GM, *et al.* Hepatic microsomal function in rats with chronic dietary iron overload. *Gastroenterology* 1986; **90**: 1844–53.

23. Britton RS, O'Neill R, Bacon BR. Chronic dietary iron overload in rats results in impaired calcium sequestration by hepatic mitochondria and microsomes. *Gastroenterology* 1991; **101**: 806–11.

24. Hershko C, Link G, Konijn AM. Cardioprotective effect of iron chelators. *Adv Exp Med Biol* 2002; **509**: 77–89.

25. Miranda CJ, Makui H, Soares RJ, *et al.* Hfe deficiency increases susceptibility to cardiotoxicity and exacerbates changes in iron metabolism induced by doxorubicin. *Blood* 2003; **102**: 2574–80.

26. Kowdley KV. Iron, hemochromatosis, and hepatocellular carcinoma. *Gastroenterology* 2004; **127**: S79–86.

27. Okada S. Iron-induced tissue damage and cancer: The role of reactive oxygen species-free radicals. *Pathol Int* 1996; **46**: 311–32.

28. Park J-W, Floyd RA. Lipid peroxidation products mediate the formation of 8-hydroxydeoxyguanosine in DNA. *Free Radic Biol Med* 1992; **12**: 245–50.

29. Zhang D, Okada S, Yu Y, Zheng P, Yamaguchi R, Kasai H. Vitamin E inhibits apoptosis, DNA modification, and cancer incidence induced by iron-mediated peroxidation in Wistar rat kidney. *Cancer Res* 1997; **57**: 2410–14.

30. Carmichael PL, Hewer A, Osborne MR, Strain AJ, Phillips DH. Detection of bulky DNA lesions in the liver of patients with Wilson's disease and primary haemochromatosis. *Mutation Res* 1995; **326**: 235–43.

31. Nair J, Carmichael PL, Fernando RC, Phillips DH, Strain AJ, Bartsch H. Lipid peroxidation-induced etheno-DNA adducts in the liver of patients with the genetic metal storage disorders Wilson's disease and primary hemochromatosis. *Cancer Epidemiol Biomarkers Prev* 1998; **7**: 435–40.

32. Hussain SP, Raja K, Amstad PA, *et al.* Increased p53 mutation load in nontumorous human liver of Wilson's disease and hemochromatosis: Oxyradical overload diseases. *Proc Natl Acad Sci USA* 2000; **97**: 12770–5.

Tests for hemochromatosis and iron overload

Iron overload and associated abnormalities can be detected by diverse biochemical and physicochemical tests. It is also possible to predict susceptibility to develop iron overload in some persons by the appropriate selection and interpretation of molecular genetic analyses. In this chapter, the clinical and laboratory assessment of iron overload is reviewed.

Transferrin and transferrin saturation

Transferrin is a ~80 kDa metal-binding glycoprotein synthesized by hepatocytes. It is the predominant iron transporter in plasma, and is responsible for the capture, transport, and distribution of free iron. Each molecule of transferrin has two high-affinity iron-binding sites, each of which can bind one ferric ion. Iron binding to transferrin is maximal at alkaline values of pH, and in the presence of bicarbonate. Transferrin binds iron absorbed via enterocytes and iron that is released by macrophages and hepatocytes. In healthy subjects, much transferrin-bound iron is delivered to erythroblasts in the bone marrow for hemoglobin synthesis via specific transferrin receptors (Chapter 2). Transferrin also transports iron to other tissues that accept iron via similar receptors. In normal subjects, approximately eight times the amount of plasma iron quantified in static measurements is delivered by transferrin to target cells each day. Transferrin also binds and transports certain non-ferrous metals (Chapter 8).

Normal subjects

The capacity of serum transferrin to bind iron is measured by automated clinical laboratory methods as the serum total iron-binding capacity (TIBC). Typically, this is calculated as the sum of the serum iron concentration and the serum unbound iron-binding capacity (UIBC). Transferrin saturation (TS) is the ratio of the serum iron concentration to the serum TIBC, expressed as a percentage. Plasma or serum levels of transferrin protein can also be measured directly using an immunoassay. The TIBC can be extrapolated from the immunoreactive transferrin level, because transferrin accounts for most of the serum (or plasma) iron-binding capacity. The TIBC estimated in this manner is usually lower than that indirectly measured by the UIBC technique.

The mean normal serum iron concentration is ~100 µg/dL (~20 µmol/L). The mean normal serum transferrin concentration is ~30 µmol/L. Thus, approximately one-third of the iron-binding capacity of transferrin is normally saturated. Approximately 40% of between-individual variation in serum transferrin (and TIBC) levels is due to genetic variations in the *TF* gene that encodes transferrin synthesis and common mutations of the *HFE* gene associated with "classic" hemochromatosis.[1] In contrast, measurement of immunoreactive transferrin has little value in the diagnosis of iron overload disorders. Mean serum iron and transferrin saturation levels are lower in persons of Asian, Native African, and Pacific Islander descent than in Caucasians,[2–4] although the genetic or physiologic basis of these differences is largely unknown.

Iron deficiency, a common disorder in most populations, induces increased transferrin synthesis and thus elevated levels of serum transferrin and TIBC. Acute or chronic inflammation, renal insufficiency, malignant neoplasms, and other common conditions are often associated with decreased transferrin synthesis and thus with decreased blood levels of serum transferrin and TIBC.

In normal individuals, transferrin saturation levels are often lowest in the early morning hours before eating. Post-prandial levels may be higher, especially after consumption of an iron-rich meal.[5,6] Serum iron and transferrin saturation levels increase approximately one hour after ingestion of iron supplements. Sustained increases may occur in persons who ingest iron supplements regularly. The intra-individual coefficient of variation for serum iron concentration and TIBC were 28.5% and 4.8%, respectively, in 13 healthy volunteers studied daily using morning samples.[7] In one study, there was diurnal variation of serum iron and transferrin saturation levels in normal subjects,[5] although other studies of normal subjects did not detect rhythmic variation in these levels.

HFE hemochromatosis

In many subjects with "classical" *HFE* hemochromatosis diagnosed in medical care, serum iron levels are typically elevated, but levels of TIBC are slightly below the corresponding lower reference limits. Consequently, measurements of TS are elevated in many adults with *HFE* hemochromatosis (Table 4.1). In some infants or children with *HFE* C282Y homozygosity, TS is elevated when iron stores are normal for age. The within-day variability of serum iron concentration, TIBC, and TS measures was studied in 43 adult hemochromatosis patients diagnosed in medical care and in normal controls; blood samples were taken at 2-h intervals for one 24-h period.[7] Serum iron levels and TS measures were constantly abnormal in the hemochromatosis patients, and revealed little variation between the mean values observed at each sample time. Accordingly, TS would appear to be a valid test for *HFE* hemochromatosis case finding in medical practice, and could permit the diagnosis of hemochromatosis before excess iron is deposited in target organs.

Screening for hemochromatosis with TS or UIBC

For hemochromatosis case finding or population screening, there are no TS threshold or cut-point levels that meet with universal agreement. Using lower TS levels increases sensitivity for detecting persons with hemochromatosis, but markedly decreases specificity due to the large number of false positives (Table 4.2). Evaluating subjects with a second TS measurement is feasible in medical practice and may increase diagnosis specificity in subjects with two elevated TS levels. In efficient population screening, the within-person biological variability of TS and

Table 4.1. Transferrin saturation in iron overload disorders

Typically elevated

Minority of *HFE* C282Y homozygotes, with or without iron overload

Hemochromatosis due to *HJV*, *TFR2*, or "gain-of-function" *SLC40A1* mutations

X-linked or refractory sideroblastic anemia, thalassemia major

Transfusion iron overload, African iron overload

Sometimes elevated

Many *HFE* C282Y homozygotes

Porphyria cutanea tarda

Ingestion of iron-rich meals or supplemental iron

Hepatocellular necrosis of diverse causes

Typically normal or decreased

Untreated *HFE* C282Y homozygotes without iron overload, especially women

Hemochromatosis due to "loss-of-function" *SLC40A1* mutations

African-American iron overload

Hereditary atransferrinemia

UIBC limits their usefulness as an initial screening test for *HFE* C282Y homozygotes who have evidence of iron overload.[8] In addition, return visits for additional testing are not feasible. In general, a TS level consistently ≥45% in women or ≥50% in men is suspicious for *HFE* hemochromatosis in either case finding or population screening. The UIBC level has also been evaluated in a similar manner; a level <24 µg/dL is suspicious for *HFE* hemochromatosis.[8,9] The most important pre-analytical factors in TS testing are ingestion of iron-containing medications, supplements, and foods, and inherent biological variability in the test results. The analytical concerns of standardization, chemical specificity, and precision have been addressed many clinical laboratories. The pre-analytical decision to order the TS test and post-analytical decision making (i.e. expertise of the clinician) are major areas that need improvement.

Many studies have evaluated the effectiveness of hemochromatosis and iron overload screening programs using TS or UIBC levels (Chapters 8, 37). One study used a UIBC cut-point of 125 µg/L for 8939

Table 4.2. Transferrin saturation in HFE hemochromatosis screening[a]

	TS decision level (%)	Detection rate	False positive rate	Likelihood ratio	Prevalence is 5 per 1000		Prevalence is 5 per 10 000	
					Positive PV	Negative PV	Positive PV	Negative PV
Men	50	0.94	0.0700	13	0.0632	0.9997	0.0067	0.9999
	55	0.91	0.0320	28	0.1250	0.9995	0.0140	0.9999
	60	0.86	0.0150	57	0.2237	0.9993	0.0279	0.9999
	65	0.79	0.0066	120	0.3756	0.9989	0.0565	0.9999
	70	0.72	0.0027	267	0.5727	0.9986	0.1177	0.9999
	75	0.64	<0.0010	640	>0.7628	0.9982	0.2425	0.9998
	no test	0.00	—	—	—	0.9950	—	0.9995
Women	50	0.82	0.0500	16	0.0761	0.9990	0.0081	0.9999
	55	0.75	0.0180	42	0.1731	0.9987	0.0204	0.9999
	60	0.67	0.0059	113	0.3633	0.9983	0.0538	0.9998
	65	0.58	0.0018	322	0.6182	0.9979	0.1388	0.9998
	70	0.48	<0.0010	480	>0.7069	0.9974	0.1936	0.9997
	no test	—	0.00	—	—	0.9950	—	0.9995

Note: [a]Adapted from Cappuccio and Phatak.[120] TS = serum transferrin saturation; PV = predictive value.

samples from 7073 people. The study identified nine persons requiring intervention and nine others whose evaluation was incomplete, but who had a reasonable likelihood to have hemochromatosis.[10] This yield is 1.3–2.6 cases per 1000 subjects screened. More recent screening studies used TS and serum ferritin phenotyping and *HFE* mutation analysis to identify C282Y and H63D alleles. In 209 previously undiagnosed *HFE* C282Y homozygotes detected in a large, primary care-based screening program, 68 homozygotes (33%) would have remained undetected by the study TS cut-points. Fifty-eight homozygotes (28%) would have been missed at the study UIBC cut-points (20 men, 38 women). There was no advantage to using fasting samples.[11] These data support the conclusion that TS has limited usefulness in screening studies to detect *HFE* C282Y homozygotes due to the wide intra-individual variation of TS. "Non-expression" of hemochromatosis further limits the value of TS or UIBC screening. In one report, 50% of female and 28% of male *HFE* C282Y homozygotes had TS levels <50%.[12]

Non-*HFE* hemochromatosis and iron overload

TS is usually elevated in persons with hemochromatosis phenotypes due to mutations in genes that encode hemojuvelin, hepcidin, and transferrin receptor-2 (Table 4.1) (Chapters 13–15). In "gain-of-function" ferroportin hemochromatosis, African iron overload, and X-linked sideroblastic anemia, TS levels are also increased (Table 4.1) (Chapters 12, 18, 25). In persons who have received multiple erythrocyte transfusions, the TS level is almost always elevated in those with iron overload sufficient to cause hyperferritinemia. TS is often normal or low in "loss-of-function" ferroportin hemochromatosis, persons of sub-Saharan Native African descent who have non-transfusion iron overload (Chapter 18), and in hereditary atransferrinemia (Table 4.1) (Chapter 19). TS levels are typically normal in persons with dysmetabolic iron overload syndrome. In a rare case, a transferrin-specific autoantibody produced circulating immune complexes that bound the majority of serum transferrin and caused an increase in serum iron levels. Immunosuppression

Table 4.3. Common causes of elevated serum ferritin levels

Primary iron overload, e.g. *HFE* hemochromatosis

Secondary iron overload, e.g. severe beta-thalassemia, chronic transfusion

Chronic alcohol consumption with increased apoferritin synthesis or secretion

Common liver disorders, e.g. viral hepatitis B and C, alcoholic liver disease, non-alcoholic fatty liver disease

Chronic renal failure

Systemic inflammatory disease, e.g. rheumatoid arthritis

Malignancies, especially hepatic metastases

Acute myocardial infarction

Serious infections

Hyperferritinemia-cataract syndrome

induced a partial remission, including a decrease in serum iron levels, an increase in free transferrin levels, disappearance of excessive iron deposited in the liver, and an increase in erythrocyte production.[13]

Serum ferritin

Ferritin, a storage molecule with cage-like morphology (Chapter 2), sequesters iron that is not required for current metabolism. Storage of iron in ferritin reduces or prevents the generation of toxic oxyradicals by reactions catalyzed by free iron. Although most cells can store iron in ferritin, hepatocytes and macrophages are particularly adapted for this function and can retain excess iron as a reserve for times of increased body iron needs (Table 4.3). Hepatocytes take up iron in different forms and act as a major site of available iron stores, and thus have a central buffering role in internal iron exchange.[14–17]

Normal subjects

Most ferritin is intracellular. Its H- and L-subunits are encoded by the *FTH1* gene (chromosome 11q12–q13) and the *FTL* gene (chromosome 19q13.3–13.4), respectively. Ferritin synthesis is controlled at the levels of transcription and translation (Chapter 2). In healthy subjects, iron exerts the strongest regulatory influence on ferritin synthesis. Most iron-associated control of ferritin synthesis is mediated at the translational level via RNA-binding iron regulatory protein (IRP) that binds to ferritin iron-responsive element (IRE), a stem–loop structure in the 5′-untranslated region of the ferritin mRNA (Chapter 2). Ferritin is synthesized primarily on free polysomes, as expected for a cytoplasmic protein; some synthesis also occurs on membrane-bound polysomes (~15% in hepatocytes). Ferritin synthesis is also stimulated at the transcriptional and translational levels by cytokines (e.g. interleukin-1, interleukin-6, and tumor necrosis factor-α), by the state of cellular differentiation, and by some hormones. A small proportion of ferritin is secreted into the plasma, although the function of secreted ferritin is unknown. Accordingly, serum ferritin levels (SF) are surrogate (but imperfect) indicators of the degree of iron repletion or overload.

In normal subjects (and in iron overload patients without tissue damage), most ferritin in plasma or serum occurs by secretion. Chronic ethanol ingestion stimulates hepatic synthesis or secretion of apoferritin in some subjects. SF levels are also increased by the injury of cells that normally contain large quantities of ferritin or apoferritin, e.g. hepatocytes or myocardium. Some neoplastic cells produce and secrete large quantities of apoferritin autonomously, although hyperferritinemia of malignancy is more often associated with the extent of organ invasion or metastasis. Thus, injured tissue is the predominant source of SF in most patients with hepatocellular damage, myocardial infarction, inflammation, or malignancy (Table 4.3).

Ferritin is the primary component of hemosiderin, an aggregate of partially degraded ferritin (including ferric hydroxide), lysosomes, and other material. Iron stored in ferritin or hemosiderin can be mobilized readily when the metabolic requirements for iron are increased. This is the basis of achieving iron depletion through phlebotomy therapy in hemochromatosis. The precise mechanisms by which iron is removed from ferritin and hemosiderin in vivo have not been elucidated. Ferritin depleted of iron is destroyed in proteasomes (Chapter 2).

SF levels of healthy persons are relatively constant, and there is little or no diurnal variation. SF levels are relatively high at birth (>300 μg/L), but fall over the first 6 months of life to levels similar to those of adults (10–200 μg/L). Some otherwise normal children or adolescents have low SF levels due to the iron demands of rapid growth and development. In men, SF levels rise slowly and progressively with age.[3]

In many healthy women of reproductive age, SF levels remain relatively low but constant. After menopause or hysterectomy, SF levels in women typically rise slowly to concentrations similar to those of men of the same age.[3] Mean SF levels are higher in persons of Asian, Native African, and Pacific Islander descent than in Caucasians matched for sex and age,[2–4] although the genetic or physiologic basis of these differences is unknown. Subnormal SF levels in the absence of iron deficiency are characteristic of neuroferritinopathy (Chapter 31). Ascorbate (vitamin C) deficiency or laboratory error sometimes cause falsely low SF levels.

There is a progressive rise in SF concentrations with increments of body iron stores. An increase in the SF concentration of 1 μg/L is equivalent to an increase in storage iron of ∼8 mg in persons who have no abnormal conditions that influence SF levels. Thus, there is a positive correlation of SF concentration and body iron stores across subjects with iron deficiency, normal iron repletion, and uncomplicated iron overload.[18]

HFE hemochromatosis and other iron overload disorders

Ferritin metabolism is fundamentally normal in most subjects with primary or secondary iron overload disorders. A low or normal level of SF (<200 μg/L in women and <300 μg/L in men) indicates that significant iron overload is not present, but such results do not substantiate the conclusion that such persons will never develop iron overload. In persons with primary iron overload disorders, the rate of accumulation of excessive iron and the age at which hyperferritinemia first occurs are determined in part by the underlying genetic abnormalities. For example, hemochromatosis associated with *HJV* or *TFR2* mutations often causes early age-of-onset iron overload. Markedly elevated SF levels may develop within the first few years of life (Table 4.3). In infants or children with hemochromatosis-associated *HFE* genotypes, in contrast, elevated SF concentrations attributable to iron overload are rare. In the majority of adult *HFE* C282Y homozygotes, SF levels increase slowly or not at all over long periods, especially in women. In the minority of *HFE* C282Y homozygotes who develop iron overload, elevated SF measures are usually detected after adolescence, typically in middle age (Table 4.3). In persons with severe thalassemia or hemoglobinopathy treated with chronic erythrocyte transfusion, SF levels due to iron overload become elevated in direct proportion to the timing and quantity of erythrocyte transfusion (Table 4.3). Regardless of the cause of iron overload, excessive iron occurs predominantly in hemosiderin, not ferritin. Measurements of ferritin-bound iron in serum can distinguish iron overload and its severity from other causes of hyperferritinemia,[19] but this test is not commercially available.

In persons with uncomplicated primary iron overload, the SF concentration is the most readily available indicator of the severity of iron overload and the risk of iron-induced organ damage. In *HFE* hemochromatosis, elevated SF concentrations first occur in the absence of architectural damage to the liver, suggesting that the initial elevation of SF is the result of enhanced ferritin secretion, rather than hepatocellular injury. The risk of hepatic cirrhosis due to iron overload is low in persons who are homozygous for *HFE* C282Y and whose SF levels are less than 1000 μg/L.[20]

All persons with severe iron overload, regardless of cause, have severe hyperferritinemia due to the combined effects of increased ferritin secretion and hepatocellular necrosis caused by iron overload. In persons with *HFE* hemochromatosis whose SF is 1000 μg/L or greater, the risk of cirrhosis is high.[20] Approximately 15% of persons with *HFE* hemochromatosis also have co-incidental viral hepatitis B or C, chronic alcohol ingestion, alcohol-induced liver injury, or non-alcoholic hepatic steatosis. These conditions may augment hyperferritinemia and hepatic injury caused by excess iron (Table 4.3). There are significant differences between the liver hemosiderins of patients with thalassemia and hemochromatosis. Such differences could play a role in the relative rates of iron mobilization in the two disorders, and in iron-related toxicity.

Distinctive clinical and laboratory abnormalities, including those of serum ferritin and iron storage, occur in persons with mutations in the *FTH1* and *FTL* genes (Chapters 16, 17).

Screening for iron overload with SF

Measurement of SF is a valid and sensitive test for iron overload case finding in medical practice and in population screening, because all persons with iron overload have elevated SF levels. As expected, an elevated SF screening criterion identifies hemochromatosis homozygotes with iron overload, but few obligate heterozygotes.[21] Nonetheless, the specificity of elevated SF levels to detect iron overload is very low, because most persons in the general population with hyperferritinemia do not have iron overload. Regardless, some persons with non-iron overload hyperferritinemia have liver or other disorders and need further evaluation and management. On the other hand, it has been traditionally held that this SF testing strategy would fail to detect persons with early iron overload due to hemochromatosis in whom timely therapy to achieve iron depletion could prevent associated organ damage.

In another SF screening approach, Waalen et al. performed retrospective analyses of white participants in a large California screening program.[22] Among 29 699 subjects, only 59 had SF levels higher than 1000 µg/L. Twenty-four of them had hemochromatosis-associated HFE genotypes; in 86% of the other subjects, the causes of elevated SF levels were excessive alcohol intake, cancer, or liver disease. It was proposed that population screening for hemochromatosis using a SF cut-point of ≥1000 µg/L would detect the majority of persons who would be "clinically affected" and could detect other significant disease in patients without hemochromatosis genotypes.[22] The major but narrow tenets of this screening approach are that liver disease is the sole subjective or objective consequence of iron overload in HFE hemochromatosis, and that no person with HFE hemochromatosis and SF <1000 µg/L will develop cirrhosis to which iron overload is a contributing factor.[23] Prospective studies are needed to evaluate this screening strategy further.[23]

In persons with hemochromatosis, SF levels can be used to estimate the number of phlebotomies required to achieve iron depletion, especially in persons without viral hepatitis B or C, chronic alcohol ingestion, alcohol-induced liver injury, or non-alcoholic hepatic steatosis. The SF level is also a useful measure of the progress of phlebotomy or iron chelation in diminishing iron overload. Most experts advocate frequent phlebotomy treatments until SF levels are in the low normal range to assure that all potentially deleterious excess iron has been removed (Chapter 36).

Serum ceruloplasmin

Ceruloplasmin is a plasma metalloprotein, an alpha-2 glycoprotein polypeptide of 1046 amino acids. It is a member of the multi-copper oxidase enzyme family. Ceruloplasmin is synthesized in hepatocytes where it binds copper, and is then secreted into plasma. It is the principal copper containing protein in plasma. About 95% of circulating plasma copper is bound to ceruloplasmin. The remainder of serum copper is bound to albumin, precuprein, and complexes of copper and amino acids. Each ceruloplasmin molecule can transport six atoms of copper. Ceruloplasmin concentration responds as an acute-phase reactant in the presence of inflammation, pregnancy, and during treatment with estrogen[24] and increases during treatment with some anticonvulsants (phenobarbital, phenytoin, carbamazepine, valproic acid).[25]

Ceruloplasmin function

Ceruloplasmin is a ferroxidase that catalyzes the oxidation of ferrous iron after it is transported out of cells (such as hepatocytes and macrophages) via ferroportin, and it is also needed to maintain ferroportin localization on cell membranes.[26] Ferric iron then becomes bound to apotransferrin and transferrin-bound iron is transported to sites of normal physiologic function, principally to the bone marrow for hemoglobin synthesis, to myoglobin, and to cytochromes. A normal physiologic function of ceruloplasmin is the prevention of lipid peroxidation. In ceruloplasmin deficiency, ferrous iron is not oxidized, so iron is not transported from storage cells into plasma. This results in accumulation of iron inside storage cells. Individuals with aceruloplasminemia develop iron overload because ceruloplasmin is not involved in iron transport from intestinal epithelia into plasma. The latter is a function of hephaestin, an intestinal multi-copper oxidase homologous to ceruloplasmin (Chapter 2).

Ceruloplasmin deficiency and iron overload

Some individuals with ceruloplasmin deficiency (e.g. Wilson disease or hereditary aceruloplasminemia) also develop iron overload. The clinical presentation and the phenotypic and genotypic tests in Wilson disease (see below) or hereditary aceruloplasminemia (Chapter 28) are quite different from those of patients who have HFE hemochromatosis. Many aspects of HFE hemochromatosis are also discussed in the current chapter. Absence of ceruloplasmin in the neurons and retina results in lipid peroxidation, that in turn causes cell damage and death, followed by organ dysfunction.

Wilson disease

Almost a century ago, Samuel Alexander Kinnier Wilson, a US-born neurologist, wrote a 210-page description of the condition that is named for him.[27] Wilson disease is caused by mutation of the *ATP7B* gene on the long arm of chromosome 13 (chromosome 13q14.3–q21.1). The gene includes 21 exons. Unlike "classical" hemochromatosis in which few *HFE* mutations account for most cases, many patients with Wilson disease have novel *ATP7B* mutations. More than 380 mutations of *ATP7B* have been reported. [28,29] Most persons with Wilson disease are compound heterozygotes, rather than homozygotes, for *ATP7B* mutations.

The *ATP7B* gene encodes a polypeptide P-type ATPase beta-polypeptide that functions as a membrane transporter of copper. ATP7B protein has 1465 amino acids, 6 copper-binding regions, and 8 transmembrane domains. In normal individuals, this ATPase causes excretion of copper into bile. In subjects with Wilson disease, the mutant ATP7B proteins fail to transport copper into bile normally, resulting in accumulation of large amounts of copper in hepatocytes. The excessive copper damages hepatocytes that consequently release copper into plasma, resulting in accumulation of copper in, and damage of, other organs. Patients with Wilson disease usually have low plasma concentrations of ceruloplasmin in plasma, but do not have *CP* mutations or qualitative abnormalities of ceruloplasmin.

The prevalence of Wilson disease varies markedly according to the population that is studied and the type of testing employed to identify abnormal homozygotes.[28,30] Using data from three published studies, an early estimate of the prevalence of Wilson disease was about 1 per 30 000.[31] More recent estimates, based on currently-available testing methods, estimated prevalences that were as high as 1 per 2600 in US[32] to 1 per 24 410 in an area of Japan.[33] In other studies from Japan, the population prevalence was estimated to be 1 per 1395 to 1 per 8055.[34,35] In a report from a study of newborns in Korea, the prevalence of Wilson disease was estimated to be 1 per 30 778.[36]

Typical clinical features of Wilson disease include: (a) Coombs'-negative hemolytic anemia due to copper-induced injury of erythrocyte membrane enzymes that becomes apparent in childhood; (b) tremor or choreiform movement disorder of limbs, dystonia, and spasticity of facial and limb muscles due to copper-induced injury of basal ganglia; (c) abnormal gait, walking on tiptoes due to spasticity of muscles; (d) dysarthria; (e) Kayser–Fleischer rings of copper accumulation in the cornea near the limbus; (f) osteoporosis; (g) renal tubular acidosis and aminoaciduria due to renal tubular injury; (h) hepatosplenomegaly due to cirrhosis with portal hypertension; and (i) hepatic failure. Intermittent episodes of hemolysis often occur in children who are later found to have Wilson disease. Facial dystonia and muscle spasticity of limb muscles occurs in many teenagers with Wilson disease. Liver failure due to cirrhosis is common in the second and third decades of life. A very small percentage of individuals with *ATP7B* genotypes consistent with Wilson disease are not diagnosed until the sixth decade of life.

The common laboratory features of Wilson disease include elevation of serum concentrations of hepatic transaminases and serum bilirubin; decreased serum concentrations of both copper and ceruloplasmin; increased urinary excretion of copper after oral administration of D-penicillamine; and a liver biopsy that reveals markedly increased stainable and biochemically measured copper (and usually cirrhosis). The serum copper level in Wilson disease is typically less than 20 µg/dL (normal >80 µg/dL). The typical serum ceruloplasmin concentration is less than 6 mg/dL (normal >20 mg/dL). Although biliary copper excretion is very low in patients with Wilson disease, this does not need to be measured. In clinical practice, mutation analysis of *ATP7B* is not needed, because the treatment for copper overload is the same for all patients, regardless of *ATP7B* genotype. For research purposes, the entire *ATP7B* gene must be sequenced to identify the two deleterious mutations in each index case.

Hepatic iron levels in Wilson disease

Hepatic storage iron is increased in some patients with Wilson disease alone,[37–40] although the increase is not as striking as it is in *HFE* hemochromatosis homozygotes with severe iron overload. In a report from Japan, liver iron levels were measured in four males with Wilson disease, aged 16 to 23 years.[39] Two of the four patients had elevated SF levels. All four individuals had stainable liver iron, but their hepatic iron indices were normal (0.5–1.1 µmol/g per y; >1.9 µmol/g per y in typical hemochromatosis homozygotes).

Co-inheritance of Wilson disease and hemochromatosis

Some persons with Wilson disease also have hemochromatosis. The frequency of *HFE* C282Y/H63D compound heterozygotes is ~20 persons per 1000 in the general US Caucasian population.[2] The expected prevalence of persons with Wilson disease and *HFE* C282Y/H63D compound heterozygosity is therefore ~20 persons per 30 000 000 general population. The frequency of homozygosity for hemochromatosis in Caucasians of European ancestry is ~4.4 per 1000.[2] Thus, it is predicted that the occurrence of both Wilson disease and hemochromatosis due to *HFE* C282Y homozygosity is very rare (~4.4 persons per 30 000 000 general population). As predicted, very few individuals have been found to have both Wilson disease and *HFE* hemochromatosis.[37,41,42]

In a recent report, a 23-year-old man with abdominal pain, ascites, hypoprothrombinemia, and elevated serum concentrations of hepatic transaminases was found to have TS >90% and SF 1188 µg/L. Liver biopsy revealed inflammation, extensive fibrosis, and increased stainable iron. His hepatic iron index was normal (1.3 µmol/g per y), whereas *HFE* C282Y homozygotes typically have hepatic iron indices greater than 1.9 µmol/g per y. DNA testing demonstrated that he had *HFE* C282Y/H63D compound heterozygosity. His serum ceruloplasmin concentration was low and his urinary excretion of copper was increased. Slit-lamp examination of his eyes revealed bilateral Kayser–Fleischer rings.[42] The authors concluded that this 23-year-old patient had both *HFE* hemochromatosis and Wilson disease. Mutation analysis of *ATP7B* or *CP* was not reported. Another patient had both Wilson disease and hemochromatosis with *HFE* C282Y homozygosity.[37]

Aceruloplasminemia

This rare heritable disorder is due to mutations of the *CP* gene located on the long arm of chromosome 3 (chromosome 3q23–q24); more than 40 *CP* deleterious mutations have been reported (Chapter 28). Aceruloplasminemia is distinguished from Wilson disease by the absence of ceruloplasmin in the serum, by the absence of excess urinary excretion of urinary copper after the administration of D-penicillamine, and by the absence of excess storage copper in the liver. This condition is one of several disorders in which iron-induced neurologic injury is prominent (Table 4.4).

Table 4.4. Characteristics of some heritable iron overload disorders

Disorder	Inheritance[a]	Gene; chromosome	Contributors to high iron phenotype
Neither neurologic abnormalities nor anemia prominent			
HFE hemochromatosis (type 1)	AR	*HFE*; 6p21.3	male sex, dietary iron content
Hemojuvelin hemochromatosis (type 2)	AR	*HJV*; 1q21	
Transferrin receptor-2 hemochromatosis (type 3)	AR	*TFR2*; 7q22	
Ferroportin hemochromatosis (type 4)	AD	*SLC40A1*; 2q32	
Porphyria cutanea tarda[b]	AD	*UROD*; 1p34	common *HFE* mutations, hepatitis C, alcohol consumption
Japanese iron overload	AD	*FTH1*; 11q12–q13	
Hereditary hyperferritinemia-cataract syndrome[c]	AD	*FTL*; 19q13.1–q13.3.3	
African iron overload	ACD	unknown	chronic consumption of traditional beer containing iron

Table 4.4. (*cont.*)

Disorder	Inheritance[a]	Gene; chromosome	Contributors to high iron phenotype
Neurologic abnormalities prominent			
Neuroferritinopathies (adult-onset basal ganglia disease)[c]	AD	*FTL*; 19q13.1–q13.3.3	
Aceruloplasminemia	AR, AD	*CP*; 3q23–q24	
Pantothenate kinase-associated neurodegeneration	AR	*PANK2*; 20p13–p12.3	
Friedreich ataxia	AR	*FXN*; 9p23–p11, 9q13	
Anemia prominent			
β-Thalassemia major	AR	*HBB*; 11p15.5	ineffective erythropoiesis with increased GDF15[d]; erythrocyte transfusions
Hereditary X-linked sideroblastic anemia	XL	*ALAS2*; Xp11.21	ineffective erythropoiesis; erythrocyte transfusions
Pyruvate kinase deficiency	AR	*PKLR*; 1q21	ineffective erythropoiesis with increased GDF15[d]; erythrocyte transfusions
Congenital dyserythropoietic anemia, type I	AR	*CDAN1*; 15q15.1–q15.3	ineffective erythropoiesis with increased GDF15[d]; erythrocyte transfusions
Congenital dyserythropoietic anemia, type II	AR	*SEC23B*; 20q11.2	ineffective erythropoiesis; erythrocyte transfusions
Atransferrinemia	AR	*TF*; 3q21	erythrocyte transfusions
DMT1 iron overload	AR	*SLC11A2*; 12q13	
Glutaredoxin-5 deficiency	AR	*GLRX5*; 14q32	
Neurologic abnormalities and anemia prominent			
X-linked sideroblastic anemia with ataxia	XL	*ABCB7*; Xq13.1–q13.3	

Notes: [a]AD = autosomal dominant; ACD = autosomal co-dominant; AR = autosomal recessive; XL = X-linked.
[b]Many patients do not have detectable UROD mutations. The contributing causes of high iron phenotypes are similar to those with heritable or sporadic porphyria cutanea tarda.
[c]In hereditary hyperferritinemia-cataract syndrome, *FTL* mutations in the nucleotides that encode the iron-responsive element result in marked hyperferritinemia without iron overload. In neuroferritinopathies, *FTL* mutations in the coding regions result in "gain-of-function" L-ferritin and abnormal protein folding; typical patients have subnormal serum ferritin levels and progressive iron deposition in basal ganglia.
[d]GDF15 = growth/differentiation factor 15.

Serum ceruloplasmin and liver copper in *HFE* hemochromatosis

The serum concentrations of ceruloplasmin are decreased in iron-loaded *HFE* hemochromatosis homozygotes, and return to normal values after iron depletion.[26] Regardless, serum ceruloplasmin measurement is not a useful phenotypic test for the diagnostic evaluation of individuals who are suspected to have hemochromatosis, nor does it provide useful prognostic or management information. Early investigators reported that levels of copper are increased in some patients who die of hemochromatosis and iron overload.[43] The pathogenesis of this phenomenon is incompletely understand. Therapeutic phlebotomy is ineffective in removing copper.

Liver biopsy

Liver biopsy continues to have a role in the clinical assessment of some patients with iron overload, especially to determine the presence and stage of fibrosis (Table 4.5).[44–49] Since the discovery of the *HFE* gene in 1996, the role of liver biopsy in the diagnosis and management of hemochromatosis has changed. With the availability of *HFE* genetic testing, fewer liver biopsies are being performed. At that time, liver biopsy was necessary to establish a diagnosis of hemochromatosis, because elevated SF and/or TS levels are frequently sensitive but non-specific for iron overload. Thus, individuals with elevated serum iron measures could have other disorders and not have iron overload: liver biopsy allowed the determination of the degree of hepatic iron loading. Many patients with non-alcoholic fatty liver disease (NAFLD), chronic viral hepatitis (B and C), or alcoholic liver disease have elevated serum iron measures in the absence of iron overload.[44–46] These three disorders (chronic viral hepatitis, NAFLD, chronic alcohol use) comprise approximately 75% of patients seen by hepatologists. Thus, it is important to be able to distinguish whether or not these patients have co-existent hemochromatosis with their other liver disease, or if they have one of these other liver diseases with mild secondary iron overload and abnormal iron studies.

With the advent of *HFE* genetic testing in the late 1990s, differentiation of *HFE* hemochromatosis and secondary iron overload disorders has improved greatly. In patients with suspected hemochromatosis, *HFE* mutation analysis should be performed prior to consideration of biopsy. In *HFE* C282Y homozygotes, liver biopsy is indicated if serum ferritin levels are greater than 1000 µg/L or if serum activities of hepatic transaminases are elevated (Table 4.5).[47–49] These guidelines are based on several studies that showed that significant fibrosis was only observed in those hemochromatosis patients who had SF levels greater than 1000 µg/L or who had elevated liver enzyme measures. Less important criteria for biopsy include the presence of hepatomegaly or age greater than 40 years.[44]

When liver biopsy is performed, a biochemical stain for iron (Perls' Prussian blue stain) should be requested. It is also reasonable to request a biochemical determination of hepatic iron concentration (HIC) (Table 4.5). With the measured HIC, the hepatic iron index (HII) can be calculated. The HII is the HIC (µmoles Fe/g liver dry weight) divided by the age of the patient (in years). Before the availability of genetic testing, HII values greater than 1.9 µmol/g per y were considered to be diagnostic of hemochromatosis. HIC determined by liver biopsy has some inherent variability, especially in cirrhotic livers.[50]

An important characteristic of liver biopsy is that it can provide an assessment of the stage of fibrosis and of other histologic abnormalities such as steatosis. From a prognostic standpoint, the presence of advanced fibrosis or cirrhosis is important to establish, because the risk of hepatocellular cancer is significantly increased in those patients who have established cirrhosis. Accordingly, as in all patients with cirrhosis, surveillance abdominal imaging is utilized to assess for the development of early hepatocellular cancer. Patients with cirrhosis should also have surveillance upper endoscopy to determine whether or not esophageal varices are present and thus, to determine whether prophylactic therapy with beta-blockers or variceal band ligation should be initiated.

Liver biopsy is a generally safe procedure, with estimated mortality rates of 1 per 1000 to 1 per 10 000 biopsies.[51] Morbidity and mortality due to liver biopsy are usually caused by uncontrolled bleeding from inadvertent capsular tear or puncture of intrahepatic or portal vessels. Furthermore, biliary peritonitis, due to puncture of the gall bladder, also has a high mortality rate.[51]

In patients with *HFE* hemochromatosis, iron deposition is first observed in periportal (zone 1) hepatocytes, and there is a periportal to pericentral gradient (Fig. 4.1).[52] Iron deposits predominate in parenchymal cells, with sparing of sinusoidal lining cells (Kupffer cells) (Fig. 4.2). With more severe iron loading, iron deposition becomes panlobular but is

Table 4.5. Liver biopsy in iron overload

Useful to determine the presence and stage of fibrosis, the pattern of iron deposition, the hepatic iron concentration, and the co-existence of other histologic changes (such as steatosis)

Indicated in *HFE* C282Y homozygotes to determine the stage of fibrosis if either serum ferritin levels exceed 1000 µg/L or if serum liver enzyme (ALT, AST) activities are elevated

Upper normal limit of hepatic iron concentration is 1500 µg/g dry weight

Generally safe, but has some morbidity and mortality primarily due to bleeding

43

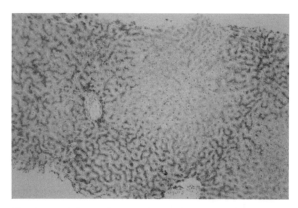

Fig. 4.1. Liver biopsy from a *HFE* C282Y homozygote shows iron deposition predominantly in periportal (zone 1) hepatocytes, with a periportal to pericentral gradient of iron (Perls' Prussian blue stain; hepatic iron concentration 5680 µg/g dry wt). See plate section for color version.

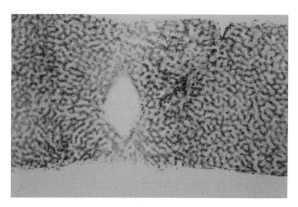

Fig. 4.2. Liver biopsy from a *HFE* C282Y homozygote shows iron deposition predominantly in hepatocytes, with sparing of Kupffer cells (Perls' Prussian blue stain; hepatic iron concentration 8085 µg/g dry wt). See plate section for color version.

(a)

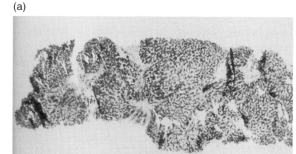

(b)

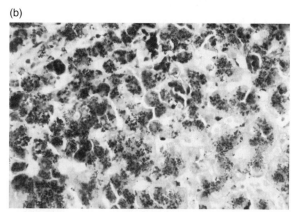

Fig. 4.3. (a) Panlobular iron deposition and micronodular cirrhosis in patient with hemochromatosis. (b) Higher magnification shows that iron is deposited predominantly in hepatocytes, despite a very high hepatic iron concentration of 40 380 µg/g dry wt (Perls' Prussian blue stain). See plate section for color version.

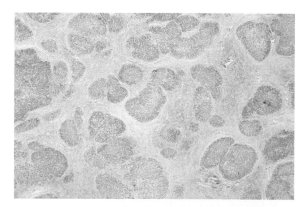

Fig. 4.4. Micronodular cirrhosis in patient with hemochromatosis and *HFE* C282Y homozygosity. The fibrous bands (stained blue) surround islands of hepatocytes (Masson trichrome stain). See plate section for color version.

still primarily in hepatocytes (Fig. 4.3). When early diagnosis is missed and treatment is not performed, manifestations can progress to micronodular cirrhosis (Fig. 4.4) and liver failure. In symptomatic patients with hemochromatosis, the HIC is typically greater than 10 000 µg/g dry weight (normal <1500 µg/g dry weight), and values as high as 40 000 µg/g dry weight have been reported. In contrast, in patients with mild secondary iron overload related to alcoholic liver disease, chronic viral hepatitis, or NAFLD, the HIC is rarely as high as 10 000 µg/g dry weight and is more commonly in the 2000–3000 µg/g dry weight range. In studies in which pre-treatment and post-treatment liver biopsies were performed, therapeutic phlebotomy was very effective in removing increased hepatic iron stores.

Liver biopsy is frequently useful in patients with secondary iron overload.[49,52] In patients with mild transfusion iron overload, the iron is stored primarily

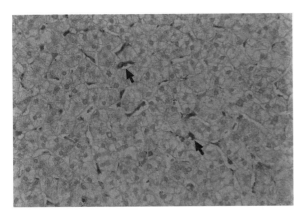

Fig. 4.5. Mild secondary iron overload due to transfusions; iron is located predominantly in Kupffer cells (Perls' Prussian blue stain). Taken from James C. Barton and Corwin Q. Edwards (eds), *Hemochromatosis: Genetics, Pathophysiology, Diagnosis and Treatment*, Cambridge University Press 2000. Reproduced with permission. See plate section for color version.

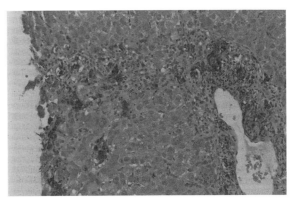

Fig. 4.6. Liver biopsy from a patient with chronic hepatitis C shows iron deposition predominantly in Kupffer cells (Perls' Prussian blue stain). Taken from James C. Barton and Corwin Q. Edwards (eds), *Hemochromatosis: Genetics, Pathophysiology, Diagnosis and Treatment*, Cambridge University Press 2000. Reproduced with permission. See plate section for color version.

in Kupffer cells (Fig. 4.5). In patients with chronic hepatitis C who have abnormal iron studies, liver biopsy can be utilized to determine the degree of iron loading. Usually, iron stains are negative or show 1+ iron deposition despite the fact that serum ferritin levels may be quite elevated (800–1000 µg/L). Iron deposition is usually panlobular, in both hepatocytes and sinusoidal lining cells, and does not have a typical hemochromatosis pattern.[52] In patients with chronic hepatitis C and secondary iron overload in whom the iron deposition is 2+ or greater, and/or the HIC is greater than 2500 µg/g dry weight, therapeutic phlebotomy may be considered prior to initiation of antiviral therapy.[53] When interferon monotherapy was the sole treatment used for treating hepatitis C, it was observed that the HIC was higher in those patients who did not respond to treatment.[53] Some studies also showed a difference in the pattern of iron deposition, in that there is greater reticuloendothelial iron in periportal regions in patients did not have a favorable response to antiviral therapy (Fig. 4.6). The importance of HIC in predicting response to treatment was diminished when better antiviral therapy with the combination of interferon and ribavirin was developed, and subsequently the combination of pegylated interferon and ribavirin. Thus, therapeutic phlebotomy in patients with chronic hepatitis C is not usually employed prior to antiviral therapy today, unless there is either severe secondary iron overload or co-existent hemochromatosis with increased iron stores.

Conventional diagnostic radiology techniques

The physical properties of iron are such that iron overload induces modifications in computed tomography attenuation and magnetic resonance signal intensity of the liver, heart, and other organs. The liver is the only iron storage compartment in which the iron content is consistently increased with increased body iron stores. The correlation of magnetic resonance signals with HIC is greater than with the serum ferritin concentration.[54] Cardiac siderosis is a major cause of death in patients with transfusion iron overload (especially beta-thalassemia major) and juvenile-onset types of hemochromatosis. This has promoted interest in developing quantitative radiologic methods for non-invasive diagnosis of iron overload in target organs, and to provide additional information about hepatocellular carcinoma arising in patients with hemochromatosis and other iron overload disorders.[54,55]

Computed tomography (CT) scanning

Due to its density, iron increases X-ray attenuation in the liver and other organs affected by iron overload. Iron is responsible for a spontaneous hyperdense liver image that produces an abnormal visualization of the portal and hepatic vascular structures. There are few in vivo studies of the quantification of hepatic iron in persons with hemochromatosis using single- or

(a)   (b)   (c)

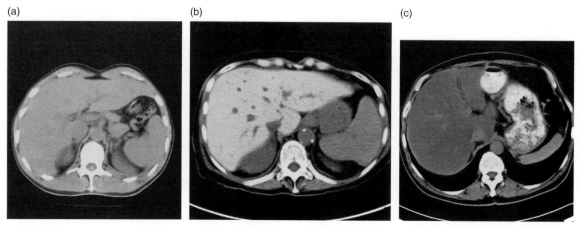

Fig. 4.7. Computed tomography (CT) scans. (a) Normal liver. Liver attenuation <70 Hounsfield units (HU). Difference between liver and spleen attenuation <20 HU. (b) Hemochromatosis. The spleen attenuation approximates normal, and the difference between liver and spleen attenuation = 35 HU. (c) Hepatic steatosis. Decreased liver attenuation (10 HU) due to massive steatosis (fatty liver). In persons who also have hemochromatosis, steatosis, which has an effect on liver attenuation that is opposite to that of iron overload, could result in false-negative results for iron quantification by CT. Reproduced from Guyader and Gandon.[54] Taken from James C. Barton and Corwin Q. Edwards (eds), **Hemochromatosis: Genetics, Pathophysiology, Diagnosis, and Treatment**, Cambridge University Press 2000. Reproduced with permission.

dual-energy CT scanning methods. Further development of these techniques was hampered because magnetic resonance techniques were more useful.[54] Nonetheless, patients with livers that appear hyperdense by CT scanning should undergo evaluation for iron overload (Fig. 4.7). Decreased attenuation of the liver can also be caused by copper overload (Wilson disease), iodine (amiodarone therapy for cardiac arrhythmias), gold (therapy for rheumatoid arthritis), and glycogen storage disorders.

Magnetic resonance imaging (MRI)

With MRI, patients are placed in a horizontal cylinder and exposed to a strong and homogeneous magnetic field by using a large magnet made by passing an electric field through superconducting coils of wire.[55] At equilibrium, hydrogen nuclei in the body normally have randomly oriented spins, but align in a direction parallel to a magnetic field. The MRI machine applies short electromagnetic pulses through a coil at a specific radio frequency (RF). An external RF coil detects the electromagnetic signals that are emitted as the hydrogen nuclei return to equilibrium. The strength of the signals varies, depending on the applied RF magnetic fields.[55] A sample returns to equilibrium in the longitudinal plane over a characteristic interval called the T1 relaxation time (the time constant for

excited nuclei to dissipate excess energy to the environment). In the transverse plane, the return to equilibrium occurs over a characteristic interval called the T2 relaxation time (the time constant for excited nuclei to go out of phase with each other). Both T1 and T2 depend on the local environments of the hydrogen nuclei.[55]

Tissue iron is detected indirectly with MRI by the effects on relaxation times of ferritin and hemosiderin iron interacting with nearby hydrogen nuclei. Paramagnetic ferritin and hemosiderin iron shorten proton relaxation times, particularly T2, although this effect is incompletely understood.[55,56] This leads to a decrease in signal intensity of the liver (and other organs with iron deposits) on T2-weighted images.[57,58] In the absence of a theoretical understanding of the effects of iron on MRI, empirical efforts to estimate HIC have used a variety of instruments, magnetic field strengths, imaging sequences (spin-echo, gradient recalled-echo (GRE)), and parameters (T1 and T2 relaxation times, and signal intensity ratios as measured in proton, T1-, T2-, or T2*-weighted images), but no standard or generally accepted method has been adopted for clinical application.[55]

The use of high magnetic field strength or the use of gradient-echo T2*-weighted sequences have greater sensitivity and detect iron overload corresponding to 80–300 μmol/g dry weight of liver.[54,59,60] GRE sequences are available on every MRI unit. According to the degree of iron overload, different sequences must be used.[54,60] Highly T2*-weighted GRE sequences give the best results for detection or quantification of mild overload ($<100\,\mu mol/g$ dry weight of liver).[54] Proton-density gradient-echo sequences give the best results in cases of moderate iron overload (HIC 100–250 $\mu mol/g$ dry weight of liver).[54] Less sensitive sequences, such as short TE spin-echo sequences, are accurate for massive iron overload with HIC $>250\,\mu mol/g$ dry weight of liver.[54] Nonetheless, the signal intensity of the liver is reduced to such an extent with increasing iron concentrations that discrimination between different concentrations becomes almost impossible with current technology.[61]

The signal intensity of the liver must be compared with a reference value. The use of reference phantoms is not always compatible with routine clinical MRI scanning.[54] Therefore, liver signal intensity is usually compared with the signal intensity of other organs on the same image not affected by iron overload. Liver/muscle (L/M) ratios are used by most observers. Liver signal intensity is averaged from several regions of interest in the right lobe of the liver. Muscle signal intensity is measured on paraspinal muscle. The L/M ratio decreases as hepatic iron overload increases. No accepted reference range exists for values of signal intensity (L/M), and threshold values differed among studies from 0.5 to 0.8 to 1.0.[54] Schematically, a liver signal intensity less than that of muscle indicates the presence of hepatic iron overload (Fig. 4.8).

MRI in iron overload disorders

Hemochromatosis due to mutations in *HFE*, *HJV*, and *TFR2* causes parenchymal iron overload and thus decreased MRI signal of the liver, pancreas, heart, and endocrine glands. In each of these types of hemochromatosis, the spleen signal is usually normal (Fig. 4.8), but may be diffusely decreased in persons with massive iron overload. MRI measurements permit accurate assignment of subjects with *HFE* hemochromatosis into hepatic fibrosis severity groups.[62] MRI technique detects differences in organ iron deposition associated with hemochromatosis caused by "gain-of-function" or "loss-of-function" ferroportin gene (*SLC40A1*) mutations.[63] MRI technique has also been used to detect cardiac siderosis in hemochromatosis, and to define alterations of cardiac high-energy phosphate metabolism in *HFE* C282Y homozygotes who have no other evidence of heart disease.[64,65]

Decreased liver or L/M signal intensity due to iron overload is not specific for hemochromatosis. Transfusion iron overload is associated with a predominance of reticuloendothelial iron overload involving the spleen, bone marrow, and Kupffer cells of the liver. In contrast to many types of hemochromatosis, transfusion iron overload therefore decreases the MRI signal in liver and in the spleen.[55] In patients with beta-thalassemia major, the presence of liver fibrosis makes estimates of HIC derived from MRI so variable that routine MRI scanning is of little practical use in the assessment and management of transfusion iron overload.[61]

Other T2 or T2* MRI techniques do have utility for evaluation of cardiac siderosis and the progress of iron chelation therapy in patients with transfusion iron overload associated with beta-thalassemia major and sickle cell disease.[66,67] In beta-thalassemia, heart T2 relaxation time appear to agree with qualitative and quantitative measures of high and low iron deposition in cardiac biopsy specimens (Fig. 4.9).[68] The degree of signal intensity reduction, measured as the pituitary-to-fat signal intensity ratio for GRE T2*-weighted images, correlates with the severity of pituitary dysfunction in patients with transfusion iron overload.[69] Iron-associated joint disease in thalassemia patients with iron overload can also be evaluated with MRI technique.[70]

Some cases of focal iron deposition have been reported.[54] Segmental wedge-shaped volumes of decreased liver signal can be related to disturbances of portal vein circulation (thrombosis or arteriovenous shunts) caused by hemodynamic factors or mild iron deposition in hepatocytes. Large regenerative nodules in otherwise iron-free cirrhotic livers may accumulate iron,[71] and some of them develop internal iron-poor foci of hyperplasia or malignancy.

Porphyria cutanea tarda, inefficient erythropoiesis, end-stage cirrhosis, dysmetabolic iron syndrome, and chronic viral hepatitis can also cause iron overload. Few studies have addressed the question of whether iron distribution that could be measured using MRI will permit a distinction of hemochromatosis to be made from these other conditions.[55] The only study that included such patients could not compare their features with those of persons with hemochromatosis, because all the hemochromatosis patients studied had massive iron overload that precluded further conclusion.[72]

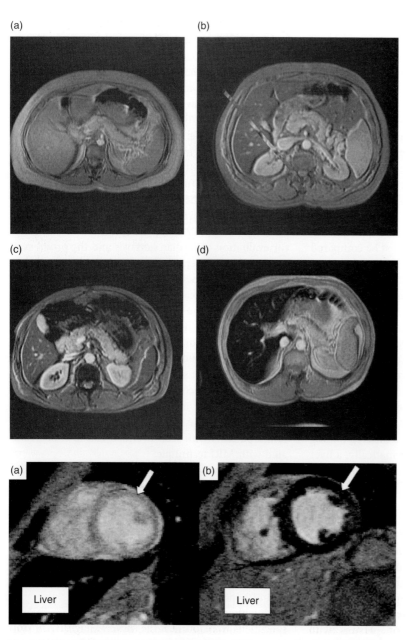

Fig. 4.8. Magnetic resonance imaging (MRI). (a) Normal liver. Signa 1.5 tesla (GEMS, Milwaukee). T2* weighted-gradient-echo sequence (TR = 120 ms; TE = 14 ms; flip angle = 20°). The liver intensity is greater than the paraspinal muscle signal intensity. (b) Hemochromatosis. Mild iron overload (hepatic iron concentration = 80 μmol/g dry weight of liver; upper limit of normal 36 μmol/g dry weight of liver). Same parameters as used for. (a) The liver signal intensity is less than the paraspinal muscle signal intensity. The signals of the pancreas and spleen are normal. (c) Hemochromatosis. Moderate iron overload (hepatic iron concentration = 146 μmol/g dry weight of liver). (d) Hemochromatosis. Severe iron overload (hepatic iron concentration = 352 μmol/g dry weight of liver). The great decrease of the hepatic signal is responsible for the appearance of a "black" liver. Reproduced from Guyader and Gandon.[54] Taken from James C. Barton and Corwin Q. Edwards (eds), **Hemochromatosis: Genetics, Pathophysiology, Diagnosis, and Treatment**, Cambridge University Press 2000. Reproduced with permission.

Fig. 4.9. Discordance of liver and myocardial iron in MRI images. In Panel A, the patient has heavy liver iron loading ("black" liver), but the heart retains signal indicating light loading (arrow). If management or myocardial iron were based on a liver biopsy in this patient, chelation treatment might be increased, but the risk of cardiac complications from iron overload is low. In Panel B, the patient has little liver iron loading ("grey" liver), but the heart has low signal indicating heavy loading (arrow). If management or myocardial iron were based on a liver biopsy in this patient, chelation treatment might be maintained at current levels or even decreased, but the risk of cardiac complications from iron overload is high. From Cohen et al.[142] Used with permission.

MRI detection of primary liver cancer

Hepatocellular carcinoma or other types of primary liver cancer is a frequent complication of *HFE* hemochromatosis, but also occurs in other iron overload disorders including beta-thalassemia major and hereditary sideroblastic anemia associated with *ALAS2* mutations.[73–75] Major risk factors for primary liver cancer in patients with *HFE* hemochromatosis and iron overload include age > 45 years, male sex, serum ferritin $>1000\,\mu g/L$, cirrhosis, alcoholism, and viral hepatitis.[76] In severe beta-thalassemia, iron overload and hepatitis C are major risk factors for hepato-cellular carcinoma.[74,75] Some patients with *HFE* hemochromatosis or beta-thalassemia without cirrhosis, viral hepatitis, or other apparent liver disorders have developed primary liver cancer.[77,78] MRI can detect small, focal cancerous lesions in cases of massive hepatic iron overload, because the decrease in liver magnetic resonance signal intensity leads to a high contrast between the tumor (devoid of iron) and the non-tumorous adjacent liver (Fig. 4.10).[79] The high frequency of malignant transformation of iron-free foci justifies the regular screening of men with *HFE* hemochromatosis aged 45 years or greater who have hepatic cirrhosis. This screening relies on regular ultrasound examinations of the liver and measurements of the serum concentration of alpha-fetoprotein, although it is unproven that this approach to surveillance will reduce death rates from primary liver cancer in persons with cirrhosis and iron overload. Although the incidence of primary liver cancer in hemochromatosis or thalassemia patients without cirrhosis is not sufficiently high to warrant routine screening, physicians should be aware that this fatal complication may rarely occur.[77]

Quantitative iron measurements using MRI

Conventional MRI measurements of tissue iron content are affected by the instrument used, the applied field strength, the repetition time used in the imaging sequence, the method used to analyze the relaxation curves, and other technical aspects of the measurement procedure.[54,55] As a consequence, comparison of absolute signal intensities from one MRI unit to another has generally been unreliable due to substantial intermachine variation.[54,55,80] Thus, MRI has been more useful as a screening technique for the detection of marked iron overload than as a means of quantitative measurement.[80]

Some advances have made it possible to quantify tissue iron more readily with MRI. Devising phantoms and other means for calibrating and validating iron concentration detected by MRI can enhance standardization between different machines and institutions.[55] A readily available, non-invasive

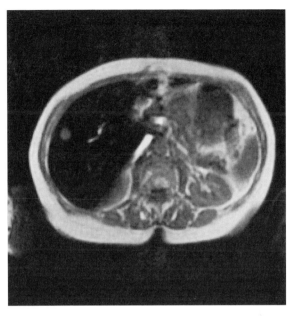

Fig. 4.10. Magnetic resonance image (MRI) of a small hepatocellular carcinoma complicating hemochromatosis. There is high contrast between the tumor (devoid of iron) and the adjacent liver (massively iron overloaded). Reproduced from Guyader and Gandon.[54] Taken from James C. Barton and Corwin Q. Edwards (eds), **Hemochromatosis: Genetics, Pathophysiology, Diagnosis, and Treatment**, Cambridge University Press 2000. Reproduced with permission.

method of measuring and imaging liver iron concentrations in vivo has been used to measure mean liver proton transverse relaxation rates (R_2; reciprocal of T2). Measurements of proton transverse relaxivity of aqueous $MnCl_2$ phantoms on 13 different magnetic resonance imaging units using the method yielded a coefficient of variation of only 2.1%.[81–83] Data are transmitted to a central location for analysis and interpretation. In 105 patients with either hemochromatosis or severe beta-thalassemia, high degrees of sensitivity and specificity of R_2 to HIC in biopsy specimens were found at the clinically significant iron concentration thresholds of 1.8, 3.2, 7.0, and 15.0 mg Fe/g dry weight. A calibration curve relating liver R_2 to HIC was deduced.[81]

T2* technique for myocardial iron was reproducible between scanners of different manufacturers, suggesting that the widespread implementation of the technique is possible for clinical assessment of cardiac siderosis in thalassemia.[84]

R2* MRI performed using 1.5T magnets was used to evaluate 43 patients with transfusion iron overload (32 sickle cell anemia, 6 beta-thalassemia major, 5 bone marrow failure).[85] Their mean serum ferritin was 2718 ± 1994 µg/L, and mean HIC was 10.9 ± 6.8 mg Fe/g dry weight. Serum ferritin levels and R2*-MRI were weakly but significantly associated (correlation coefficients 0.41–0.48 across three reviewers; all $P <0.01$). R2* MRI was strongly associated with HIC according to all three reviewers (correlation coefficients 0.96–0.98; all $P <0.001$). These results support the proposal that R2* MRI has clinical utility for predicting HIC in transfusion iron overload.[85]

Superconducting quantum interference device (SQUID)

Magnetic susceptibility can be used to measure hepatic iron stores non-invasively, based on the paramagnetic property of iron stored in ferritin and hemosiderin (Table 4.6).[55,86] This approach has been likened to performing an "automated magnetic biopsy" of liver ferritin and hemosiderin iron.[55] SQUID technique uses a low-power magnetic field and a sensitive detector that measures the interference of iron within the field. The sensor of the SQUID requires cooling in liquid helium. In the seminal clinical report, Brittenham *et al.* used this technique in 20 normal subjects and 110 patients with liver disease, iron deficiency, hereditary hemochromatosis, or transfusion iron overload.[86] Magnetic in vivo measurements of liver iron were highly correlated with chemical in vitro measurements in liver biopsy specimens ($r = 0.98$). SQUID methodology for magnetic measurement of hepatic iron stores has been validated in subsequent studies.[55,87–89] SQUID technique currently does not have sufficient spatial or temporal resolution to evaluate myocardial iron levels.[89]

The clinical availability of biomagnetic susceptometry has been limited by the high cost and complexity of SQUIDs, and their restricted utility to measure iron content only in the liver or spleen. Currently, SQUIDs are used clinically in only four locations: Columbia University (New York, NY); Children's Hospital and Research Center (Oakland, CA); University of Hamburg (Germany); and University of Turin (Italy).[89] These machines have been employed in numerous investigational studies of chelation therapy in patients with transfusion iron overload.[55,87–89]

Table 4.6. Hepatic iron measurement using SQUID[a]

Magnetic susceptibility can be used to measure hepatic iron stores using a SQUID

SQUID technique is non-invasive, safe, and accurate

SQUID is currently not capable of measuring cardiac iron content

Clinical accessibility has been limited by the high cost and complexity of SQUID

Four SQUIDs are operating worldwide

Note: [a]Superconducting Quantum Interference Device.

Quantitative phlebotomy

Quantitative phlebotomy is the preferred treatment for iron overload of diverse etiologies in patients who are not transfusion dependent, and can be used to measure total body iron stores. Although quantitative phlebotomy is generally acceptable only if the procedure provides therapeutic benefit, it can be used to evaluate carefully selected patients for the presence of iron overload. Patient selection, performance, and other phlebotomy-associated issues are presented in Chapter 36.

Measuring iron using phlebotomy

Phlebotomy observations for each treatment should be recorded in the medical chart on a standard chart form designed for this purpose. The record should include date, pre- and post-phlebotomy vital signs, current hemoglobin or hematocrit values, recent serum ferritin values, volume of blood removed, phlebotomy technique, and favorable or adverse events associated with the current phlebotomy session. A serum ferritin level is the most convenient (although indirect) means to assess iron stores and the progress of therapy, but has limited value to predict iron stores before phlebotomy or to quantify iron removed by phlebotomy. Likewise, serum iron levels and transferrin saturation values are not useful. Phlebotomy to induce iron depletion should be discontinued when the serum ferritin level is less than 20 µg/L, when the hemoglobin concentration is less than 11.0 g/dL (110 g/L), or when the hematocrit is less than 33% (0.33) for more than 3 weeks (in patients without chronic anemia).

The approximate amount of iron removed (mg) with each phlebotomy treatment is expressed as:

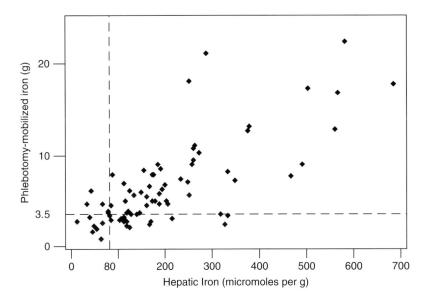

Fig. 4.11. Correlation between hepatic iron and phlebotomy-mobilized iron. Phlebotomy-mobilized iron in grams is plotted against hepatic iron in μmol/g dry weight ($r = 0.74$). The dotted lines depict the conventional cut-point of 80 μmol/g and the corresponding cut-point of 3.5 g mobilizable iron calculated using the regression equation. From Phatak and Barton.[90] Used with permission.

current hematocrit (percent) × blood removed (mL)

or

current hemoglobin (g/dL) × blood removed (mL) × 0.0347.

Some clinicians prefer to total the volume of blood removed over the entire course of treatment. In this case, 1 unit of blood (450–500 mL) is approximately equivalent to 200 mg of iron in patients without anemia. Phlebotomy-mobilized iron accurately mirrors liver iron content in hemochromatosis patients with C282Y homozygosity (Fig. 4.11).[90]

Slightly more precise quantitative phlebotomy measurements can be obtained in adults with hemochromatosis by deducting the amount of iron absorbed daily (typically 1 mg) over the entire course of phlebotomy from the amount of iron removed by phlebotomy. In juvenile hemochromatosis cases, iron absorbed daily often approaches 3 mg. At best, these "corrections" for absorbed iron are estimates, because daily iron absorption varies widely. Nonetheless, they are fairly accurate if intervals between phlebotomy treatments are not long, and if phlebotomy has not induced iron deficiency.

Blood and bone marrow examination technique

Examination of blood and bone marrow cells with light microscopy is sometimes useful to evaluate patients with iron overload disorders, because some iron overload disorders are associated with anemia (often with microcytosis) (Table 4.4). Specimens should be prepared with Wright/Giemsa and Perls' (Prussian blue) techniques to enhance general cytologic detail and non-heme ferric iron deposits, respectively. Finer examination of subcellular detail in marrow specimens can be accomplished with smear or imprint preparations than with tissue sections of paraffin-embedded biopsy specimens. Non-heme ferric iron is retained in smear or touch preparations, but is often removed from biopsy specimens treated with hydrochloric acid or EDTA for decalcification. The morphology of blood and marrow cells should be assessed, and the iron positivity of marrow macrophages and erythroid cells should be described or semi-quantified using a grading system. In unusual cases, electron microscopy techniques can provide additional information.

Interpretation of blood specimens

Types of anemia associated with iron overload often have characteristic morphologic abnormalities of erythrocytes. These include: beta-thalassemia (marked anisocytosis and poikilocytosis, microcytosis, target cells (leptocytes), basophilic stippling); sideroblastic anemia (dimorphic erythrocyte populations, Pappenheimer bodies); and hereditary spherocytosis (spherocytes, polychromatophilia). Perls' staining of blood smears sometimes reveals iron-positive erythrocyte inclusions in sideroblastic anemia. In pyruvate kinase deficiency, small dense echinocytes are sometimes present, but the appearance of most erythrocytes is normal. Persons with untreated primary iron overload due to hereditary atransferrinemia or mutations in the divalent metal transporter-1 (*SLC11A2*) gene have hypochromic, microcytic anemia. In *HFE* hemochromatosis, macrocytosis (usually mild) is often present, but anemia is uncommon. One unusual patient who had both congenital dyserythropoietic anemia type II and *HFE* C282Y homozygosity had anemia with macrocytosis.

Interpretation of bone marrow specimens

Macrophages phagocytose senescent or damaged erythroblasts and erythrocytes, and recover their iron using heme oxygenase. Macrophages also acquire iron from transferrin and lactoferrin via specific cell surface receptors, and from haptoglobin-hemoglobin and hemopexin-heme complexes via surface CD32+ surface scavenger receptors. In normal subjects, macrophages incorporate iron into ferritin or hemosiderin (partially degraded ferritin) for storage. Iron is returned to the circulation by macrophages via ferroportin under the regulation of hepcidin. Macrophage iron in specimens prepared with Perls' technique appears as dense, irregularly shaped, spherical, or granular particles, or as diffuse cytoplasmic staining. In the centers of smear preparations, macrophages ruptured by smear preparation may leave behind their characteristic iron-positive hemosiderin particles.

Iron overload disorders in which hepcidin levels are absolutely or relatively high are characterized by increased iron in macrophages of the marrow (and spleen and liver). These conditions include iron overload due to "loss-of-function" ferroportin (*SLC40A1*) mutations, African iron overload, some cases of African American iron overload, and transfusion iron overload. Iron overload disorders in which hepcidin levels are absolutely or relatively low are characterized by decreased or absent macrophage iron. These conditions include hemochromatosis associated with pathogenic *HFE*, *TFR2*, *HJV*, *HAMP*, or "gain-of-function" ferroportin (*SLC40A1*) genotypes.

Erythroblasts acquire iron from transferrin via cell surface receptors, and synthesize heme via intra- and extra-mitochondrial reactions. In normal subjects, some erythroblast iron detectable by light microscopy occurs in ferritin molecules dispersed throughout the cytoplasm. Erythroblasts that contain granular aggregates that appear as iron-positive cytoplasmic inclusions are termed sideroblasts. These comprise 20%–50% of marrow erythroblasts in normal subjects. Iron overload disorders in which hepcidin levels are absolutely or relatively high are often associated with decreased delivery of iron to erythroblasts and sometimes with mild anemia. Iron overload disorders in which hepcidin levels are absolutely or relatively low are characterized by increased delivery of iron to erythroblasts, and with mildly elevated hemoglobin levels and increased mean corpuscular volume in some cases. These conditions include hemochromatosis associated with pathogenic *HFE*, *TFR2*, *HJV*, *HAMP*, or "gain-of-function" ferroportin (*SLC40A1*) genotypes. Regardless, morphologic changes in erythroblasts in either of these groups of disorders are often so subtle that marrow examination by light microscopy is usually not helpful for diagnosis or monitoring treatment.

Congenital dyserythropoietic anemia, type I, is characterized by megaloblastic erythroid precursors and incompletely divided nuclear segments. In congenital dyserythropoietic anemia type II, characteristic late erythroblasts contain 2–7 normal-appearing nuclei. Increased macrophage iron stores due to ineffective erythropoiesis or erythrocyte transfusion are usually present in each of these types, whereas stainable erythroblast iron is usually not increased. Iron overload is very rare in congenital dyserythropoietic anemia, type III.

Among iron overload disorders, bone marrow examination is most useful for the diagnosis and evaluation of sideroblastic anemias of many causes. In these disorders, variable proportions of erythroblasts have iron-laden mitochondria that assume a perinuclear orientation (ringed sideroblasts); these cells are readily visualized in smear or imprint specimens prepared with Perls' technique. In sideroblastic anemia associated with mutations in the X-linked erythroid-specific ALA synthase gene (*ALAS2*), systemic iron overload (including increased marrow macrophage iron) is often present. A majority of erythroblasts are ringed sideroblasts, macrophage iron is often increased, and non-erythroid cells typically have normal morphology (Chapter 25). Marrow findings in X-linked sideroblastic anemia due to mutations in the ATP-binding cassette gene *ABCB7* resemble those of *ALAS2* sideroblastic anemia.

Anemia with ringed sideroblasts (often less than 50% of erythroblasts) and dysmorphism of one or more marrow cell lines are typical manifestations of myelodysplasia. Some patients with myelodysplasia and ringed sideroblasts develop iron overload, due in part to increased iron absorption in the absence of explanatory *HFE* genotypes and to erythrocyte transfusion. Ringed sideroblasts are present in relatively small numbers in the marrow of some patients beta-thalassemia major. Sideroblastic anemia can also occur due to exposure to a variety of drugs and chemicals. In these cases, the percentage of erythroblasts that appear as ringed sideroblasts is usually low, morphology of other marrow cells is typically normal, and most patients do not have or develop systemic iron overload.

Deferoxamine-induced urinary iron excretion

Iron is not very soluble in water, and less than 50 µg of iron is excreted each 24 hours in the urine of either iron-loaded or normal individuals. Deferoxamine (synonym desferrioxamine) is an injectable chelator derived from bacteria that binds iron, creating a complex of iron-deferoxamine that is water soluble and undergoes urinary excretion. The amount of 24-hour urinary iron excretion that occurs after the intramuscular injection of deferoxamine provides some insight into the magnitude of body iron stores.

Measurement of urinary iron excretion

This test requires the intramuscular administration of 15 mg deferoxamine/kg body weight. Because deferoxamine is not very water soluble, each 500 mg vial of lyophilized deferoxamine must be dissolved in a relatively large volume (2 mL) of sterile injectable water. For example, a person who weighs 147 pounds (67 kg) would receive 1000 mg of deferoxamine dissolved in 4 mL sterile water. One-half of this volume (2 mL) must be injected into each hip. Heavily iron-loaded individuals typically excrete more than 2 mg of urinary iron in 24 hours after such a deferoxamine injection. Normal subjects and hemochromatosis homozygotes who are not iron-loaded do not excrete increased quantities of urinary iron after receiving intramuscular deferoxamine.

Major problems with the deferoxamine challenge test include parenteral administration, pain largely due to the large volume of the injected solution, the time and attention required to obtain a complete 24-hour urine collection, and the need to send the urine to a reference laboratory to measure the excreted iron. Measurement of serum ferritin concentration is both fast and simple for the patient, physician, nurse, and laboratory, and has replaced the deferoxamine challenge in estimating body iron stores. *HFE* genotyping is widely available to demonstrate whether or not an individual is homozygous for the C282Y hemochromatosis-associated mutation.

Cobalt absorption/excretion test

The increased gastrointestinal absorption of orally administered inorganic radiocobalt (isotopes ^{57}Co or ^{60}Co as Co^{2+}) and its subsequent excretion and measurement in the urine are the basis of a presumptive diagnostic test for hemochromatosis (and iron deficiency).[91–93] Intestinal absorption of inorganic iron and cobalt in hemochromatosis homozygotes diagnosed in medical care is 1.5–3 times greater than that in normal control subjects. Increased absorption of cobalt occurs in men and women with hemochromatosis, and is not affected by the presence or absence of iron overload, hepatic cirrhosis, or diabetes mellitus.[91,93] The renal excretion of absorbed inorganic cobalt is rapid and quantitative.[92,93] Altogether, persons with hemochromatosis absorb greater quantities of orally administered inorganic radiocobalt than normal subjects, and thus supranormal quantities of radiocobalt are recovered in their urine at the conclusion of the test. The cobalt absorption test has been used to identify persons with hemochromatosis among the family members of hemochromatosis index patients.[94]

The physiologic and molecular bases of cobalt absorption test and its outcomes are largely understood. Divalent metal transporter-1 (DMT1) expressed on the luminal surfaces of absorptive enterocytes is the major Fe^{2+} transporter that mediates cellular iron uptake. DMT1 is upregulated in *HFE* hemochromatosis (and iron deficiency) and binds inorganic cobalt. Absorbed cobalt binds transferrin and enters cells via transferrin receptors.[95,96] Absorbed cobalt is not incorporated into ferritin, consistent with its rapid excretion after absorption. It is not detectable in multiple tissues of hemochromatosis patients.[95]

The cobalt absorption test is infrequently used today due to the availability of serum iron measures, *HFE* genotyping, and other superior means to diagnose hemochromatosis and iron overload.

Genotype testing

Many heritable disorders are associated with iron overload, and each is caused by mutation(s) of a different gene (Table 4.4). Some persons with acquired iron overload disorders also have mutations in iron- or anemia-related genes that increase their risk to develop iron overload (Table 4.7). Mutations identify individuals at risk to develop iron overload on a one-time testing basis, whether or not iron loading is present at the time of evaluation. Specimens of genomic DNA are first extracted from blood (buffy coat leukocytes), buccal swabs, or other sources. The copy numbers of DNA in the specimens are amplified using the polymerase chain reaction (PCR). Mutation-specific molecular genetics techniques are then applied to identify known mutations of certain genes and corresponding genotypes, especially those of *HFE*.

HFE hemochromatosis

The *HFE* gene (chromosome 6p21.3; H = hemochromatosis; FE = iron) comprises seven exons, the seventh of which is untranslated. Human HFE protein predicted from the cDNA sequence is composed of 343 amino acids and has a molecular weight of ~48 kDa; multiple splice variants have been described. HFE is a human leukocyte antigen (HLA)-like protein that associates with β_2-microglobulin, modulates transferrin binding to transferrin receptor, and may modulate hepatic expression of hepcidin. Many non-synonymous mutations of the *HFE* gene have been reported (Table 4.8). The majority of the known *HFE* mutations occur in exons (coding regions); most of these are missense mutations (due to the substitution of a single nucleotide). Others are nucleotide deletions, with or without resulting premature stop-codon triplets. *HFE* splice errors have been found in exons and introns. *HFE* hemochromatosis is usually caused by co-inheritance of a paternal and a maternal chromosome 6, each of which bears a deleterious *HFE* mutation. Many hemochromatosis patients have homozygosity for a single deleterious *HFE* mutation. Others are heterozygous for each of two deleterious *HFE* mutations (compound heterozygosity). It is rare

Table 4.7. Characteristics of some acquired iron overload disorders

Disorder	Source, cause of iron overload
Transfusion iron overload	Multiple erythrocyte transfusions
Refractory anemia with ringed sideroblasts (myelodysplasia)[a]	Ineffective erythropoiesis with increased GDF15[b]; erythrocyte transfusion
Porphyria cutanea tarda (sporadic)[a]	Common *HFE* mutations, hepatitis C, alcohol consumption
Portocaval shunt	Excessive iron absorption
Neonatal hemochromatosis	Increases transplacental iron transport due to maternal alloimmunity against fetal liver determinant
Medicinal iron overload[a]	Excessive oral iron supplements or parenteral iron (usually in parenteral nutrition formulas)
Hematite-associated iron overload	Inhalation, accidental ingestion of hematite (Fe_2O_3) dust during mining, ore processing

Notes: [a]Some patients have *HFE* hemochromatosis or other common *HFE* genotypes, beta-thalassemia minor, or other mutations that may enhance iron absorption.
[b]GDF15 = growth differentiation factor 15.

for a single chromosome 6 to bear more than one deleterious *HFE* mutation.

The majority of iron-loaded patients with *HFE* hemochromatosis are homozygous for a *HFE* missense mutation (nt.845G→A) that is common in western European whites. This mutation results in alteration of the HFE protein such that the normal cysteine at the 282 position of the HFE polypeptide chain is replaced by tyrosine (C282Y), disrupting HFE binding to β_2-microglobulin. Two other common *HFE* mutations are sometimes associated with iron overload that is usually mild. These are H63D (nt.187C→G; normal histidine 63 is replaced by aspartate) and S65C (nt. 193A→T; normal serine 65 is replaced by cysteine). Commercial testing is widely available to identify these three most common pathogenic *HFE* mutations (C282Y, H63D, S65C) (Table 4.8). Most other deleterious *HFE* mutations are rare, occur only in specific

Table 4.8. Mutations of the hemochromatosis gene (*HFE*)[a]

cDNA nucleotide substitution	Amino acid substitution[b]	Phenotype[c]	Reference
88C→T	L30L	0	121
128G→A + 187C→G	G43D + H63D	1	122
138T→G	L46W	1	123
157G→A	V53M	0	124
175G→A	V59M	0	124
187C→G	H63D	1	105
189T→C	H63H	0	124
193A→T	S65C	1	125
196C→T	R66C	2	121
211C→T	R74X	2	126
277G→C	G93R	1	127
277del	G93fs	2	128
314T→C	I105T	1	127
381A→C	Q127H	0	124
385G→A	D129N	0	123
414T→G	Y138X	2	123
471del	A158fs	2	129
478del	P160fs	2	130
502G→C	E168Q	1	131
502G→T	E168X	2	132
506G→A	W169X	2	132
636G→C	V212V	0	133
671G→A	R224G	2	121
689A→T	Y230F	2	123
696C→T	P232P	0	121
814G→T	V272L	0	134
829G→A	E277K	0	133
845G→A	C282Y	2	105
845G→C	C282S	2	135
848A→C	Q283P	2	136
867C→G	L289L	0	121
989G→T	R330M	2	124
IVS2 (+4) T→C	—	0	137
IVS3 (+1) G→T	(null allele)	2	138
IVS3 (+21) T→C	—	0	121
IVS4 (+37) A→G	—	0	124
IVS4 (+109) A→G	—	0	124
IVS4 (+115) T→C	—	0	124
IVS5 (+1) G→A	—	0	139

Notes: [a]Deletion of *HFE* (Chr6 g.(26 175 442)_g.(26 208 186)del) in French and Sardinian subjects is associated with a phenotype that is similar to that of *HFE* C282Y homozygotes.[140,141]
[b]Designated using international abbreviations for respective amino acids.
[c]Phenotype: 0 = none known; 1 = probably weak effect on iron homeostasis; 2 = probably strong effect on iron homeostasis.

families ("private" mutations), and are not detected by routine allele-specific mutation analyses available through most reference laboratories. It is likely that additional pathogenic *HFE* mutations will be found in the future, but they will almost certainly be uncommon.

Non-*HFE* hemochromatosis

Mutations in other genes (e.g. *SLC40A1*, *HJV*, *HAMP*, *TFR2*) also cause iron overload disorders (Chapters 12–15). Relative to *HFE* hemochromatosis, these disorders are rare, and many persons with these disorders have novel or rare mutations not typically detected in members of the general population. In some patients or kinships, an entire gene(s) must be evaluated to identify novel or unusual mutations responsible for the iron overload phenotype. DNA scanning using denaturing high-performance liquid chromatography, followed by direct nucleotide sequencing, is often used to evaluate such cases. Thus, mutation analyses of these genes are not commercially practical in the US. DNA sequencing or testing for specific rare mutations in these genes (or for unusual *HFE* alleles) may be available from interested research scientists, although the results of such testing is not useful in formulating and monitoring treatment for patients.

Human Leukocyte Antigen (HLA) typing in *HFE* hemochromatosis

Studies of the short arm of chromosome 6 (chromosome 6p) in hemochromatosis patients localized the hemochromatosis gene to this region of the genome, and permitted an investigational strategy that led to the identification of the *HFE* gene. Today, studies of chromosome 6p are the fundamental basis of understanding the age and population distributions of the common hemochromatosis mutation *HFE* C282Y, and an important adjunct to identifying "modifier" genes that may affect phenotype heterogeneity of C282Y homozygotes.

Hemochromatosis haplotypes

A haplotype is a chromosome or chromosome segment inherited from a single parent that is defined or characterized by one or more markers encoded in gene(s) on the haplotype. HLA proteins, like HFE protein, are encoded in genes of the major histocompatibility complex (MHC) on chromosome 6p. HLA genes are polymorphic, i.e. many alleles and corresponding protein serotypes exist normally within populations. HLA typing can be used to characterize chromosome 6p haplotypes that carry *HFE* hemochromatosis mutations.

Founders are individuals in whom a new mutation of interest occurred on a older haplotype. After a new mutation occurs, it may be transmitted from generation to generation as part of the original or ancestral haplotype.[97,98] Subsequently, the mutation may become situated on different haplotypes due either to subsequent mutations and translocations involving the ancestral haplotype, or to identical *de novo* mutations on other haplotypes of the same chromosome. Due to migrations of individuals and populations, haplotypes may eventually appear in persons or populations far away from the geographic region of the founder.

In the mid 1970s, Simon and colleagues described the association of hemochromatosis in subjects in Brittany with the antigens HLA-A and -B (especially HLA-A*03 and also -B*07 and -*B14) and confirmed that hemochromatosis iron overload phenotypes were inherited as an autosomal recessive disorder.[99] They correctly assigned the hemochromatosis gene to the short arm of chromosome 6 by demonstrating its linkage to the MHC that includes the HLA-A and -B genes.[99,100] Alleles in a haplotype are said to be in positive linkage disequilibrium when the observed frequency of a haplotype is greater than the frequency expected from random encounter of the alleles. Thus, HLA-B*07 and -B*14 were observed more frequently in association with HLA-A*03 than would be expected by chance.[101] The important conclusion from Simon's analyses was that HLA-A*03 was the only independent marker significantly associated with hemochromatosis. Simon initiated a positional cloning strategy ("recombinant haplotype mapping") based on the search for maximal allelic association and the analysis of hemochromatosis-associated haplotypes, both ancestral and recombinants, under the assumption of a strong founder effect.[101] This strategy permitted the correct prediction that the hemochromatosis gene was located on chromosome 6p, distal to HLA-A locus.[99,100]

Subsequent studies confirmed the association of HLA-A*03 with hemochromatosis in other European and derivative countries and regions including the United Kingdom, Germany, Sweden, Canada, the US, and Australia.[102,103] For example, the HLA-A*03, B*07 haplotype predominates in hemochromatosis cases in France, Canada, Germany, and the US. The haplotype HLA-A*03, B*14 is common in France, England, Ireland, and Scotland. The HLA-A*03, B*35 haplotype occurs largely in northeast Italy. Using analyses of microsatellites (polymorphic alleles scattered throughout the genome), it became possible to define the ancestral haplotype beyond HLA-A and HLA-B. Microsatellite characterization of hemochromatosis chromosomes in several populations indicated that: (a) the gene for hemochromatosis was associated with different haplotypes, but that the predominant (ancestral) haplotype carried HLA-A*03; (b) the ancestral haplotype extended at least 4 Mb telomeric to HLA-A; (c) the same ancestral haplotype was recognized in all hemochromatosis populations examined; and (d) the ancestral haplotype was exclusively associated with hemochromatosis. These data provided convincingly supported Simon's earlier proposal that hemochromatosis arose by a single mutation in a single ancestral individual.[101,104]

Simon's positional cloning strategy led to the discovery of the previously unknown HLA class I *HFE* gene on chromosome 6p21.3 by Feder and colleagues in 1996. *HFE* is widely accepted as the "classical" hemochromatosis gene of European whites[105] (Chapter 6). The core of the ancestral haplotype comprises ~250 kb around the *HFE* gene. This region, highly conserved, is still found on the vast majority of chromosomes carrying *HFE* C282Y. Extensive analyses of the geographic and race/ethnicity distribution of *HFE* C282Y have shown that this mutation is a western Caucasian allele. The highest frequency of *HFE* C282Y is found in Ireland, where one of ten chromosomes 6p bear this mutation.

Age and origin of *HFE* C282Y

The age and population of origin of *HFE* C282Y have been the topics of many debates. After the identification of *HFE,* Distante *et al.* estimated that the *HFE* C282Y mutation occurred in mainland Europe before 4000 BC.[106] In contrast, Ajioka *et al.* estimated that the C282Y mutation arose 60–80 generations ago.[107] Assuming an average generation time of 20 years, this estimate places the age of the origin of the mutation at 800–1200 years ago.

The geographical locations of *HFE* C282Y in Europe have been used to support the proposal that a single C282Y mutational event occurred in an ancient Celt. The Celts arose in Middle Europe and their numbers then expanded throughout northern Europe in a pattern consistent with the appearance of *HFE* C282Y, although it is unknown whether a cohesive Celtic civilization ever existed. It has been suggested that the Celts arrived in the area of the present United Kingdom ca. 4500 BC. If the age of *HFE* C282Y were relatively more recent than the ca. 4500 BC estimate, the timing of its introduction and spread throughout northern Europe are also consistent with the hypothesis that the *HFE* C282Y founder was a Viking. The main Viking invasions of Europe occurred *c.* 800 AD and involved the countries of northern Europe where hemochromatosis is now found in high frequency. For example, the highest frequencies (5.1%–9.7%) of the C282Y mutation are observed in populations in the northern part of Europe, i.e. Denmark, Norway, Sweden, Faeroe Islands, Iceland, eastern part of England (Danelaw), and the Dublin area, all Viking homelands and settlements. The highest allele frequencies are reported among populations living along the coastlines. The frequencies of the C282Y mutation decline from northern to southern europe. Intermediate allele frequencies (3.1%–4.8%) are seen in the populations in central Europe, the original Celtic homeland. Allele frequencies are relatively low (0%–3.1%) in populations in southern Europe and the Mediterranean.[108] Perhaps the only unequivocal demonstration of the geographic/population origin of *HFE* hemochromatosis will come from the identification of the C282Y mutation in ancient remains that are either Celtic or Viking in origin. Regardless of the population of origin of C282Y, it seems likely that its spread in Europe is attributable to Viking exploration.

Diagnosis of *HFE* hemochromatosis using HLA-A*03 and HLA haplotypes

HLA testing is useful to study first-degree family members of *HFE* hemochromatosis homozygotes diagnosed using strict phenotype criteria or ascertained by mutation analyses that demonstrate *HFE* C282Y homozygosity. HLA identity of hemochromatosis probands with their full siblings demonstrates that the siblings are also hemochromatosis homozygotes (Fig. 4.12). First-degree family members who are one-haplotype matches with proven homozygotes are typically C282Y heterozygotes. Because the prevalence of *HFE* C282Y is relatively great in western European whites, HLA criteria cannot be used to exclude C282Y homozygosity in parents or children of homozygous probands. The present commercial availability of *HFE* mutation analyses to identify C282Y obviates the need to perform HLA typing in most routine clinical situations.

HLA testing is not useful to identify persons with *HFE* hemochromatosis in routine clinical practice or in population screening. For example, approximately 1 in 165 Alabama whites are C282Y homozygotes. HLA-A*03 was detected in 74.8% of hemochromatosis probands, whereas 27.4% of control Alabama whites also had HLA-A*03.[103] Regarding HLA-A*03, B*07, 29.7% of hemochromatosis chromosomes had this haplotype, whereas 3.3% of no. 6 chromosomes in control whites also had this haplotype. Taken together, these examples demonstrate that most whites with HLA-A*03 or HLA-A*03,B*07 do not have hemochromatosis, although some are heterozygous for C282Y.

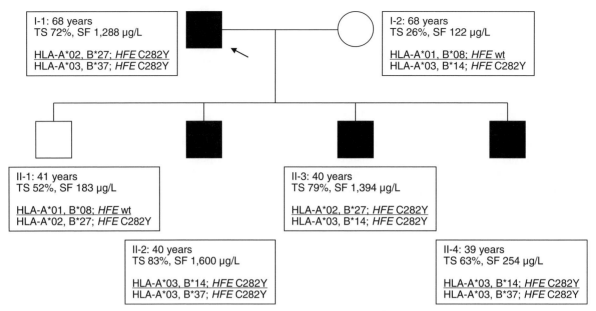

Fig. 4.12. Pedigree illustrating the mating of a *HFE* C282Y homozygote and a C282Y heterozygote. The proband is indicated by an arrow; filled figures indicate diagnosis of hemochromatosis. TS = transferrin saturation; SF = serum ferritin; HLA = human leukocyte antigen; and wt = wild-type, defined as absence of *HFE* C282Y, H63D, and S65C. The iron phenotype of brother II-1 did not strongly suggest hemochromatosis, and he shared only one HLA haplotype (A*02, B*27) with one other brother who had a hemochromatosis phenotype (II-3). The HLA identity of brothers II-2 and II-4 established that both have hemochromatosis, although the iron phenotype of brother II-4 alone did not strongly suggest hemochromatosis. Brother II-3 has a hemochromatosis phenotype, but he shares a single HLA haplotype (A*03, B*14) with brothers II-2 and II-4 who have hemochromatosis. Hemochromatosis diagnoses and haplotype assignments in this kinship were confirmed by *HFE* mutation analysis. Adapted from Barton *et al.*[143]

Clinical expression of *HFE* hemochromatosis and the ancestral haplotype

Expression of iron phenotypes among individuals homozygous for *HFE* C282Y mutation is very heterogeneous. Some early data suggest that individuals with hemochromatosis and the ancestral haplotype may have more severe disease expression. In Australian families, hemochromatosis homozygotes who had two copies of the ancestral haplotype had significantly greater iron overload than hemochromatosis patients with one or no copy of the ancestral haplotype.[109] In addition, some hemochromatosis heterozygotes also had partial clinical expression of hemochromatosis and this expression was influenced by the presence of the ancestral haplotype in women, but not in men.[109] Similar observations linking the presence of the ancestral haplotype to severe iron loading measured using quantitative phlebotomy were subsequently reported in American and Italian hemochromatosis cohorts.[110,111] In the American cohort, phlebotomy requirements to achieve iron

depletion were higher in hemochromatosis patients homozygous for HLA-A3 and D6S105 allele 8, two of the markers found on the ancestral haplotype.[110] In the Italian population, the amount of iron removed by phlebotomy was divided by age, and the resulting value was categorized as either mild or severe hemochromatosis. The ancestral haplotype was significantly associated with a severe phenotype; seven of eight patients categorized as having a severe phenotype were homozygous for the ancestral haplotype.[111] Another study reported evidence that a "modifier" gene(s) may exist on chromosome 6p.[112] Each of these studies comprised relatively small numbers of subjects, selection bias may have influenced the choice of subjects, and most statistical analyses were univariate.

In a subsequent analysis of 141 consecutive Alabama hemochromatosis probands with C282Y homozygosity diagnosed in medical care, multivariate analyses revealed that there are disparate frequencies of HLA haplotypes A*03-B*07 and A*03-B*14 in men and women, and that HLA-A*03 and HLA-A*03-B*07 are not independent variables associated with iron overload severity.[113] There is a significant inverse relationship of total blood lymphocyte counts and severity of iron overload in hemochromatosis probands with *HFE* C282Y homozygosity. In univariate and multivariate analyses, total blood lymphocyte counts were significantly lower in probands with the HLA-A*01-B*08 haplotype than in probands without this haplotype.[114] Alleles of the gene that encodes tumor necrosis factor-alpha (*TNF*; chromosome 6p21.3) may also contribute to phenotype heterogeneity in C282Y homozygotes.[115,116] In a genome linkage scan of probands with hemochromatosis or evidence of elevated iron stores and their family members, however, no quantitative trait locus for serum iron measures was identified on chromosome 6 after adjustments for age, gender, race/ethnicity, and *HFE* genotype were made.[117] Cumulatively, these data suggest that the phenotypic variation in hemochromatosis is associated with hemochromatosis haplotype and may thus be determined partly by genetic factors. Mutations in the gene that encodes bone morphogenetic protein 6 (*BMP6*; chromosome 6p24–p23) may cause iron overload in humans[118,119] and account for some observations regarding the ancestral haplotype and chromosome 6p hemochromatosis "modifier" mutations.

HLA types in non-*HFE* hemochromatosis

Mutation in genes other than *HFE* can lead to distinct inherited forms of iron overload. None of these genes, with the exception of *BMP6*, occurs on chromosome 6p. Consequently, there is no particular relevance of HLA haplotypes to most types of non-*HFE* hemochromatosis.

References

1. Benyamin B, McRae AF, Zhu G, *et al.* Variants in *TF* and *HFE* explain approximately 40% of genetic variation in serum-transferrin levels. *Am J Hum Genet* 2009; **84**: 60–5.

2. Adams PC, Reboussin DM, Barton JC, *et al.* Hemochromatosis and iron overload screening in a racially diverse population. *N Engl J Med* 2005; **352**: 1769–78.

3. Barton JC, Acton RT, Dawkins FW, *et al.* Initial screening transferrin saturation values, serum ferritin concentrations, and *HFE* genotypes in whites and blacks in the Hemochromatosis and Iron Overload Screening Study. *Genet Test* 2005; **9**: 231–41.

4. Harris EL, McLaren CE, Reboussin DM, *et al.* Serum ferritin and transferrin saturation in Asians and Pacific Islanders. *Arch Intern Med* 2007; **167**: 722–6.

5. Edwards CQ, Griffen LM, Kaplan J, Kushner JP. Twenty-four hour variation of transferrin saturation in treated and untreated haemochromatosis homozygotes. *J Intern Med* 1989; **226**: 373–9.

6. Torti FM, Torti SV. Regulation of ferritin genes and protein. *Blood* 2002; **99**: 3505–16.

7. Witte DL, Crosby WH, Edwards CQ, Fairbanks VF, Mitros FA. Practice guideline development task force of the College of American Pathologists. Hereditary hemochromatosis. *Clin Chim Acta* 1996; **245**: 139–200.

8. Adams PC, Bhavana V. Unsaturated iron-binding capacity: a screening test for C282Y hemochromatosis? *Clin Chem* 2000; **46**: 1870–1.

9. Adams PC, Kertesz AE, McLaren CE, Barr R, Bamford A, Chakrabarti S. Population screening for hemochromatosis: a comparison of unbound iron-binding capacity, transferrin saturation, and C282Y genotyping in 5211 voluntary blood donors. *Hepatology* 2000; **31**: 1160–64.

10. Witte DL. Mild liver enzyme abnormalities: eliminating hemochromatosis as cause. *Clin Chem* 1997; **43**: 1535–38.

11. Adams PC, Reboussin DM, Press RD, *et al.* Biological variability of transferrin saturation and unsaturated iron-binding capacity. *Am J Med* 2007; **120**: 999. e1–7.

12. Beutler E, Felitti VJ, Koziol JA, Ho NJ, Gelbart T. Penetrance of 845G>A (C282Y) *HFE* hereditary haemochromatosis mutation in the USA. *Lancet* 2002; **359**: 211–18.

13. Westerhausen M, Meuret G. Transferrin-immune complex disease. *Acta Haematol* 1977; **57**: 96–101.

14. Harrison PM, Arosio P. The ferritins: molecular properties, iron storage function and cellular regulation. *Biochim Biophys Acta* 1996; **1275**: 161–203.

15. Worwood M. Serum ferritin. *CRC Crit Rev Clin Lab Sci* 1979; **10**: 171–204.

16. Worwood M. Serum ferritin. *Clin Sci (Lond)* 1986; **70**: 215–20.

17. Worwood M. Ferritin. *Blood Rev* 1990; **4**: 259–69.

18. Worwood M. The diagnostic value of serum ferritin determinations for assessing iron status. *Haematologia (Budap)* 1987; **20**: 229–35.

19. Herbert V, Jayatilleke E, Shaw S, *et al.* Serum ferritin iron, a new test, measures human body iron stores unconfounded by inflammation. *Stem Cells* 1997; **15**: 291–6.

20. Morrison ED, Brandhagen DJ, Phatak PD, *et al.* Serum ferritin level predicts advanced hepatic fibrosis among US patients with phenotypic hemochromatosis. *Ann Intern Med* 2003; **138**: 627–33.

21. Beaumont C, Simon M, Fauchet R, *et al.* Serum ferritin as a possible marker of the hemochromatosis allele. *N Engl J Med* 1979; **301**: 169–74.

22. Waalen J, Felitti VJ, Gelbart T, Beutler E. Screening for hemochromatosis by measuring ferritin levels: a more effective approach. *Blood* 2008; **111**: 3373–6.

23. Barton JC. Ferritin >1000: grand for hemochromatosis screening? *Blood* 2008; **111**: 3309.

24. Cox DW. Factors influencing serum ceruloplasmin levels in normal individuals. *J Lab Clin Med* 1966; **68**: 893–904.

25. Tutor-Crespo MJ, Hermida J, Tutor JC. Assessment of copper status in epileptic patients treated with anticonvulsant drugs by measuring the specific oxidase activity of ceruloplasmin. *Epilepsy Res* 2003; **56**: 147–53.

26. de Domenico I, Word DM, di Patti MC *et al.* Ferroxidase activity is required for the stability of cell surface ferroportin in cells expressing EPI-ceruloplasmin. *EMBO J* 2007; **26**; 2823–31.

27. Wilson SAK. Progressive lenticular degeneration. A familial nervous disease associated with cirrhosis of the liver. *Brain* 1912; **34**: 295–309.

28. Davies LP, Macintyre G, Cox DW. New mutations in the Wilson disease gene, *ATP7B*: implications for molecular testing. *Genet Test* 2008; **12**: 139–45.

29. Davies L, Kenney S, Cox DW. *Wilson Disease Mutation Database*. University of Alberta. 01/23/2010.

30. Mak CM, Lam CW. Diagnosis of Wilson's disease: a comprehensive review. *Crit Rev Clin Lab Sci* 2008; **45**: 263–90.

31. Scheinberg I, Sternlieb AI. Wilson's disease. *Major Probl Intern Med* 1984; **23**: 1–24.

32. Olivarez L, Caggana M, Pass KA, Ferguson P, Brewer GJ. Estimate of the frequency of Wilson's disease in the US Caucasian population: a mutation analysis approach. *Ann Hum Genet* 2001; **65**: 459–63.

33. Owada M, Suzuki K, Fukushi M, Yamauchi K, Kitagawa T. Mass screening for Wilson's disease by measuring urinary holoceruloplasmin. *J Pediatr* 2002; **140**: 614–16.

34. Ohura T, Abukawa D, Shiraishi H, *et al.* Pilot study of screening for Wilson's disease using dried blood spots obtained from children seen at outpatient clinics. *J Inherit Metab Dis* 1999; **22**: 74–80.

35. Yamaguchi Y, Aoki T, Arashima S, *et al.* Mass screening for Wilson's disease: results and recommendations. *Pediatr Int* 1999; **41**: 405–8.

36. Kim GH, Yang JY, Park JY, Lee JJ, Kim JH, Yoo HW. Estimation of Wilson's disease incidence and carrier frequency in the Korean population by screening *ATP7B* major mutations in newborn filter papers using the SYBR green intercalator method based on the amplification refractory mutation system. *Genet Test* 2008; **12**: 395–9.

37. Walshe JM, Cox DW. Effect of treatment of Wilson's disease on natural history of haemochromatosis. *Lancet* 1998; **352**: 112–13.

38. Hafkemeyer P, Schupp M, Storch M, Gerok W, Haussinger D. Excessive iron storage in a patient with Wilson's disease. *Clin Investig* 1994; **72**: 134–6.

39. Shiono Y, Wakusawa S, Hayashi H, *et al.* Iron accumulation in the liver of male patients with Wilson's disease. *Am J Gastroenterol* 2001; **96**: 3147–51.

40. Hayashi H, Yano M, Fujita Y, Wakusawa S. Compound overload of copper and iron in patients with Wilson's disease. *Med Mol Morphol* 2006; **39**: 121–6.

41. Fasano A, Bentivoglio AR, Colosimo C. Movement disorder due to aceruloplasminemia and incorrect diagnosis of hereditary hemochromatosis. *J Neurol* 2007; **254**: 113–14.

42. Abuzetun JY, Hazin R, Suker M, Porter J. A rare case of hemochromatosis and Wilson's disease coexisting in the same patient. *J Natl Med Assoc* 2008; **100**: 112–14.

43. Sheldon JH. *Haemochromatosis*. London, Oxford University Press, 1935.

44. Bacon BR. Hemochromatosis: diagnosis and management. *Gastroenterology* 2001; **120**: 718–25.

45. Tavill AS. Diagnosis and management of hemochromatosis. *Hepatology* 2001; **33**: 1321–8.

46. Powell LW. Diagnosis of hemochromatosis. *Semin Gastrointest Dis* 2002; **13**: 80–8.

47. Tavill AS, Adams PC. A diagnostic approach to hemochromatosis. *Can J Gastroenterol* 2006; **20**: 535–40.

48. Wheeler CJ, Kowdley KV. Hereditary hemochromatosis: a review of the genetics, mechanism, diagnosis, and treatment of iron overload. *Compr Ther* 2006; **32**: 10–16.

49. Deugnier Y, Brissot P, Loreal O. Iron and the liver: update 2008. *J Hepatol* 2008; **48** Suppl 1: S113–123.

50. Emond MJ, Bronner MP, Carlson TH, Lin M, Labbe RF, Kowdley KV. Quantitative study of the variability of hepatic iron concentrations. *Clin Chem* 1999; **45**: 340–6.

51. Shah S, Mayberry JF, Wicks AC, Rees Y, Playford RJ. Liver biopsy under ultrasound control: implications for training in the Calman era. *Gut* 1999; **45**: 628–29.

52. Brunt EM. Pathology of hepatic iron overload. *Semin Liver Dis* 2005; **25**: 392–401.

53. Alla V, Bonkovsky HL. Iron in non-hemochromatotic liver disorders. *Semin Liver Dis* 2005; **25**: 461–72.

54. Guyader D, Gandon Y. Computed tomography and magnetic resonance imaging in the diagnosis of hemochromatosis. In: Barton JC, Edwards CQ, eds. *Hemochromatosis. Genetics, Pathophysiology, Diagnosis and Treatment.* Cambridge, Cambridge University Press. 2000; 219–25.

55. Brittenham GM, Badman DG. Non-invasive measurement of iron: report of an NIDDK workshop. *Blood* 2003; **101**: 15–19.

56. Gossuin Y, Roch A, Muller RN, Gillis P. Relaxation induced by ferritin and ferritin-like magnetic particles: the role of proton exchange. *Magn Reson Med* 2000; **43**: 237–43.

57. Brasch RC, Wesbey GE, Gooding CA, Koerper MA. Magnetic resonance imaging of transfusional hemosiderosis complicating thalassemia major. *Radiology* 1984; **150**: 767–71.

58. Stark DD, Moseley ME, Bacon BR, *et al.* Magnetic resonance imaging and spectroscopy of hepatic iron overload. *Radiology* 1985; **154**: 137–42.

59. Ernst O, Sergent G, Bonvarlet P, Canva-Delcambre V, Paris JC, L'Hermine C. Hepatic iron overload: diagnosis and quantification with MR imaging. *Am J Roentgenol* 1997; **168**: 1205–8.

60. Gandon Y, Guyader D, Heautot JF, *et al.* Hemochromatosis: diagnosis and quantification of liver iron with gradient-echo MR imaging. *Radiology* 1994; **193**: 533–38.

61. Angelucci E, Giovagnoni A, Valeri G, *et al.* Limitations of magnetic resonance imaging in measurement of hepatic iron. *Blood* 1997; **90**: 4736–42.

62. Olynyk JK, St Pierre TG, Britton RS, Brunt EM, Bacon BR. Duration of hepatic iron exposure increases the risk of significant fibrosis in hereditary hemochromatosis: a new role for magnetic resonance imaging. *Am J Gastroenterol* 2005; **100**: 837–41.

63. Pietrangelo A, Corradini E, Ferrara F, *et al.* Magnetic resonance imaging to identify classic and non-classic forms of ferroportin disease. *Blood Cells Mol Dis* 2006; **37**: 192–6.

64. Ptaszek LM, Price ET, Hu MY, Yang PC. Early diagnosis of hemochromatosis-related cardiomyopathy with magnetic resonance imaging. *J Cardiovasc Magn Reson* 2005; **7**: 689–92.

65. Schocke MF, Zoller H, Vogel W, *et al.* Cardiac phosphorus-31 two-dimensional chemical shift imaging in patients with hereditary hemochromatosis. *Magn Reson Imaging* 2004; **22**: 515–21.

66. He T, Gatehouse PD, Kirk P, *et al.* Black-blood T2* technique for myocardial iron measurement in thalassemia. *J Magn Reson Imaging* 2007; **25**: 1205–9.

67. Wood JC, Tyszka JM, Carson S, Nelson MD, Coates TD. Myocardial iron loading in transfusion-dependent thalassemia and sickle cell disease. *Blood* 2004; **103**: 1934–6.

68. Mavrogeni SI, Markussis V, Kaklamanis L, *et al.* A comparison of magnetic resonance imaging and cardiac biopsy in the evaluation of heart iron overload in patients with beta-thalassemia major. *Eur J Haematol* 2005; **75**: 241–7.

69. Sparacia G, Iaia A, Banco A, D'Angelo P, Lagalla R. Transfusional hemochromatosis: quantitative relation of MR imaging pituitary signal intensity reduction to hypogonadotropic hypogonadism. *Radiology* 2000; **215**: 818–23.

70. Karimi M, Jamalian N, Rasekhi A, Kashef S. Magnetic resonance imaging (MRI) findings of joints in young beta-thalassemia major patients: fluid surrounding the scaphoid bone: a novel finding, as the possible effect of secondary hemochromatosis. *J Pediatr Hematol Oncol* 2007; **29**: 393–8.

71. Zhang J, Krinsky GA. Iron-containing nodules of cirrhosis. *NMR Biomed* 2004; **17**: 459–64.

72. Rocchi E. [Magnetic resonance and hepatic siderosis]. *Recenti Prog Med* 1994; **85**: 447–51.

73. Barton JC, Lee PL. Disparate phenotypic expression of *ALAS2* R452H (nt 1407 G>A) in two brothers, one with severe sideroblastic anemia and iron overload, hepatic cirrhosis, and hepatocellular carcinoma. *Blood Cells Mol Dis* 2006; **36**: 342–6.

74. Borgna-Pignatti C, Vergine G, Lombardo T, *et al.* Hepatocellular carcinoma in the thalassaemia syndromes. *Br J Haematol* 2004; **124**: 114–17.

75. Mancuso A, Sciarrino E, Renda MC, Maggio A. A prospective study of hepatocellular carcinoma incidence in thalassemia. *Hemoglobin* 2006; **30**: 119–24.

76. Deugnier YM, Guyader D, Crantock L, *et al.* Primary liver cancer in genetic hemochromatosis: a clinical, pathological, and pathogenetic study of 54 cases. *Gastroenterology* 1993; **104**: 228–34.

77. Hiatt T, Trotter JF, Kam I. Hepatocellular carcinoma in a non-cirrhotic patient with hereditary hemochromatosis. *Am J Med Sci* 2007; **334**: 228–30.

78. Mancuso A, Rigano P, Renda D, *et al.* Hepatocellular carcinoma on cirrhosis-free liver in a HCV-infected thalassemic. *Am J Hematol* 2005; **78**: 158–9.

79. Guyader D, Gandon Y, Sapey T, *et al.* Magnetic resonance iron-free nodules in genetic hemochromatosis. *Am J Gastroenterol* 1999; **94**: 1083–6.

80. Bonkovsky HL, Rubin RB, Cable EE, Davidoff A, Rijcken TH, Stark DD. Hepatic iron concentration: non-invasive estimation by means of MR imaging techniques. *Radiology* 1999; **212**: 227–34.

81. St Pierre TG, Clark PR, Chua-anusorn W, *et al.* Non-invasive measurement and imaging of liver iron concentrations using proton magnetic resonance. *Blood* 2005; **105**: 855–61.

82. St Pierre TG, Clark PR, Chua-anusorn W. Single spin-echo proton transverse relaxometry of iron-loaded liver. *NMR Biomed* 2004; **17**: 446–58.

83. Clark PR, Chua-anusorn W, St Pierre TG. Proton transverse relaxation rate (R2) images of liver tissue; mapping local tissue iron concentrations with MRI. *Magn Reson Med* 2003; **49**: 572–5.

84. Westwood MA, Anderson LJ, Firmin DN, *et al.* Interscanner reproducibility of cardiovascular magnetic resonance T2* measurements of tissue iron in thalassemia. *J Magn Reson Imaging* 2003; **18**: 616–20.

85. Hankins JS, McCarville MB, Loeffler RB, *et al.* R2* magnetic resonance imaging of the liver in patients with iron overload. *Blood* 2009; **113**: 4853–5.

86. Brittenham GM, Farrell DE, Harris JW, *et al.* Magnetic-susceptibility measurement of human iron stores. *N Engl J Med* 1982; **307**: 1671–5.

87. Nielsen P, Fischer R, Engelhardt R, Tondury P, Gabbe EE, Janka GE. Liver iron stores in patients with secondary haemosiderosis under iron chelation therapy with deferoxamine or deferiprone. *Br J Haematol* 1995; **91**: 827–33.

88. Brittenham GM, Sheth S, Allen CJ, Farrell DE. Non-invasive methods for quantitative assessment of transfusional iron overload in sickle cell disease. *Semin Hematol* 2001; **38**: 37–56.

89. Wood JC. Diagnosis and management of transfusion iron overload: the role of imaging. *Am J Hematol* 2007; **82**: 1132–5.

90. Phatak PD, Barton JC. Phlebotomy-mobilized iron as a surrogate for liver iron content in hemochromatosis patients. *Hematology* 2003; **8**: 429–32.

91. Olatunbosun D, Corbett WE, Ludwig J, Valberg LS. Alteration of cobalt absorption in portal cirrhosis and idiopathic hemochromatosis. *J Lab Clin Med* 1970; **75**: 754–62.

92. Sorbie J, Olatunbosun D, Corbett WE, Valberg LS. Cobalt excretion test for the assessment of body iron stores. *Can Med Assoc J* 1971; **104**: 777–82.

93. Valberg LS, Ludwig J, Olatunbosun D. Alteration in cobalt absorption in patients with disorders of iron metabolism. *Gastroenterology* 1969; **56**: 241–51.

94. Miller A, Zimelman A, Brauer MJ. A family study of a patient with idiopathic hemochromatosis. *Am J Hematol* 1977; **2**: 41–6.

95. Barton JC. The absorption and metabolism of non-ferrous metals in hemochromatosis. *Hemochromatosis: Genetics, Pathophysiology, Diagnosis and Treatment.* Cambridge, Cambridge University Press. 2000; 131–3.

96. Smith TA. Human serum transferrin cobalt complex: stability and cellular uptake of cobalt. *Bioorg Med Chem* 2005; **13**: 4576–9.

97. Simon M, Le Mignon L, Fauchet R, *et al.* A study of 609 HLA haplotypes marking for the hemochromatosis gene: (1) mapping of the gene near the HLA-A locus and characters required to define a heterozygous population; and (2) hypothesis concerning the underlying cause of hemochromatosis-HLA association. *Am J Hum Genet* 1987; **41**: 89–105.

98. Simon M, Yaouanq J, Fauchet R, Le Gall JY, Brissot P, Bourel M. Genetics of hemochromatosis: HLA association and mode of inheritance. *Ann N Y Acad Sci* 1988; **526**: 11–22.

99. Simon M, Bourel M, Fauchet R, Genetet B. Association of HLA-A3 and HLA-B14 antigens with idiopathic haemochromatosis. *Gut* 1976; **17**: 332–4.

100. Simon M, Alexandre JL, Bourel M, Le Marec B, Scordia C. Heredity of idiopathic haemochromatosis: a study of 106 families. *Clin Genet* 1977; **11**: 327–41.

101. Yaouanq J. Human leukocyte antigen (HLA) association and typing in hemochromatosis. In: Barton JC, Edwards CQ, eds. *Hemochromatosis: Genetics, Pathophysiology, Diagnosis and Treatment.* Cambridge, Cambridge University Press. 2000; 63–74.

102. Porto G, de Sousa M. Variation of hemochromatosis prevalence and genotype in national groups. In: Barton JC, Edwards CQ, eds. *Hemochromatosis: Genetics, Pathophysiology, Diagnosis and Treatment.* Cambridge, Cambridge University Press. 2000; 51–62.

103. Barton JC, Acton RT. HLA-A and -B alleles and haplotypes in hemochromatosis probands with *HFE* C282Y homozygosity in central Alabama. *BMC Med Genet* 2002; **3**: 9.

104. Jazwinska EC. The ancestral haplotype in hemochromatosis. In: Barton JC, Edwards CQ, eds. *Hemochromatosis: Genetics, Pathophysiology, Diagnosis and Treatment.* Cambridge, Cambridge University Press. 2000; 91–8.

105. Feder JN, Gnirke A, Thomas W, *et al.* A novel MHC class I-like gene is mutated in patients with hereditary haemochromatosis. *Nat Genet* 1996; **13**: 399–408.

106. Distante S, Robson KJ, Graham-Campbell J, Arnaiz-Villena A, Brissot P, Worwood M. The origin and spread of the *HFE*-C282Y haemochromatosis mutation. *Hum Genet* 2004; **115**: 269–79.

107. Ajioka RS, Jorde LB, Gruen JR, et al. Haplotype analysis of hemochromatosis: evaluation of different linkage-disequilibrium approaches and evolution of disease chromosomes. *Am J Hum Genet* 1997; **60**: 1439–47.

108. Milman N, Pedersen P. Evidence that the Cys282Tyr mutation of the *HFE* gene originated from a population in southern Scandinavia and spread with the Vikings. *Clin Genet* 2003; **64**: 36–47.

109. Crawford DHG, Powell LW, Leggett BA, *et al.* Evidence that the ancestral haplotype in Australian hemochromatosis patients may be associated with a common mutation in the gene. *Am J Hum Genet* 1995; **57**: 362–7.

110. Barton JC, Harmon L, Rivers C, Acton RT. Hemochromatosis: association of severity of iron overload with genetic markers. *Blood Cells Mol Dis* 1996; **22**: 195–204.

111. Piperno A, Arosio C, Fargion S, *et al.* The ancestral hemochromatosis haplotype is associated with a severe phenotype expression in Italian patients. *Hepatology* 1996; **24**: 43–6.

112. Barton JC, Shih WW, Sawada-Hirai R, *et al.* Genetic and clinical description of hemochromatosis probands and heterozygotes: evidence that multiple genes linked to the major histocompatibility complex are responsible for hemochromatosis. *Blood Cells Mol Dis* 1997; **23**: 135–45.

113. Barton JC, Wiener HW, Acton RT, Go RC. HLA haplotype A*03-B*07 in hemochromatosis probands with *HFE* C282Y homozygosity: frequency disparity in men and women and lack of association with severity of iron overload. *Blood Cells Mol Dis* 2005; **34**: 38–47.

114. Barton JC, Wiener HW, Acton RT, Go RC. Total blood lymphocyte counts in hemochromatosis probands with *HFE* C282Y homozygosity: relationship to severity of iron overload and HLA-A and -B alleles and haplotypes. *BMC Blood Disord* 2005; **5**: 5.

115. Krayenbuehl PA, Maly FE, Hersberger M, *et al.* Tumor necrosis factor-alpha -308G>A allelic variant modulates iron accumulation in patients with hereditary hemochromatosis. *Clin Chem* 2006; **52**: 1552–8.

116. Fargion S, Valenti L, Dongiovanni P, *et al.* Tumor necrosis factor alpha promoter polymorphisms influence the phenotypic expression of hereditary hemochromatosis. *Blood* 2001; **97**: 3707–12.

117. Acton RT, Snively BM, Barton JC, *et al.* A genome-wide linkage scan for iron phenotype quantitative trait loci: the HEIRS Family Study. *Clin Genet* 2007; **71**: 518–29.

118. Meynard D, Kautz L, Darnaud V, Canonne-Hergaux F, Coppin H, Roth MP. Lack of the bone morphogenetic protein BMP6 induces massive iron overload. *Nat Genet* 2009; **41**: 478–81.

119. Andriopoulos B, Jr., Corradini E, Xia Y, *et al.* BMP6 is a key endogenous regulator of hepcidin expression and iron metabolism. *Nat Genet* 2009; **41**: 482–7.

120. Cappuccio J, Phatak PD. Cost-effectiveness of screening for hemochromatosis. In: Barton JC, Edwards CQ, eds. *Hemochromatosis: Genetics, Pathophysiology, Diagnosis and Treatment.* Cambridge, Cambridge University Press. 2000; 525–34.

121. Biasiotto G, Belloli S, Ruggeri G, *et al.* Identification of new mutations of the *HFE*, hepcidin, and transferrin receptor 2 genes by denaturing HPLC analysis of individuals with biochemical indications of iron overload. *Clin Chem* 2003; **49**: 1981–8.

122. Dupradeau FY, Pissard S, Coulhon MP, *et al.* An unusual case of hemochromatosis due to a new compound heterozygosity in *HFE* (p.[Gly43Asp; His63Asp]+[Cys282Tyr]): structural implications with respect to binding with transferrin receptor 1. *Hum Mutat* 2008; **29**: 206.

123. Mendes AI, Ferro A, Martins R, et al. Non-classical hereditary hemochromatosis in Portugal: novel mutations identified in iron metabolism-related genes. *Ann Hematol* 2009; **88**: 229–34.

124. de Villiers JN, Hillermann R, Loubser L, Kotze MJ. Spectrum of mutations in the *HFE* gene implicated in haemochromatosis and porphyria. *Hum Mol Genet* 1999; **8**: 1517–22.

125. Henz S, Reichen J, Liechti-Gallati S. *HLA-H* gene mutations and haemochromatosis: the likely association of H63D with mild phenotype and the detection of S65C, a novel variant in exon 2 [abstract]. *J Hepatol* 1997; 26: **57A**.

126. Beutler E, Griffin MJ, Gelbart T, West C. A previously undescribed nonsense mutation of the *HFE* gene. *Clin Genet* 2002; **61**: 40–2.

127. Barton JC, Sawada-Hirai R, Rothenberg BE, Acton RT. Two novel missense mutations of the *HFE* gene (I105T and G93R) and identification of the S65C mutation in Alabama hemochromatosis probands. *Blood Cells Mol Dis* 1999; **25**: 147–55.

128. Barton JC, West C, Lee PL, Beutler E. A previously undescribed frameshift deletion mutation of *HFE* (c.del277; G93fs) associated with hemochromatosis

and iron overload in a C282Y heterozygote. *Clin Genet* 2004; **66**: 214–16.

129. Cukjati M, Koren S, Curin S, V, Vidan-Jeras B, Rupreht R. A novel homozygous frameshift deletion c.471del of *HFE* associated with hemochromatosis. *Clin Genet* 2007; **71**: 350–3.

130. Pointon JJ, Lok CY, Shearman JD, *et al.* A novel *HFE* mutation (c.del478) results in nonsense-mediated decay of the mutant transcript in a hemochromatosis patient. *Blood Cells Mol Dis* 2009; **43**: 194–8.

131. Oberkanins C, Moritz A, de Villiers JN, Kotze MJ, Kury F. A reverse-hybridization assay for the rapid and simultaneous detection of nine *HFE* gene mutations. *Genet Test* 2000; **4**: 121–4.

132. Piperno A, Arosio C, Fossati L, *et al.* Two novel nonsense mutations of *HFE* gene in five unrelated italian patients with hemochromatosis. *Gastroenterology* 2000; **119**: 441–5.

133. Bradbury R, Fagan E, Payne SJ. Two novel polymorphisms (E277K and V212V) in the haemochromatosis gene *HFE*. *Hum Mutat* 2000; **15**: 120.

134. A simple genetic test identifies 90% of UK patients with haemochromatosis. The UK Haemochromatosis Consortium. *Gut* 1997; **41**: 841–4.

135. Rosmorduc O, Poupon R, Nion I, *et al.* Differential *HFE* allele expression in hemochromatosis heterozygotes. *Gastroenterology* 2000; **119**: 1075–86.

136. Le Gac G, Dupradeau FY, Mura C, *et al.* Phenotypic expression of the C282Y/Q283P compound

heterozygosity in *HFE* and molecular modeling of the Q283P mutation effect. *Blood Cells Mol Dis* 2003; **30**: 231–7.

137. Beutler E, West C. New diallelic markers in the HLA region of chromosome 6. *Blood Cells Mol Dis* 1997; **23**: 219–29.

138. Wallace DF, Dooley JS, Walker AP. A novel mutation of *HFE* explains the classical phenotype of genetic hemochromatosis in a C282Y heterozygote. *Gastroenterology* 1999; **116**: 1409–12.

139. Steiner M, Ocran K, Genschel J, *et al.* A homozygous *HFE* gene splice site mutation (IVS5+1 G/A) in a hereditary hemochromatosis patient of Vietnamese origin. *Gastroenterology* 2002; **122**: 789–95.

140. Le Gac G, Gourlaouen I, Ronsin C, *et al.* Homozygous deletion of *HFE* produces a phenotype similar to the *HFE* p.C282Y/p.C282Y genotype. *Blood* 2008; **112**: 5238–40.

141. Pelucchi S, Mariani R, Bertola F, Arosio C, Piperno A. Homozygous deletion of *HFE*: the Sardinian hemochromatosis? *Blood* 2009; **113**: 3886.

142. Cohen AR, Galanello R, Pennell DJ, Cunningham MJ, Vichinsky E. Thalassemia. *Hematology Am Soc Hematol Educ Program* 2004; 14–34.

143. Barton JC, Rothenberg BE, Bertoli LF, Acton RT. Diagnosis of hemochromatosis in family members of probands: a comparison of phenotyping and *HFE* genotyping. *Genet Med* 1999; **1**: 89–93.

Complications of hemochromatosis and iron overload

Liver disease

Iron and the liver

The liver is the major site of iron storage in the body, and iron overload can cause hepatic fibrosis, cirrhosis, and hepatocellular carcinoma.[1–7] (Table 5.1) In hereditary hemochromatosis, a pathologic expansion of body iron stores can occur due to excessive absorption of dietary iron (Chapters 2, 8). The excess iron is preferentially deposited in parenchymal cells of the liver and other organs.[2–4,6] When storage mechanisms are overwhelmed, iron in low-molecular weight forms can catalyze free radical reactions (Chapter 3). The resulting oxyradicals have the potential to damage cellular lipids, nucleic acids, proteins, and carbohydrates, resulting in wide-ranging impairment in hepatocyte function and integrity[2–4,6] (Chapter 3). Damage can result in increased hepatic fibrogenesis, micronodular cirrhosis, and hepatocellular carcinoma.[2–4,6] Important co-factors of iron-induced liver injury include chronic hepatitis C, excess alcohol consumption, and steatosis.[1,5,7] Liver fibrogenesis shows a concordance with hepatic iron concentration and the duration of exposure to high iron levels.[1,5,7,8] Phlebotomy therapy can reverse iron-induced hepatic fibrosis, but cirrhosis is less amenable to phlebotomy treatment.[5]

In disorders of erythropoiesis, increased iron absorption and tissue iron deposition can occur.[8] (Chapters 21–25). A common factor in iron-loading anemias is refractory anemia with a hypercellular bone marrow and ineffective erythropoiesis.[8] These conditions include β-thalassemia, sideroblastic anemias, congenital dyserythropoietic anemias, and pyruvate kinase deficiency. In these syndromes, clinical and pathologic consequences similar to those seen in *HFE* hemochromatosis can occur.[5,8] In disorders of erythropoiesis in which there are concomitant blood transfusions, the iron burden can increase very rapidly through the combined impact of increased iron absorption and

transfusion-derived iron (administered as hemoglobin). Therefore, these patients may present with iron-induced hepatic fibrosis earlier than patients with *HFE* hemochromatosis[5,8] (Fig. 5.1). Many patients with other common liver diseases (e.g. chronic viral hepatitis, alcoholic liver disease, and non-alcoholic fatty liver disease) also develop secondary iron overload of mild or moderate severity.[9,10]

Iron also plays a key role in the pathogenesis of porphyria cutanea tarda (Chapter 10). Iron-dependent oxidation of uroporphyrinogen produces uroporphomethene, an inhibitor of uroporphyrinogen decarboxylase that causes porphyria cutanea tarda.[11] The prevalence of common *HFE* mutations (C282Y or H63D) in porphyria cutanea tarda patients is high, and achieving iron depletion with phlebotomy is used to treat porphyria cutanea tarda.[9,10,12]

In the past, hemochromatosis was recognized by a constellation of symptoms and physical findings related to significant iron loading in the liver, pancreas, heart, skin, and pituitary gland. Since the 1990s, most individuals with hemochromatosis diagnosed in medical care are asymptomatic.[13,14] This is because they are usually identified as the result of screening blood tests obtained during routine health physical examinations, or by testing for *HFE* mutations during family screening. In such persons with hemochromatosis, phlebotomy treatment can be started before there are any significant manifestations of iron overload.

A useful definition of the various stages of *HFE* hemochromatosis was identified at a consensus conference of the European Association for the Study of Liver Disease.[15] These stages are defined as:

- Stage 1: hemochromatosis-associated *HFE* genotypes with no increase in iron stores;
- Stage 2: hemochromatosis-associated *HFE* genotypes with phenotypic evidence of iron overload but no tissue or organ damage;

Table 5.1. Liver disease in iron overload

Hepatic iron overload can cause hepatic fibrosis, cirrhosis, and hepatocellular carcinoma

Liver fibrogenesis is concordant with hepatic iron concentration and duration of exposure to high iron levels

Chronic alcohol consumption, chronic viral hepatitis, and steatosis are co-factors in iron-induced fibrogenesis

Population screening studies suggest that the prevalence of cirrhosis in *HFE* C282Y homozygotes has a strong male predominance, and ranges from 3%–18% in males and 0.3%–5% in females

Cirrhosis is very rare in *HFE* C282Y homozygotes with serum ferritin values less than 1000 µg/L and normal serum liver enzyme levels

The risk of hepatocellular carcinoma is increased in hemochromatosis patients with cirrhosis, even after excess iron has been removed by phlebotomy

Therapeutic phlebotomy can reverse iron-induced hepatic fibrosis

- Stage 3: hemochromatosis-associated *HFE* genotypes, iron overload, and iron deposition to the degree that tissue and organ damage occurs.

This recognition is important to allow clinicians to categorize patients who have positive genetic test results for *HFE* mutations.

Prevalence of liver disease in C282Y homozygotes

Liver disease that is associated with iron overload, and especially with cirrhosis and hepatocellular carcinoma, has a high morbidity. Thus, there is particular interest in the incidence of liver disease in *HFE* C282Y homozygotes. Liver disease in C282Y homozygotes has a strong male predominance.[16–19] An Australian population study showed that the prevalence of hepatic fibrosis was 13.5% and that of cirrhosis was 2.7% (2 of 74 subjects) in male C282Y homozygotes; the prevalence of hepatocellular carcinoma was similar to that of cirrhosis.[19] One of the two subjects with cirrhosis had consumed more than 100 g of alcohol daily, consistent with a previous report that excessive alcohol consumption increased the risk of cirrhosis in C282Y homozygotes.[20] In three other studies that identified

(a)

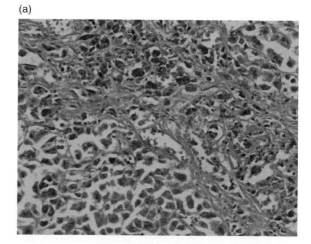

(b)

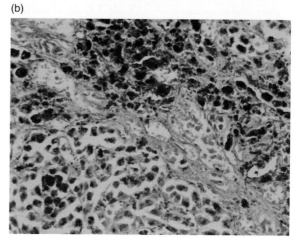

Fig. 5.1. Liver biopsy specimens from woman with pure red cell aplasia treated with numerous transfusions. Hematoxylin and eosin staining reveals brown pigment (hemosiderin) in hepatocytes; an adjacent section stained with Perls' technique reveals grade 4 blue-black intrahepatocytic iron. Original magnification 400×. See plate section for color version.

C282Y homozygotes on the basis of population screening,[18] health assessment,[17] or family studies,[16] the prevalence of cirrhosis in men (4.2%, 5.6%, and 18%, respectively) and women (0.3%, 1.9%, and 5%, respectively) were higher than those observed in the Australian study,[19] perhaps due to population variation.

Diagnosis of liver disease in hemochromatosis

Large population screening studies have revealed that only about 60%–80% of *HFE* C282Y homozygotes have an elevated serum ferritin level, and many

C282Y homozygotes do not have "classical" symptoms previous associated with hemochromatosis (Chapter 8). Nonetheless, it is important for clinicians to be aware of the symptoms that individuals with hemochromatosis may report. The diagnosis of hemochromatosis should be considered patients complain of fatigue, right upper quadrant abdominal pain, arthralgias, impotence, decreased libido, or symptoms of heart failure or diabetes mellitus.[1,5,7] Similarly, physical findings of an enlarged heart, particularly in the presence of cirrhosis, extrahepatic manifestations of chronic liver disease, testicular atrophy, signs of congestive heart failure, increased skin pigmentation, or arthritis should raise a suspicion of hemochromatosis.[1,5,7] Many of these signs and symptoms are also associated with conditions other than hemochromatosis, but clinicians should evaluate patients with these symptoms for hemochromatosis and iron overload.

Liver biopsy has become less critical in establishing the diagnosis of hemochromatosis since genetic testing for *HFE* mutations has become widely available. Currently, if a patient is a *HFE* C282Y homozygote or a compound heterozygote (*HFE* C282Y/H63D) with normal liver enzyme activities (alanine aminotransferase (ALT) or aspartate aminotransferase (AST)) and abnormal iron measures, then the patient has *HFE* hemochromatosis and phlebotomy therapy can be initiated. If serum levels of ALT and AST activities are elevated, or if the serum ferritin level is greater than 1000 μg/L, then it should be considered if the patient needs a liver biopsy (Chapter 4). This is recommended to identify patients with advanced fibrosis and cirrhosis. The biopsy specimen should be stained with Perls' Prussian blue stain to visualize iron, and it is reasonable to determine the hepatic iron concentration (Chapter 4). In *HFE* hemochromatosis, iron deposition begins in periportal (zone 1) hepatocytes, and there is a periportal to pericentral (zone 3) gradient.[21,22] At higher power, iron is seen predominantly in hepatocytes; there is very little iron staining in Kupffer cells. With severe iron loading, the zonal gradient of iron deposition is diminished, iron deposition is observed in bile duct epithelial cells, and increased fibrosis is found in the periportal region.[21,22]

Liver biopsy will also provide information about: (1) the degree of fibrosis; (2) the presence or absence of cirrhosis; and (3) the presence or absence of other histologic abnormalities such as steatosis (Chapter 4). For prognosis, it is important to determine if there is advanced fibrosis or cirrhosis, because the risk of hepatocellular carcinoma is significantly increased in patients with cirrhosis. In patients with advanced liver disease, cirrhosis is typically micronodular.[21,22] In symptomatic patients, the hepatic iron concentration is typically greater than 10 000 μg/g dry weight (normal <1500 μg/g dry weight), and values as high as 40 000 μg/g dry weight can occur but are uncommon.[1,5,7]

Iron and *HFE* mutations in non-hemochromatosis liver diseases

Many patients with liver disease have abnormalities of serum markers of iron metabolism.[9,10] These abnormalities are detected more commonly in patients with hepatocellular liver disease than in those with cholestatic liver disease. Approximately 50% of patients with alcoholic liver disease, chronic viral hepatitis (B or C), and non-alcoholic fatty liver disease have abnormalities in serum iron measures. Elevation of serum ferritin level is the most characteristic abnormality, but some patients also have elevated transferrin saturation levels.[9,10] Liver biopsies in these patients reveal increased iron deposition in a panlobular (rather than a periportal) distribution, and iron is deposited in both hepatocytes and Kupffer cells (rather than predominantly in hepatocytes).[21,22] The hepatic iron concentration is rarely as high as 10 000 μg/g dry weight, and is commonly in the range of 2000–3000 μg/g dry weight.[9,10] Genetic testing can distinguish whether these patients have either *HFE* hemochromatosis and another liver disease, or a primary liver disease complicated by secondary iron overload.

In patients with alcoholic liver disease, the prevalence of either *HFE* C282Y or H63D is not significantly higher than that in a control population.[23,24] Furthermore, there is no increase in the prevalence of common *HFE* mutations in patients with alcoholic liver disease who have increased hepatic fibrosis. Thus, the abnormal iron studies seen in most patients with alcoholic liver disease are probably due to mechanisms other than *HFE* mutations. Alcohol decreases the expression of hepcidin in the liver, and this could increase iron absorption and hepatic iron deposition.[25]

In chronic hepatitis C, a relationship between elevated hepatic iron concentrations and treatment response to interferon monotherapy has been reported.[26–29] Patients with chronic hepatitis C who failed to respond to interferon monotherapy had a higher hepatic iron concentration than those who responded to the treatment.[26-29] Accordingly, therapeutic phlebotomy was used to deplete iron stores in an effort to enhance the response to interferon therapy in such patients. Iron reduction by phlebotomy decreased serum levels of ALT and AST, but did not improve rates of sustained virologic response to interferon therapy.[30-33] When similar studies were performed in chronic hepatitis C patients treated with dual therapy (interferon/ribavirin or pegylated-interferon/ribavirin), there was no significant relationship between hepatic iron concentration and response to antiviral therapy.[34]

In patients with chronic hepatitis C, the prevalence of *HFE* C282Y and H63D mutations does not differ significantly from that in control subjects (as seen in alcoholic liver disease).[9,10] Nonetheless, most studies have shown that patients with *HFE* mutations have increased iron stores seen histologically, and some studies have shown synergism of increased hepatic iron levels with hepatitis C on hepatic fibrogenesis.[35-38] Currently, it is recommended that *HFE* mutation analysis be performed in patients with chronic hepatitis C and abnormal iron studies.[9] It is also recommended that iron staining and quantitative measurement of iron be performed on liver biopsy samples (in addition to grading of inflammation and staging of fibrosis). If iron stores are increased, it is reasonable to perform therapeutic phlebotomy to deplete excess iron before initiating antiviral treatment.[9]

In patients with non-alcoholic fatty liver disease, the prevalence of the *HFE* C282Y mutation (usually in heterozygous configuration) is significantly higher than that control subjects.[39-42] It remains controversial whether increased hepatic iron levels are associated with the enhanced development of fibrosis in non-alcoholic fatty liver disease, and thus further investigation in this area is warranted.[9,10] Iron depletion of patients with non-alcoholic fatty liver disease may lead to decreased levels of serum ALT and reduced insulin resistance (Chapter 6).

In porphyria cutanea tarda, iron plays an important role in catalyzing the production of an inhibitor of uroporphyrinogen decarboxylase,[11] and iron depletion by phlebotomy is used as a treatment.[12] There is an increased prevalence of *HFE* mutations in patients with porphyria cutanea tarda that may contribute to increased iron availability in the liver.[2,9,10,12] Many porphyria cutanea tarda patients are infected with hepatitis C virus or consume excessive amounts of alcohol; both of these latter conditions may decrease hepcidin expression and thereby increase iron accumulation.[25,43] Therefore, serum iron measures, *HFE* mutation analysis, and hepatitis C virus studies should be performed in patients with porphyria cutanea tarda.

Hepatocellular cancer in hemochromatosis

The incidence of hepatocellular carcinoma is increased in hemochromatosis patients.[44-48] The relative risk is at least 11-fold greater in hemochromatosis patients than in control populations.[48] Hepatocellular carcinoma is one of the most common causes of death in hemochromatosis patients with phenotypic expression.[44,46,47] Most hemochromatosis patients who develop hepatocellular carcinoma are males aged more than 50 years who have cirrhosis.[44-48] In hemochromatosis patients without cirrhosis, hepatocellular carcinoma appears to be uncommon; only about a dozen cases have been reported.[47] High hepatic iron concentrations and longer duration of exposure to iron overload both contribute to an increased risk of hepatocellular carcinoma.[46,47] Other risk factors include concomitant infection with either hepatitis B or C, alcoholism, and tobacco smoking. Even after excess iron has been removed by phlebotomy, the risk of hepatocellular carcinoma remains increased in hemochromatosis patients with cirrhosis.[46,47]

The pathogenesis of hepatocellular carcinoma in hemochromatosis may be due in part to iron-induced DNA damage (Chapter 3) and liver progenitor cell proliferation.[49] Nodules of proliferative hepatocytes, called iron-free foci, are sometimes observed in liver biopsies taken from hemochromatosis patients with heavy iron overload. This strongly suggests that iron-free foci are proliferative, pre-neoplastic lesions, and their detection should trigger enhanced surveillance for hepatocellular carcinoma.[50,51]

The prognosis of patients with hepatocellular carcinoma is poor, largely because many patients have an advanced tumor burden at the time of diagnosis.[46,47] This precludes resection or transplant as definitive treatment modalities. Therefore, regular screening with abdominal imaging is recommended for hemochromatosis patients with cirrhosis to detect early hepatocellular carcinoma that can be definitively treated with resection or liver transplantation.[46,47] If hemochromatosis can be detected and treated before cirrhosis develops, the incidence of hepatocellular carcinoma should decrease markedly.

Cardiac abnormalities

Early investigators reported serious cardiac abnormalities in early clinical and autopsy case studies of persons with hemochromatosis.[52–54] Clinical correlates regarding severe cardiac siderosis made then are similar to those of today: most such patients are adolescents or young adults who also have cirrhosis and hypogonadism. Arthropathy occurs in many patients. This rare syndrome, often called juvenile or early age-of-onset hemochromatosis, is typically due to homozygosity or compound heterozygosity for deleterious mutation(s) of the *HJV* gene that encodes hemojuvelin (Chapter 13); even rarer cases may be due to mutations in other genes (Chapters 12, 14, 15). Iron deposition in the heart is usually advanced before abnormalities of cardiac rhythm control and pump function cause symptoms. In persons with severe beta-thalassemia, progressive systemic iron overload develops as a consequence of both increased absorption and chronic erythrocyte transfusion to alleviate severe anemia. Cardiac iron overload is the leading cause of death in patients with beta-thalassemia major (Chapter 21), and its cardiac manifestations are similar to those in patients with juvenile hemochromatosis. In contrast, complications of *HFE* hemochromatosis due to cardiac iron overload are rare; heart disease is much more likely to be caused by coronary atherosclerosis or other non-iron causes than by siderosis. In this section, the diagnosis and management of cardiac iron overload are discussed in the context of an informative presentation of the case of a young woman that exemplifies this unusual complication of severe iron overload and suggests approaches to its diagnosis and management.[55]

Case presentation

A 35-year-old Caucasian woman sought medical attention at an emergent care center on the day of hospitalization. Her chief complaint was "I'm having trouble breathing" for the past 2 days. She reported having progressive dyspnea accompanied by forceful palpitations. She became short of breath at rest and felt as if she had to work to breathe. Her ankles had become swollen recently. In the previous 4–6 weeks, she had gained 15 pounds (6.8 kg) despite having a poor appetite, and she had experienced increasing fatigue, weakness, and difficulty sleeping.

She had no history of cardiac problems. She had been treated for amenorrhea by a reproductive endocrinologist for 6–8 years. She had panhypopituitarism of undetermined cause with hypothyroidism, adrenal insufficiency, amenorrhea, and infertility, accompanied by decreased serum or plasma concentrations of thyroid-stimulating hormone, free T_3, free T_4, cortisol, follicle-stimulating hormone, luteinizing hormone, and estradiol. She had an episode of iritis a few years earlier. She took replacement thyroid, glucocorticoid, and estrogen medications for panhypopituitarism, and ibuprofen for arthralgias of knees and ankles. She did not have a history of liver disease, or a history of diabetes mellitus. She reported having no recent respiratory tract infection. She did not drink alcohol or use tobacco products. She reported no family history of heart disease or of iron overload, although her mother had adult-onset diabetes mellitus and arthritis of unknown type.

Physical examination revealed that she had mild respiratory distress while sitting. Heart rate was 238 beats/minute and regular; blood pressure was 106/64 mm/Hg; temperature was normal; and oxygen saturation by pulse oximetry was 97% while wearing a 100% O_2 non-rebreathing mask. Her skin color was ashen to pale. Jugular venous pressure was elevated (>15 cm of H_2O); there was no thyromegaly or lymph node enlargement. Chest was non-tender to percussion. Lungs revealed bibasilar crackles. The left ventricular apical impulse was displaced laterally, and enlarged and sustained. A prominent S3 gallop was present; there was a grade III/VI holosystolic murmur heard best at the apex. Abdomen was soft and bowel sounds were present. Liver was palpable 4 cm below the right costal margin in the mid-clavicular line; there was no abdominal tenderness. Extremities were cool and cyanotic, with 1–2+ pitting edema in the lower legs and ankles. Neurologic examination revealed no focal abnormalities.

Laboratory data included leukocytes 10 300/μL, hemoglobin 15 g/dL, and platelets 186 000/μL. Serum chemistry measurements included Na 141 mmol/L, K 5.4 mmol/L, blood urea nitrogen 17 mg/dL, creatinine 0.7 mg/dL, total cholesterol 201 mg/dL, aspartate aminotransferase 85 U/L, alanine aminotransferase 91 U/L, and glucose 203 mg/dL. A portable chest X-ray revealed findings interpreted as pulmonary edema due to congestive heart failure (Fig. 5.2). Her electrocardiogram revealed atrial flutter with 1:1 conduction, a heart rate of 239 beats/minute, and other abnormalities (Fig. 5.3).

69

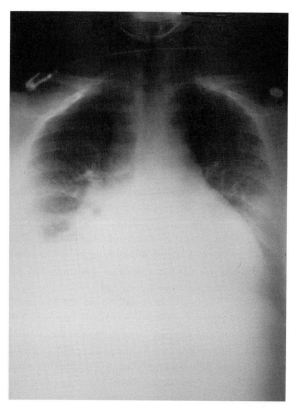

Fig. 5.2. Chest X-ray (upright position) of patient with cardiac siderosis due to hemochromatosis presented in this case study. The heart is markedly enlarged and there are alveolar infiltrates, perihilar hazy infiltrates, right pleural effusion, widening of the superior mediastinal vessels, and increased blood flow in the vessels of the superior lung fields, all compatible with pulmonary edema. From Muhlestein.[55] Taken from James C. Barton and Corwin Q. Edwards (eds), **Hemochromatosis: Genetics, Pathophysiology, Diagnosis and Treatment,** Cambridge University Press 2000. Reproduced with permission.

The initial working diagnosis was pulmonary edema and atrial flutter with 1:1 conduction due to viral myocarditis or idiopathic cardiomyopathy. The attending physicians also considered autoimmune disorders, amyloidosis, and hemochromatosis as possible unifying explanations for her cardiomyopathy, panhypopituitarism, arthralgias and glucose intolerance.

She was treated in the emergency room with intravenous ibutilide; this converted her rapid atrial flutter to sinus tachycardia for a short period. In the intensive care unit, her rhythm reverted to atrial flutter, so she was given intravenous diltiazem for rate control, but her rhythm soon deteriorated to atrial fibrillation with a rapid ventricular response. In an attempt to convert her rhythm from atrial fibrillation to sinus rhythm, she was given intravenous procainamide but there was

no response. She underwent unsuccessful attempts at electrical cardioversion using 50 joules followed by 360 joules. The procainamide therapy was discontinued, and intravenous amiodarone was started, but again cardioversion was not successful.

She underwent echocardiography to evaluate the functional anatomy of her heart. Her echocardiogram revealed a markedly dilated left ventricle with normal wall thickness (Fig. 5.4). There was severe reduction in global contractility of the left ventricle, and a markedly decreased ejection fraction of <30%. The size and thickness of the right ventricle was normal, but there was moderate reduction in global function. There was mild-moderate enlargement of the left and right atrial chambers. The anatomy of all cardiac valves was normal, but she had mild mitral regurgitation and moderate tricuspid regurgitation. The inferior vena cava was distended, consistent with intravascular volume overload. The remainder of her echocardiography, including evaluation of the aortic root and the pericardium, appeared normal. She did not have a pericardial effusion.

She also was treated for pulmonary edema and congestive heart failure, using continuous intravenous infusions of furosemide and captopril. Her clinical condition continued to deteriorate. She required more than 50% oxygen by face mask to maintain an arterial oxygen percent saturation of about 80%. Milrinone, an intravenous positive inotropic agent, was administered in an attempt to improve her cardiac output, but without success.

Her condition continued to deteriorate, and thus right heart catheterization was performed. This documented very low cardiac output of 2.4 L/minute and a cardiac index of 1.6 L/min/m^2 (normal 2.6–3.5 L/min/m^2), despite an elevated pulmonary capillary wedge pressure of 25 mm Hg. An endomyocardial biopsy was obtained. Atrial fibrillation with a rapid ventricular response persisted, so atrio-ventricular nodal radiofrequency ablation was performed, followed by implantation of a cardiac pacemaker. The ablation procedure slowed her rapid ventricular rate, but she remained hypoxemic and developed progressive hypotension.

She underwent endotracheal intubation to improve oxygenation and implantation of an intra-aortic balloon pump to improve her hemodynamic status, but she developed cardiac asystole during the procedures. She underwent prolonged resuscitation, transfer to the thoracic intensive care unit in the hopes of finding a cardiac transplant donor, and for consideration of

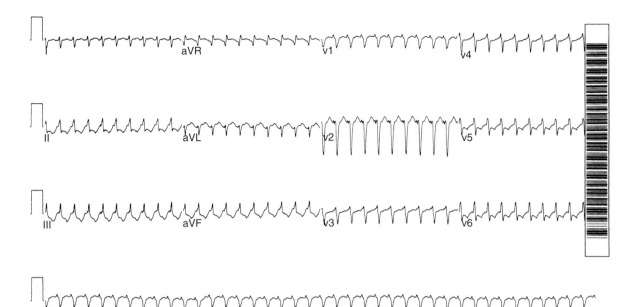

Fig. 5.3. Admission 12-lead electrocardiogram of the patient with cardiac hemochromatosis presented in this case study. The arrhythmia is atrial flutter with 1:1 contraction at a rate of 233 beats per minute. A non-specific interventricular conduction delay is present in all leads, and T-wave abnormalities are present in leads II, III, AVF, and V_{5-6}, suggestive of inferolateral ischemia. There is slow R-wave progression in precordial leads V_{1-4}. From Muhlestein.[55] Taken from James C. Barton and Corwin Q. Edwards (eds), **Hemochromatosis: Genetics, Pathophysiology, Diagnosis and Treatment**, Cambridge University Press 2000. Reproduced with permission.

placement of a total artificial heart. Nonetheless, she expired 48 hours after presentation.

Results of blood iron measures were returned after her death. Serum ferritin was 5350 μg/L (normal females <81 μg/L). Electron microscopy performed on the endomyocardial biopsy sample revealed iron-laden myocardial cells, confirming the diagnosis of hemochromatosis. Her siblings were advised to seek medical evaluation for possible hemochromatosis.

Comments on case presentation

This course of this patient's illness demonstrates the importance of establishing an early diagnosis of hemochromatosis before end-stage, intractable complications of iron overload occur. Her secondary amenorrhea led to the diagnosis of hypopituitarism 6–8 years before she developed cardiac decompensation. At that time, it is presumed that her serum ferritin level was elevated, and that she had liver abnormalities consistent with iron overload. If iron overload had been considered as a possible cause of her secondary amenorrhea and panhypopituitarism, the diagnosis of hemochromatosis could have been established, and performing iron depletion therapy could have prevented the development of lethal cardiac complications.

Diagnosis in this patient

This patient probably had juvenile hemochromatosis, not *HFE* hemochromatosis. Her early age-of-onset arthralgias, amenorrhea, panhypopituitarism, dilated cardiomyopathy, and life-threatening intractable arrhythmias are all compatible with and strongly suggest the diagnosis of juvenile hemochromatosis. The severe clinical illness caused by juvenile hemochromatosis typically occurs 20–30 years earlier than that of *HFE* hemochromatosis. It is likely that this patient's intractable heart failure was caused by iron deposition in cardiac myocytes, as demonstrated by electron microscopic analysis of her endomyocardial biopsy, and was exacerbated by a tachycardia-induced systolic dysfunction.

Treatment of iron overload cardiomyopathy then (1996) and now (2010)

Medications

Some treatments that were available in 1996 for the treatment of this patient are still used now. Ibutilide is often considered to be the drug of choice for the treatment of atrial flutter with a very fast ventricular rate. Diltiazem is still used to slow the heart rate in patients with atrial

(a)

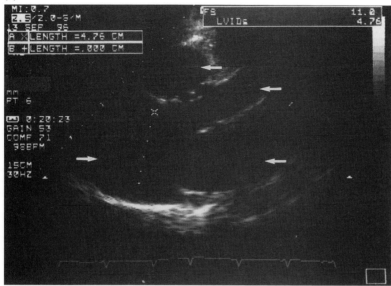

(b)

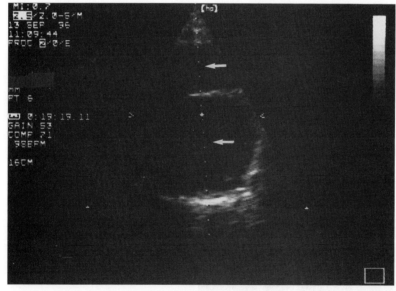

Fig. 5.4. Echocardiogram (2-D and M-mode) of patient with cardiac siderosis due to hemochromatosis in this case study. (a) Parasternal long axis view: top center arrow indicates right ventricle; bottom left arrow indicates markedly enlarged left ventricle; top right arrow indicates aorta; bottom right arrow indicates left atrium; (b) short axis view: top arrow incates right ventricle; bottom arrow indicates markedly enlarged left ventricle; (c) M-mode tracing includes five arrows: top arrow points to anterior wall of right ventricle; second arrow points to moderately enlarged right ventricle; middle arrow refers to marked hypokinesis of interventricular septum; fourth arrow points to markedly enlarged left ventricle; bottom arrow refers to marked hypokinesis of posterior wall of left ventricle; and (d) top left arrow points to right ventricle; bottom left arrow points to right atrium; top right arrow points to left ventricle (cross-hatched area) with large volume of end-systolic blood; the calculated ejection fraction from this apical four-chamber view is very low 32% (normal; 55%–78%); bottom right arrow points to left atrium. From Muhletein.[55]

flutter. Amiodarone is still used to try to convert atrial fibrillation to sinus rhythm. Furosemide and captopril, or a different angiotensin-converting enzyme inhibitor or an angiotensin receptor blocker, are still used in the treatment of patients who have heart failure. It is much more convenient for a patient to take a single daily dose of a angiotensin converting enzyme inhibitor such as benazepril that has long half-life rather than multiple daily doses of captopril. Milrinone is still used for its positive inotropic effect in patients with hypotension and decreased cardiac output. Procainamide is not used now to convert atrial fibrillation to sinus rhythm. It is not very effective and it has a negative inotropic effect, an undesirable attribute for use in patients with heart failure.

Defibrillators then (1996) and now (2010)

The defibrillators that were available in 1996 were monophasic. This means that all of the energy that was discharged from the defibrillator paddles flowed

(c)

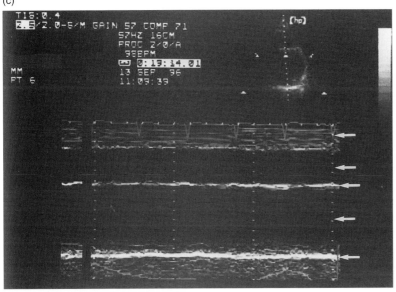

Fig. 5.4. *(cont.)*

(d)

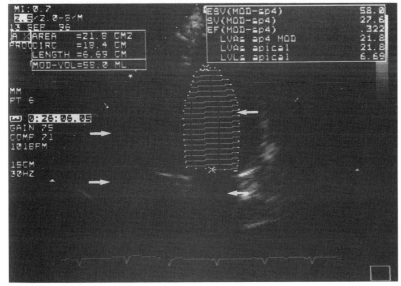

through the chest wall in one direction, from front to back. Frequently, the energy setting on the defibrillator had to be increased, usually starting at 50 joules, increasing to a maximum (very rarely) of 360 joules. Defibrillators in common use today are biphasic; their energy is delivered from both paddles on the chest wall. The energy is directed in more of a side-to-side pattern, rather than front to back. This is considered to be an improvement for patients who need to undergo electrical cardioversion. If the patient's physicians were to treat her today, they may have opted for early cardioversion using improved defibrillators, rather than using cardioversion only after attempts at chemical cardioversion failed. It is also possible that the early use of biphasic defibrillation may not have converted the current patient's arrhythmias to sinus rhythm.

Chelation therapy then (1996) and now (2010)

The current patient was hemodynamically unstable and thus phlebotomy therapy was not feasible. Had she lived longer, her physicians may have treated her with intravenous deferoxamine to remove iron from her cardiac myocytes. This could have reduced her risk of death due to intractable heart failure and arrhythmia. Some young patients with heart failure and cardiac arrhythmias due to juvenile hemochromatosis have survived after receiving iron chelation therapy that was given early after presentation. Combined use of two types of iron chelators may be more effective than single-agent chelation therapy to deplete iron deposited in the heart (Chapter 36). If she were treated today, her physicians would probably use intravenous deferoxamine and oral deferasirox. In some countries, the oral iron chelation drug deferiprone is available.

Mechanical support of cardiac output then (1996) and now (2010)

In 1996, the use of an intra-aortic balloon pump or total cardiopulmonary bypass were the final measures that were available for mechanical circulatory support. Usually, they provided little increase in cardiac output although some patients are still treated with intra-aortic balloon pumps. Today, the present patient would probably have been treated with an implantable left ventricular assist device (LVAD). An LVAD can be used long term as so-called destination therapy, or used short term as temporary, bridging therapy. LVADs serve as destination therapy for patients who refuse transplantation, or for patients who are not candidates for a transplant. LVADs serve as temporary bridging therapy for patients awaiting heart transplant.

The LVAD consists of two flexible synthetic conduits, one on each side of a pump. One conduit is sutured to the left ventricle and the other into the supravalvular aorta. Blood flows from the left ventricle through the pump into the aorta. One or more drive lines pass through the anterior abdominal wall to connect to a control module. The patient wears packs that contain the control module and rechargeable battery packs. The LVAD typically provides a cardiac output of 3–4 L/min. Some patients are able to return to work and recreational activities. LVADs can only be implanted in an operating room. The pumps of some early versions were bulky, weighed 2–3 pounds, and were placed in the abdomen. The control modules of older LVAD models were quite noisy; they were also very heavy and were thus placed on carts with wheels. The pumps of some newer LVADs are small and weigh about 10 ounces.

Another device that is now available is a percutaneous ventricular assist device (pVAD). Some models provide a cardiac output of about 4 L/min. A pVAD is designed to provide temporary, bridging, mechanical support of the circulation for 5–7 days until the patient's cardiac output improves or until a donor heart becomes available for transplantation. It is an external pump that has an external computerized control system and external power source. A large-bore catheter is inserted into a femoral vein, a catheter is passed into the right atrium, then across the inter-atrial septum where oxygenated blood is pumped from the left atrium into one or both femoral arteries. The pVAD device can be deployed in a cardiac catheterization laboratory, rather than only in the operating room.

Symptoms

The symptoms of heart disease due to severe iron overload typically are related to the area of the heart where the greatest quantities of iron have accumulated. The most common cardiac symptom is the sensation of extra beats or irregular heart rhythm. In patients whose iron overload has been present for decades, dyspnea and decreased exercise tolerance may reflect the development of heart failure. Heart failure is common at the time of diagnosis of the syndrome of heart failure and endocrinopathy in very young people who have juvenile hemochromatosis. A patient with iron overload who has palpitations can be tested easily by electrocardiography to identify atrial or ventricular premature contractions, atrial fibrillation or flutter, or ventricular tachycardia or fibrillation. Of these, the most common abnormality in iron-loaded individuals is frequent atrial premature contractions; alone, this manifestation is usually innocuous. Nonetheless, most patients with hemochromatosis or other causes of iron overload do not have cardiac symptoms attributable to cardiac siderosis.

Physical examination findings

The most common abnormality is an irregular rhythm, usually due to atrial premature contractions; the second most common is intermittent ventricular premature contractions. Persons with atrial fibrillation typically have irregularly irregular cardiac rhythm. Examination may also detect pulmonary crackles, dullness to chest percussion due to a pleural effusion, an S3 gallop due to decreased compliance of the left ventricle, and increased weight associated with ankle edema. Tachycardia is usually due to sinus tachycardia or atrial fibrillation with a rapid ventricular response. Nonetheless, the cardiac examination in many patients with iron overload is normal.

Diagnosis of iron-related cardiac disease

The diagnosis of cardiac dysfunction in patients with severe iron overload is based on an evaluation that is similar to that appropriate for patients with heart disease of other causes. Serum iron measures obtainable within hours can specifically distinguish between iron overload cardiomyopathy and other types of heart disease. It is expected that the percent saturation of serum transferrin and the serum ferritin concentration will be elevated in almost all patients with heart disease due to severe iron overload. Other informative tests yield informative but non-specific information. These include a standard 12-lead electrocardiogram and a posterior-anterior and lateral chest X-ray views. Electrocardiograms in iron-loaded patients with palpitations may show non-specific findings atrial or ventricular premature contractions, or atrial fibrillation or flutter, or ventricular tachycardia or fibrillation. Of these, the most common abnormality in iron-loaded individuals is frequent atrial premature contractions, which alone are usually innocuous. It usually is important to investigate the functional anatomy of the heart using transthoracic echocardiography to measure chamber sizes, estimate wall motion and contractility, measure wall thickness, examine valvular diameter and function and blood flow, estimate pressures, and detect any pericardial effusion.

If a liver biopsy has not been or cannot be performed, a myocardial biopsy should be obtained during cardiac catheterization. The presence of cardiac iron loading is established by staining a myocardial biopsy for the presence of iron using Perls' (Prussian blue) technique. The specimen can evaluated using electron microscopy, if viral myocarditis is a consideration in the differential diagnosis of congestive heart failure. Often a right heart catheterization is sufficient. If patient age and presentation suggest the likelihood of coronary artery atherosclerosis, a left heart catheterization can be performed instead.

Treatment of iron-related cardiac disease

In patients with life-threatening arrhythmias due to severe myocardial siderosis, the initial management must be directed to reversal of the arrhythmia, stabilization of cardiac output, and support of left ventricular function. The definitive long-term treatment of iron-induced heart disease is depletion of excessive iron stores. In hemochromatosis patients, phlebotomy therapy is nearly always the most efficient method of iron depletion. In patients who have chronic anemia and iron overload, phlebotomy therapy is not a treatment option. These patients can be treated with injectable deferoxamine or with an oral iron chelator, such as deferiprone.

Response of cardiac disease to iron depletion

During iron depletion therapy, iron is mobilized from cardiac myocytes, just as it is mobilized from storage sites in the liver and other organs. Cardiac arrhythmias and even congestive heart failure may improve after successful depletion of excess cardiac storage iron. In the patient whose course was herein, atrial arrhythmias, and ventricular function were insufficiently stable to permit therapeutic phlebotomy, iron chelation therapy with deferoxamine, or combined phlebotomy and chelation management.

Many patients with increased iron absorption due to ineffective erythropoiesis and chronic erythrocyte transfusion, such as those with β-thalassemia major, accumulate more myocardial iron than patients with hemochromatosis. There is some evidence that iron acquired by erythrocyte transfusion may be preferentially deposited in the heart. Patients with severe β-thalassemia should avoid vitamin C supplements, because vitamin C may increase iron release from ferritin, cause myocardial irritability, and result in life-threatening ventricular arrhythmias.

Arthropathy
History and physical examination findings

The complaint of arthralgias and the physical examination finding of arthropathy are among the most common abnormalities in hemochromatosis homozygotes. In one series, about 44 percent of hemochromatosis patients had arthralgias or arthritis.[16] Heavily iron-loaded individuals are more likely to develop hemochromatosis arthropathy than those who have only modestly or moderately increased body iron stores. In two large screening studies, the self-reported frequency of arthritis was no greater among *HFE* C282Y homozygotes than among study participants who did not have *HFE* mutations.

Arthropathy typically appears in patients with hemochromatosis and severe iron overload during the fourth or fifth decade of life (Figs. 5.5, 5.6). Hemochromatosis arthropathy has distinctive synovial membrane changes, a typical distribution of involved joints, and characteristic radiographic findings. The arthritis of hemochromatosis is a symmetrical polyarticular arthritis that typically begins in the hands. It may lead to the early diagnosis and management of hemochromatosis before the development of irreversible injury of the liver, heart, endocrine organs, and joints.

Pathophysiology

Iron is deposited in cartilage and synovial cells. Iron accumulation causes degenerative changes of articular cartilage. In synovium, iron accumulates principally within the synovial type B synthetic cells. Less iron accumulates in the phagocytic type A synovioctyes. Iron can accumulate in joint macrophages, especially in patients with heavy iron overload. Iron can also accumulate in joint macrophages in persons who have rheumatoid arthritis, osteoarthritis, or hemarthrosis of any cause. Joints in hemochromatosis patients can accumulate

crystals of calcium pyrophosphate that can cause acute, painful attacks of pseudogout, a condition clinically similar to acute gouty arthritis. Calcium apatite crystals can also accumulate in joints affected by hemochromatosis.

Natural history

The natural history of the arthropathy of hemochromatosis begins with arthralgias, usually in the second and third metacarpal-phalangeal (MCP) joints. In any individual, the specific joints, the number of joints affected, and the sequence of involvement may vary. Many patients who later develop the hemochromatosis arthropathy usually state that they experience gradual worsening of discomfort in their MCP joints, while they retain normal range of motion and full function of their hands. During a period of years, the arthralgias are followed by slowly progressive enlargement of the MCP joints, associated with a quite gradual loss of range of motion, followed by the inability to make a tight fist or to hold small objects in their palms, and then a loss of grip strength. A distinctive difference between hemochromatosis and other types of osteoarthritis is that hemochromatosis patients may not have swelling of the proximal or distal interphalangeal joints. Some patients have both the arthropathy of hemochromatosis and Heberden nodes in the distal interphalangeal joints of the hand that are characteristic of osteoarthritis.

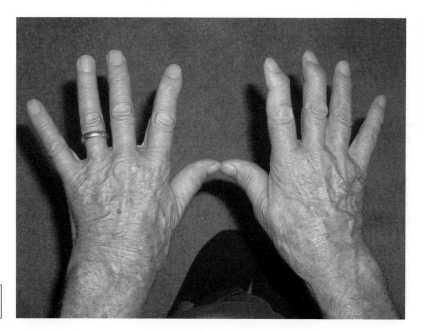

Fig. 5.5. Hands of a 68-year-old Caucasian man with hemochromatosis homozygosity and arthropathy. There is enlargement of the second and third metacarpophalangeal joints of both hands; degenerative changes are present in the right second and third distal interphalangeal joints. Skin bronzing is visible. Courtesy of Scott M. Stevens, MD, Internal Medicine, Salt Lake City, 2004.

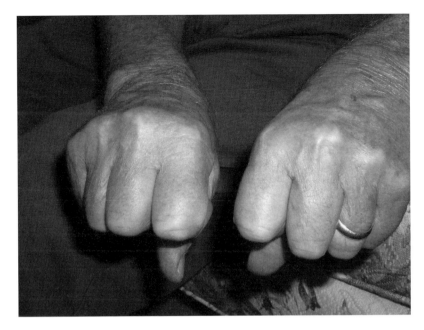

Fig. 5.6. Hands of a 68-year-old Caucasian man with hemochromatosis homozygosity and arthropathy (same patient as in Fig. 5.5). Bony hypertrophy caused loss of the normal depression between the second and third metacarpophalangeal joints of each hand; there was no tenderness or synovitis. Courtesy of Scott M. Stevens, MD, Internal Medicine, Salt Lake City, 2004.

On physical examination, the MCP joints appear enlarged, there is loss of the visible natural dip between the distal ends of metacarpal bones, the joints are hard, the fingers cannot be curled into a claw or a tight fist, and grip strength is decreased due to decreased range of motion. The physical appearance becomes typical of hand osteoarthritis of other causes. Affected individuals can usually continue to take performed required activities of daily living, and most continue to pursue their work and other activities of interest.

In some hemochromatosis patients, the onset of arthritis in the hands may simulate new-onset rheumatoid arthritis, with pain, erythema of the overlying skin, and synovitis. An important physical exam difference from rheumatoid arthritis is that in hemochromatosis, the arthropathy does not progress to rapid-onset restricted range of motion, and it does not progress to cause ulnar deviation.

Among hemochromatosis homozygotes, the knees are the second most commonly involved joints. These joints may appear normal, even when they ache, and even when there is radiographic evidence of arthropathy. Arthralgias and arthritis can also occur in the shoulders, hips, ankles, and back. Some patients experience severe restriction in the range of motion or functional ability of the knees, hips, or shoulders. Some develop enough disability that they become unable to perform activities of daily life, to perform their work, and to participate in some hobbies, physical exercise, recreation or other activities. These patients require joint replacement to restore adequate or full functional ability.

Laboratory studies for evaluation of arthritis
Serologic tests

Rheumatoid factor testing distinguishes hemochromatosis arthropathy from seropositive rheumatoid arthritis. Some patients diagnosed to have seronegative rheumatoid arthritis actually have hemochromatosis arthropathy. Some persons have both hemochromatosis and seropositive rheumatoid arthritis, but such cases are uncommon. In a study of the prevalence of *HFE* C282Y homozygosity in English Caucasians, 5 of 1000 study participants in both the inflammatory arthritis group and in a normal control group were hemochromatosis homozygotes.[56] This is consistent with the independent occurrence of the C282Y mutation and rheumatoid arthritis.

The H63D mutation of *HFE* is more prevalent in rheumatoid arthritis patients who have an HLA-DRB1 QKRAA/QKRAA epitope than in normal subjects. This HLA-D epitope and the H63D mutation independently convey increased risk for the development of rheumatoid arthritis. Serologic tests for other immunologic disorders typically are negative in hemochromatosis. As expected, some patients with hemochromatosis develop another type of arthritis that is not causally related to *HFE* C282Y or to iron overload.

Radiographic tests

Radiographs of the hands of patients with hemochromatosis arthropathy often reveal loss of joint space between the second and third metacarpal and phalangeal bones, and periarticular demineralization of the MCP joints, subchondral bone cysts, formation of beak-like osteophytes on the distal metacarpal heads, and flattening of the metacarpal heads. Although the second and third MCP joints are most frequently affected (Fig. 5.7),[57] all joints of the hands can be involved.

Chondrocalcinosis, especially that of the knees, occurs in approximately one-third of patients who have hemochromatosis. In knee radiographs, chondrocalcinosis is recognizable as a faint white horizontal line of calcium in the joint space between the distal femur and the proximal tibial plateau (Fig. 5.8), whereas this space in normal knees appears dark.[57] In the wrist, chondrocalcinosis occurs in the radio-carpal cartilage distal to the radial styloid process (radial collateral ligament), and in the ulnar collateral (triangular) ligament. Chondrocalcinosis may also be seen in the cartilage of hip joints. Knees and hips can undergo considerable joint destruction. Osteoporosis complicated by fractures can occur in hemochromatosis patients, whether or not hypogonadism is present.

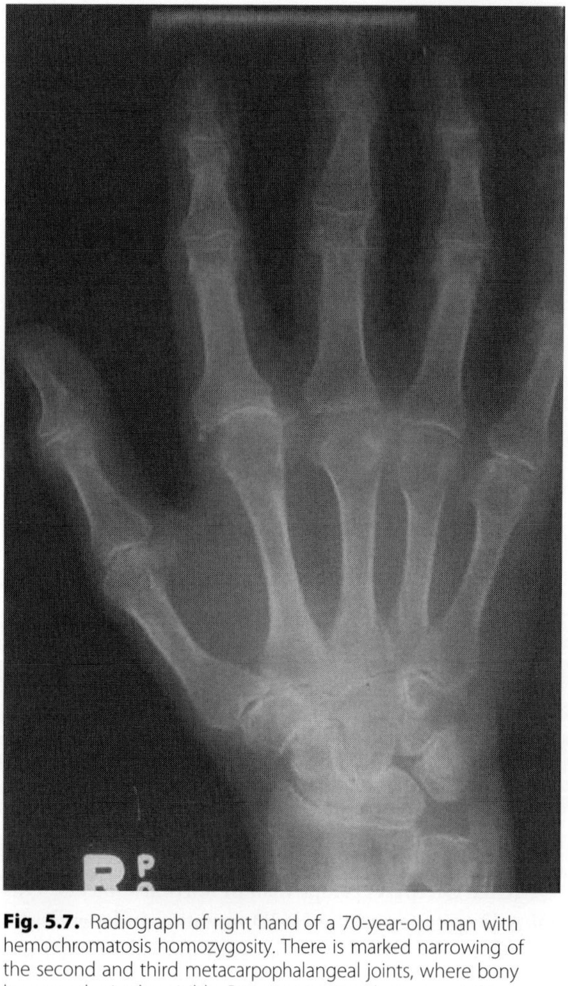

Evaluation of joint aspirates

Individuals who experience painful flare-ups of acute joint pain may have crystal-induced arthritis or bacterial infection, such as that due to *Yersinia* sp. or *Staphylococcus* sp. At the first occurrence of a flare-up of

Fig. 5.7. Radiograph of right hand of a 70-year-old man with hemochromatosis homozygosity. There is marked narrowing of the second and third metacarpophalangeal joints, where bony hypertrophy is also visible. Prominent osteophytes are visible in the second through fifth metacarpophalangeal joints. Similar abnormalities are present in the proximal interphalangeal joint of the thumb. Demineralization of periarticular bones of the metacarpophalangeal joints also is apparent. From Stevens and Edwards.[57]

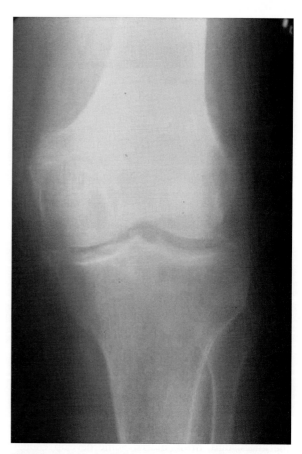

Fig. 5.8. Radiograph of left knee of a 56-year-old man with hemochromatosis homozygosity. Abundant chondrocalcinosis is visible in the medial cartilage between the distal femur and the proximal tibia.

synovitis, it is reasonable to perform joint aspiration to demonstrate the presence of calcium pyrophosphate (pseudogout) or urate (gout) crystals, and to prove the absence of bacteria by Gram stain and joint fluid culture. The leukocyte count in synovial fluid during a flare of crystal-induced arthritis is often exceeds 100 000 cells/μL, mostly polymorphonuclear neutrophils.

Treatment

General measures

Heat, modest or moderate exercise, physical therapy, and occupational therapy may help patients with hemochromatosis to maintain independent function, similar to patients with arthritis of other causes.

Medications

Many patients need medications for relief of arthralgias. As in patients with other causes of liver disease, renal insufficiency, gastrointestinal bleeding, diabetes mellitus, or anticoagulation, or in older individuals, it is important to adjust medications appropriately for each patient. Hemochromatosis patients are just as likely to experience symptomatic relief of pain from non-steroidal anti-inflammatory agents as patients with degenerative arthritis of other causes. Arthritis symptoms and signs in most patients responds to therapy with salicylates, acetaminophen, ibuprofen, or inhibitors of cyclooxygenase type 2. If a patient does not experience relief from one class of medication, it is useful to switch to a medication of a different class. Some oral non-steroidal anti-inflammatory agents, and the observed effect on joint pain following their use by hemochromatosis patients are displayed in Table 5.2.[58]

Acute attacks of pseudogout often respond to therapy with oral medications such as non-steroidal anti-inflammatory agents, indomethacin, prednisone, or colchicine. If joint aspiration reveals calcium pyrophosphate crystals and there are no stainable bacteria, crystal-induced synovitis will respond to intra-articular injection of a steroid such as triamcinolone combined with a long-acting local anesthetic such as bupivicaine.

Joint replacement

Patients whose arthropathy progresses to end-stage joint injury may require total joint replacement of the knees, shoulders, or hips. Joint infection by *Yersinia* sp. is more likely to occur after joint

Table 5.2. Effect of non-steroidal anti-inflammatory drugs (NSAIDs) on relief of joint symptoms in hemochromatosis patients[a]

Medication	Symptoms improved		Symptoms not improved	
	No. of subjects	%	No. of subjects	%
Aspirin	57/63	90	6/63	10
Indomethacin	13/14	93	1/14	7
Other NSAIDs	32/42	76	10/32	24

Note: [a]Modified from Schumacher *et al.*[58]

replacement in hemochromatosis patients than in persons without iron overload.

Phlebotomy

If phlebotomy therapy is started before end-stage arthropathy is present, iron depletion may improve arthralgias. After phlebotomy therapy in patients who report arthralgias, about one-third of patients experience improvement in symptoms; about one-third experience worsening of arthralgias; and about one-third don't experience a change in their symptoms. Even so, favorable responses may not become evident until weeks or months after iron depletion has been achieved.

Diabetes mellitus

The original descriptions of hemochromatosis included the occurrence of diabetes mellitus.[54] For nearly 100 years, it was considered that the presence of diabetes was necessary to establish the diagnosis of so-called "bronze cirrhosis," or hemochromatosis. Segregation analysis that was conducted and published in the 1970s revealed that diabetes and hemochromatosis segregated independently, as genetic traits. If diabetes were present within a family, an individual who had hemochromatosis was also likely to have diabetes. If diabetes were not present in other family members, an individual who had hemochromatosis usually did not have diabetes.

Hemochromatosis homozygotes who have diabetes mellitus usually are overweight or obese and have decreased insulin secretory capacity.[59,60] These findings also occur in mouse models of hemochromatosis.[61] Compared to non-blood donors, people who donate blood have greater insulin sensitivity, along with the expected decreased amounts of storage iron and lower average serum ferritin concentration.[62]

79

Prevalence of diabetes in hemochromatosis patients

Most patients with hemochromatosis and end-stage iron overload nearly always have diabetes mellitus. Similarly, patients with hemochromatosis and hepatic cirrhosis usually have diabetes. Hemochromatosis homozygotes who have neither heavy iron overload nor hepatic cirrhosis usually do not have diabetes.

The prevalence of diabetes among 2653 hemochromatosis patients from eight studies is displayed in Table 5.3.[16,54,63–68] In these studies, the prevalence of diabetes ranged from 9.5% to 82%. This enormous variation is due to the differences in method of ascertainment. The very low prevalence of diabetes was found among healthy homozygotes who were only identified because they participated in a screening study. The very high prevalence of diabetes was found among homozygotes who were heavily iron-loaded, were sick, and had severe iron overload.

The largest hemochromatosis screening study ever performed is the Hemochromatosis and Iron Overload Screening (HEIRS Study). In the HEIRS Study, the prevalence of self-reported diabetes among newly-diagnosed *HFE* C282Y homozygotes did not differ significantly from that of study participants without common *HFE* mutations.[69] In another large study, 8.4% of normal control subjects and 5.6% of hemochromatosis homozygotes reported that they had diabetes.[70]

Effect of method of ascertainment on prevalence of diabetes

The prevalence of diabetes mellitus among 505 hemochromatosis homozygotes in Utah studies, segregated by method of ascertainment and by gender, is displayed in Table 5.4.[16] In these studies, homozygotes were ascertained in three ways: sick probands were diagnosed during evaluation of illness; healthy, usually young probands were identified only because they participated in screening studies; and homozygous relatives were only identified during pedigree studies after a sick or a healthy proband was identified in the family. Of 184 sick probands, 24% of the men and 13% of the women had diabetes. In contrast, diabetes was rare among the healthy screening probands: 3% of asymptomatic men and none of the women. Among the clinically-unselected homozygotes (relatives

Table 5.3. Prevalence of diabetes mellitus in 2653 hemochromatosis patients from eight studies

Author (reference)	No. of patients	Patients with diabetes, *n*	Patients with diabetes, (%)
Sheldon[54]	311	255	82
Finch[63]	707	551	78
Dymock[64]	115	72	63
Saddi[65]	96	66	69
Niederau[44]	251	120	48
Yaouanq[67]	474	190	40
Adams[68]	194	47	24
Bulaj[16]	505	48	9.5
All cases	2653	1349	51

found to have hemochromatosis only because they participated in family studies), 3% and 6% percent of men and women, respectively, had diabetes.[16]

Prevalence of hemochromatosis in persons with diabetes

The estimated prevalence of hemochromatosis or *HFE* mutations among persons with diabetes is about the same as in background populations.[71–81] In some areas of the world, the prevalence of hemochromatosis or *HFE* gene mutations is higher than in the background population.[48,82–86] In a study of 418 persons with diabetes in south Australia, four individuals had hemochromatosis proven by biopsy. That is consistent with an estimated prevalence of hemochromatosis in 9.6 per 1000 persons with diabetes.[86] Considered together, the data from many studies demonstrate that the prevalence of hemochromatosis among persons with diabetes varies among populations, and varies according to methods of ascertainment.

Glucose tolerance, insulin requirement, and cirrhosis

Among hemochromatosis patients who have cirrhosis, the proportion with diabetes mellitus is as high as 87%. The prevalence of glucose intolerance, an established diagnosis of diabetes, and insulin dependence in a cohort of 251 hemochromatosis patients (142 with and 109 without cirrhosis) is displayed in Table 5.5.[87] In this

Table 5.4. Prevalence of diabetes mellitus in 505 hemochromatosis homozygotes in Utah[a]

Sick probands	Screening probands, clinically unselected		
Identified due to illness	Identified by elevated transferrin saturation		Homozygous relatives
Men $n = 136$ 24% diabetes	$n = 66$ 3% diabetes		$n = 113$ 3% diabetes
Women $n = 48$ 13% diabetes	$n = 41$ 0% diabetes		$n = 101$ 6% diabetes

Note: [a]Adapted from Bulaj et al.[16]

Table 5.5. Glucose intolerance and insulin dependence in 251 hemochromatosis patients[a]

Glucose metabolism	All patients ($n = 251$)	Cirrhosis ($n = 142$)	No cirrhosis ($n = 109$)	Value of P by z-test
	Percent of group (n)			
Normal glucose tolerance	39 (98)	20 (28)	73 (80)	0.001
Abnormal glucose tolerance[b]	13 (33)	13 (18)	14 (15)	NS[c]
Diabetes mellitus[d]	18 (120)	72 (102)	17 (18)	0.001
Non-insulin dependent diabetes mellitus	20 (51)	28 (39)	11 (12)	0.01
Insulin-dependent diabetes mellitus	27 (69)	44 (63)	6 (6)	0.001

Notes: [a]From Strohmeyer and Niederau.[87]
[b]Abnormal glucose tolerance was defined as a plasma glucose increase >200 mg/dL 2 h after oral intake of 75 g glucose.
[c]NS = not significant at 0.05 level of significance.
[d]Diabetes mellitus was defined according to World Health Organization criteria: fasting or postprandial plasma glucose >120 mg/dL or 200 mg/dL, respectively.

study, 72% of hemochromatosis patients with cirrhosis had diabetes, whereas only 17% of hemochromatosis patients without cirrhosis had diabetes (P <0.001). Similarly, insulin dependence was more prevalent among hemochromatosis patients with cirrhosis and diabetes (28%) than in hemochromatosis patients without cirrhosis (28% vs. 11%, respectively; P <0.01). The relationship of cirrhosis and non-cirrhosis in hemochromatosis patients with or without diabetes is displayed in Table 5.6.

Iron stores in hemochromatosis patients with diabetes

Hemochromatosis patients who have diabetes typically have severe iron overload; this finding has been reported in numerous studies. Among 474 hemochromatosis patients in France, 191 patients who also had diabetes had twice as much phlebotomy-mobilizable storage iron as the 283 patients who did not have diabetes.[67] The amount of iron that was removed by

Table 5.6. Relationship between hepatic cirrhosis and diabetes mellitus in 251 hemochromatosis patients in Germany

Cirrhosis	Diabetes mellitus present	Diabetes mellitus absent	Total
Present	102 (71.8%)	40 (28.2%)	142 (56.6%)
Absent	18 (16.5%)	91 (83.5%)	109 (43.3%)
Total	120 (47.8%)	131 (52.2%)	251 (100%)

Note: [a]These data represent observations in 251 patients at diagnosis of hemochromatosis. Chi-square analysis of the figures revealed: $X^2 = 73.4$; $p < 0.9 \times 10^{-15}$. From Strohmeyer and Niederau.[87]

phlebotomy therapy from groups of hemochromatosis patients with and without diabetes is displayed in Table 5.7. The mean quantity of iron removed to achieve iron depletion was much greater in hemochromatosis patients with than in those without diabetes (26 g vs. 16 g, respectively). Mean amounts of iron

Table 5.7. Amounts of iron removed by therapeutic phlebotomy in 185 hemochromatosis patients[a]

Characteristic	Presence of characteristic	Absence of characteristic	Value of P
Liver cirrhosis	25.7 ± 1.7	14.8 ± 1.5	0.001
Diabetes mellitus	26.3 ± 1.7	16.5 ± 1.5	0.001
Arthropathy	21.4 ± 1.7	20.9 ± 1.8	>0.2
Survival	19.4 ± 1.7 ($n = 150$)	29.1 ± 2.6 ($n = 35$)	0.01

Note: [a]The amount of iron removed was calculated by assuming that 1 liter of blood contained ~500 mg of iron. Results are expressed as grams of iron and are displayed as mean $\pm$ S.E. for patients in whom iron depletion was documented by repeated hepatic biopsy. The mean quantity of iron removed from the 185 patients was 21.2 ± 1.1 g. From Strohmeyer and Niederau.[87]

removed were greater in hemochromatosis patients with cirrhosis than in those without cirrhosis (25.7 g vs. 14.8 g, respectively) (Table 5.7).

Pathophysiology of diabetes mellitus

Iron overload

Diabetes in hemochromatosis is thought to be caused by two main conditions: (1) damage of insulin-secreting pancreatic islet beta-cells; and (2) insulin insensitivity or resistance. Many hemochromatosis patients without cirrhosis have normal fasting serum glucose concentrations. After a meal, or during a glucose tolerance test, their plasma insulin concentration values rise about twice as high as those of persons without hemochromatosis (60–80 µIU/mL vs. 20–40 µIU/mL, respectively). During the same test, the plasma C-peptide concentration remains normal even though the plasma insulin concentrations become markedly elevated. This suggests that hepatocytes in hemochromatosis patients do not take up or metabolize plasma insulin properly. Glucagon secretion from pancreatic alpha cells is normal in hemochromatosis patients without cirrhosis.

Hemochromatosis patients who have hepatic cirrhosis also have massive pancreatic iron overload, principally in the beta-cells. In far-advanced hemochromatosis, beta-cells secrete less insulin than is needed, leading to worsening glucose intolerance. Eventually, such patients develop insulin-dependent diabetes. Even in hemochromatosis with advanced iron overload, glucagon secretion is normal, indicating that the pancreatic alpha cells are not damaged by iron overload, whereas beta-cells undergo extensive damage and dropout.

Genetic factors

Heritable factors probably do not contribute greatly to the etiology of diabetes mellitus in hemochromatosis patients with cirrhosis. The prevalence of diabetes in hemochromatosis homozygotes without iron overload is very low. The majority of hemochromatosis patients with heavy iron overload also have diabetes. Relatives of hemochromatosis patients with diabetes do not have a higher-than-expected prevalence of diabetes. Hemochromatosis patients with cirrhosis have a much greater prevalence of diabetes than patients with cirrhosis due to non-hemochromatosis causes. Taken together, these observations suggest that iron overload of pancreatic beta-cells and of hepatocytes is the major cause of the diabetes that occurs in hemochromatosis.

Complications of diabetes

Hemochromatosis patients who have had diabetes for more than 10 years experience the same vascular and end-organ complications typical of diabetes as patients who do not have hemochromatosis. Loss of sensation to touch and vibration confer risk of skin breakdown, infection and ulceration, and in some patients, the joint dislocation and destruction characteristic of Charcot foot. Untreated proliferative retinopathy with hemorrhage and macular injury lead to impaired vision or blindness. Renal insufficiency leads to hypertension, renal failure, and dependence on peritoneal or hemodialysis, or kidney transplantation. Large-vessel peripheral vascular disease is associated with carotid stenosis or claudication of legs. Coronary artery atherosclerosis is common. Autonomic neuropathy results in gastroparesis, problems with bowel control, and loss of erectile function.

Overall, about 65 percent of hemochromatosis patients who also had diabetes develop complications of diabetes.[64,87] These results are similar to those of non-hemochromatosis patients who have diabetes for more than 10 years. The most common complications of diabetes in subjects with hemochromatosis were hypertension, coronary or peripheral vascular atherosclerosis, diabetic retinopathy, and renal insufficiency, each of which affected more than 20 percent of patients (Fig. 5.9).[87]

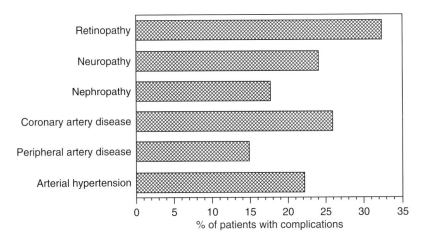

Fig. 5.9. Frequency of vascular complications of insulin-dependent diabetes mellitus among hemochromatosis patients in Düsseldorf. The mean duration of diabetes was 12 ± 5 years.[87] From Strohmeyer and Niederau.[87] Taken from James C. Barton and Corwin Q. Edwards (eds), **Hemochromatosis: Genetics, Pathophysiology, Diagnosis, and Treatment**, Cambridge University Press 2000. Reproduced with permission.

Management of diabetes in hemochromatosis patients

General principles

The principles of management of diabetes mellitus type 1 and type 2 apply to patients who have hemochromatosis and diabetes. These patients should control their weight, increase their exercise, as tolerated, and monitor fingerstick glucose measurements at home. It is very important for patients with diabetes to protect their feet. They should examine their shoes inside and out to remove any foreign bodies to prevent skin punctures and infection. Evaluation and on-going management of foot and nail condition by a podiatrist can help to prevent foot ulceration and infection.

The patient's physician should arrange systematic monitoring of serum creatinine, blood urea nitrogen, urinary specific gravity, and urinary protein excretion. This provides information about renal function. Measurement of glycosylated hemoglobin (HbA1c) provides an estimate of the overall glucose control during the previous 2–3 months. Yearly ophthalmoscopic examinations allow the early detection of retinal microaneurysms or small hemorrhages. When a retinal abnormality is identified, evaluation and management by an ophthalmologist is critical for treatment to preserve vision.

Medications

Hemochromatosis patients who have type 2 diabetes mellitus are likely to respond to therapy with metformin and oral hypoglycemic agents. Individuals whose glycosylated HbA1c values remain elevated may benefit from the addition of 10–15 u/d of a peakless insulin, such as glargine. The use of an angiotensin-converting enzyme inhibitor is recommended to help preserve renal function. Hypertension may also respond to the same therapy. If hypertension persists, an additional medication(s) is advisable. Diabetes mellitus is considered to be a coronary artery atherosclerosis equivalent. The probability that individuals with peripheral atherosclerosis to have coronary artery atherosclerosis is about 50%.

A recommendation of the US National Cholesterol Education Program (NCEP 2003) is that serum cholesterol levels in persons with diabetes should be less than 130 mg/dL. The Adult Treatment Panel III of the NCEP indicated that diabetes is considered to be a coronary artery atherosclerosis equivalent, and that it may be advisable to achieve LDL cholesterol levels less than 100 mg/dL, the desired range for persons who have experienced myocardial infarction. The reason that diabetes is considered to be a coronary artery atherosclerosis equivalent is that persons diagnosed to have diabetes have a high risk of myocardial infarction within 10 years, and that the survival rate of persons with diabetes mellitus who suffer myocardial infarction is low.

The enzyme 3-hydroxy-3-methyl-glutaryl-CoEnzymeA reductase (HMGCoAR) is the rate-limiting enzyme in cholesterol synthesis. Medications that inhibit the activity of HMGCoAR (so-called "statins") can lower serum cholesterol levels. Another desirable effect of statins is to decrease inflammation in arterial plaques. This could protect against plaque rupture and occlusion of coronary arteries. Nicotinic acid (niacin, vitamin B_3) therapy lowers serum triglyceride and cholesterol levels, but worsens hyperglycemia. Therefore, it may not be advisable to use nicotinic acid to treat hypertriglyceridemia and hypercholesterolemia in persons with diabetes.

Table 5.8. Changes in characteristics of diabetes mellitus in 182 hemochromatosis homozygotes after iron depletion[a]

Characteristic	At diagnosis	After iron depletion		
		Improved	Unchanged	Worsened
	Percent of group (n)			
Diabetes mellitus (n = 81)	*44 (81)*	*41 (33)*	*53 (43)*	*6 (5)*
Insulin-dependent	25 (46)	41 (19)[b]	50 (23)	10 (4)
Non-insulin dependent	19 (35)	40 (14)	57 (20)	3 (1)
Glucose tolerance (n = 101)	*56 (101)*	*10 (10)*	*87 (88)*	*3 (3)*
Impaired	15 (27)	37 (10)	56 (15)	7 (2)
Normal	40 (74)	—	99 (73)	1 (1)

Note: [a]Data were obtained from a 6-month interval after the end of the initial phlebotomy. From Strohmeyer and Niederau.[87]
[b]The daily insulin dose could be reduced in 19 of the 46 insulin-dependent patients, but insulin dependency was not abolished in any patient.

Hemochromatosis patients with type 1 diabetes need insulin replacement therapy. Some patients with type 2 diabetes may also need treatment with insulin. It is also advisable to treat patients with diabetes with an angiotensin-converting enzyme inhibitor and a "statin" drug, unless they have contraindications to taking these medications.

Phlebotomy therapy

It is important to pursue phlebotomy therapy to achieve iron-limited erythropoiesis, which provides a non-invasive estimate of adequate iron depletion. The hope that is extended by phlebotomy therapy is that target organs not permanently damaged by iron overload may maintain normal function, or may experience some improvement. Hemochromatosis patients who have glucose intolerance, and who undergo phlebotomy therapy, may experience improvement in glucose tolerance if the pancreatic islet beta-cells have not been irreversibly damaged. About 40 percent of hemochromatosis patients with insulin-dependent diabetes can decrease their insulin requirement by a few units daily. The majority of patients with either type 1 or type 2 diabetes did not experience improvement of their diabetes following therapy (Table 5.8). Iron depletion of hemochromatosis patients with insulin-dependent diabetes is not expected to eliminate the need for insulin replacement.

Prognosis

Three known factors influence the survival prognosis for hemochromatosis patients: (1) achieving iron depletion; (2) the presence or absence of diabetes mellitus; and (3) the presence or absence of hepatic cirrhosis. Patients with heavy iron overload due to far-advanced hemochromatosis, who for any reason do not achieve adequate iron depletion, may only live for about 18 months, on the average.[66–68,87–89] Persons with hemochromatosis who have neither diabetes mellitus nor hepatic cirrhosis have an expected survival that is similar to that of persons in the normal background population.

Overall, hemochromatosis patients who have either diabetes or cirrhosis are likely to live about 10 years less than persons with hemochromatosis who do not have diabetes or cirrhosis. A comparison of the survival of three groups of people in Germany is displayed in Fig. 5.10[87,89]: (1) 120 individuals with hemochromatosis and diabetes; (2) 131 people with hemochromatosis without diabetes; and (3) the background German population. The hemochromatosis patients who did not have diabetes had a survival rate that was the same as that of the background population. The survival of hemochromatosis patients who had diabetes was significantly lower than that of the other two groups ($P < 0.01$).[89]

Hypogonadism
Classification and prevalence

The second most common endocrinopathy that occurs in hemochromatosis patients is hypogonadism. The prevalence of hypogonadism in series of hemochromatosis patients varies according to the

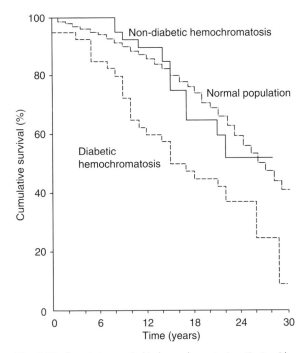

Fig. 5.10. Cumulative survival in hemochromatosis patients with ($n = 120$) and without ($n = 131$) diabetes mellitus. Survival was less in patients with diabetes than in patients without diabetes ($P < 0.01$, log-rank test). The survival of patients without diabetes was similar to that of sex- and age-matched normal control subjects (broken line), whereas patients with diabetes had reduced survival (expected survival rates outside the confidence intervals are not shown). From Strohmeyer and Niederau.[87] Taken from James C. Barton and Corwin Q. Edwards (eds), **Hemochromatosis: Genetics, Pathophysiology, Diagnosis and Treatment**, Cambridge University Press 2000. Reproduced with permission.

methods employed to define hypogonadism and the reasons for identifying patients. In groups of patients who were found to have hypogonadism because they sought medical attention, the prevalence of hypogonadism ranged from 10%–47% of men and 0%–10% of women. Among asymptomatic homozygotes who were identified only because they or their relative participated in a population screening study, 0%–2% of men and women had hypogonadism.[16] Hypogonadism usually occurs only in patients who have had heavy iron overload for decades.

Of hemochromatosis patients who have hypogonadism, 80% or more have the secondary type, hypogonadotrophic hypogonadism. Primary hypogonadism occurs in a smaller proportion of hemochromatosis patients. It is likely that the majority of the hemochromatosis patients who are thought to have tertiary hypogonadism (hypothalamic injury) actually have the secondary type (pituitary injury).

Unless prolonged, adequate stimulation of the pituitary is performed (2–4 weeks of daily pulsed gonadotrophic releasing hormone, GnRH) to allow adequate time for a dormant pituitary to regain responsiveness, an inadequate pituitary response can be misinterpreted as failure of the hypothalamus to secrete luteinizing hormone-releasing hormone, LHRH.[90,91] If the pituitary does not respond after 2–4 weeks of adequate stimulation with GnRH, secondary hypogonadism is present, rather than the tertiary type.

Most studies of hypogonadism were conducted in a small number of patients. In a survey of hypogonadism among 191 hemochromatosis patients, 6 percent of men and 5 percent of women had hypogonadism.[91] In a study of 505 homozygotes, 6 percent of men and 2 percent of women had hypogonadism.[16] In a study of hypogonadism in a group of 141 hemochromatosis patients, 6% (9 individuals) had abnormally low testosterone levels. Of these 9 patients, 8 (89%) also had low values of luteinizing hormone and follicle-stimulating hormone. These findings are characteristic of the hypogonadotrophic hypogonadism that occurs in some heavily iron-loaded hemochromatosis patients.[91]

Women may develop hypogonadism that is due to hemochromatosis, but this occurs much less frequently than among men with hemochromatosis. The great majority of women with hemochromatosis do not experience premature menopause. When hypogonadism does occur in women with hemochromatosis, it is usually of the secondary, hypogonadotrophic type. In young women, secondary hypogonadism presents as premature loss of menses, secondary amenorrhea, in the third to fifth decade. In women who experience menopause at age 45–55 years, this could represent physiologic age-related menopause, or it could be due to pituitary injury.

The prevalence of hypogonadism that can be ascribed to iron overload among male and female hemochromatosis homozygotes in 10 studies is displayed in Table 5.9.[16,90–99] The results of evaluation for hypogonadism among 505 hemochromatosis homozygotes who were evaluated during hemochromatosis studies in Utah are displayed in Table 5.10.[16]

Pathology

The pituitary gland is a site of iron deposition in heavily iron-loaded hemochromatosis homozygotes. Iron stores can be estimated by light microscopy

Table 5.9. Prevalence of hypogonadism among hemochromatosis patients from 10 studies

Author (reference)	Men (n)	Women, (n)	Hypogonadotrophic hypogonadism, % (n)	Primary hypogonadism, % (n)
Walsh[98]	12	0	17% M (2/12)	0
Bezwoda[92]	10	2	80% M (8/10); 100% F (2/2)	0
Charbonnel[93]	36	0	47% M (17/36)	0
Walton[99]	8	4	63% M (5/8); 50% F (2/4)	13% M (1/8); 0% F
Kelly[94]	41	23	10% M (4/41); 0% F	2.4% M (1/41); 0% F
Lufkin[95]	11	0	64% M (7/11)	0
Piperno[97]	7	0	100% M (7/7)	0
Duranteau[90]	7	0	100% M (7/7)	0
Bulaj[16]	315	190	6% M (19/315); 1.6% F (3/190)	<1% M (1/315); <1% F (1/190)
McDermott[91]	144	47	6% M (9/141); 5% F (2/38)	<1% M (1/141); 0% F

Table 5.10. Prevalence of hypogonadotrophic hypogonadism in 505 hemochromatosis homozygotes in Utah[a]

Sick Probands (136 men, 48 women)		Screening probands (66 men, 41 women)		Homozygous relatives (113 men, 101 women)	
Men, % (n)	Women, % (n)	Men, % (n)	Women, % (n)	Men, % (n)	Women, % (n)
12 (16)	6 (3)	0 (0)	2.4 (1)	4 (4)	0 (0)

Note: [a]Modified from Bulaj et al.[16]

using the usual iron stain (Perls' Prussian blue technique). The hormone-producing cells in the anterior pituitary gland can be distinguished from each other by light microscopy, using immunohistochemical stains that react specifically with follicle-stimulating hormone (FSH), luteinizing hormone (LH), thyroid-stimulating hormone (TSH), prolactin (PRL), or adrenocorticotrophic hormone (ACTH).

Autopsy series that were performed in iron-loaded homozygotes who died before iron depletion demonstrated that the majority of pituitary iron accumulated in the gonadotroph cells in the anterior pituitary. Typically, the cells that stored TSH, PRL, or ACTH contained much less iron than the gonadotroph cells. In an autopsy study of 57 patients who had hemochromatosis, 49 (86%) had iron deposits in the anterior pituitary.[96]

Pathophysiology

Excessive iron stores in gonadotroph cells causes cellular injury and decreased synthesis, storage and secretion of FSH and LH. The result of inadequate

FSH and LH stimulus in men is that the Leydig cells of the testicles do not produce an adequate amount of testosterone (T). In turn, a decreased amount of testosterone substrate is presented to the 5-α-reductase enzyme in hepatocytes, so there is inadequate production of the 5-α-reduced, dihydrogenated type of testosterone (dihydrotestosterone, DHT).

In women, hypogonadism due to iron overload may occur 10–20 years later than among men with hemochromatosis. Measurement of plasma hormones may be the only way to determine if natural age-related menopause occurred, of if menopause is due to the loss of pituitary trophic hormones (secondary hypogonadism). In physiologic, age-related menopause, women have decreased plasma estradiol (E2) and markedly elevated values of FSH and LH. Women whose menopause is due to iron overload and hypogonadotrophic hypogonadism have very low values of plasma E2, FSH, and LH.

Dihydrotestosterone is the hormone that is responsible for stimulation of libido and of the growth of midline structures and hair (including facial, chest, axillary, arm, and pubic hair), testicular size, sperm production, and prostate growth. Insufficient plasma concentrations of T and DHT cause decreased need to shave, loss of libido, inadequate penile erectile function, and impotence in men who have hypogonadism due to hemochromatosis.

Laboratory diagnosis of hypogonadism

Secondary hypogonadism

This is the most common type of hypogonadism that occurs in hemochromatosis homozygotes. Men with secondary hypogonadism have decreased plasma concentrations of T, DHT, FSH, and LH due to an abnormality in the gonadotroph cells. These hormonal test results are the same as in tertiary hypogonadism. Subjects with secondary hypogonadism also have an elevated plasma concentration of gonadotrophin-releasing hormone (LHRH, gonadorelin, GnRH), which usually is not measured.

In a patient the test for GnRH concentration cannot be performed, the patient can be tested with a GnRH challenge to establish the diagnosis of secondary versus the tertiary type of hypogonadism. When a patient with secondary hypogonadism is given a challenge with GnRH (0.1 mg intravenously or subcutaneously), the pituitary gland does not respond appropriately—there is no appropriate rise in plasma FSH and LH during the 90 minutes following the administration of GnRH, because the gonadotroph cells have been damaged and are unable to synthesize or release more FSH and LH.

Tertiary hypogonadism

Tertiary hypogonadism occurs as a result of injury of hypothalamus cells that synthesize GnRH. Tertiary hypogonadism is not common in hemochromatosis, but it is known to occur in a small proportion of subjects. These individuals have decreased plasma concentrations of T, DHT, FSH, and LH, plus a decreased plasma GnRH concentration.

In a patient with tertiary hypogonadism, the pituitary gland responds appropriately to a GnRH challenge–plasma FSH and LH rise appropriately. If the patient is tested with human chorionic gonadotrophin (β-HCG), T and DHT increase in men and E2 rises in women. These responses demonstrate that the endocrine abnormality is in the hypothalamus, not in the pituitary gland, testes or ovaries. As described above, tertiary hypogonadism is very uncommon in hemochromatosis. When a hemochromatosis patient with

hypogonadism is given 2 to 4 weeks of daily pulsed GnRH stimulation, and the FSH, LH, T, and DHT do not increase, the patient has secondary hypogonadism, not the tertiary type.

Primary hypogonadism

This is the second most common type of hypogonadism in hemochromatosis patients. It is thought to occur as a result of direct testicular injury by iron. These individuals have elevated concentrations of GnRH, FSH, and LH. They also have low T and DHT concentrations. The testicular injury prevents the normal response to abundant trophic hormones in the plasma.

Endocrine failure and heart failure syndrome

A syndrome of severe endocrine failure and congestive heart failure occurs in a small percentage of young hemochromatosis patients during adolescence. Teenage girls may fail to undergo menarche, or may experience secondary amenorrhea soon after the onset of menarche. Males and females with this syndrome may present with congestive heart failure and life-threatening ventricular tachycardia or ventricular fibrillation. This severe endocrine-cardiac syndrome occurs much more frequently in patients with juvenile hemochromatosis (typically due to mutations in *HJV* but also in *HAMP* or *TFR2*) than among subjects who have *HFE* hemochromatosis. The endocrinopathy and heart failure associated with *HJV* hemochromatosis are more prevalent and severe than the endocrinopathy and heart failure that occur in older men and women with *HFE* hemochromatosis.

Treatment

After a hemochromatosis patient is found to have hypogonadism that is not caused by a mass in the pituitary gland or the hypothalamus, treatment typically is the same, whether the hypogonadism is of the secondary, primary, or tertiary type: replacement of testosterone or estradiol.

Hormone replacement with estradiol

The principles of estrogen replacement in women with hypogonadism due to hemochromatosis are similar to replacement in women who experience physiologic menopause. The benefits and possible risks of estrogen replacement are expected to apply equally to women with and without hemochromatosis, based on age and other conditions that affect health. Due to controversy and emerging medical literature, it is important to follow accepted guidelines for estrogen replacement, including interval evaluation for complications of replacement.

Hormone replacement with testosterone

Hormone replacement therapy in men may cause improvement in strength, sense of well-being, libido, and erectile function, and it may also stimulate erythropoiesis in patients with or without anemia. Testosterone can be self-administered intramuscularly or transcutaneously by a patch that is applied on the skin. Intramuscular testosterone enanthate or cypionate can be prescribed. Testosterone enanthate usually has an effective duration of action of about 2 weeks. Testosterone skin patches should be replaced at 1-week intervals.

Phlebotomy therapy

Women with hemochromatosis who experience age-related physiologic menopause, rather than secondary amenorrhea due to iron overload, do not experience return of menses, ovulation, or fertility after iron depletion with phlebotomy.

Most men whose hypogonadism is due to hemochromatosis have heavy organ iron overload and advanced complications. Most of these men do not experience reversal of hypogonadism and return of normal sexual function following iron depletion therapy with phlebotomy. About 20% of men with hypogonadism due to iron overload do experience the return of normal function of the pituitary gonadotroph cells after iron depletion with phlebotomy.[94] This usually occurs in younger men without iron overload that has been present for several decades. If normal gonadotroph function returns, plasma FSH and LH concentrations rise and plasma testosterone levels increase.

Thyroid disease

Prevalence

The prevalence of hypothyroidism in adult populations is about 1–3 percent. Hyperthyroidism is present in about 0.1 percent of adults. Hypothyroidism and hyperthyroidism have been described in iron-loaded hemochromatosis patients.[100] Hyperthyroidism has been reported, but does not occur frequently in hemochromatosis patients.[100] Some studies of hemochromatosis patients did not find an increased frequency of hypothyroidism.

Hypothyroidism in iron-loaded hemochromatosis patients

In a tabulation of hypothyroidism from 9 reports, 8 percent of 171 iron-loaded hemochromatosis patients had hypothyroidism.[100] The majority of the hypothyroid hemochromatosis patients were men. Authors of a recent publication discussed the possibility that iron-induced organ injury might cause an autoimmune response that could result in thyroid injury.[101] In other studies conducted by experienced investigators, there was no difference in the prevalence of hemochromatosis patients compared to the background population.[102–105] In a study of 154 hemochromatosis patients in Ireland, hypothyroidism was not more prevalent among hemochromatosis patients compared to normal subjects.[105]

Hypothyroidism in hemochromatosis homozygotes in screening studies

The Hemochromatosis and Iron Overload Screening (HEIRS) Study is the largest hemochromatosis screening study ever performed. As a part of this study, 176 C282Y homozygotes were tested for thyroid disorders using TSH and T_4. The results of thyroid testing among these newly-diagnosed homozygotes were compared to the results among 312 individuals who did not have the C282Y or H63D mutations.[106] The prevalence of hypothyroidism was similar among the newly diagnosed homozygotes and the normal individuals.[106] A large screening study of 65 717 people in Norway found that 297 participants were C282Y homozygotes.[107] Of the women under age 50 years who were hemochromatosis homozygotes, 12.5 percent had hypothyroidism compared to 3 percent of the corresponding group of normal women in the population.

Based on the data that are presented here, it is obvious that the prevalence of hypothyroidism varies among studies. The differences are believable and still have not yet been fully explained. Heavy iron loading may be the cause of some of the differences in the results in sick homozygotes compared to homozygotes who were only identified because they participated in hemochromatosis screening studies.[100,101]

Diagnosis of thyroid disorders

Individuals who have complaints of fatigue or lethargy that is disproportionate to their life circumstances, intolerance to cold, decreased frequency of bowel movements, change in hair texture or distribution, or coarsening of skin may have hypothyroidism. Primary hypothyroidism (injury of thyroid gland) is associated with decreased concentrations of free-T_3 and free-T_4, and elevated values of TSH. Secondary hypothyroidism is associated with low values of free-T_3, free-T_4, and TSH.

A thyroid hormone-releasing hormone (THRH) challenge test can be performed to distinguish secondary hypothyroidism (pituitary injury) from tertiary hypothyroidism (injury of the hypothalamus). Following subcutaneous injection of THRH, the thyroid gland of a patient with secondary hypothyroidism cannot respond appropriately—it fails to secrete TSH into plasma. The thyroid gland of a patient with tertiary hypothyroidism responds to THRH by secreting TSH.

Treatment

Hypothyroidism is by far the easiest endocrine disorder to treat. A young patient with new onset hypothyroidism with minimal or no symptoms is likely to tolerate a full replacement dosage of l-thyroxine, which usually is 150 µg (0.15 mg) by mouth once each day. This dosage usually causes reversal of the symptoms of hypothyroidism, and a gradual rise in body temperature, and an increased heart rate, as well as normalization of an elevated TSH value. In a person who has known or suspected heart disease, it is advisable to start thyroid replacement at a quite low dose, such as 25 µg (0.025 mg) of l-thyroxine by mouth each day. If this dosage is tolerated without problem, the dosage can be increased at 3–4 week intervals.[105]

In normal persons, the half-life of thyroxine in plasma is about 1 week. Due to the abnormally low metabolic rate in a hypothyroid person, the plasma half-life of thyroxine is about 2 weeks. Because of this long half-life, it is reasonable to wait about 6 weeks (3 half-lives) before measuring the plasma free T_4 and TSH levels. The dosage of l-thyroxine can be adjusted modestly up or down to maintain the TSH concentration between 1 and 4 µIU/mL. If the person has hypothyroidism due to pituitary injury, TSH values are not useful in long-term follow-up and management decisions. In this case, adequacy of thyroid hormone replacement is based on the serum concentration of free-T_3 or free-T_4.

Thyroid hormone acts on nuclear receptors, resulting in stimulation of the sodium-potassium ATPase cell membrane pump. This increases both oxygen consumption and the basal metabolic rate. In a patient with coronary artery disease, a sudden increase in oxygen consumption and basal metabolic rate could cause cardiac angina.

There are no large randomized controlled trials to guide whether to accept or reject one of these treatment regimens over the other. Some authors favor the use of T_4 as initial thyroid hormone replacement, while others advocate starting with T_3. In patients who have coronary artery disease, it seems reasonable to initiate thyroid hormone replacement at a low dose.

Hormone replacement can be started using T_3 or T_4. Both T_3 and T_4 have advantages and disadvantages. T_3 has the advantage of a very rapid onset (minutes) and duration of action (hours) compared to T_4, which has a delayed onset (hours) and a prolonged duration of action (7 to 14 days). For example, if thyroid hormone replacement with T_3 causes a patient to experience cardiac angina, the duration of effect of T_3 will be short, compared to the prolonged duration of action of T_4. Conversely, a person with underlying coronary artery disease may be less likely to experience cardiac angina during thyroid hormone replacement if started with T_4, which has a quite slow onset of action. Whether the initial hormone replacement regimen is T_3 or T_4, the development of hypotension may signal the occurrence of acute myocardial infarction.

If T_3 is used for initial thyroid hormone replacement, a low-dose regimen (triiodothyronine 12.5 µg orally three times daily) may be chosen for the first week before converting to long-term maintenance replacement with l-thyroxine (T_4). If T_4 is selected as the initial thyroid hormone replacement, a low dose such as 0.05 mg (50 µg) orally each day can be given for the first week, followed by 0.1 mg orally each day for 1 week, followed by full dosage replacement of 0.15 mg orally each day.

In a hypothyroid patient whose temperature is lower than normal, body temperature usually begins to rise within 24 hours of starting thyroid hormone replacement. Heart rate often rises within 24 hours. Improvement in other symptoms usually begins after 7–14 days. Normalization of TSH may not occur until an equilibrium of plasma and tissue thyroid hormone is reached (4–6 weeks).

In patients with profound hypothyroidism, it is prudent to pre-treat them with cortisol to prevent the occurrence of adrenal crisis, unless testing already performed demonstrated a normal pituitary-adrenal axis. Cortisol replacement is discussed below in the section on adrenal insufficiency.

Panhypopituitarism

A very small proportion of hemochromatosis patients have panhypopituitarism. Heavily iron-loaded men are more likely to have this complication than women or men who have iron overload that is less severe. Patients with panhypopituitarism usually feel very weak, develop smooth facial skin, lose body hair, have to shave infrequently, may have cold intolerance, and have decreased libido and erectile function.

In hemochromatosis, panhypopituitarism is the result of iron accumulation in and injury of multiple types of trophic cells in the anterior pituitary. Panhypopituitarism can also be caused by injury of the hypothalamus that results in inadequate synthesis and secretion of releasing hormones that should stimulate the pituitary to secrete follicle-stimulating hormone (FSH), luteinizing hormone (LH), thyroid-stimulating hormone (TSH), prolactin (PRL), and adrenocorticotrophic hormone (ACTH).

Diagnosis

Patients with panhypopituitarism have decreased plasma concentrations of FSH, LH, estradiol (E_2, in women), testosterone (T), and dihydrotestosterone (DHT) (in men), TSH, free triiodothyronine (T_3), free thyroxine (T_4), ACTH, and cortisol. Stimulatory tests can establish that the pituitary gland fails to respond to stimulation by GnRH, THRH, and corticotrophin-stimulating hormone (such as Cortrosyn®).

GnRH test

The GnRH test involves measurement of FSH and LH just before the intravenous or subcutaneous injection of gonadorelin 0.1 mg. This is followed by measurement of FSH and LH 30 or 45 minutes after injection. The normal pituitary responds to this test by secreting increased amounts of FSH and LH into plasma. A patient with hypopituitarism does not experience the expected normal rise in FSH and LH following the GnRH injection.

THRH test

In this test, blood is drawn for measurement of TSH before the intravenous injection of THRH 0.1 mg. This is followed by drawing blood for measurement of TSH 30 and 60 minutes after injection of the THRH. The normal pituitary responds to this challenge by secreting increased amounts of TSH into plasma. A patient with hypopituitarism does not experience a rise in TSH after injection of THRH.

Corticotropin stimulation test

At the start of the test, blood is drawn for measurement of ACTH. Thereafter, synthetic corticotrophin 0.25 units is injected intravenously. Blood for measurement of plasma ACTH is drawn 30, 60, 90, and 120 minutes after the injection. ACTH is unstable in a warm test tube, so all of the samples are drawn in heparin (green top tubes), placed on ice, and taken to the laboratory immediately after the final blood sample is drawn, so the cold blood can be processed and frozen until the ACTH assay batch can be run. The normal pituitary gland responds to this test by secreting increased amounts of ACTH into plasma. A patient with hypopituitarism does not experience a rise in ACTH following the injection of corticotropin.

Evaluation for other hormone deficiencies

It is important to evaluate hemochromatosis patients with a subnormal plasma concentration of one hormone for other endocrine abnormalities. For example, if a hemochromatosis patient is found to have hypothyroidism, the patient is likely to have hypogonadism, because the gonadotroph cells are usually are the first cells in the anterior pituitary to be injured by iron accumulation. Similarly, if a hemochromatosis patient has adrenal insufficiency due to iron overload, it is likely that the individual also has hypogonadism and hypothyroidism, because the gonadotroph and thyrotroph cells are usually the first and second trophic cells types that are damaged by iron overload, and the corticotroph cells are damaged much less frequently.

Patients with adrenal insufficiency and hypothyroidism

It is important to first treat a person who has both hypothyroidism and adrenal insufficiency with hydrocortisone before adding thyroxine replacement. Treatment of a hypo-adrenal, hypothyroid patient with thyroxine alone can markedly worsen the adrenal insufficiency, precipitating a life-threatening adrenal crisis. It is estimated that about 1 of 2000 people in the general population have co-existent secondary hypothyroidism and secondary adrenal insufficiency.

For many years it was thought that the adrenal glands of a normal adult secreted about 25 mg of cortisol per day. Recently, more accurate methods of measurement indicate that normal adrenal glands in adults secrete about 18 mg of cortisol per day. Cortisol replacement therapy in a person who has adrenal insufficiency should be started at about 3–4 times the daily requirement of normal people. This corresponds to an oral hydrocortisone replacement dosage schedule of about 50 mg two or three times per day for a few days, if the person is not septic and does not have other severe, acute illness. Mortality risk of patients with sepsis and adrenal insufficiency might decrease if the patients are treated with oral or intravenous hydrocortisone every six hours for a few days. Massive doses of corticosteroid replacement (e.g. hydrocortisone 100 mg four to six times daily or methylprednisolone 1 g or more daily) may induce greater morbidity and mortality risks than a replacement regimen that is only moderately higher than normal adrenal cortisol secretion.

After an initial 1 or 2 weeks of hydrocortisone replacement therapy, the dosage can be converted to a long-term regimen of cortisol 15–20 mg orally each morning plus 5–10 mg orally each evening, assuming the patient is doing well. The dosage should be doubled if serious intercurrent illness develops. If prednisone is used instead of hydrocortisone, a reasonable dosage regimen is 7.5 mg orally each day. This dosage provides about the same glucocorticoid effect as hydrocortisone 25 mg per day.

Cutaneous manifestations

History

Cutaneous manifestations occur predominantly in persons with severe iron overload.[108,109] Early clinicians and pathologists reported that cutaneous hyperpigmentation associated with excessive melanin and iron deposition is common in patients with severe iron overload due to hemochromatosis.[54,110] The term "bronze diabetes with cirrhosis" is derived from Troisier's 1871 account of "*diabète bronzé et cirrhose pigmentaire*" (Chapter 1).[110] The "classic" triad of skin hyperpigmentation, diabetes mellitus, and cirrhosis is observed only in patients with advanced iron overload, but is infrequently seen today because the proportion of persons with *HFE* hemochromatosis who also have severe iron overload is small.[13] Chevrant-Breton and colleagues described the skin manifestations of hemochromatosis and iron overload in 100 patients with

hemochromatosis diagnosed in medical care.[111] This section reviews the skin abnormalities associated with iron overload in hemochromatosis and related disorders.

Skin pigmentation

The appearance of hyperpigmentation is insidious, and it is sometimes unrecognized by patients, family members, or physicians. In other cases, especially in patients whose relatives have fair skin, hyperpigmentation may be noticed before other manifestations of iron overload become apparent. The discoloration ranges from metallic gray to brown, although the presence and severity of hyperpigmentation are largely subjective, and depend on race/ethnicity of the patient, season, sun exposure, and ambient lighting under which physical examination is performed. Hyperpigmentation tends to occur on sun-exposed areas, but may be generalized and thus involve areas unexposed to sun. In some cases, hyperpigmentation may be especially noticeable on external genitalia, scars, flexion folds, conjunctivae, and buccal mucosa (Figs. 5.11, 5.12).[112]

Hyperpigmentation is a marker of severe iron overload, and thus it is more frequently observed in patients who have other manifestations of severe iron overload such as cirrhosis and diabetes mellitus. Accordingly, the prevalence of hyperpigmentation in case series of adult-onset hemochromatosis has declined because diagnostic criteria have changed and permit earlier diagnosis. In a case series from 1977, 98% of patients had hyperpigmentation.[111] In a series of symptomatic patients diagnosed during the interval 1950–1985, 72% had hyperpigmentation.[113] In two 1997 series, 5%–58% of patients had hyperpigmentation.[114,115] The prevalence of hyperpigmentation in early age-of-onset ("juvenile") hemochromatosis remains high, because severe iron overload is present at diagnosis in most index patients. Among 29 young patients, 74% had cutaneous hyperpigmentation.[116]

Skin biopsy was positive for excessive melanin in 57% of cases and for hemosiderin iron in 67% of adults who presented with symptoms attributable to iron overload.[113] Brownish hyperpigmentation is largely due to increased melanin in the basal layer of the epidermis.[54,111–113] Brownish hyperpigmentation occurred on the margins of the eyelids in 21% of patients with hemochromatosis; most of them also had generalized hyperpigmentation.[117] In some patients with hyperpigmentation, increased iron as hemosiderin is deposited

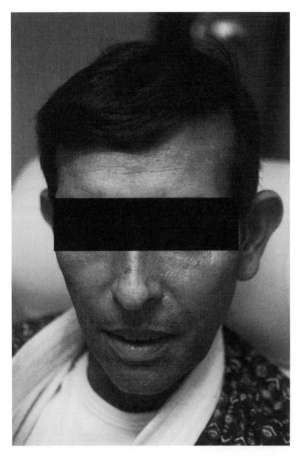 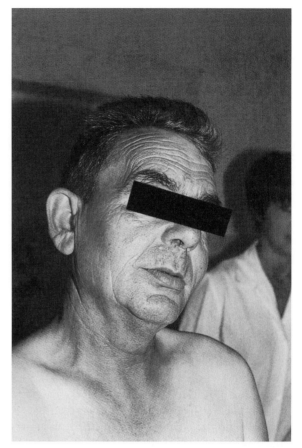

Figs. 5.11 and 5.12. Cutaneous pigmentation in hemochromatosis: grayish hue; brown hue. From Chevrant-Breton.[112] Taken from James C. Barton and Corwin Q. Edwards (eds), **Hemochromatosis: Genetics, Pathophysiology, Diagnosis and Treatment**, Cambridge University Press 2000. Reproduced with permission. See plate section for color version.

within and around the eccrine sweat glands and in dermal macrophages.[54,112,113]

Melanin hyperpigmentation also occurs in chronic liver disorders unassociated with iron overload, especially primary biliary cirrhosis.[118] Thus, the occurrence of hyperpigmentation in persons with cirrhosis is not diagnostic of hemochromatosis or iron overload. In both hemochromatosis and primary biliary cirrhosis, plasma or serum levels of melanocyte-stimulating hormone are normal.[118,119] This suggests that hyperpigmentation in these disorders may be due to increased numbers of melanocytes or to decreased degradation of melanin. Local cutaneous toxicity of iron has been proposed as a mechanism to explain melanin hyperpigmentation and hair loss in persons with hemochromatosis. HFE protein is not expressed in skin structures,[120,121] and thus probably does not participate directly in the pathogenesis of hyperpigmentation.

Other cutaneous signs of hemochromatosis

Chevrant-Breton and colleagues reported that 42% of patients had cutaneous atrophy.[111,112] The shins are predominantly affected, but skin atrophy is generalized in some cases. Most histologic changes appear in the epidermis, but may also involve the dermis and connective tissue. An icthyosis-like skin condition was reported to occur in about one-half of patients (Fig. 5.13).[111,112] Total hair loss occurred in 12% and partial hair loss in 62% of patients with hemochromatosis. Hair loss is usually associated with hypogonadism and cirrhosis.[111,112]

Koilonychia or platonychia, particularly involving first three digits, is common in patients with hemochromatosis and severe iron overload.[112] Marked spooning of the nails (Fig. 5.14) was present in one-quarter of cases.[111,112] Paradoxically, koilonychia also

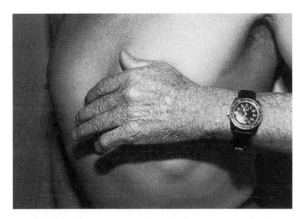

Fig. 5.13. Skin atrophy and icthyosis in hemochromatosis. From Chevrant-Breton.[112] Taken from James C. Barton and Corwin Q. Edwards (eds), **Hemochromatosis: Genetics, Pathophysiology, Diagnosis and Treatment**, Cambridge University Press 2000. Reproduced with permission.

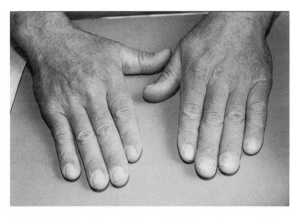

Fig. 5.14. Koilonychia and leukonychia in hemochromatosis. From Chevrant-Breton.[112] Taken from James C. Barton and Corwin Q. Edwards (eds), **Hemochromatosis: Genetics, Pathophysiology, Diagnosis and Treatment**, Cambridge University Press 2000. Reproduced with permission.

occurs in iron deficiency. More than 10% of patients develop leukonychia.[112] This abnormality also occurs in some patients with cirrhosis due to causes other than iron overload. Spider angiomata and palmar erythema sometimes occur in patients with hemochromatosis, but these manifestations are related to the presence of cirrhosis and are not a direct consequence of iron overload.

Diagnosis and management

The value of skin biopsy in the overall assessment of hemochromatosis is limited.[112] Endocrinologic evaluation of patients with partial or complete hair loss should be performed to identify possible hypogonadism. Hyperpigmentation and nail changes often diminish or resolve with depletion of iron stores by phlebotomy (Chapter 36). Recurrence of hyperpigmentation usually indicates that excessive quantities of iron have re-accumulated.

Porphyria cutanea tarda, hemochromatosis, and skin manifestations

Porphyria cutanea tarda is caused by the deficiency of uroporphyrinogen decarboxylase (UROD). In persons with typical familial porphyria cutanea tarda, all tissues have deficient UROD activity; others have deficient UROD activity only in the liver. In persons with sporadic porphyria cutanea tarda, deficient UROD activity occurs only in hepatocytes (Chapter 10). Cutaneous manifestations of porphyria cutanea tarda include blisters and erosions on sun-exposed skin (particularly on the face and dorsum of the hands). The healing of these blisters is associated with scars, milia, and extreme skin fragility. Some patients develop malar hypertrichosis. Other uncommon symptoms are scleroderma-like changes of the face and upper body, diffuse hyperpigmentation, alopecia, and chronic ulcers. The diagnosis of porphyria cutanea tarda can be established by pathologic examination of a skin biopsy specimen that shows characteristic bullae. Increased hemosiderin deposition is not characteristic of such biopsy specimens. The biochemical derangement typical of PCT is the presence of increased urinary porphyrin (Chapter 10).

Most patients with porphyria cutanea tarda have evidence of abnormal iron metabolism, including the presence of increased deposition of hemosiderin in the periportal hepatocytes, similar to that observed in *HFE* hemochromatosis. The pathophysiologic relationship between PCT and iron overload may be related in part to the ability of ferrous iron to inhibit UROD activity.[122] Persons with porphyria cutanea tarda are more likely than persons in the general population to be heterozygous or homozygous for the common *HFE* mutations C282Y and H63D.[123–127] Other factors that precipitate porphyria cutanea tarda are alcohol ingestion, drugs (especially estrogens and related compounds), workplace exposure to certain chemicals, and viral infections (including those of hepatitis B and C, and human immunodeficiency viruses). Altogether, these observations suggest that hemochromatosis-related mutations, perturbed iron metabolism, iron overload of variable degrees, and certain drugs, chemicals, and infections contribute significantly to the clinical and laboratory findings observed in persons with PCT.[123–127]

Many patients with porphyria cutanea tarda have mild or moderate iron overload, and achieving iron depletion by therapeutic phlebotomy usually results in remission of cutaneous photosensitivity and typical skin lesions (Chapters 10, 36). In some cases, skin lesions recur with the re-accumulation of relatively small amounts of iron.

Miscellaneous symptoms

Many patients diagnosed to have hemochromatosis in medical care report symptoms that are not readily attributable to specific body systems or are not typical of specific disorders. The most common of these are fatigue and lack of physical endurance.[115,128,129] In many patients, their onset is insidious, and they progress slowly. Many patients diagnosed in medical care to have hemochromatosis report that they have palpitations. In a large hemochromatosis screening program, the prevalence of each of these symptoms did not differ significantly in untreated participants found to have *HFE* C282Y homozygosity and in control participants matched for age and sex.[130] A small proportion of patients diagnosed in medical care report symptoms that suggest neurologic abnormalities, such as generalized weakness, loss of muscle strength, poor co-ordination, areas of decreased sensation, loss of memory, incalculia, declining hearing or vision, or somnolence, may be symptoms of hemochromatosis or iron overload. In unusual cases, patients report the sensation of unpleasant or metallic tastes or odors, or loss of taste or smell. One woman with hemochromatosis reported severe headache.[131]

Symptoms of restless legs syndrome have been reported to occur in patients with hemochromatosis,[132,133] and these symptoms may be exacerbated by phlebotomy therapy to achieve iron depletion.[132] Restless legs syndrome occurs as a sporadic disorder, especially in persons with iron deficiency; in other cases, this disorder appears to be heritable.[134] Restless legs syndrome has been associated with subnormal levels of iron in certain parts of the brain, and with subnormal concentrations of ferritin in cerebrospinal fluid.[134] In persons with hemochromatosis and restless legs syndrome, levels of iron in substantia nigra, red nucleus, and pallidum were low, a finding typical of patients with restless legs syndrome who do not have hemochromatosis.[135] These results indicate that local brain iron deficiency may occur in patients with hemochromatosis, and are consistent with a role for brain iron metabolism in the pathophysiology of restless legs syndrome.

Performing cardiac, pulmonary, and neurologic evaluation, assessing endocrine function (measurement of glucose tolerance, sex hormone levels, thyroid hormones, and pituitary trophic hormones), or making general health and metabolism appraisals is appropriate in patients with hemochromatosis who have seemingly non-specific symptoms, but investigation does not reveal a satisfying cause for the complaints in many patients. Nonetheless, many patients experience relief of symptoms after they achieve iron depletion, suggesting that at least some of their symptoms are caused by iron overload.[115,131]

Right upper quadrant pain in persons with hemochromatosis is sometimes related to hepatic iron overload. Primary liver cancer, portal vein thrombosis, gallbladder disease, lesions in the hepatic flexure, or nephrolithiasis can also cause right upper quadrant pain. A small percentage of patients report increased frequency or severity of infections, usually of the upper or lower respiratory tract; some of these patients have heritable antibody deficiency.[136] Rarely, persons presenting with hemochromatosis report having survived a life-threatening bacterial infection.[137]

Morbidity and mortality

Consideration of estimates of morbidity or mortality among groups of individuals who have iron overload first requires an understanding of terms germane to such estimates. Because these terms are often understood or used differently, we adapted definitions of these terms from dictionaries of genetic terms that seem both authoritative and reasonable.

The term *penetrance* refers to the proportion of people with a specified genotype who have an abnormal phenotype due to that genotype. This is often recorded as a ratio or as a percentage, such as 10 per 1000 (1%), or 250 per 1000 (25%). The term *expressivity* refers to the consistency of the manifestations of a genetic disorder. Expressivity is typically referred to

Table 5.11. Clinical observations of morbidity in hemochromatosis patients[a]

Observation	Sheldon 1935[54]	Finch 1966[63]	Milder 1980[142]	Edwards 1982[143]	Adams 1991[13]	Milman 1991[113]	Fargion 1992[144]	Niederau 1996[66]	Moirand 1997[145]
Number of patients	311	787	34	41	118	179	212	251	352
Men	298	711	34	26	94	140	181	224	176
Women	16	76		15	24	39	31	27	176
Symptoms (percentage of patients)									
Weakness	13	70	73	22	9	79		82	54
Weight loss		44	53	7			69		
Arthralgias			47	56	13	44		44	40
Abdominal pain	26	29	50	20	6	34		56	
Loss of libido and/or impotence	6	14	56	24[b]	1	41		36	
Amenorrhea						10		15	
Cardiac complaints		33	35	39					
Asymptomatic			15	37	18				
Physical and laboratory findings (percentage of patients)									
Skin pigmentation	84	85	82	49		70	35	72	52
Hepatomegaly	92	93	76	54		84	75	81	
Abnormal hepatic enzyme tests			54	61	13	92			
Cirrhosis	92		94	41		84	69	57	20
Primary liver cancer	6	14	18	2.4			12		
Splenomegaly	55	50	38	37		12		10	
Diabetes mellitus	79	82	53	12	10	47	30		12

Table 5.11. (cont.)

Observation	Sheldon 1935[54]	Finch 1966[63]	Milder 1980[142]	Edwards 1982[143]	Adams 1991[13]	Milman 1991[113]	Fargion 1992[144]	Niederau 1996[66]	Moirand 1997[145]
Testicular atrophy		16	50	20					
Hypogonadism, documented			40[b]	20[b]			20[b]		
Hypogonadotrophic hypogonadism			100[b]	80[b]					
Arthropathy			44	68			13		
Cardiac arrhythmia		35	26	7			20	35	14
Congestive heart failure		33	35	2.4	15				

Notes: [a]These symptoms of illness, abnormal physical examination findings, and laboratory abnormalities were observed in patients in nine studies from seven countries.[13,54,63,66,113,142–145] Results expressed as percent. From Edwards et al.[146]
[b]Findings in males only; not all males were studied.

as being high or low. There is usually much variation in the manifestations of a genetic disorder that has low expressivity. The term *expression* refers to the translation of information from a gene into mRNA, and its subsequent transcription to synthesize a protein.

The term *incidence* refers to the number of people with a new diagnosis of a disorder within a specific population within a discrete period of time. This is often presented as a ratio, such as 300 cases per 100 000 persons per year. The term *prevalence* refers to the number of people who have a disorder divided by the number of people in the background population at a point in time. This is typically expressed as a proportion or as a percentage. The term *bias* refers to a point of view that prevents impartial judgment, and that can lead to an incorrect conclusion about data under consideration. The term *ascertainment bias* refers to a systematic use of non-impartial criteria in the selection of individuals for participation in a study. *Observer bias* is an effect introduced by an observer on the data that are collected, or on conclusion(s) drawn from the data.

Morbidity of hemochromatosis

Morbidity refers to an abnormality, illness, or complication that is caused by some condition or disorder. The complications that occur in hemochromatosis patients constitute the morbidity of the disorder. There is much variation in the reported prevalence of complications of hemochromatosis, as described below. An explanation for some of the differences is ascertainment bias. For example, sick patients who seek medical attention and are tested for complications of iron overload are expected to have symptoms or signs caused by iron overload. Thus, these patients are selected for the presence of morbidity. At the opposite extreme, people who are only tested because they participated in a population screening study of healthy young blood donors are very unlikely to have iron overload and morbidity. These individuals are selected to have good health.

When the methods and definitions and inclusion criteria are stated clearly and followed appropriately in a report, ascertainment bias does not imply any degree of dishonesty or any deficit of ability. In fact, one may draw the opposite conclusion: the investigators clearly and adequately described their definitions, methods, and study population. This allows other investigators

Table 5.12. Complications of hemochromatosis in 212 patients in Italy grouped by presence or absence of cirrhosis[a]

Characteristics	No cirrhosis (*n* = 66)	Cirrhosis (*n* = 146)
Men: women	54: 12 (82%: 18%)	127: 19 (87%: 13%)
Age, y[b]	46 ± 12 (24–70)	53 ± 10 (26–79)
Alcohol abuse	3 (5%)	28 (19%)
HB$_s$Ag positivity[c]	6 (9%)	13 (9%)
Anti-HCV positive[d]	9 of 54 (17%)	26 of 91 (29%)
β-thalassemia trait	9 (14%)	15 (10%)
Hepatomegaly	33 (50%)	127 (87%)
Skin pigmentation	10 (15%)	65 (45%)
Diabetes mellitus	7 (11%)	56 (38%)
Cardiac involvement	3 (5%)	39 (27%)
Joint involvement	3 (5%)	25 (17%)
Hypogonadism (men)	6 (11%)	37 (29%)
Portal hypertension	1 (1%)	46 (31%)
Child class B/C	—	29/6 (20%/4%)

Notes: [a]Table adapted from Fargion *et al.*[144]
[b]Mean ± S.D.; range given in parentheses.
[c]Anti-HB$_s$Ag = antibody to hepatitis B virus surface Ag.
[d]Anti-HCV = antibody to hepatitis C virus.

to study and understand the results, and to follow the same methods in the analysis of another population. In turn, this should allow investigators to corroborate or reject independently the findings and conclusions of other studies. Usually, all investigators neither use exactly the same methods as other observers nor use the same definitions in their study population. The effect (symptoms, physical examination findings, and laboratory results) of studying groups of hemochromatosis homozygotes whose ascertainment was biased either for illness or for good health is evident in tables displayed in this chapter.

Observer bias can cause an investigator either to over-report or to under-report a finding, based on other things he/she knows or believes to be present in a patient or a dataset, thus directly affecting the results. For example, observer bias could possibly

Table 5.13. Disease-related morbidity in three groups of subjects with hemochromatosis: Utah study of 505 homozygotes

Characteristic	Sick probands identified due to illness (*n* = 184; men: women)	Screening probands identified by elevated transferrin saturation (*n* = 107; men: women)	Clinically unselected homozygous relatives of probands (*n* = 214; men: women)
Liver biopsies	136: 48	66: 41	113: 101
Disease-related conditions (n)[b]	123: 44	54: 33	78: 40
Cirrhosis	55: 10	3: 2	14: 2
Hepatic fibrosis	32: 9	6: 2	13: 4
Elevated serum aminotransferase activity	16: 7	9: 7	11: 2
Arthropathy	5: 3	1: 3	5: 2
Subjects with at least one disease-related, condition, n (%)	108 (79%): 29 (60%)	19 (29%): 14 (34%)	43 (38%): 10 (10%)
Other clinical findings			
Diabetes mellitus	32: 6	2: 0	3: 5
Hypogonadotrophic hypogonadism	16: 3	0: 1	4: 0
Cardiac arrhythmia[c]	21: 5	2: 1	10: 3
Portal hypertension with splenomegaly	25: 4	0: 0	9: 2
Hepatocellular carcinoma	14: 0	0: 0	2: 0
Porphyria cutanea tarda	10: 9	0: 0	1: 1

Notes: [a]Adapted from Bulaj *et al.* and Edwards.[16,147]
[b]Subjects who had more than one of the first four conditions listed (cirrhosis, hepatic fibrosis, elevated serum aminotransferase activity, arthropathy) were classified as having only the condition listed first.
[c]Arrhythmia was documented by electrocardiography.

occur if an investigator who is grading the amount of stainable iron in hepatocytes (a subjective scoring system) knows that the patient's serum ferritin concentration is greater than 1000 µg/L. An experienced observer might know that patients whose ferritin values are greater than 1000 µg/L typically have high-grade stainable iron in hepatocytes (grade 4 on a scale of 0–4). If the liver biopsy shows that about 33 percent of hepatocytes are iron-loaded, the observer could record the stainable iron grade as grade 4, rather than as grade 3. Based on a published scoring method that included adequate detail, the correct grade for this patient's hepatocellular stainable iron is grade 3.[138] When this type of bias occurs in a scientific investigation, the observer has directly affected the results. In medical care delivery, the same biased interpretation of the liver iron grade may influence a physician's conclusions about the patient's condition and the development of plans for management for that patient.

Observer bias could occur in the interpretation of radiographs of the hands or knees. For example, if the physician interpreting the radiographs knows that the patient complains of arthralgias in the hands and in

Table 5.14. Age, iron phenotype, and complications in 194 hemochromatosis homozygotes in Canada[a]

Characteristic	Men, discovered cases: probands	Women, discovered cases: probands	Normal values
Number	46: 95	28: 25	
Age	48: 53	54: 63	
Mean transferrin saturation, %	70: 83	68: 72	<55
Mean serum ferritin, µg/L	876: 658	524: 1555	M <300; F <200
Mean hepatic iron concentration, µmol/g dry weight	225: 321	208: 292	<35
Mean hepatic iron index	4.7: 6.6	4.1: 5.0	<1.9
Weakness, %	72: 60	67: 59	
Skin pigmentation, %	9: 49	4: 36	
Hepatomegaly, %	12: 60	9: 61	
Arthritis, %	26: 42	25: 52	
Testicular atrophy, %	7: 24	—	
Cardiac failure, %	6: 15	4: 35	
Diabetes mellitus, %	14: 36	8: 22	
Liver disease, %	3: 46	8: 48	
Cardiac arrhythmia, %	3: 20	0: 29	
Hepatocellular carcinoma, %	1: 5	0: 5	

Note: [a]These data include observations on 120 probands and 74 other homozygotes discovered during evaluation of relatives or during screening, not due to illness. Adapted from Edwards et al.[146] Frequency (%) values were estimated from bar graphs; numerical data not presented in original text.[68]

the knees; has physical exam evidence of arthropathy in those joints; has an elevation of serum ferritin; has increased amounts of stainable iron in hepatocytes; and has joint space narrowing, the physician might conclude that the patient has the arthropathy of hemochromatosis. This type of observer bias can occur without any implication of dishonesty or intent to falsify data.

Controversy about morbidity and penetrance

There is variable penetrance and expressivity in hemochromatosis. Some homozygotes have heavy and others have near-normal (or even subnormal) iron stores. Some hemochromatosis patients have multiple morbid complications of iron overload, whereas others never become iron-loaded, and never develop morbidity. An area of great interest for

investigators is to identify "modifier" genes that interact in some way with mutations of *HFE*, resulting in heavy iron overload and severe morbidity. It is possible that in the absence of "modifier" genes, *HFE* mutations may not cause massive iron loading and severe morbidity. Conversely, "modifier" genes could preclude the development of severe iron overload. To date, some putative "modifier" genes have been identified in *HFE* C282Y homozygotes whose iron overload was either more severe than was observed in other C282Y homozygotes in the same kinship, or occurred at an earlier age than expected. These "modifier" genes comprise mutations in non-*HFE* iron-related genes. In most cases, in vivo expression models have not been utilized to corroborate that the "modifier" genes are likely to have the biological effect on iron absorption ascribed to them, although there are exceptions.[139] Further, population studies have not identified sufficient numbers of such "modifier" genes or mutations to account for most of the variable penetrance and expressivity characteristic of *HFE* C282Y homozygotes with either high- or low-iron phenotypes.[140]

Penetrance of hemochromatosis

Three very large studies have been performed in order to determine the prevalence of the *HFE* C282Y homozygous genotype in defined populations, and to estimate of the prevalence of complications among the discovered homozygotes. In these studies, 99 711 people in North America, 41 038 Americans, and 65 238 Norwegians were screened for C282Y homozygosity, and for the presence of complications.[69,70,141] The estimates of population frequency of the *HFE* C282Y/C282Y genotype in these studies were similar to the estimates made during screening studies that were published before the *HFE* gene was identified.[138] About 4 to 6 per 1000 Caucasians whose ancestry was of northern, central or western European origin were C282Y homozygotes.

The complications that were observed in many different studies of hemochromatosis patients identified in medical care or diagnosed as a part of family studies are displayed in Tables 5.11–5.14.[13,16,54,63,66,68,113,142–147] Complications were identified in 10–50 percent of individuals who had hemochromatosis. The frequency of observed complications in these subjects was much higher than was found in large screening studies where penetrance estimates of 1 percent or less were reported.[69,70,141] The types of subjects who were studied, the study design, the definitions, and the follow-up evaluation of homozygotes in these studies varied widely, and could account for much of the apparent differences in outcomes of the studies.

Additional work continues in this important area of inquiry that has yielded disparate results, conclusions, and recommendations. Scholarly discussions have been published about honorable differences of opinion in the interpretation of data about morbidity, penetrance, ascertainment bias, and observer bias in hemochromatosis studies. Interested readers are referred to a series of discussions and interpretations of the differing results that have been reported.[148–150]

Mortality of hemochromatosis

The results of survival analysis from research centers in the UK, Italy, Germany, and Canada provide substantial

information about mortality among persons with hemochromatosis. In general, survival probability is lower in persons whose iron overload is great at diagnosis than in those with iron overload that is less severe. Longevity is decreased in patients with severe iron overload who do not undergo phlebotomy to achieve iron depletion, or in those whose iron overload is so severe that iron depletion cannot be achieved within 1 year after diagnosis. Longevity is decreased in many patients with cirrhosis or diabetes mellitus.

Among 111 hemochromatosis patients in England, the average survival of 85 patients who underwent phlebotomy therapy was 72 months. Among the 16 patients who did not undergo iron depletion, the mean survival was only 14 months. The investigators concluded that a major determinant of survival was whether or not their patients underwent phlebotomy therapy to achieve iron depletion.[88]

The clinical features and disease-related complications of hemochromatosis that occurred in 212 Italian patients are displayed in Table 5.12.[144] The frequency of the complications of hemochromatosis was much higher in the 146 patients who had hepatic cirrhosis than in the 66 patients who did not have cirrhosis. In this series, the most common cause of death was hepatocellular carcinoma (20 of 44 patients; 45%), followed by liver failure in 10 of 44 patients

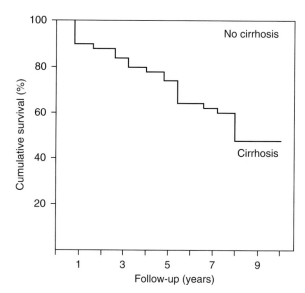

Fig. 5.15. Survival of 212 hemochromatosis patients in Italy grouped by the presence (*n* = 146) or absence (*n* = 66) of cirrhosis. From Fargion *et al.*[144]; reprinted with permission from John Wiley & Sons, Inc.

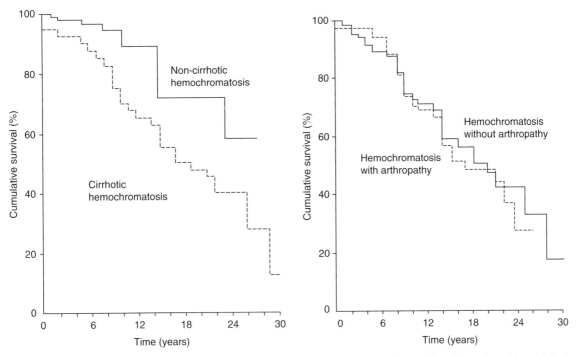

Fig. 5.16. Survival of 251 hemochromatosis patients in Germany grouped by the presence ($n = 142$) or absence ($n = 109$) of cirrhosis. Adapted from Niederau *et al.*[89] Taken from James C. Barton and Corwin Q. Edwards (eds), **Hemochromatosis: Genetics, Pathophysiology, Diagnosis and Treatment**, Cambridge University Press 2000. Reproduced with permission.

(23%). Multivariate analysis revealed that alcohol abuse, elevated serum concentration of gammaglobulins (>2 g/dL), and Child-Pugh (classification of severity of liver disease) class B or C had a negative prognostic effect on survival. The survival of the hemochromatosis patients who had hepatic cirrhosis (50% survival at 8 years) was much lower than that of the hemochromatosis patients who did not have cirrhosis (100% survival at 10 years) (Fig. 5.15).[144]

In a study of 251 hemochromatosis patients in Germany, the survival of 142 patients who had hepatic cirrhosis was compared with that of the 109 patients without cirrhosis. Survival in the group that had cirrhosis was significantly lower than that of the group that did not have cirrhosis (Fig. 5.16).[89] The same authors studied the survival of their 251 hemochromatosis patients grouped by the presence or absence of diabetes mellitus. Survival among the group of 120 patients who had diabetes was lower than among the 131 who did not have diabetes (Fig. 5.10).[89]

Multivariate analysis of observations in 277 *HFE* C282Y homozygotes in Canada revealed that cirrhosis and diabetes mellitus were the major factors that decreased survival.[151] The risk ratios for decreased

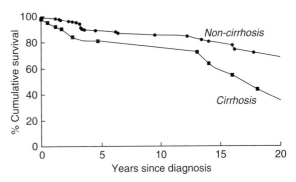

Fig. 5.17. Cumulative survival in 277 C282Y hemochromatosis homozygotes in Canada grouped by the presence ($n = 40$) or absence ($n = 237$) of cirrhosis. From Wojcik[151]; used with permission.

survival due to cirrhosis and diabetes were 3.95 and 2.92, respectively. The survival of 40 C282Y homozygotes with cirrhosis was about 80% at 5 years, 70% at 10 years, and about 30% at 20 years. Among the 237 C282Y homozygotes without cirrhosis, the survival at 5 years was about 90%, 85% at 10 years, and about 70% at 20 years.[151] Kaplan–Meier survival curves for these patients are displayed in Fig. 5.17.

101

References

1. Bacon BR. Hemochromatosis: diagnosis and management. *Gastroenterology* 2001; **120**: 718–25.

2. Brissot P. Clinical spectrum of hepatic disease in hemochromatosis. In: Barton JC, Edwards CQ, eds. *Hemochromatosis: Genetics, Pathophysiology, Diagnosis and Treatment*. Cambridge, Cambridge University Press. 2000; 250–7.

3. Britton RS. Mechanisms of iron toxicity. In: Barton JC, Edwards CQ, eds. *Hemochromatosis: Genetics, Pathophysiology, Diagnosis and Treatment*. Cambridge, Cambridge University Press. 2000; 229–38.

4. Papanikolaou G, Pantopoulos K. Iron metabolism and toxicity. *Toxicol Appl Pharmacol* 2005; **202**: 199–211.

5. Powell LW. Hereditary hemochromatosis and iron overload diseases. *J Gastroenterol Hepatol* 2002; **17** Suppl: S191–5.

6. Ramm GA, Ruddell RG. Hepatotoxicity of iron overload: mechanisms of iron-induced hepatic fibrogenesis. *Semin Liver Dis* 2005; **25**: 433–49.

7. Tavill AS. Diagnosis and management of hemochromatosis. *Hepatology* 2001; **33**: 1321–8.

8. Bottomley SS. Secondary iron overload disorders. *Semin Hematol* 1998; **35**: 77–86.

9. Harrison SA, Bacon BR. Hereditary hemochromatosis: update for 2003. *J Hepatol* 2003; **38** Suppl 1: S14–S23.

10. Alla V, Bonkovsky HL. Iron in nonhemochromatotic liver disorders. *Semin Liver Dis* 2005; **25**: 461–72.

11. Phillips JD, Bergonia HA, Reilly CA, Franklin MR, Kushner JP. A porphomethene inhibitor of uroporphyrinogen decarboxylase causes porphyria cutanea tarda. *Proc Natl Acad Sci USA* 2007; **104**: 5079–84.

12. Lambrecht RW, Thapar M, Bonkovsky HL. Genetic aspects of porphyria cutanea tarda. *Semin Liver Dis* 2007; **27**: 99–108.

13. Adams PC, Kertesz AE, Valberg LS. Clinical presentation of hemochromatosis: a changing scene. *Am J Med* 1991; **90**: 445–9.

14. Bacon BR, Sadiq SA. Hereditary hemochromatosis: presentation and diagnosis in the 1990s. *Am J Gastroenterol* 1997; **92**: 784–9.

15. Adams P, Brissot P, Powell LW. EASL International Consensus Conference on Haemochromatosis. *J Hepatol* 2000; **33**: 485–504.

16. Bulaj ZJ, Ajioka RS, Phillips JD, *et al.* Disease-related conditions in relatives of patients with hemochromatosis. *N Engl J Med* 2000; **343**: 1529–35.

17. Powell LW, Dixon JL, Ramm GA, *et al.* Screening for hemochromatosis in asymptomatic subjects with or without a family history. *Arch Intern Med* 2006; **166**: 294–301.

18. Asberg A, Hveem K, Kannelonning K, Irgens WO. Penetrance of the C28Y/C282Y genotype of the *HFE* gene. *Scand J Gastroenterol* 2007; **42**: 1073–7.

19. Allen KJ, Gurrin LC, Constantine CC, *et al.* Iron-overload-related disease in *HFE* hereditary hemochromatosis. *N Engl J Med* 2008; **358**: 221–30.

20. Fletcher LM, Dixon JL, Purdie DM, Powell LW, Crawford DHG. Excess alcohol greatly increases the prevalence of cirrhosis in hereditary hemochromatosis. *Gastroenterology* 2002; **122**: 281–9.

21. Brunt EM. Pathology of hepatic iron overload. *Semin Liver Dis* 2005; **25**: 392–401.

22. Deugnier Y, Turlin B. Pathology of hepatic iron overload. *World J Gastroenterol* 2007; **13**: 4755–60.

23. Grove J, Daly AK, Burt AD, *et al.* Heterozygotes for *HFE* mutations have no increased risk of advanced alcoholic liver disease. *Gut* 1998; **43**: 262–6.

24. Lauret E, Rodriguez M, Gonzalez S, *et al. HFE* gene mutations in alcoholic and virus-related cirrhotic patients with hepatocellular carcinoma. *Am J Gastroenterol* 2002; **97**: 1016–21.

25. Harrison-Findik DD, Schafer D, Klein E, *et al.* Alcohol metabolism-mediated oxidative stress down-regulates hepcidin transcription and leads to increased duodenal iron transporter expression. *J Biol Chem* 2006; **281**: 22974–82.

26. Van Thiel DH, Friedlander L, Fagiuoli S, Wright HI, Irish W, Gavaler JS. Response to interferon alpha therapy is influenced by the iron content of the liver. *J Hepatol* 1994; **20**: 410–15.

27. Olynyk JK, Reddy KR, Di Bisceglie AM, *et al.* Hepatic iron concentration as a predictor of response to interferon alfa therapy in chronic hepatitis C. *Gastroenterology* 1995; **108**: 1104–9.

28. Piperno A, Sampietro M, D'Alba R, *et al.* Iron stores, response to alpha-interferon therapy, and effects of iron depletion in chronic hepatitis C. *Liver* 1996; **16**: 248–54.

29. Fargion S, Fracanzani AL, Sampietro M, *et al.* Liver iron influences the response to interferon alpha therapy in chronic hepatitis C. *Eur J Gastroenterol Hepatol* 1997; **9**: 497–503.

30. Fong TL, Han SH, Tsai NC, *et al.* A pilot randomized, controlled trial of the effect of iron depletion on long-term response to alpha-interferon in patients with chronic hepatitis C. *J Hepatol* 1998; **28**: 369–74.

31. Fontana RJ, Israel J, LeClair P, *et al.* Iron reduction before and during interferon therapy of chronic hepatitis C: results of a multicenter, randomized, controlled trial. *Hepatology* 2000; **31**: 730–6.

32. Di Bisceglie AM, Bonkovsky HL, Chopra S, *et al.* Iron reduction as an adjuvant to interferon therapy in patients with chronic hepatitis C who have previously not responded to interferon: a multicenter, prospective, randomized, controlled trial. *Hepatology* 2000; **32**: 135–8.

33. Yano M, Hayashi H, Wakusawa S, *et al.* Long term effects of phlebotomy on biochemical and histological parameters of chronic hepatitis C. *Am J Gastroenterol* 2002; **97**: 133–7.

34. Rulyak SJ, Eng SC, Patel K, McHutchison JG, Gordon SC, Kowdley KV. Relationships between hepatic iron content and virologic response in chronic hepatitis C patients treated with interferon and ribavirin. *Am J Gastroenterol* 2005; **100**: 332–7.

35. Beinker NK, Voigt MD, Arendse M, Smit J, Stander IA, Kirsch RE. Threshold effect of liver iron content on hepatic inflammation and fibrosis in hepatitis B and C. *J Hepatol* 1996; **25**: 633–8.

36. Smith BC, Gorve J, Guzail MA, *et al.* Heterozygosity for hereditary hemochromatosis is associated with more fibrosis in chronic hepatitis C. *Hepatology* 1998; **27**: 1695–9.

37. Martinelli AL, Franco RF, Villanova MG, *et al.* Are haemochromatosis mutations related to the severity of liver disease in hepatitis C virus infection? *Acta Haematol* 2000; **102**: 152–6.

38. Negro F, Samii K, Rubbia-Brandt L, *et al.* Hemochromatosis gene mutations in chronic hepatitis C patients with and without liver siderosis. *J Med Virol* 2000; **60**: 21–7.

39. George DK, Goldwurm S, MacDonald GA, *et al.* Increased hepatic iron concentration in non-alcoholic steatohepatitis is associated with increased fibrosis. *Gastroenterology* 1998; **114**: 311–18.

40. Bonkovsky HL, Jawaid Q, Tortorelli K, *et al.* Non-alcoholic steatohepatitis and iron: increased prevalence of mutations of the *HFE* gene in non-alcoholic steatohepatitis. *J Hepatol* 1999; **31**: 421–9.

41. Chitturi S, Weltman M, Farrell GC, *et al.* HFE mutations, hepatic iron, and fibrosis: ethnic-specific association of NASH with C282Y but not with fibrotic severity. *Hepatology* 2002; **36**: 142–9.

42. Valenti L, Dongiovanni P, Fracanzani AL, *et al.* Increased susceptibility to non-alcoholic fatty liver disease in heterozygotes for the mutation responsible for hereditary hemochromatosis. *Dig Liver Dis* 2003; **35**: 172–8.

43. Nishina S, Hino K, Korenaga M, *et al.* Hepatitis C virus-induced reactive oxygen species raise hepatic iron level in mice by reducing hepcidin transcription. *Gastroenterology* 2008; **134**: 226–38.

44. Niederau C, Fischer R, Sonnenberg A, Stremmel W, Trampisch HJ, Strohmeyer G. Survival and causes of death in cirrhotic and in noncirrhotic patients with primary hemochromatosis. *N Engl J Med* 1985; **313**: 1256–62.

45. Deugnier YM, Loreal O. Iron as a carcinogen. In: Barton JC, Edwards CQ, eds. *Hemochromatosis: Genetics, Pathophysiology, Diagnosis and Treatment.* Cambridge, Cambridge University Press. 2000; 239–49.

46. Kowdley KV. Iron, hemochromatosis, and hepatocellular carcinoma. *Gastroenterology* 2004; **127**: S79–S86.

47. Harrison SA, Bacon BR. Relation of hemochromatosis with hepatocellular carcinoma: epidemiology, natural history, pathophysiology, screening, treatment, and prevention. *Med Clin North Am* 2005; **89**: 391–409.

48. Ellervik C, Birgens H, Tybjaerg-Hansen A, Nordestgaard BG. Hemochromatosis genotypes and risk of 31 disease endpoints: meta-analyses including 66 000 cases and 226 000 controls. *Hepatology* 2007; **46**: 1071–80.

49. Lowes KN, Brennan BA, Yeoh GC, Olynyk JK. Oval cell numbers in human chronic liver diseases are directly related to disease severity. *Am J Pathol* 1999; **154**: 537–41.

50. Deugnier YM, Charalambous P, Le Quilleuc D, *et al.* Preneoplastic significance of hepatic iron-free foci in genetic hemochromatosis: a study of 185 patients. *Hepatology* 1993; **18**: 1363–9.

51. Deugnier YM, Guyader D, Crantock L, *et al.* Primary liver cancer in genetic hemochromatosis: a clinical, pathological, and pathogenetic study of 54 cases. *Gastroenterology* 1993; **104**: 228–34.

52. Bezançon F, de Gennes I, Delarue J, Oumensky V. *Cirrhose pigmentaire avec infantilisme et insuffisance cardiaque et aplasie endocriniennes multiples. Bull Mém Soc Méd Hôp Paris* 1932; **48**: 967.

53. de Vericourt R. *Le syndrome endocrino-hepato-myocardiaque (sur un aspect des cirrhoses pigmentaires).* Paris. 1935.

54. Sheldon JH. *Haemochromatosis.* London, Oxford University Press, 1935.

55. Muhlestein JB. Cardiac abnormalities in hemochromatosis. In: Barton JC, Edwards CQ, eds. *Hemochromatosis: Genetics, Pathophysiology, Diagnosis and Treatment.* Cambridge, Cambridge University Press. 2000; 297–311.

103

56. Willis G, Scott DG, Jennings BA, Smith K, Bukhari M, Wimperis JZ. *HFE* mutations in an inflammatory arthritis population. *Rheumatology (Oxford)* 2002; **41**: 176–9.

57. Stevens SM, Edwards CQ. Identifying and managing hemochromatosis arthropathy. *J Musculoskel Med* 2009; **26**: 15–24.

58. Schumacher HR, Straka PC, Krikker MA, Dudley AT. The arthropathy of hemochromatosis. Recent studies. *Ann NY Acad Sci* 1988; **526**: 224–33.

59. McClain DA, Abraham D, Rogers J, *et al*. High prevalence of abnormal glucose homeostasis secondary to decreased insulin secretion in individuals with hereditary haemochromatosis. *Diabetologia* 2006; **49**: 1661–9.

60. Wilson JG. Iron and glucose homeostasis: new lessons from hereditary haemochromatosis. *Diabetologia* 2006; **49**: 1459–61.

61. Cooksey RC, Jouihan HA, Ajioka RS, *et al*. Oxidative stress, beta-cell apoptosis, and decreased insulin secretory capacity in mouse models of hemochromatosis. *Endocrinology* 2004; **145**: 5305–12.

62. Fernández-Real JM, López-Bermejo A, Ricart W. Iron stores, blood donation, and insulin sensitivity and secretion. *Clin Chem* 2005; **51**: 1201–5.

63. Finch SC, Finch CA. Idiopathic hemochromatosis, an iron storage disease. *Medicine* 1966; **34**: 381–430.

64. Dymock IW, Cassar J, Pyke DA, Oakley WG, Williams R. Observations on the pathogenesis, complications and treatment of diabetes in 115 cases of haemochromatosis. *Am J Med* 1972; **52**: 203–10.

65. Saddi R, Feingold J. Idiopathic hemochromatosis and diabetes mellitus. *Clin Genet* 1974; **5**: 242–7.

66. Niederau C, Fischer R, Purschel A, Stremmel W, Haussinger D, Strohmeyer G. Long-term survival in patients with hereditary haemochromatosis. *Gastroenterology* 1996; **110**: 1107–19.

67. Yaouanq JM. Diabetes and haemochromatosis: current concepts, management, and prevention. *Diabete Metab* 1995; **21**: 319–29.

68. Adams PC, Valberg LS. Evolving expression of hereditary hemochromatosis. *Semin Liver Dis* 1996; **16**: 47–54.

69. Adams PC, Reboussin DM, Barton JC, *et al*. Hemochromatosis and iron-overload screening in a racially diverse population. *N Engl J Med* 2005; **352**: 1769–78.

70. Beutler E, Felitti VJ, Koziol JA, Ho NJ, Gelbart T. Penetrance of 845G–> A (C282Y) *HFE* hereditary haemochromatosis mutation in the USA. *Lancet* 2002; **359**: 211–18.

71. Braun J, Donner H, Plock K, Rau H, Usadel KH, Badenhoop K. Hereditary haemochromatosis mutations (*HFE*) in patients with type 2 diabetes mellitus. *Diabetologia* 1998; **41**: 983–4.

72. Davis TM, Beilby J, Davis WA, *et al*. Prevalence, characteristics, and prognostic significance of *HFE* gene mutations in type 2 diabetes: the Fremantle Diabetes Study. *Diabetes Care* 2008; **31**: 1795–801.

73. Dubois-Laforgue D, Larger E, Timsit J. [Is diabetes mellitus a sufficient condition to suspect hemochromatosis?] *Diabetes Metab* 2000; **26**: 318–21.

74. Fernández-Real JM, Vendrell J, Baiget M, Gimferrer E, Ricart W. C282Y and H63D mutations of the hemochromatosis candidate gene in type 2 diabetes. *Diabetes Care* 1999; **22**: 525–6.

75. Frayling T, Ellard S, Grove J, Walker M, Hattersley AT. C282Y mutation in *HFE* (haemochromatosis) gene and type 2 diabetes. *Lancet* 1998; **351**: 1933–4.

76. Habeos IG, Psyrogiannis A, Kyriazopoulou V, Psilopanagiotou A, Papavassiliou AG, Vagenakis AG. The role of hemochromatosis C282Y and H63D mutations in the development of type 2 diabetes mellitus in Greece. *Hormones (Athens)* 2003; **2**: 55–60.

77. Hahn JU, Steiner M, Bochnig S, Schmidt H, Schuff-Werner P, Kerner W. Evaluation of a diagnostic algorithm for hereditary hemochromatosis in 3500 patients with diabetes. *Diabetes Care* 2006; **29**: 464–6.

78. Halsall DJ, McFarlane I, Luan J, Cox TM, Wareham NJ. Typical type 2 diabetes mellitus and *HFE* gene mutations: a population-based case-control study. *Hum Mol Genet* 2003; **12**: 1361–5.

79. Singh BM, Grunewald RA, Press M, Muller BR, Wise PH. Prevalence of haemochromatosis among patients with diabetes mellitus. *Diabet Med* 1992; **9**: 730–1.

80. Turnbull AJ, Mitchison HC, Peaston RT, *et al*. The prevalence of hereditary haemochromatosis in a diabetic population. *Q J Med* 1997; **90**: 271–5.

81. Vantyghem MC, Fajardy I, Dhondt F, *et al*. Phenotype and *HFE* genotype in a population with abnormal iron markers recruited from an Endocrinology Department. *Eur J Endocrinol* 2006; **154**: 835–41.

82. Conte D, Manachino D, Colli A, *et al*. Prevalence of genetic hemochromatosis in a cohort of Italian patients with diabetes mellitus. *Ann Intern Med* 1998; **128**: 370–3.

83. Ellervik C, Mandrup-Poulsen T, Nordestgaard BG, *et al*. Prevalence of hereditary haemochromatosis in late-onset type 1 diabetes mellitus: a retrospective study. *Lancet* 2001; **358**: 1405–9.

84. Kwan T, Leber B, Ahuja S, Carter R, Gerstein HC. Patients with type 2 diabetes have a high frequency of

the C282Y mutation of the hemochromatosis gene. *Clin Invest Med* 1998; **21**: 251–7.

85. Moczulski DK, Grzeszczak W, Gawlik B. Role of hemochromatosis C282Y and H63D mutations in *HFE* gene in development of type 2 diabetes and diabetic nephropathy. *Diabetes Care* 2001; **24**: 1187–91.

86. Phelps G, Chapman I, Hall P, Braund W, Mackinnon M. Prevalence of genetic haemochromatosis among diabetic patients. *Lancet* 1989; **2**: 233–4.

87. Strohmeyer G, Niederau C. Diabetes mellitus and hemochromatosis. In: Barton JC, Edwards CQ, eds. *Hemochromatosis: Genetics, Pathophysiology, Diagnosis and Treatment.* Cambridge, Cambridge University Press. 2000; 269–74.

88. Bomford A, Williams R. Long-term results of venesection therapy in idiopathic haemochromatosis. *Q J Med* 1976; **45**: 611–23.

89. Niederau C, Strohmeyer G. Survival in hemochromatosis. In: Barton JC, Edwards CQ, eds. *Hemochromatosis: Genetics, Pathophysiology, Diagnosis and Treatment.* Cambridge, Cambridge University Press. 2000; 359–68.

90. Duranteau L, Chanson P, Blumberg-Tick J, *et al.* Non-responsiveness of serum gonadotropins and testosterone to pulsatile GnRH in hemochromatosis suggesting a pituitary defect. *Acta Endocrinol (Copenh)* 1993; **128**: 351–4.

91. McDermott JH, Walsh CH. Hypogonadism in hereditary hemochromatosis. *J Clin Endocrinol Metab* 2005; **90**: 2451–5.

92. Bezwoda WR, Bothwell TH, Van Der Walt LA, Kronheim S, Pimstone BL. An investigation into gonadal dysfunction in patients with idiopathic haemochromatosis. *Clin Endocrinol (Oxf)* 1977; **6**: 377–85.

93. Charbonnel B, Chupin M, Le Grand A, Guillon J. Pituitary function in idiopathic haemochromatosis: hormonal study in 36 male patients. *Acta Endocrinol (Copenh)* 1981; **98**: 178–83.

94. Kelly TM, Edwards CQ, Meikle AW, Kushner JP. Hypogonadism in hemochromatosis: reversal with iron depletion. *Ann Intern Med* 1984; **101**: 629–32.

95. Lufkin EG, Baldus WP, Bergstralh EJ, Kao PC. Influence of phlebotomy treatment on abnormal hypothalamic-pituitary function in genetic hemochromatosis. *Mayo Clin Proc* 1987; **62**: 473–9.

96. MacDonald RA, Mallory GK. Hemochromatosis and hemosiderosis. *Arch Intern Med* 1960; **105**: 686–700.

97. Piperno A, Rivolta MR, D'Alba R, *et al.* Preclinical hypogonadism in genetic hemochromatosis in the early stage of the disease: evidence of hypothalamic dysfunction. *J Endocrinol Invest* 1992; **15**: 423–28.

98. Walsh CH, Wright AD, Williams JW, Holder G. A study of pituitary function in patients with idiopathic hemochromatosis. *J Clin Endocrinol Metab* 1976; **43**: 866–72.

99. Walton C, Kelly WF, Laing I, Bu'lock DE. Endocrine abnormalities in idiopathic haemochromatosis. *Q J Med* 1983; **52**: 99–110.

100. Edwards CQ, Kelly TM, Ellwein G, Kushner JP. Thyroid disease in hemochromatosis. Increased incidence in homozygous men. *Arch Intern Med* 1983; **143**: 1890–3.

101. Tamagno G, De Carlo E, Murialdo G, Scandellari C. A possible link between genetic hemochromatosis and autoimmune thyroiditis. *Minerva Med* 2007; **98**: 769–72.

102. Hempenius LM, van Dam PS, Marx JJ, Koppeschaar HP. Mineralocorticoid status and endocrine dysfunction in severe hemochromatosis. *J Endocrinol Invest* 1999; **22**: 369–76.

103. Murphy MS, Walsh CH. Thyroid function in haemochromatosis. *Ir J Med Sci* 2004; **173**: 27–9.

104. Paris I, Hermans M, Buysschaert M. [Endocrine complications of genetic hemochromatosis.] *Acta Clin Belg* 1999; **54**: 334–45.

105. Walsh CH. Non-diabetic endocrinopathy in hemochromatosis. In: Barton JC, Edwards CQ, eds. *Hemochromatosis: Genetics, Pathophysiology, Diagnosis and Treatment.* Cambridge, Cambridge University Press. 2000; 278–89.

106. Barton JC, Leiendecker-Foster C, Reboussin DM, Adams PC, Acton RT, Eckfeldt JH. Thyroid-stimulating hormone and free thyroxine levels in persons with *HFE* C282Y homozygosity, a common hemochromatosis genotype: the HEIRS Study. *Thyroid* 2008; **18**: 831–8.

107. Asberg A, Hveem K, Kruger O, Bjerve KS. Persons with screening-detected haemochromatosis: as healthy as the general population? *Scand J Gastroenterol* 2002; **37**: 719–24.

108. Cawley EP, Hsu YT, Wood BT, Weary PE. Hemochromatosis and the skin. *Arch Dermatol* 1969; **100**: 1–6.

109. Edwards CQ, Cartwright GE, Skolnick MH, Amos DB. Homozygosity for hemochromatosis: clinical manifestations. *Ann Intern Med* 1980; **93**: 519–25.

110. Troisier M. Diabète sucré. *Bull Soc Anat Paris* 1871; **16**: 231–35.

111. Chevrant-Breton J, Simon M, Bourel M, Ferrand B. Cutaneous manifestations of idiopathic

105

hermochromatosis. Study of 100 cases. *Arch Dermatol* 1977; **113**: 161–5.

112. Chevrant-Breton J. Cutaneous manifestations of hemochromatosis. In: Barton JC, Edwards CQ, eds. *Hemochromatosis: Genetics, Pathophysiology, Diagnosis and Treatment*, Cambridge, Cambridge University Press. 2000; 290–6.

113. Milman N. Hereditary haemochromatosis in Denmark 1950–1985. Clinical, biochemical and histological features in 179 patients and 13 preclinical cases. *Dan Med Bull* 1991; **38**: 385–93.

114. Bacon BR, Sadiq SA. Hereditary hemochromatosis: presentation and diagnosis in the 1990s. *Am J Gastroenterol* 1997; **92**: 784–9.

115. Barton JC, Barton NH, Alford TJ. Diagnosis of hemochromatosis probands in a community hospital. *Am J Med* 1997; **103**: 498–503.

116. De Gobbi M, Roetto A, Piperno A, *et al*. Natural history of juvenile haemochromatosis. *Br J Haematol* 2002; **117**: 973–9.

117. Davies G, Dymock I, Harry J, Williams R. Deposition of melanin and iron in ocular structures in haemochromatosis. *Br J Ophthalmol* 1972; **56**: 338–42.

118. Mills PR, Skerrow CJ, MacKie RM. Melanin pigmentation of the skin in primary biliary cirrhosis. *J Cutan Pathol* 1981; **8**: 404–10.

119. Smith AG, Shuster S, Bomford A, Williams R. Plasma immunoreactive beta-melanocyte-stimulating hormone in chronic liver disease and fulminant hepatic failure. *J Invest Dermatol* 1978; **70**: 326–27.

120. Byrnes V, Ryan E, O'Keane C, Crowe J. Immunohistochemistry of the Hfe protein in patients with hereditary hemochromatosis, iron deficiency anemia, and normal controls. *Blood Cells Mol Dis* 2000; **26**: 2–8.

121. Parkkila S, Parkkila AK, Waheed A, *et al*. Cell surface expression of HFE protein in epithelial cells, macrophages, and monocytes. *Haematologica* 2000; **85**: 340–5.

122. Mukerji SK, Pimstone NR. In vitro studies of the mechanism of inhibition of rat liver uroporphyrinogen decarboxylase activity by ferrous iron under anaerobic conditions. *Arch Biochem Biophys* 1986; **244**: 619–29.

123. Young LC. Porphyria cutanea tarda associated with Cys282Tyr mutation in *HFE* gene in hereditary hemochromatosis: a case report and review of the literature. *Cutis* 2007; **80**: 415–18.

124. Syn WK, Ahmed MM. Genetic haemochromatosis presenting as porphyria cutanea tarda. *Int J Clin Pract Suppl* 2005; 48–50.

125. Mehrany K, Drage LA, Brandhagen DJ, Pittelkow MR. Association of porphyria cutanea tarda with hereditary hemochromatosis. *J Am Acad Dermatol* 2004; **51**: 205–11.

126. Lambrecht RW, Bonkovsky HL. Hemochromatosis and porphyria. *Semin Gastrointest Dis* 2002; **13**: 109–19.

127. Bulaj ZJ, Phillips JD, Ajioka RS, *et al*. Hemochromatosis genes and other factors contributing to the pathogenesis of porphyria cutanea tarda. *Blood* 2000; **95**: 1565–71.

128. Witte DL, Crosby WH, Edwards CQ, Fairbanks VF, Mitros FA. Practice guideline development task force of the College of American Pathologists. Hereditary hemochromatosis. *Clin Chim Acta* 1996; **245**: 139–200.

129. Adams PC, Deugnier Y, Moirand R, Brissot P. The relationship between iron overload, clinical symptoms, and age in 410 patients with genetic hemochromatosis. *Hepatology* 1997; **25**: 162–6.

130. Waalen J, Felitti V, Gelbart T, Ho NJ, Beutler E. Prevalence of hemochromatosis-related symptoms among individuals with mutations in the *HFE* gene. *Mayo Clin Proc* 2002; **77**: 522–30.

131. Stovner LJ, Hagen K, Waage A, Bjerve KS. Hereditary haemochromatosis in two cousins with cluster headache. *Cephalalgia* 2002; **22**: 317–19.

132. Barton JC, Wooten VD, Acton RT. Hemochromatosis and iron therapy of restless legs syndrome. *Sleep Med* 2001; **2**: 249–51.

133. Shaughnessy P, Lee J, O'Keeffe ST. Restless legs syndrome in patients with hereditary hemochromatosis. *Neurology* **2005**; 64: 2158.

134. Earley CJ. Hemochromatosis and iron therapy of restless legs syndrome. *Sleep Med* 2001; **2**: 181–3.

135. Haba-Rubio J, Staner L, Petiau C, Erb G, Schunck T, Macher JP. Restless legs syndrome and low brain iron levels in patients with haemochromatosis. *J Neurol Neurosurg Psychiatry* 2005; **76**: 1009–10.

136. Barton JC, Bertoli LF, Acton RT. Common variable immunodeficiency and IgG subclass deficiency in central Alabama hemochromatosis probands homozygous for *HFE* C282Y. *Blood Cells Mol Dis* 2003; **31**: 102–11.

137. Barton JC, Acton RT. Hemochromatosis and *Vibrio vulnificus* wound infections. *J Clin Gastroenterol* 2009; **43**: 890–3.

138. Edwards CQ, Carroll M, Bray P, Cartwright GE. Hereditary hemochromatosis. Diagnosis in siblings and children. *N Engl J Med* 1977; **297**: 7–13.

139. Island ML, Jouanolle AM, Mosser A, *et al*. A new mutation in the hepcidin promoter impairs its BMP response and contributes to a severe phenotype in *HFE* related hemochromatosis. *Haematologica* 2009; **94**: 720–4.

140. Barton JC, LaFreniere SA, Leiendecker-Foster C, *et al*. *HFE*, *SLC40A1*, *HAMP*, *HJV*, *TFR2*, and *FTL* mutations detected by denaturing high-performance liquid chromatography after iron phenotyping and

HFE C282Y and H63D genotyping in 785 HEIRS Study participants. *Am J Hematol* 2009; **84**: 710–14.

141. Asberg A, Hveem K, Thorstensen K, *et al.* Screening for hemochromatosis: high prevalence and low morbidity in an unselected population of 65 238 persons. *Scand J Gastroenterol* 2001; **36**: 1108–15.

142. Milder MS, Cook JD, Stray S, Finch CA. Idiopathic hemochromatosis, an interim report. *Medicine (Baltimore)* 1980; **59**: 34–49.

143. Edwards CQ, Dadone MM, Skolnick MH, Kushner JP. Hereditary haemochromatosis. *Clin Haematol* 1982; **11**: 411–35.

144. Fargion S, Mandelli C, Piperno A, *et al.* Survival and prognostic factors in 212 Italian patients with genetic hemochromatosis. *Hepatology* 1992; **15**: 655–9.

145. Moirand R, Adams PC, Bicheler V, Brissot P, Deugnier Y. Clinical features of genetic hemochromatosis in women compared with men. *Ann Intern Med* 1997; **127**: 105–10.

146. Edwards CQ, Griffen LM, Bulaj ZS, Ajioka RS, Kushner JP. Estimate of the frequency of morbid complications of hemochromatosis. In: Barton JC, Edwards CQ, eds. *Hemochromatosis: Genetics, Pathophysiology, Diagnosis and Treatment.* Cambridge, Cambridge University Press. 2000; 312–17.

147. Edwards CQ. Hemochromatosis. In: Greer JP, Foerster J, Rodgers GM, *et al.*, eds. *Wintrobe's Clinical Hematology* 12th edn. Philadelphia, Lippincott Williams and Wilkins. 2009; 857–80.

148. Beutler E. The *HFE* Cys282Tyr mutation as a necessary but not sufficient cause of clinical hereditary hemochromatosis. *Blood* 2003; **101**: 3347–50.

149. Ajioka RS, Kushner JP. Clinical consequences of iron overload in hemochromatosis homozygotes. *Blood* 2003; **101**: 3351–3.

150. McCune A, Worwood M. Penetrance in hereditary hemochromatosis. *Blood* 2003; **102**: 2696–7.

151. Wojcik JP, Speechley MR, Kertesz AE, Chakrabarti S, Adams PC. Natural history of C282Y homozygotes for hemochromatosis. *Can J Gastroenterol* 2002; **16**: 297–302.

Insulin resistance and iron overload

Elevated serum ferritin levels and increased body iron stores are now recognized as features that sometimes occur in the insulin resistance syndrome (IRS; also known as the metabolic syndrome) and type 2 diabetes mellitus.[1–7] A key component of IRS is abdominal obesity. Other metabolic risk factors may also accompany IRS, including atherogenic dyslipidemia, hypertension, a pro-thrombotic state, and a pro-inflammatory state.[8,9] Some persons are genetically predisposed to IRS.[9–11] Acquired factors, such as excess body fat and physical inactivity, can elicit IRS in some persons.[8,9,11] The incidence of IRS is increasing, and it is estimated about 25% of adult Americans have IRS.[10,11] Approximately 15% of individuals with IRS have increased ferritin levels.[6] Increased hepatic iron has been found in as many as one-third of patients with non-alcoholic fatty liver disease (NAFLD).[12] NAFLD, a manifestation of IRS, is characterized by hepatic insulin resistance.[13–16] The molecular mechanisms underlying the interrelationship between insulin resistance, NAFLD, and iron metabolism remain unclear.[17–21]

Clinical manifestations

In 1997, Moirand et al. described a new syndrome of moderate hepatic iron overload with normal transferrin saturation.[1] It is now considered that most of these patients, and those in a subsequent study by the same group,[3] had IRS with iron overload.[2–6] In the first study, Moirand et al. described 65 patients who had been referred for further evaluation of suspected iron overload.[1] These patients were referred either for an evaluation of fatigue and arthralgias or hyperferritinemia. Six of the 65 patients had serum ferritin levels >1000 µg/L. They differed from typical patients with hemochromatosis because they had normal transferrin saturation value on at least two occasions. The authors excluded patients who

reported that they drank excess amounts of alcohol, those who had changes of alcoholic liver disease on biopsy, those who consumed excess amounts of iron or ascorbic acid, and those who had repeated blood transfusions, porphyria cutanea tarda, chronic hepatitis B or C, or a chronic inflammatory condition.[1]

Liver biopsies revealed iron deposition in both hepatocytes and Kupffer cells. Hepatic iron concentration was measured either by direct analysis of liver biopsy tissue or by magnetic resonance imaging (MRI), or both. The patients had elevated hepatic iron concentrations (normal <36 µmol Fe/g dry weight of liver). The hepatic iron index (ratio of hepatic iron concentration to patient's age) was >1.9 in 22 of the 65 patients (33.8%). Thus, the typical increases in hepatic iron concentration were mild or moderate. Human leukocyte antigen (HLA) type was determined in 62 of the 65 patients. The frequency of HLA-A*03 was similar to that of the general population.[1]

These patients were treated with therapeutic phlebotomy. On the average, 2.5 g of iron was removed (range 1.2–10 g). The mean quantity of iron removed by phlebotomy to achieve iron depletion from a control group of typical hemochromatosis patients was 5 g (range 2–20 g). The majority (72%) of the IRS patients had an elevated body mass index >25 kg/m², 65% had elevated serum lipid levels, 43% had abnormal glucose metabolism, and 19% had hypertension. The authors concluded that they had identified a new, non-HLA-linked iron overload syndrome characterized by normal transferrin saturation and IRS (increased body mass index, abnormal glucose homeostasis, hyperlipidemia, and hypertension). Quantitative phlebotomy revealed that the amount of iron removed was greater than that expected to be stored in normal adults, but less than that removed from typical hemochromatosis patients.[1]

A follow-up study of a larger group of patients was published in 1999 by the same investigators after the availability of *HFE* mutation analysis.[3] Therein, the authors reported 161 patients with IRS in whom *HFE* mutation analysis had been performed; they excluded subjects who were homozygous for *HFE* C282Y. The patients were predominantly male and middle-aged. All had unexplained iron overload, and most (94%) had one or more of the following: body mass index $>25 \text{ kg/m}^2$; abnormal glucose metabolism; hyperlipidemia; and hypertension. Transferrin saturation was elevated in 35% of these patients, a finding that differs from that of the original report.[1] The median hepatic iron concentration was elevated (90 μmol Fe/g dry weight of liver; range 38–332 μmol Fe/g dry weight).[3]

The investigators reported that 20% of the patients had *HFE* C282Y, and that 30% had *HFE* H63D (9% of controls had C282Y and 17% had H63D); their respective differences were significant. Nonetheless, there was no significant difference in the severity of iron overload in patients with or without *HFE* mutations. As in the previous study, iron deposits in the liver appeared in both hepatocytes and Kupffer cells, unlike the predominance of hepatocyte iron deposition typical of hemochromatosis.[22] Approximately 25% of the IRS patients had hepatic steatosis alone, and 27% of patients had both steatosis and inflammation, hallmarks of non-alcoholic steatohepatitis (NASH). Periportal fibrosis was present in 62% of patients and was usually observed in association with steatosis, inflammation, and greater age.[22] Serum ferritin levels were higher in patients with NASH than in those without NASH, but hepatic iron concentration and the frequency of *HFE* C282Y and H63D were similar in the two groups.

Taken together, the results of these two studies[1,3] and subsequent reports by others[2,4–6,14,15] indicate that some patients with IRS have elevated ferritin levels and moderate hepatic iron overload. Many of these patients also have co-existing NAFLD, and some have NASH.[3,13–19]

Current diagnostic criteria

The diagnostic criteria for IRS of the American Heart Association and the National Heart, Lung, and Blood Institute[8] are displayed in Table 6.1. These criteria are more rigorous than those used by Moirand *et al.* in their 1999 study of IRS with iron overload.[3] The

Table 6.1. Diagnostic criteria for insulin resistance syndrome (metabolic syndrome)

Presence of three or more of these criteria:
1. Elevated waist circumference (men $\geq$40 inches (102 cm); women $\geq$35 inches (88 cm))
2. Elevated triglycerides ($\geq$150 mg/dL)
3. Reduced HDL cholesterol (men $<$ 40 mg/dL; women $<$ 50 mg/dL)
4. Elevated blood pressure ($\geq$130/85 mm Hg)
5. Elevated fasting glucose ($\geq$100 mg/dL)

concurrence of IRS in patients with an elevated serum ferritin level suggests that they may have IRS with iron overload. This diagnostic possibility is more likely after exclusion of possible co-existing conditions such as hemochromatosis, excess alcohol consumption, chronic viral hepatitis, hematological abnormalities, blood transfusions, porphyria cutanea tarda, and a condition associated with chronic inflammation.[3] The presence of iron overload is confirmed by liver biopsy (with iron quantification or histologic scoring), MRI, or quantitative phlebotomy. Liver biopsy will also reveal if steatosis, NASH, or fibrosis is present.[3,13,16]

Treatment
General management

The suggested treatment of patients with IRS and iron overload is summarized in Table 6.2.[3,8,9,13,16] Weight loss, achieved gradually, is recommended to achieve a body mass index $<25 \text{ kg/m}^2$. A weight loss program should stress healthy eating habits that include reduced intake of saturated fat, trans-fat, and cholesterol. Patients should also be encouraged to exercise, with at least 30 minutes of moderate-intensity activity per day. In addition, treatment with therapeutic phlebotomy may be considered, based on reports that iron removal by phlebotomy decreases hyperinsulinemia, hyperglycemia, and improves liver function in patients with IRS and NAFLD.[17–19] One study used a phlebotomy protocol of 1 unit of blood removed every 2 weeks to decrease serum ferritin <80 μg/L, followed by maintenance phlebotomy to keep ferritin levels <100 μg/L.[19] In patients with NASH, clinical trials are underway to test the efficacy of pioglitazone (a peroxisome proliferator-activated receptor gamma

Table 6.2. Treatment of insulin resistance syndrome with iron overload

Gradual weight loss to achieve body mass index <25 kg/m²
Reduced intake of saturated fat, trans-fat, and cholesterol
Increased physical activity (≥30 minutes of moderate-intensity activity daily)
Consider phlebotomy (1 unit every 2 weeks until serum ferritin <80 µg/L), then maintenance phlebotomy to keep ferritin levels <100 µg/L

ligand) and vitamin E (an antioxidant) against hepatic injury.[23]

Iron depletion

Iron removal by phlebotomy has been reported to decrease both hyperinsulinemia and hyperglycemia, and to decrease elevated serum levels of hepatic transaminases in patients with IRS and NAFLD.[17–19] One study evaluated 128 NAFLD patients who had elevated serum ferritin or alanine aminotransferase levels. All patients were counseled regarding the importance of modifying their lifestyle, and 64 also underwent phlebotomy for 8 months.[19] No adverse effects were observed during phlebotomy treatment. There was a positive correlation of pre-phlebotomy serum ferritin levels and iron removed by phlebotomy. Iron depletion by phlebotomy was associated with a significantly greater decrease in insulin resistance than lifestyle modification alone. Larger multicenter trials are warranted to validate this therapeutic approach in IRS patients with iron overload.

References

1. Moirand R, Mortaji AM, Loreal O, Paillard F, Brissot P, Deugnier Y. A new syndrome of liver iron overload with normal transferrin saturation. *Lancet* 1997; **349**: 95–7.

2. Fernandez-Real JM, Ricart-Engel W, Arroyo E, *et al.* Serum ferritin as a component of the insulin resistance syndrome. *Diabetes Care* 1998; **21**: 62–8.

3. Mendler MH, Turlin B, Moirand R, *et al.* Insulin resistance-associated hepatic iron overload. *Gastroenterology* 1999; **117**: 1155–63.

4. Fargion S, Mattioli M, Fracanzani AL, *et al.* Hyperferritinemia, iron overload, and multiple metabolic alterations identify patients at risk for non-alcoholic steatohepatitis. *Am J Gastroenterol* 2001; **96**: 2448–55.

5. Wrede CE, Buettner R, Bollheimer LC, Scholmerich J, Palitzsch KD, Hellerbrand C. Association between serum ferritin and the insulin resistance syndrome in a representative population. *Eur J Endocrinol* 2006; **154**: 333–40.

6. Bozzini C, Girelli D, Olivieri O, *et al.* Prevalence of body iron excess in the metabolic syndrome. *Diabetes Care* 2005; **28**: 2061–3.

7. Dongiovanni P, Valenti L, Ludovica FA, Gatti S, Cairo G, Fargion S. Iron depletion by deferoxamine up-regulates glucose uptake and insulin signaling in hepatoma cells and in rat liver. *Am J Pathol* 2008; **172**: 738–47.

8. Grundy SM. A constellation of complications: the metabolic syndrome. *Clin Cornerstone* 2005; **7**: 36–45.

9. Reaven GM. The insulin resistance syndrome: definition and dietary approaches to treatment. *Annu Rev Nutr* 2005; **25**: 391–406.

10. Grundy SM. Metabolic syndrome pandemic. *Arterioscler Thromb Vasc Biol* 2008; **28**: 629–36.

11. Batsis JA, Nieto-Martinez RE, Lopez-Jimenez F. Metabolic syndrome: from global epidemiology to individualized medicine. *Clin Pharmacol Ther* 2007; **82**: 509–24.

12. Valenti L, Dongiovanni P, Fracanzani AL, *et al.* Increased susceptibility to non-alcoholic fatty liver disease in heterozygotes for the mutation responsible for hereditary hemochromatosis. *Dig Liver Dis* 2003; **35**: 172–8.

13. Harrison SA, Neuschwander-Tetri BA. Non-alcoholic fatty liver disease and non-alcoholic steatohepatitis. *Clin Liver Dis* 2004; **8**: 861–79, ix.

14. Marchesini G, Brizi M, Morselli-Labate AM, *et al.* Association of non-alcoholic fatty liver disease with insulin resistance. *Am J Med* 1999; **107**: 450–5.

15. Marchesini G, Brizi M, Bianchi G, *et al.* Non-alcoholic fatty liver disease: a feature of the metabolic syndrome. *Diabetes* 2001; **50**: 1844–50.

16. Neuschwander-Tetri BA. Fatty liver and the metabolic syndrome. *Curr Opin Gastroenterol* 2007; **23**: 193–8.

17. Aigner E, Theurl I, Theurl M, *et al.* Pathways underlying iron accumulation in human non-alcoholic fatty liver disease. *Am J Clin Nutr* 2008; **87**: 1374–83.

18. Facchini FS, Hua NW, Stoohs RA. Effect of iron depletion in carbohydrate-intolerant patients with

clinical evidence of non-alcoholic fatty liver disease. *Gastroenterology* 2002; **122**: 931–9.

19. Valenti L, Fracanzani AL, Dongiovanni P, *et al.* Iron depletion by phlebotomy improves insulin resistance in patients with non-alcoholic fatty liver disease and hyperferritinemia: evidence from a case-control study. *Am J Gastroenterol* 2007; **102**: 1251–8.

20. Fernandez-Real JM, Lopez-Bermejo A, Ricart W. Cross-talk between iron metabolism and diabetes. *Diabetes* 2002; **51**: 2348–54.

21. Swaminathan S, Fonseca VA, Alam MG, Shah SV. The role of iron in diabetes and its complications. *Diabetes Care* 2007; **30**: 1926–33.

22. Turlin B, Mendler MH, Moirand R, Guyader D, Guillygomarc'h A, Deugnier Y. Histologic features of the liver in insulin resistance-associated iron overload. A study of 139 patients. *Am J Clin Pathol* 2001; **116**: 263–70.

23. Non-alcoholic steatohepatitis clinical research network. *Hepatology* 2003; **37**: 244.

Infections and immunity

Persons with hemochromatosis or other iron overload conditions are susceptible to infection by some organisms that rarely cause illness in people with normal body iron stores (Table 7.1). Bacteria require iron for their own metabolism. Hosts with iron overload may thus have increased susceptibility to infection with certain bacteria. *Vibrio vulnificus*[1-14] and *Yersinia* species[11,15-28] are well-known causes of life-threatening infections in persons with iron overload. *Listeria monocytogenes*[11,29-36] and organisms associated with zygomycosis[11,37-39] sometimes cause severe infections in persons who have hemochromatosis, other types of liver disease, diabetes mellitus, immunodeficiency, or skin wounds. Infections with *Escherichia coli* are common in persons without iron overload,[11,40-42] although unusually severe *E. coli* infections have been reported in some patients who had hemochromatosis or iron overload.[40,44] Infections with these organisms also occur in patients without iron overload, many of whom have non-iron conditions that may increase their susceptibility to infection.[2,45-51] Some persons with hemochromatosis or iron overload have abnormal phagocyte function, low levels of one or more blood lymphocyte subsets, or selective deficiency of immunoglobulin isotypes.

Vibrio vulnificus infections

Epidemiology

V. vulnificus is a motile, halophilic, free-living Gram-negative bacillus that grows as normal marine flora and is distributed worldwide in warm, coastal waters. It can cause very serious infections in persons with iron overload, cirrhosis, or decreased immunity.[1-14] *V. vulnificus* causes three major categories of infections: (1) primary septicemia occurs due to ingestion of uncooked oysters or other raw shellfish (or of cooked food contaminated with seawater drippings); (2) wound infections develop after contact of superficial wounds with seawater that contains *V. vulnificus*; and (3) gastroenteritis, associated with raw shellfish consumption, is accompanied by vomiting, diarrhea, abdominal pain, and positive stool cultures for *V. vulnificus*, but blood cultures are negative and there is no associated wound.[45]

In the US, relatively high seawater temperatures promote growth of *V. vulnificus* during late spring and summer months. This is also the time of year in the US when many persons visit ocean regions and consume fresh shellfish. Thus, the majority of marine *Vibrio* infections in the US occurs between April and October, with a peak incidence in September and August.[51,52] The risk of non-food-borne *Vibrio* infections is two to threefold greater in persons who reside in or visit the region of the Gulf of Mexico than the Atlantic or Pacific coast regions; the proportion of cases that occur in inland regions is small.[1,51,52] Other coastal regions where the seawater temperature, salinity, and other factors favor the growth of *V. vulnificus* include coastal areas of Japan, Taiwan, Korea, and Australia.[14]

Host factors markedly increase risk of infection with *V. vulnificus* and other marine vibrios. These include consumption of raw shellfish, contact with seawater during vocational and recreational activities, male sex, and age. Co-morbid conditions that increase risk for infection include liver disease or alcoholism, renal disease or dependency on dialysis, decreased cellular or humoral immunity, malignancy, heart disease, and diabetes mellitus.[6,51,52] Agents that reduce gastric acidity may increase risk of *V. vulnificus* primary septicemia. Nonetheless, approximately one-quarter of persons with non-gastroenteritis *V. vulnificus* infections have no reported co-morbid condition.

Clinical manifestations

Primary septicemia or wound infection due to *V. vulnificus* is usually accompanied by the rapid

Table 7.1. Infections and iron overload disorders

Organism or infection	Iron overload disorder	Typical manifestations	Comments
Vibrio vulnificus	Hemochromatosis, thalassemia	Septicemia, wound infection, extensive tissue necrosis, necrotizing fasciitis; rapid progression; high fatality rate	Common in Gulf of Mexico, Taiwan, Japan, and Australia; most cases due to eating raw shellfish or contact of wounds with seawater; cirrhosis is major risk factor for death
Yersinia enterocolitica	Thalassemia, hemochromatosis, sickle cell disease	Liver abscess, ileocolitis, other abdominal infection	Often occurs during iron chelation therapy
Listeria monocytogenes	Hemochromatosis, other iron overload disorders	Meningitis	Many cases in young children
Escherichia coli	Hemochromatosis	Peritonitis, septicemia; rapid progression; high fatality rate	Cirrhosis is major risk factor
Zygomycosis	Hemochromatosis, other iron overload disorders	Primary site in paranasal sinuses, nose, orbit, face, or brain; arterial invasion, emboli common; rapid progression; high fatality rate	Diabetes mellitus, immune suppression, iron chelation therapy common
Hepatitis B and C viruses	Thalassemia, hemochromatosis, porphyria cutanea tarda	Elevated liver transaminase levels, liver fibrosis, cirrhosis	Major factors in pathogenesis of cirrhosis, primary liver cancer
Tuberculosis	African iron overload	Lung involvement	Role of iron overload not clear

onset and progression of fever, nausea and vomiting, cellulitis, pain, and cutaneous bullae. Almost all patients need hospitalization within a few hours after the onset of symptoms. Blood or tissue cultures are positive in most cases. Management of tissue necrosis and ulceration of the extremities and necrotizing fasciitis may require surgical debridement or amputation. Shock may cause death within hours of presentation. Death occurs in approximately 50% of persons with primary septicemia and about 17% of those with non-foodborne *V. vulnificus* infections.[51,53] The most common co-morbid condition associated with death due to non-gastroenteritis *V. vulnificus* infections is cirrhosis or other liver disease.[6,53]

Early case series of *V. vulnificus* primary septicemia included subjects who also had hemochromatosis.[1,45] A man who had *HFE* C282Y heterozygosity and cirrhosis died of *V. vulnificus* primary septicemia,[7] Three patients with hemochromatosis had *V. vulnificus* wound infections; two different authors reported accounts of one case.[2,10,12,14] Some patients with severe thalassemia have developed *V. vulnificus* infections.[54–57,58] A man treated with chronic hemodialysis developed *V. vulnificus* primary septicemia soon after he was treated with intravenous iron.[8] Diverse liver disorders and renal conditions that perturb iron metabolism may increase risk for *V. vulnificus* infections.[8,59–63] Nonetheless, there are no reports of a case-by-case evaluation for iron overload disorders in large series of *V. vulnificus* infections. In an analysis of a US series of 428 *V. vulnificus* non-foodborne infections, it was not possible to assess hemochromatosis as a risk factor.[51]

Iron and *V. vulnificus* infections

Abundant iron in the blood of humans (especially those with hemochromatosis) and other mammals promotes rapid growth of *V. vulnificus*.[5,6,64–66]. The presence of deferoxamine enhances the in vitro growth and proliferation of *V. vulnificus*.[68] Invasive *V. vulnificus* thrive in tissue from which the bacteria obtain iron from erythrocytes or blood contamination of wounds, or directly from blood, especially that with an elevated iron content. Characteristics of persons with iron overload and related disorders could contribute to serious skin and wound infections.[14] An increased amount of iron is present in skin structures of patients who have iron overload from hemochromatosis or some other condition. Men with C282Y homozygosity have mean hemoglobin values about 6 percent higher than whites without this genotype.[68] Among 299 C282Y homozygotes diagnosed during the HEIRS screening study, transferrin saturation was elevated in 84% of men and 73% of women. In the same study, serum ferritin concentration was increased in 88% and 57% of men and women, respectively.[69] *HFE* C282Y homozygotes with iron overload have decreased expression of hepcidin, an antimicrobial peptide produced by hepatocytes (Chapter 2).[59] It is plausible that decreased amounts of hepcidin contribute to the increased susceptibility to infections by *V. vulnificus* in persons with untreated iron overload,[59] although this is unproven.

Local factors are important in the pathogenesis of *V. vulnificus* wound infection.[70] A metalloprotease in the bacterium damages skin proteins, destroys basement membranes and capillaries, and permits extravasation of blood.[71] The organism produces a cholesterol-binding hemolysin that lyses erythrocytes and releases hemoglobin. This allows the bacteria to use iron from hemoglobin, from heme, or from hematin via the heme receptor HupA.[72] In the presence of extravasated blood, the bacterium could also acquire iron from ferritin.[5,6] *V. vulnificus* also produces the siderophore vulnibactin that may permit the bacterium to acquire iron from transferrin and lactoferrin.[73] *V. vulnificus* can survive as long as 24 hours on skin. This may contribute to the development of wound infections.[74]

There are pathogenic *Vibrio* species other than *V. vulnificus*, including *V. cholerae*, *V. alginolyticus*, *V. parahaemolyticus*, and others. In general, serious morbidity and mortality are less likely to occur in patients with infections due to these species than in patients who have *V. vulnificus* infections. Further, non-*vulnificus Vibrio* infections do not seem to be as closely associated with hosts who have hemochromatosis or iron overload as *V. vulnificus* infections.

Streptococcus pyogenes is the usual bacterium that causes necrotizing fasciitis. There are increasing numbers of reports of patients, some with and others without iron overload, who developed necrotizing fasciitis due to *V. vulnificus* infections.[8,10,12,14,50,51] In a report of 13 patients with necrotizing fasciitis due to *Vibrio* infections, the patients had liver disease, and/or diabetes mellitus, hepatocellular carcinoma, renal insufficiency, or corticosteroid replacement for adrenal insufficiency.[50] The authors did not report information about iron stores in these cases. The patients required urgent fasciotomy and debridement, and some required limited or proximal amputations of digits or limbs.[50]

Prevention

Physicians who treat patients with hemochromatosis, iron overload, liver disease, or other risk factors should educate their patients about *V. vulnificus* infections. Notices at points of sale of seafood, required by law in some areas, should advise consumers of the risks associated with contact with and consumption of raw seafood. Two expert hemochromatosis management groups recommended that patients diagnosed to have hemochromatosis or iron overload should not consume raw shellfish.[75,76] It is also prudent that persons diagnosed to have hemochromatosis or iron overload prevent contact of wounds with seawater, and avoid direct handling of uncooked saltwater finfish or shellfish.[14] Thoroughly cooked seafood uncontaminated with seawater drippings does not contain viable *V. vulnificus*, and is thus safe for consumption. All patients who develop either primary septicemia or wound infections due to *V. vulnificus* should be evaluated for hemochromatosis, iron overload, and liver disorders.[14,76]

Treatment

V. vulnificus can cause fulminant septicemia or damage to skin and limbs; shock and death may occur within a few hours. If infection is suspected, it is advisable to obtain expert consultation urgently to help determine the best possible antibiotic therapy and assessment for possible debridement/fasciotomy. The antibiotics of choice for management of patients with severe *V. vulnificus* infections include intravenous administration of a third-generation cephalosporin such ceftazidime in combination with intravenous or oral doxycycline. An alternative antibiotic choice is combined therapy with cefotaxime and doxycycline. The organism may also be sensitive to ciprofloxacin.[77] Bacterial sensitivity and resistance to different antibiotics may vary from one area to another.

Tetracycline, minocycline, doxycycline, ceftazidime, and levofloxacin are widely regarded as effective antibiotics for *V. vulnificus* infections.[77] Only 14% of patients with non-foodborne vibrio infection received a presumably effective antibiotic at the time treatment was started.[51] In all, only 31% of patients received an antibiotic at any time that was considered to be effective.[51] Persons with *V. vulnificus* infection may die within hours to 6 days after presentation. Thus, one or more presumably effective antibiotics should be administered empirically and without delay, after which antibiotic sensitivity and resistance of the involved vibrio can be determined in vitro. Debridement, fasciotomy, or amputation may be required immediately in some patients with either primary septicemia or wound infections.

Yersinia species infections

Epidemiology

Y. enterocolitica is a Gram-negative bacillus of the family *Enterobacteriaceae*. It often causes fever, septicemia, gastroenteritis, ileocolitis, hepatic abscesses, or bloody diarrhea. Usually, *Y. enterocolitica* is ingested in contaminated water, pork, milk, bean sprouts, or chocolate;[23–25] in one unusual case, *Y. enterocolitica* infection occurred in a patient who had been exposed to raw pork intestines (chitterlings).[78] Whereas *Vibrio* is usually present in warm coastal waters, *Yersinia* is often present in colder climates or as a contaminant in any climate. Approximately 80% of persons with iron overload and *Y. enterocolitica* infections are children less than 5 years of age.[79] Iron chelation therapy with deferoxamine promotes *Yersinia* infections, because these organisms can utilize iron bound to this siderophore derived from *Streptomyces pilosus*.[80–82] It has been reported that the in vivo proliferation of *Y. enterocolitica* is greater in the presence of deferoxamine than deferiprone, an oral iron chelation drug (Chapter 36).[82] Regardless, some patients with severe beta-thalassemia developed *Y. enterocolitica* infection during treatment with deferiprone.[80] Other patients developed *Y. enterocolitica* infection when they were not receiving chelation therapy.[80]

Clinical manifestations

Yersinia can cause severe infections in patients with hemochromatosis,[5,6] including bacteremia[23] and multiple hepatic abscesses.[21,22,25,26] The reports of 46 cases of hepatic abscesses caused by *Yersinia* were reviewed in 2001,[24] and additional cases have been reported.[28] A man with hemochromatosis and cirrhosis developed peritonitis due to *Y. enterocolitica*.[83] A patient with hemochromatosis and diabetes mellitus presented with *Y. pseudotuberculosis* septicemia and serological evidence of concomitant infection with *Y. enterocolitica*.[16]

Y. enterocolitica infections are relatively common in persons with severe beta-thalassemia.[80,84–88] Regional manifestations include abdominal pain, ileocolitis, intussusception, bowel perforation and abscess, mesenteric lymphadenitis, peritonitis, and liver abscess.[80,84–89] Septicemia, osteomyelitis, arthritis, pharyngitis, and meningitis have also been reported.[57,79,80,85,90–92] One child with severe thalassemia developed septicemia due to *Y. pseudotuberculosis*.[93] Iron-loaded patients with beta-thalassemia are at greatly increased risk for severe yersiniosis, even when their body iron burden (as indicated by the serum ferritin level) is only moderately elevated and they are not receiving iron-chelating therapy with deferoxamine.[80]

Some patients with sickle cell disease and iron overload have also developed *Yersinia* infections; some were undergoing iron chelation therapy with deferoxamine.[78,94,95] A patient with Blackfan-Diamond syndrome and transfusion iron overload developed infection with *Y. enterocolitica* while receiving deferoxamine chelation therapy.[96]

Treatment

Antibiotics of choice for the treatment of infections caused by *Yersinia enterocolitica* include the combination of doxycycline and an aminoglycoside such as tobramycin or gentamicin. Second-line antibiotic choices include trimethoprim-sulfamethoxazole or a fluoroquinolone.[77] A longer course of treatment for patients with septicemia or other severe manifestations of infection is needed than for other patients.[85] It is important to verify the in vitro sensitivity and resistance of the *Yersinia* isolate(s), so that the patient can be treated with the most effective antibiotic(s). Bacterial sensitivity and resistance to different antibiotics may vary significantly across cases. Chelation therapy should be discontinued if infection is suspected and not resumed until after antibiotic therapy has been completed.[85]

Listeria monocytogenes infections

Epidemiology and clinical manifestations

Listeria monocytogenes is a Gram-positive bacterium that is widely distributed in the soil, sewage, silage, and feces of healthy humans and animals. L. monocytogenes can cause meningitis or encephalitis, endocarditis, and septic abortion, although infections with this organism are uncommon. L. monocytogenes usually causes infections in children less than 3 years of age, in adults older than age 50 years, and in immunosuppressed individuals of any age. There are a few reports of Listeria meningitis in patients with hemochromatosis or other iron overload disorders.[29,30,32,35] The severity of Listeria infections and its predilection to cause meningitis in persons with iron overload demand that it be considered as a possible pathogen in persons with iron overload who have otherwise unexplained evidence of infection. There are a few reports of listeriosis that occurred in dialysis patients, some of whom had iron overload.[31,33,34,36,47]

Treatment

The antibiotic of first choice for Listeria meningitis is ampicillin. A reasonable second choice antibiotic is trimethoprim-sulfamethoxazole.[77] As is the case in all infections, optimal therapy requires initial suspicion that Listeria is the pathogen, appropriate empiric management, and subsequent adjustment of antibiotic therapy based on evidence of sensitivity or resistance of cultured bacteria to an array of antibiotics.

Escherichia coli infections

Epidemiology

E. coli is a Gram-negative enteric bacillus that is a common cause of urinary tract infections in normal people, in hospitalized patients with urethral catheters, and in men who have urethral obstruction due to prostate hypertrophy. E. coli sepsis from bladder or other urogenital sources is also relatively common. E. coli is a common cause of spontaneous peritonitis, sometimes with septicemia, in persons with cirrhosis of diverse causes.

Host factors in persons with iron overload could increase the risk for serious E. coli infections because this bacterium requires iron for growth.[97-99] Transferrin, ovotransferrin, or lactoferrin unsaturated with iron, or the presence of iron chelators, inhibit E. coli growth in vitro.[100-106] Accordingly, it is plausible that elevated transferrin saturation typical of untreated persons with hemochromatosis and some other forms of iron overload could promote E. coli growth in serum or plasma. Such a phenomenon has been proposed to explain susceptibility of patients with hemochromatosis for V. vulnificus bacteremia.[89] E. coli is also a serious pathogen in persons with thalassemia and iron overload,[57,107-109] and in infants treated with intravenous iron dextran.[110] Nonetheless, no differences were found in the growth rate of E. coli in sera from individuals representing the entire range of transferrin saturation found in humans.[102] One patient with hemochromatosis was treated with phlebotomy before E. coli infection occurred.[111] E. coli is a very common cause of infection in adults, and but it is unknown whether this organism may cause infection more frequently in persons with iron overload than in those without iron overload.

Clinical manifestations

Rapidly progressive E. coli infection, especially bacteremia that arises from a peritoneal source in the absence of frank peritonitis or bowel perforation, occurs in some patients with hemochromatosis or other non-thalassemia iron overload. In addition to iron overload, many patients had or were suspected to have cirrhosis.[112-117] Most of them had a syndrome that is otherwise similar to that of spontaneous bacterial peritonitis that occurs in association with cirrhosis due to non-iron overload causes.[112-117] In the latter circumstances, E. coli is also a common pathogen.[112,117-119] It has been reported that other patients with hemochromatosis or other non-thalassemia iron overload disorders died after presenting with fever, abdominal pain, and shock, although no causative organisms were detected.[40,111,120-122] E. coli infection could explain illness in these patients,[111] although spontaneous Yersinia peritonitis and bacteremia also occur in persons with hemochromatosis or iron overload.[83,123] One patient with E. coli bacteremia also developed E. coli meningitis.[43]

Treatment

The resistance of E. coli to antibiotics is increasing. Resistance to trimethoprim-sulfamethoxazole

(>25% of isolates in some areas) and ampicillin and amoxicillin (50% resistance in some centers) is so great that these antibiotics are not appropriate choices for initial treatment. Increasing resistance of *E. coli* to levofloxacin and ciprofloxacin is also occurring in some areas. Possible antibiotics of choice for management of severe *E. coli* infections include a combination of ampicillin and gentamicin; of piperacillin and tazobactam; and of ticarcillin and clavulanate. Single-agent treatment with imipenem or meropenem may also be satisfactory.[77] If the resistance of *E. coli* isolates in a region or in a specific medical center is known to be relatively low, ciprofloxacin, levofloxacin, or gatifloxacin may be reasonable initial antibiotic choices. The director of the local microbiology laboratory may be able to provide useful data about the sensitivity/resistance to antibiotics that would guide the selection of initial therapy. Typically, results of culture and sensitivity data are available within 48 hours after cultures are established. The initial choice of antibiotic(s) can be adjusted based on these results. We found no comprehensive reports of the characteristics of pathogenic *E. coli* strains isolated from patients with hemochromatosis and iron overload.

Zygomycosis
Epidemiology

The term zygomycosis denotes infections due to any member of the zygomycetes family of fungi. These are fast-growing saprophytic fungi of worldwide distribution; more than 660 species have been described. The fungi or their manifestations that have been reported as pathogens in persons with hemochromatosis or other iron overload disorders are known as *Cunninghamella* and mucormycosis.[37–39,124] Overall, most affected patients have diabetes mellitus, immunosuppression, organ transplant, or lymphoma or leukemia. Many patients who develop zygomycosis are receiving corticosteroid or azathioprine treatment when infection occurs. Some patients who were being treated with deferoxamine chelation therapy to alleviate iron overload have developed zygomycosis. Some patients treated with bone marrow transplantation for management of severe thalassemia have developed mucormycosis.[125]

Clinical manifestations

Sites of infection typically include the paranasal sinuses, nose, orbit, face, or brain; in some cases, the primary infection occurs in the lungs, gastrointestinal tract, or skin. Zygomycetes often invade arteries, thus leading to embolization and necrosis of adjacent or distal tissues. The infection may be fulminant and lethal, even when the diagnosis is established quickly and antifungal therapy is initiated promptly.

Treatment

Posaconazole and lipid formulations of amphotericin may be the best initial antibiotics of choice to treat zygomycosis/mucormycosis.[77] Surgical debridement is also often required.

Helicobacter pylori infections

Strong associations have been found between infection with *H. pylori* and iron deficiency in children. Accordingly, it was plausible to hypothesize that *H. pylori* could cause iron depletion or deficiency in persons with *HFE* C282Y homozygosity and act as a "modifier" of the expression of hemochromatosis homozygotes by decreasing the amount of storage iron. This hypothesis was tested in a comparison of hemoglobin concentration, erythrocyte mean corpuscular volume, transferrin saturation, serum ferritin concentration, and serial phlebotomy therapy in 76 women and 79 men with C282Y homozygosity, subgrouped as men and women who were seropositive or seronegative for *H. pylori*. The results of the study revealed no significance difference between the same-sex groups of seronegative and seropositive homozygotes. The authors concluded that *H. pylori* infection does not modify the iron stores of C282Y homozygotes.[126]

Other infections

Bacterial infections due to diverse organisms other than those reviewed above are major causes of morbidity and mortality in patients with severe beta-thalassemia and iron overload.[57,127–129] Chronic viral hepatitis B and C, common in persons with severe beta-thalassemia due predominantly to chronic erythrocyte transfusion, increase risks for cirrhosis and primary liver cancer.[130] In Italian patients with porphyria cutanea tarda, the prevalence of hepatitis C virus infection is high, and hepatitis C is probably the main pathogenetic factor of the liver disease in such patients.[131] In contrast, hepatitis G infection was unrelated to liver injury in most patients with thalassemia and iron overload.[132] Chronic hepatitis B and C occur as coincidental infections in patients with hemochromatosis,[133] and also increase risks for cirrhosis and primary liver cancer.[134] Tuberculosis is a common infection in Native Africans with iron overload due to chronic ingestion of traditional beer.[135–137] Increased iron may play a role in the pathogenesis of tuberculosis in such subjects.[135–137] Elevated surrogate measures of body iron may be associated with adverse outcomes of human immunodeficiency virus-1 infection.[138]

Phagocytes

Neutrophils

Lactoferrin is an iron-binding glycoprotein synthesized largely by neutrophils and localized in cytoplasmic granules (Chapter 2).[139] Neutrophils employ lactoferrin to deprive ingested microbes of iron, and to kill them with oxyradicals generated from the iron. In hemochromatosis, the lactoferrin content of blood neutrophils (regardless of the presence or absence of cirrhosis) measured by diverse techniques is slightly decreased.[139–144] Histochemical and flow cytometric analyses of neutrophils in persons with hemochromatosis suggest that the decreased lactoferrin content of these cells could be explained by a lactoferrin-deficient subpopulation of neutrophils.[139,143] Whether this is due to decreased lactoferrin synthesis, to neutrophil degranulation, or to other causes is unknown.[139] The lactoferrin content of neutrophils, the molecular weight and isoelectric point of the protein, the dissociation of its complex with iron at acidic pH, its binding to isolated monocytes, and its uptake by the mouse reticuloendothelial system were similar in patients with hemochromatosis and in control subjects.[142] After therapeutic phlebotomy to achieve iron depletion, neutrophil lactoferrin concentrations in persons with hemochromatosis are reduced further, as they are in non-hemochromatosis subjects with iron deficiency.[140] This could be explained by structural, biosynthetic, or functional changes in neutrophils that occur in iron deficiency.[139]

Deferoxamine alters microbicidal properties of neutrophils and modulates their interaction with *Y. enterocolitica*. This could explain in part the dual role of deferoxamine in the pathogenesis of *Yersinia* infection, namely growth support of the pathogen and modulation of the antimicrobial host response.[81] Deferoxamine did not alter calcium signaling in neutrophils but transiently increased phagocytosis of *Y. enterocolitica*. Higher counts of viable bacteria in neutrophils and increased chemiluminescence signals after stimulation with *Y. enterocolitica* were observed in the presence of neutrophils. Deferoxamine reduced the chemiluminescence signal elicited individually by zymosan, phorbol myristate acetate, and formyl-met-leu-phe. Comparison of plasmid-cured with plasmid-harboring *Y. enterocolitica* revealed that plasmid-encoded determinants modulate phagocytosis, chemiluminescence signal, and bactericidal properties of neutrophils.[81]

The mean phagocytic capacity for *Staphylococcus aureus* and the mean chemotactic responsiveness of neutrophils from 16 patients with hemochromatosis were significantly lower than those of control subjects.[145] Phagocytosis of *S. aureus* by neutrophils of another patient with hemochromatosis was similar to that of control subjects. In this subject, addition of iron in vitro decreased the phagocytic capacity of the neutrophils.[30]

Monocytes and macrophages

Lactoferrin released from neutrophils can transport iron to monocytes and macrophages that express surface lactoferrin receptors.[139] Monocyte surface and cytoplasmic lactoferrin evaluated using immunofluorescence and flow cytometry is less prominent in persons with hemochromatosis than it is in control subjects.[146] This could be an indirect consequence of the decreased quantities of neutrophil lactoferrin in hemochromatosis, or to other abnormalities.[139] The ability of macrophages from patients with hemochromatosis and control subjects to bind and ingest lactoferrin and to process the iron bound to the protein were similar.[142]

The mean phagocytic capacity for *S. aureus* and the mean bactericidal activity of monocytes from 15 patients with hemochromatosis were significantly lower than those of control subjects.[145] In another study, the capacity of monocytes and macrophages of patients with hemochromatosis to phagocytose *Staphylococcus aureus* was decreased. The phagocytosis defect was observed in all patients studied, and was independent of the magnitude of iron overload, age, or extent of liver injury.[147] The abnormal phagocytosis in vitro cannot be attributed to a different level of expression of receptors involved in phagocytosis or to Fc gamma RIIa polymorphism.[148] The monocytes of a patient with hemochromatosis who developed *L. monocytogenes* meningitis also had reduced phagocytic capacity for *S. aureus*. Phagocytic function returned to normal after a series of therapeutic phlebotomies, and the addition of iron in vitro decreased the phagocytic capacity of the monocytes.[30]

Blood lymphocyte subsets and iron phenotype

In humans, numbers of blood CD8+ T-lymphocytes in humans are linked to the HLA class I region on the short arm of chromosome 6.[149,150] In normal persons and in C282Y homozygotes, CD8+ and total blood lymphocyte counts are significantly associated with certain common HLA–A and –B alleles and haplotypes.[151,152] Persons with hemochromatosis have significantly different CD8+ blood T-lymphocyte subsets than control subjects,[153] and high CD4+/CD8+ lymphocyte ratios precede the development of severe iron overload in hemochromatosis.[154,155] CD8+ and total blood lymphocyte counts at diagnosis in C282Y homozygotes are negatively associated with serum ferritin levels at diagnosis, degree of iron overload, and hepatic cirrhosis.[151] Lymphocyte surface and cytoplasmic lactoferrin evaluated using immunofluorescence and flow cytometry is less prominent in persons with hemochromatosis than it is in control subjects.[146]

Interleukin-6, produced predominantly by lymphocytes and macrophages, induces expression of hepcidin, a potent inhibitor of iron absorption. Although levels of hepcidin are significantly decreased in persons with *HFE* hemochromatosis,[156] any direct role of lymphocytes in hepcidin regulation in hemochromatosis is unreported. It is possible that there is an interaction between HLA and *HFE* in CD8+ T-lymphocytes, although evidence that *HFE* is expressed in lymphocytes is conflicting.[157–160] In HfeRag1(-/-) and beta2mRag1(-/-) double knockout mice, blood lymphocyte numbers were significantly associated with iron overload severity in the absence of functional HFE protein.[161] Using analyses of extended chromosome 6p haplotypes, however, a candidate region associated with blood CD8+ T-lymphocyte numbers has been identified that may also contain a gene that modifies the phenotype of C282Y homozygotes.[152] Such haplotypes may contain alleles of a putative gene(s) suggested by linkage disequilibrium and genome scan techniques,[162,163] but it is improbable

that the HLA alleles or lymphocyte counts themselves directly determine iron phenotypes.[151,152]

Humoral immunity

Severe infections due to a variety of bacteria have been reported to occur in patients with hemochromatosis. In some C282Y homozygotes, increased susceptibility to infections is associated with deficiencies of serum IgG typical of common variable immunodeficiency (CVID) or selective immunoglobulin (Ig) G subclass deficiency (IgGSD).[164] Thirty percent of unselected Alabama C282Y homozygous probands had CVID or IgGSD characterized by various Ig isotype deficiency patterns involving IgG_1, IgG_3, and IgG_4 subclasses.[164] IgG_2 deficiency or IgA deficiency was not observed,[164] although hemochromatosis and IgA deficiency have been reported to occur in different members of the same family.[165] IgM deficiency occurs in ~2% of C282Y homozygotes.[164] There has been little study of the prevalence of positivity for specific antibody activity in persons with hemochromatosis. In one study, the prevalence of anti-*Yersinia* antibodies in patients with hemochromatosis and *HFE* C282Y homozygosity was not increased.[166]

Approximately 10% of hemochromatosis probands with CVID or IgGSD phenotypes had frequent, severe, or recurrent infections, especially bacterial infections of the upper and lower respiratory tract or *Varicella* zoster, whereas no probands without CVID or IgGSD reported having such infections.[164] Male: female ratios and mean values of age, transferrin saturation and serum ferritin levels at diagnosis and units of phlebotomy to induce iron depletion were similar in probands with or without CVID or IgGSD. Phlebotomy had no apparent effect on IgG levels in probands with CVID or IgGSD.[164] There was concordance of Ig and hemochromatosis phenotypes in probands and respective HLA-identical siblings.[164] The prevalence of C282Y homozygosity is also significantly greater in CVID and IgGSD index cases than in control subjects.[164]

These observations can be explained by the significantly greater frequencies of the common "ancestral" hemochromatosis haplotype HLA-A*03, B*07, and the haplotype HLA-A*01, B*08 in C282Y homozygotes, and in CVID and IgGSD index patients than in control subjects, and by the common occurrence of putative CVID or IgGSD allele(s) on haplotypes bearing *HFE* C282Y.[164,167,168] There are multiple distinct susceptibility loci on chromosome 6p, especially in the HLA class II and III regions, that correspond to specific patterns of Ig deficiency, and each has an independent effect on the Ig deficiency phenotype; some are recessive and others are dominant.[169–172] Although there are at least two IgA deficiency susceptibility loci on chromosome 6p,[171,173,174] these may occur infrequently on chromosome 6p haplotypes that include *HFE* C282Y because IgA deficiency was not observed in C282Y homozygotes with CVID or IgGSD phenotypes.[164] Mutations in the tumor necrosis factor receptor superfamily gene *TNFRSF13B* (chromosome 17p11.2) that encodes TACI are also associated with CVID and IgA deficiency phenotypes,[175,176] and mannose-binding lectin (*MBL2*) alleles on chromosome 10q11.2–q21 are associated with earlier age of onset of manifestations of antibody deficiency and increased risk of autoimmunity.[177] To date, *TNFRSF13B* or *MBL2* mutations have not been reported in persons with hemochromatosis.

Serum IgG subclass levels should be quantified in *HFE* C282Y homozygotes, especially those with frequent, severe, or recurrent infections or autoimmune disorders. Monthly replacement therapy with intravenous IgG should be considered in those found to have CVID or IgGSD phenotypes.[164] Therapeutic phlebotomy to achieve and maintain low body iron stores may reduce the risk of certain infections due to its salutary effects on serum iron and ferritin levels, leukocyte lactoferrin content, and T-lymphocyte subsets.[151] Indicated vaccinations, appropriate management of diabetes mellitus and hepatic disorders, and avoiding consumption of raw shellfish may also reduce infection risks.[76]

References

1. Blake PA, Merson MH, Weaver RE, Hollis DG, Heublein PC. Disease caused by a marine *Vibrio*. Clinical characteristics and epidemiology. *N Engl J Med* 1979; **300**: 1–5.

2. Bonner JR, Coker AS, Berryman CR, Pollock HM. Spectrum of *Vibrio* infections in a Gulf Coast community. *Ann Intern Med* 1983; **99**: 464–9.

3. McManus R, Gordon RS. Highly invasive new bacterium isolated from US East Coast waters. *JAMA* 1984; **251**: 323–5.

4. Muench KH. Hemochromatosis and infection: alcohol and iron, oysters and sepsis. *Am J Med* 1989; **87**: 40N–3N.

5. Bullen JJ, Spalding PB, Ward CG, Gutteridge JM. Hemochromatosis, iron, and septicemia caused by *Vibrio vulnificus*. *Arch Intern Med* 1991; **151**: 1606–9.

6. Bullen JJ. Bacterial infections in hemochromatosis. In: Barton JC, Edwards CQ, eds. *Hemochromatosis: Genetics, Pathophysiology, Diagnosis, and Treatment*. Cambridge, Cambridge University Press. 2000; 381–6.

7. Gerhard GS, Levin KA, Price GJ, Wojnar MM, Chorney MJ, Belchis DA. *Vibrio vulnificus* septicemia in a patient with the hemochromatosis *HFE* C282Y mutation. *Arch Pathol Lab Med* 2001; **125**: 1107–9.

8. Barton JC, Coghlan ME, Reymann MT, Ozbirn TW, Acton RT. *Vibrio vulnificus* infection in a hemodialysis patient receiving intravenous iron therapy. *Clin Infect Dis* 2003; **37**: e63–e67.

9. Barton JC, Ratard RC. *Vibrio vulnificus* bacteremia associated with chronic lymphocytic leukemia, hypogammaglobulinemia, and hepatic cirrhosis: relation to host and exposure factors in 252 *V. vulnificus* infections reported in Louisiana. *Am J Med Sci* 2006; **332**: 216–20.

10. Byrnes JM. Necrotizing fasciitis: a common problem in Darwin. *Int J Low Extrem Wounds* 2006; **5**: 271–76.

11. Khan FA, Fisher MA, Khakoo RA. Association of hemochromatosis with infectious diseases: expanding spectrum. *Int J Infect Dis* 2007; **11**: 482–7.

12. Ralph A, Currie BJ. *Vibrio vulnificus* and *V. parahaemolyticus* necrotising fasciitis in fishermen visiting an estuarine tropical northern Australian location. *J Infect* 2007; **54**: e111–14.

13. Kim DM, Cho HS, Kang JI, Kim HS, Park CY. Deferasirox plus ciprofloxacin combination therapy after rapid diagnosis of *Vibrio vulnificus* sepsis using real-time polymerase chain reaction. *J Infect* 2008; **57**: 489–92.

14. Barton JC, Acton RT. Hemochromatosis and *Vibrio vulnificus* wound infections. *J Clin Gastroenterol* 2009; **43**: 890–3.

15. Robins-Browne RM, Rabson AR, Koornhof HJ. Generalized infection with *Yersinia enterocolitica* and the role of iron. *Contrib Microbiol Immunol* 1979; **5**: 277–82.

16. Abbott M, Galloway A, Cunningham JL. Haemochromatosis presenting with a double *Yersinia* infection. *J Infect* 1986; **13**: 143–5.

17. Conway SP, Dudley N, Sheridan P, Ross H. Haemochromatosis and aldosterone deficiency presenting with *Yersinia pseudotuberculosis* septicaemia. *Postgrad Med J* 1989; **65**: 174–6.

18. Olesen LL, Ejlertsen T, Paulsen SM, Knudsen PR. Liver abscesses due to *Yersinia enterocolitica* in patients

with haemochromatosis. *J Intern Med* 1989; **225**: 351–4.

19. Munoz MT, Garcia PJ, Collazos GJ, de Miguel PJ. [*Yersinia enterocolitica* bacteremia and hemochromatosis.] *Rev Clin Esp* 1991; **189**: 92.

20. Vadillo M, Corbella X, Pac V, Fernandez-Viladrich P, Pujol R. Multiple liver abscesses due to *Yersinia enterocolitica* discloses primary hemochromatosis: three cases reports and review. *Clin Infect Dis* 1994; **18**: 938–41.

21. Collazos J, Guerra E, Fernandez A, Mayo J, Martinez E. Miliary liver abscesses and skin infection due to *Yersinia enterocolitica* in a patient with unsuspected hemochromatosis. *Clin Infect Dis* 1995; **21**: 223–4.

22. Abdelli N, Thiefin G, Chevalier P, Zeitoun P. [Spontaneously regressive liver abscess caused by *Yersinia enterocolitica* revealing genetic hemochromatosis: a second case.] *Gastroenterol Clin Biol* 1996; **20**: 212–13.

23. Piroth L, Meyer P, Bielefeld P, Besancenot JF. [*Yersinia* bacteremia and iron overload.] *Rev Med Interne* 1997; **18**: 932–8.

24. Bergmann TK, Vinding K, Hey H. Multiple hepatic abscesses due to *Yersinia enterocolitica* infection secondary to primary haemochromatosis. *Scand J Gastroenterol* 2001; **36**: 891–5.

25. Hopfner M, Nitsche R, Rohr A, Harms D, Schubert S, UR Folsch. *Yersinia enterocolitica* infection with multiple liver abscesses uncovering a primary hemochromatosis. *Scand J Gastroenterol* 2001; **36**: 220–4.

26. Mennecier D, Lapprand M, Hernandez E, *et al.* [Liver abscesses due to *Yersinia pseudotuberculosis* discloses a genetic hemochromatosis.] *Gastroenterol Clin Biol* 2001; **25**: 1113–15.

27. Benbrika S, Boukari L, Stirnemann J, *et al.* [A case of yersiniasis with multiple liver abscesses.] *Rev Med Interne* 2005; **26**: 151–2.

28. Crosbie J, Varma J, Mansfield J. *Yersinia enterocolitica* infection in a patient with hemochromatosis masquerading as proximal colon cancer with liver metastases: report of a case. *Dis Colon Rectum* 2005; **48**: 390–2.

29. Sinkovics JG, Cormia F, Plager C. Hemochromatosis and *Listeria* infection. *Arch Intern Med* 1980; **140**: 284.

30. van Asbeck BS, Verbrugh HA, van Oost BA, Marx JJ, Imhof HW, Verhoef J. *Listeria monocytogenes* meningitis and decreased phagocytosis associated with iron overload. *Br Med J (Clin Res Ed)* 1982; **284**: 542–4.

31. Mossey RT, Sondheimer J. Listeriosis in patients with long-term hemodialysis and transfusional iron overload. *Am J Med* 1985; **79**: 397–400.

32. Henrion J, de Neve A, Heller F. [Bacterial septicemia: an unrecognized complication of hemochromatosis. Study of 3 cases and review of the literature.] *Acta Clin Belg* 1986; **41**: 10–17.

33. Calubiran OV, Horiuchi J, Klein NC, Cunha BA. *Listeria monocytogenes* meningitis in a human immunodeficiency virus-positive patient undergoing hemodialysis. *Heart Lung* 1990; **19**: 21–3.

34. Hoen B, Kessler M. [Infectious risks in patients with renal failure on hemodialysis. Importance of iron overload and deferoxamine.] *Presse Med* 1991; **20**: 681–2.

35. Manso C, Rivas I, Peraire J, Vidal F, Richart C. Fatal *Listeria* meningitis, endocarditis and pericarditis in a patient with haemochromatosis. *Scand J Infect Dis* 1997; **29**: 308–9.

36. Seeger W, Hugo F, Heine C, Handrick W. [Listeriosis in a patient with hemodialysis and iron overload.] *Med Klin (Munich)* 2007; **102**: 483–5.

37. Brennan RO, Crain BJ, Proctor AM, Durack DT. *Cunninghamella*: a newly recognized cause of rhinocerebral mucormycosis. *Am J Clin Pathol* 1983; **80**: 98–102.

38. Van Johnson E, Kline LB, Julian BA, Garcia JH. Bilateral cavernous sinus thrombosis due to mucormycosis. *Arch Ophthalmol* 1988; **106**: 1089–92.

39. McNab AA, McKelvie P. Iron overload is a risk factor for zygomycosis. *Arch Ophthalmol* 1997; **115**: 919–21.

40. MacSween RNM. Acute abdominal crises, circulatory collapse and sudden death in haemochromatosis. *Q J Med* 1966; **35**: 589–98.

41. Christopher GW. *Escherichia coli* bacteremia, meningitis, and hemochromatosis. *Arch Intern Med* 1985; **145**: 1908.

42. Corke PJ, McLean AS, Stewart D, Adams S. Overwhelming Gram-negative septic shock in haemochromatosis. *Anaesth Intensive Care* 1995; **23**: 346–9.

43. Christopher GW. *Escherichia coli* bacteremia, meningitis, and hemochromatosis. *Arch Intern Med* 1985; **145**: 1908.

44. Corke PJ, McLean AS, Stewart D, Adams S. Overwhelming Gram-negative septic shock in haemochromatosis. *Anaesth Intensive Care* 1995; **23**: 346–9.

45. Klontz KC, Lieb S, Schreiber M, Janowski HT, Baldy LM, Gunn RA. Syndromes of *Vibrio vulnificus* infections. Clinical and epidemiologic features in Florida cases, 1981–1987. *Ann Intern Med* 1988; **109**: 318–23.

46. Kumamoto KS, Vukich DJ. Clinical infections of *Vibrio vulnificus*: a case report and review of the literature. *J Emerg Med* 1998; **16**: 61–6.

47. Bufano G, Ceruti T, Ferrari L, Pecchini F. Listeriosis in a patient with long-term hemodialysis but without iron overload. *Nephron* 1995; **69**: 356.

48. Mead PS, Slutsker L, Dietz V, *et al.* Food-related illness and death in the United States. *Emerg Infect Dis* 1999; **5**: 607–25.

49. Johnson RW, Arnett FC. A fatal case of *Vibrio vulnificus* presenting as septic arthritis. *Arch Intern Med* 2001; **161**: 2616–18.

50. Tsai YH, Hsu RW, Huang KC, *et al.* Systemic *Vibrio* infection presenting as necrotizing fasciitis and sepsis. A series of 13 cases. *J Bone Joint Surg Am* 2004; **86-A:** 2497–502.

51. Dechet AM, Yu PA, Koram N, Painter J. Non-foodborne *Vibrio* infections: an important cause of morbidity and mortality in the United States, 1997–2006. *Clin Infect Dis* 2008; **46**: 970–6.

52. Hlady WG, Klontz KC. The epidemiology of *Vibrio* infections in Florida, 1981–1993. *J Infect Dis* 1996; **173**: 1176–83.

53. Hlady WG, Mullen RC, Hopkin RS. *Vibrio vulnificus* from raw oysters. Leading cause of reported deaths from foodborne illness in Florida. *J Fla Med Assoc* 1993; **80**: 536–8.

54. Shih YT, Peng CT, Tsai CH, Tsai FJ. [Beta-thalassemia major complicated with *Vibrio vulnificus* septicemia: report of one case.] *Zhonghua Min Guo Xiao Er Ke Yi Xue Hui Za Zhi* 1994; **35**: 84–9.

55. Chang JJ, Sheen IS, Peng SM, Chen PC, Wu CS, Leu HS. *Vibrio vulnificus* infection–report of 8 cases and review of cases in Taiwan. *Changgeng Yi Xue Za Zhi* 1994; **17**: 339–46.

56. Kuo CH, Dai ZK, Wu JR, Hsieh TJ, Hung CH, Hsu JH. Septic arthritis as the initial manifestation of fatal *Vibrio vulnificus* septicemia in a patient with thalassemia and iron overload. *Pediatr Blood Cancer* 2009; **53**: 1156–8.

57. Wang SC, Lin KH, Chern JP, *et al.* Severe bacterial infection in transfusion-dependent patients with thalassemia major. *Clin Infect Dis* 2003; **37**: 984–8.

58. Katz BZ. *Vibrio vulnificus* meningitis in a boy with thalassemia after eating raw oysters. *Pediatrics* 1988; **82**: 784–6.

59. Ashrafian H. Hepcidin: the missing link between hemochromatosis and infections. *Infect Immun* 2003; **71**: 6693–700.

60. Gholami P, Lew SQ, Klontz KC. Raw shellfish consumption among renal disease patients. A risk factor for severe Vibrio vulnificus infection. *Am J Prev Med* 1998; **15**: 243–5.

61. Stabellini N, Camerani A, Lambertini D, *et al.* Fatal sepsis from *Vibrio vulnificus* in a hemodialyzed patient. *Nephron* 1998; **78**: 221–4.

62. Wang SM, Liu CC, Chiou YY, Yang HB, Chen CT. *Vibrio vulnificus* infection complicated by acute respiratory distress syndrome in a child with nephrotic syndrome. *Pediatr Pulmonol* 2000; **29**: 400–3.

63. Ruiz CC, Agraharkar M. Unusual marine pathogens causing cellulitis and bacteremia in hemodialysis patients: report of two cases and review of the literature. *Hemodial Int* 2003; **7**: 356–9.

64. Wright AC, Simpson LM, Oliver JD. Role of iron in the pathogenesis of *Vibrio vulnificus* infections. *Infect Immun* 1981; **34**: 503–7.

65. Hor LI, Chang TT, Wang ST. Survival of *Vibrio vulnificus* in whole blood from patients with chronic liver diseases: association with phagocytosis by neutrophils and serum ferritin levels. *J Infect Dis* 1999; **179**: 275–8.

66. Hor LI, Chang YK, Chang CC, Lei HY, Ou JT. Mechanism of high susceptibility of iron-overloaded mouse to *Vibrio vulnificus* infection. *Microbiol Immunol* 2000; **44**: 871–8.

67. Neupane GP, Kim DM. Comparison of the effects of deferasirox, deferiprone, and deferoxamine on the growth and virulence of *Vibrio vulnificus*. *Transfusion* 2009; **49**: 1762–9.

68. Barton JC, Bertoli LF, Rothenberg BE. Peripheral blood erythrocyte parameters in hemochromatosis: evidence for increased erythrocyte hemoglobin content. *J Lab Clin Med* 2000; **135**: 96–104.

69. Adams PC, Reboussin DM, Barton JC, *et al.* Hemochromatosis and iron-overload screening in a racially diverse population. *N Engl J Med* 2005; **352**: 1769–78.

70. Beckman EN, Leonard GL, Castillo LE, Genre CF, Pankey GA. Histopathology of marine vibrio wound infections. *Am J Clin Pathol* 1981; **76**: 765–72.

71. Shinoda S. [Pathogenic factors of vibrios with special emphasis on *Vibrio vulnificus*.] *Yakugaku Zasshi* 2005; **125**: 531–47.

72. Litwin CM, Byrne BL. Cloning and characterization of an outer membrane protein of *Vibrio vulnificus* required for heme utilization: regulation of expression and determination of the gene sequence. *Infect Immun* 1998; **66**: 3134–41.

73. Kim CM, Park RY, Park JH, *et al. Vibrio vulnificus* vulnibactin, but not metalloprotease VvpE, is essentially required for iron-uptake from human holotransferrin. *Biol Pharm Bull* 2006; **29**: 911–18.

74. Colodner R, Chazan B, Kopelowitz J, Keness Y, Raz R. Unusual portal of entry of *Vibrio vulnificus*: evidence of its prolonged survival on the skin. *Clin Infect Dis* 2002; **34**: 714–15.

75. Witte DL, Crosby WH, Edwards CQ, Fairbanks VF, Mitros FA. Practice guideline development task force of the College of American Pathologists. Hereditary hemochromatosis. *Clin Chim Acta* 1996; **245**: 139–200.

76. Barton JC, McDonnell SM, Adams PC, *et al.* Management of hemochromatosis. Hemochromatosis Management Working Group. *Ann Intern Med* 1998; **129**: 932–9.

77. Gilbert DN, Moellering RC, Eliopoulos GM, Sande MA, eds. *The Sanford Guide to Antimicrobial Therapy*, 38th edn. Sperryville, Antimicrobial Therapy Inc. 2008.

78. Stoddard JJ, Wechsler DS, Nataro JP, Casella JF. *Yersinia enterocolitica* infection in a patient with sickle cell disease after exposure to chitterlings. *Am J Pediatr Hematol Oncol* 1994; **16**: 153–5.

79. Lafleur L, Hammerberg O, Delage G, Pai CH. *Yersinia enterocolitica* infection in children: 4 years experience in the Montreal urban community. *Contrib Microbiol Immunol* 1979; **5**: 298–303.

80. Adamkiewicz TV, Berkovitch M, Krishnan C, Polsinelli C, Kermack D, Olivieri NF. Infection due to *Yersinia enterocolitica* in a series of patients with beta-thalassemia: incidence and predisposing factors. *Clin Infect Dis* 1998; **27**: 1362–6.

81. Ewald JH, Heesemann J, Rudiger H, Autenrieth IB. Interaction of polymorphonuclear leukocytes with *Yersinia enterocolitica*: role of the *Yersinia* virulence plasmid and modulation by the iron-chelator desferrioxamine B. *J Infect Dis* 1994; **170**: 140–50.

82. Lesic B, Foulon J, Carniel E. Comparison of the effects of deferiprone versus deferoxamine on growth and virulence of *Yersinia enterocolitica*. *Antimicrob Agents Chemother* 2002; **46**: 1741–5.

83. Capron JP, Capron-Chivrac D, Tossou H, Delamarre J, Eb F. Spontaneous *Yersinia enterocolitica* peritonitis in idiopathic hemochromatosis. *Gastroenterology* 1984; **87**: 1372–5.

84. Green NS. *Yersinia* infections in patients with homozygous beta-thalassemia associated with iron overload and its treatment. *Pediatr Hematol Oncol* 1992; **9**: 247–54.

85. Cherchi GB, Pacifico L, Cossellu S, *et al.* Prospective study of *Yersinia enterocolitica* infection in thalassemic patients. *Pediatr Infect Dis J* 1995; **14**: 579–84.

86. Hansen MG, Pearl G, Levy M. Intussusception due to *Yersinia enterocolitica* enterocolitis in a patient with beta-thalassemia. *Arch Pathol Lab Med* 2001; **125**: 1486–8.

87. Pallister C, Rotstein OD. *Yersinia enterocolitica* as a cause of intra-abdominal abscess: the role of iron. *Can J Surg* 2001; **44**: 135–6.

88. Greco L, Marino F, Gentile A, Catalano G, Angilletta D. *Yersinia enterocolitica* ileocolitis in beta-thalassemic patients. *Colorectal Dis* 2006; **8**: 525.

89. Bullen JJ, Spalding PB, Ward CG, Gutteridge JM. Hemochromatosis, iron and septicemia caused by *Vibrio vulnificus*. *Arch Intern Med* 1991; **151**: 1606–9.

90. Hewstone AS, Davidson GP. *Yersinia enterocolitica* septicaemia with arthritis in a thalassaemic child. *Med J Aust* 1972; **1**: 1035–8.

91. Thirumoorthi MC, Dajani AS. *Yersinia enterocolitica* osteomyelitis in a child. *Am J Dis Child* 1978; **132**: 578–80.

92. De Virgiliis S, Dessi S, Melis R, Cao A. Fatal *Yersinia enterocolitica* meningitis in thalassemia major. *Boll Ist Sieroter Milan* 1984; **63**: 171–2.

93. Gordts B, Rummens E, deMeirleir L, Butzler JP. *Yersinia pseudotuberculosis* septicaemia in thalassaemia major. *Lancet* 1984; **1**: 41–2.

94. Pierron H, Gillet R, Perrimond H, Broudeur JC, Soudry G. [*Yersinia* infection and hemoglobin disorder. Apropos of 4 cases.] *Pediatrie* 1990; **45**: 379–82.

95. Blei F, Puder DR. *Yersinia enterocolitica* bacteremia in a chronically transfused patient with sickle cell anemia. Case report and review of the literature. *Am J Pediatr Hematol Oncol* 1993; **15**: 430–4.

96. Kruger N, Kraus C, Tillmann W, Schroter W. [Frequent occurrence of *Yersinia* infection in hemosiderosis.] *Monatsschr Kinderheilkd* 1985; **133**: 876–8.

97. Stuart SJ, Greenwood KT, Luke RK. Iron-suppressible production of hydroxamate by *Escherichia coli* isolates. *Infect Immun* 1982; **36**: 870–5.

98. Neilands JB. Parallels in the mode of regulation of iron assimilation in all living species. In: Ponka P, Schulman HM, Woodworth RC, eds. *Iron Transport and Storage*. Boca Raton, CRC Press, Inc. 1990; 42–54.

99. Ouyang Z, Isaacson R. Identification and characterization of a novel ABC iron transport system, fit, in *Escherichia coli*. *Infect Immun* 2006; **74**: 6949–56.

100. Bullen JJ. Iron-binding proteins and other factors in milk responsible for resistance to *Escherichia coli*. *Ciba Found Symp* 1976; 149–69.

101. Rogers HJ. Ferric iron and the antibacterial effects of horse 7S antibodies to *Escherichia coli* O111. *Immunology* 1976; **30**: 425–33.

102. Baltimore RS, Shedd DG, Pearson HA. Effect of iron saturation on the bacteriostasis of human serum: in vivo does not correlate with in vitro saturation. *J Pediatr* 1982; **101**: 519–23.

103. Rivier D, Page N, Isliker H. Synergism between iron chelators and complement for bactericidal activity. *Ann Immunol (Paris)* 1983; **134C**: 25–30.

104. Chart H, Buck M, Stevenson P, Griffiths E. Iron regulated outer membrane proteins of *Escherichia coli*: variations in expression due to the chelator used to restrict the availability of iron. *J Gen Microbiol* 1986; **132**: 1373–8.

105. Rainard P. Bacteriostasis of *Escherichia coli* by bovine lactoferrin, transferrin, and immunoglobulins (IgG1, IgG2, IgM) acting alone or in combination. *Vet Microbiol* 1986; **11**: 103–15.

106. Brock JH, Liceaga J, Kontoghiorghes GJ. The effect of synthetic iron chelators on bacterial growth in human serum. *FEMS Microbiol Immunol* 1988; **1**: 55–60.

107. Peng CT, Tsai CH, Wang JH, Chiu CF, Chow KC. Bacterial infection in patients with transfusion-dependent beta-thalassemia in central Taiwan. *Acta Paediatr Taiwan* 2000; **41**: 318–21.

108. Wanachiwanawin W. Infections in E-beta-thalassemia. *J Pediatr Hematol Oncol* 2000; **22**: 581–7.

109. Alebouyeh M, Moussavi F. Occurrence of overwhelming Gram-negative infections in splenectomised patients with thalassaemia major. *Eur J Pediatr* 2003; **162**: 637–8.

110. Becroft DM, Dix MR, Farmer K. Intramuscular iron-dextran and susceptibility of neonates to bacterial infections. In vitro studies. *Arch Dis Child* 1977; **52**: 778–81.

111. Zala G. [Acute abdomen with irreversible shock, a rare but typical complication of hemochromatosis.] *Schweiz Med Wochenschr* 1985; **115**: 1461–5.

112. Jain AP, Chandra LS, Gupta S, Gupta OP, Jajoo UN, Kalantri SP. Spontaneous bacterial peritonitis in liver cirrhosis with ascites. *J Assoc Physicians India* 1999; **47**: 619–21.

113. Dinis-Ribeiro M, Cortez-Pinto H, Marinho R, *et al.* Spontaneous bacterial peritonitis in patients with hepatic cirrhosis: evaluation of a treatment protocol at specialized units. *Rev Esp Enferm Dig* 2002; **94**: 473–81.

114. Thanopoulou AC, Koskinas JS, Hadziyannis SJ. Spontaneous bacterial peritonitis (SBP): clinical, laboratory, and prognostic features. A single-center experience. *Eur J Intern Med* 2002; **13**: 194–8.

115. Caruntu FA, Benea L. Spontaneous bacterial peritonitis: pathogenesis, diagnosis, treatment. *J Gastrointestin Liver Dis* 2006; **15**: 51–6.

116. van Erpecum KJ. Ascites and spontaneous bacterial peritonitis in patients with liver cirrhosis. *Scand J Gastroenterol Suppl* 2006; 79–84.

117. Ribeiro TC, Chebli JM, Kondo M, Gaburri PD, Chebli LA, Feldner AC. Spontaneous bacterial peritonitis: How to deal with this life-threatening cirrhosis complication? *Ther Clin Risk Manag* 2008; **4**: 919–25.

118. Bert F, Panhard X, Johnson J, *et al.* Genetic background of *Escherichia coli* isolates from patients with spontaneous bacterial peritonitis: relationship with host factors and prognosis. *Clin Microbiol Infect* 2008; **14**: 1034–40.

119. Cereto F, Herranz X, Moreno E, *et al.* Role of host and bacterial virulence factors in *Escherichia coli* spontaneous bacterial peritonitis. *Eur J Gastroenterol Hepatol* 2008; **20**: 924–9.

120. Desforges G. Abdominal pain in hemochromatosis. *N Engl J Med* 1949; **241**: 485–7.

121. Jones NL. Irreversible shock in haemochromatosis. *Lancet* 1962; **1**: 569–72.

122. Garvie WH, Caridis DT. Idiopathic hemochromatosis presenting as "acute abdomen": a report of two cases. *Can J Surg* 1970; **13**: 262–6.

123. Cuenca-Moron B, Solis-Herruzo JA, Moreno D, Guijarro C, Gentil AA, Castellano G. Spontaneous bacterial peritonitis due to *Yersinia enterocolitica* in secondary alcoholic hemochromatosis. *J Clin Gastroenterol* 1989; **11**: 675–8.

124. Rex JH, Ginsberg AM, Fries LF, Pass HI, Kwon-Chung KJ. *Cunninghamella bertholletiae* infection associated with deferoxamine therapy. *Rev Infect Dis* 1988; **10**: 1187–94.

125. Gaziev D, Baronciani D, Galimberti M, *et al.* Mucormycosis after bone marrow transplantation: report of four cases in thalassemia and review of the literature. *Bone Marrow Transplant* 1996; **17**: 409–14.

126. Beutler E, Gelbart T. *Helicobacter pylori* infection and *HFE* hemochromatosis. *Blood Cells Mol Dis* 2006; **37**: 188–91.

127. de Montalembert M, Girot R. Infections in thalassemic patients (hepatitis and bone marrow transplantation-related infections excluded). *Prog Clin Biol Res* 1989; **309**: 231–8.

128. Wanachiwanawin W. Infections in E-beta-thalassemia. *J Pediatr Hematol Oncol* 2000; **22**: 581–7.

129. Rahav G, Volach V, Shapiro M, Rund D, Rachmilewitz EA, Goldfarb A. Severe infections in thalassaemic patients: prevalence and predisposing factors. *Br J Haematol* 2006; **133**: 667–74.

130. De Virgiliis S, Fiorelli G, Fargion S, *et al.* Chronic liver disease in transfusion-dependent thalassaemia: hepatitis B virus marker studies. *J Clin Pathol* 1980; **33**: 949–53.

131. Fargion S, Piperno A, Cappellini MD, *et al.* Hepatitis C virus and porphyria cutanea tarda: evidence of a strong association. *Hepatology* 1992; **16**: 1322–6.

132. Sampietro M, Corbetta N, Cerino M, *et al.* Prevalence and clinical significance of hepatitis G virus infection

in adult beta-thalassaemia major patients.
Br J Haematol 1997; **97**: 904–7.

133. Edwards CQ, Griffen LM, Kushner JP. Coincidental hemochromatosis and viral hepatitis. *Am J Med Sci* 1991; **301**: 50–4.

134. Piperno A, Fargion S, D'Alba R, *et al.* Liver damage in Italian patients with hereditary hemochromatosis is highly influenced by hepatitis B and C virus infection. *J Hepatol* 1992; **16**: 364–8.

135. Strachan AS. *Haemosiderosis and haemochromatosis in South African natives with a comment on the etiology of haemochromatosis. MD Thesis.* University of Glasgow, 1929.

136. Kasvosve I, Gangaidzo IT, Gomo ZA, Gordeuk VR. African iron overload. *Acta Clin Belg* 2000; **55**: 88–93.

137. Boelaert JR, Vandecasteele SJ, Appelberg R, Gordeuk VR. The effect of the host's iron status on tuberculosis. *J Infect Dis* 2007; **195**: 1745–53.

138. Gordeuk VR, Delanghe JR, Langlois MR, Boelaert JR. Iron status and the outcome of HIV infection: an overview. *J Clin Virol* 2001; **20**: 111–15.

139. Barton JC, Bertoli LF. Histochemistry of iron and iron proteins. In: Barton JC, Edwards CQ, eds. *Hemochromatosis: Genetics, Pathophysiology, Diagnosis and Treatment.* Cambridge, Cambridge University Press. 2000; 200–218.

140. de Vet BJ, ten Hoopen CH. Lactoferrin in human neutrophilic polymorphonuclear leukocytes in relation to iron metabolism. *Acta Med Scand* 1978; **203**: 197–203.

141. Chung S, Hayward C, Brock DJ, Van Heyningen V. A monoclonal antibody-based immunoassay for human lactoferrin. *J Immunol Methods* 1985; **84**: 135–41.

142. Moguilevsky N, Masson PL, Courtoy PJ. Lactoferrin uptake and iron processing into macrophages: a study in familial haemochromatosis. *Br J Haematol* 1987; **66**: 129–36.

143. Butler TW, Heck LW, Huster WJ, Grossi CE, Barton JC. Assessment of total immunoreactive lactoferrin in hematopoietic cells using flow cytometry. *J Immunol Methods* 1988; **108**: 159–70.

144. Barton JC, Huster WJ, Parmley RT. Iron-binding reactivity in mature neutrophils: relative cell content quantification by cytochemical scoring. *J Histochem Cytochem* 1988; **36**: 649–58.

145. van Asbeck BS, Marx JJ, Struyvenberg A, Verhoef J. Functional defects in phagocytic cells from patients with iron overload. *J Infect* 1984; **8**: 232–40.

146. Butler TW, Heck LW, Berkow R, Barton JC. Radioimmunometric quantification of surface

lactoferrin in blood mononuclear cells. *Am J Med Sci* 1994; **307**: 102–7.

147. Moura E, Verheul AF, Marx JJ. A functional defect in hereditary haemochromatosis monocytes and monocyte-derived macrophages. *Eur J Clin Invest* 1998; **28**: 164–73.

148. Moura E, Verheul AF, Marx JJ. Evaluation of the role of Fc gamma and complement receptors in the decreased phagocytosis of hereditary haemochromatosis patients. *Scand J Immunol* 1997; **46**: 399–405.

149. Amadori A, Zamarchi R, De Silvestro G, *et al.* Genetic control of the CD4/CD8 T-cell ratio in humans. *Nat Med* 1995; **1**: 1279–83.

150. Hall MA, Ahmadi KR, Norman P, *et al.* Genetic influence on peripheral blood T lymphocyte levels. *Genes Immun* 2000; **1**: 423–7.

151. Barton JC, Wiener HW, Acton RT, Go RC. Total blood lymphocyte counts in hemochromatosis probands with *HFE* C282Y homozygosity: relationship to severity of iron overload and HLA-A and -B alleles and haplotypes. *BMC Blood Disord* 2005; **5**: 5.

152. Cruz E, Vieira J, Almeida S, *et al.* A study of 82 extended HLA haplotypes in *HFE*-C282Y homozygous hemochromatosis subjects: relationship to the genetic control of CD8+ T-lymphocyte numbers and severity of iron overload. *BMC Med Genet* 2006; **7**: 16.

153. Arosa FA, Oliveira L, Porto G, *et al.* Anomalies of the CD8+ T cell pool in haemochromatosis: HLA-A3-linked expansions of CD8+. *Clin Exp Immunol* 1997; **107**: 548–54.

154. Reimao R, Porto G, de Sousa M. Stability of CD4/CD8 ratios in man: new correlation between CD4/CD8 profiles and iron overload in idiopathic haemochromatosis patients. *C R Acad Sci III* 1991; **313**: 481–7.

155. Porto G, Reimao R, Goncalves C, Vicente C, Justica B, de Sousa M. Haemochromatosis as a window into the study of the immunological system: a novel correlation between CD8+ lymphocytes and iron overload. *Eur J Haematol* 1994; **52**: 283–90.

156. Nemeth E, Valore EV, Territo M, Schiller G, Lichtenstein A, Ganz T. Hepcidin, a putative mediator of anemia of inflammation, is a type II acute-phase protein. *Blood* 2003; **101**: 2461–3.

157. Feder JN, Gnirke A, Thomas W, *et al.* A novel MHC class I-like gene is mutated in patients with hereditary haemochromatosis. *Nat Genet* 1996; **13**: 399–408.

158. Parkkila S, Parkkila AK, Waheed A, *et al.* Cell surface expression of HFE protein in epithelial cells, macrophages, and monocytes. *Haematologica* 2000; **85**: 340–5.

159. Chitambar CR, Wereley JP. Expression of the hemochromatosis (*HFE*) gene modulates the cellular uptake of [67]Ga. *J Nucl Med* 2003; **44**: 943–6.

160. Feeney GP, Carter K, Masters GS, Jackson HA, Cavil I, Worwood M. Changes in erythropoiesis in hereditary hemochromatosis are not mediated by HFE expression in nucleated red cells. *Haematologica* 2005; **90**: 180–7.

161. Miranda CJ, Makui H, Andrews NC, Santos MM. Contributions of beta2-microglobulin-dependent molecules and lymphocytes to iron regulation: insights from HfeRag1(-/-) and beta2mRag1(-/-) double knockout mice. *Blood* 2004; **103**: 2847–9.

162. Pratiwi R, Fletcher LM, Pyper WR, *et al.* Linkage disequilibrium analysis in Australian haemochromatosis patients indicates bipartite association with clinical expression. *J Hepatol* 1999; **31**: 39–46.

163. Acton RT, Snively BM, Barton JC, *et al.* A genome-wide linkage scan for iron phenotype quantitative trait loci: the HEIRS Family Study. *Clin Genet* 2007; **71**: 518–29.

164. Barton JC, Bertoli LF, Acton RT. Common variable immunodeficiency and IgG subclass deficiency in central Alabama hemochromatosis probands homozygous for *HFE* C282Y. *Blood Cells Mol Dis* 2003; **31**: 102–11.

165. Joske RA, Traub M. Haemochromatosis, active chronic hepatitis, and familial IgA deficiency. *Digestion* 1975; **12**: 32–8.

166. Jolivet-Gougeon A, Ingels A, Danic B, *et al.* No increased seroprevalence of anti-*Yersinia* antibodies in patients with type 1 (C282Y/C282Y) hemochromatosis. *Scand J Gastroenterol* 2007; **42**: 1388–9.

167. Barton JC, Acton RT. HLA-A and -B alleles and haplotypes in hemochromatosis probands with *HFE* C282Y homozygosity in central Alabama. *BMC Med Genet* 2002; **3**: 9.

168. Barton JC, Bertoli LF, Acton RT. HLA-A and -B alleles and haplotypes in 240 index patients with common variable immunodeficiency and selective IgG subclass deficiency in central Alabama. *BMC Med Genet* 2003; **4**: 3.

169. Spickett GP, Farrant J, North ME, Zhang JG, Morgan L, Webster AD. Common variable immunodeficiency: how many diseases? *Immunology Today* 1997; **18**: 325–8.

170. Alper CA, Marcus-Bagley D, Awdeh Z, *et al.* Prospective analysis suggests susceptibility genes for deficiencies of IgA and several other immunoglobulins on the [HLA-B8, SC01, DR3] conserved extended haplotype. *Tissue Antigens* 2000; **56**: 207–16.

171. Vorechovsky I, Cullen M, Carrington M, Hammarstrom L, Webster AD. Fine mapping of is in IgA deficiency and common variable immunodeficiency: identification and characterization of haplotypes shared by affected members of 101 multiple-case families. *J Immunol* 2000; **164**: 4408–16.

172. Kralovicova J, Hammarstrom L, Plebani A, Webster AD, Vorechovsky I. Fine-scale mapping at IGAD1 and genome-wide genetic linkage analysis implicate HLA-DQ/DR as a major susceptibility locus in selective IgA deficiency and common variable immunodeficiency. *J Immunol* 2003; **170**: 2765–75.

173. Volanakis JE, Zhu ZB, Schaffer FM, *et al.* Major histocompatibility complex class III genes and susceptibility to immunoglobulin A deficiency and common variable immunodeficiency. *J Clin Invest* 1992; **89**: 1914–22.

174. De la Concha EG, Fernandez-Arquero M, Gual L, *et al.* MHC susceptibility genes to IgA deficiency are located in different regions on different HLA haplotypes. *J Immunol* 2002; **169**: 4637–43.

175. Castigli E, Wilson SA, Garibyan L, *et al.* TACI is mutant in common variable immunodeficiency and IgA deficiency. *Nat Genet* 2005; **37**: 829–34.

176. Salzer U, Chapel HM, Webster AD, *et al.* Mutations in *TNFRSF13B* encoding TACI are associated with common variable immunodeficiency in humans. *Nat Genet* 2005; **37**: 820–8.

177. Mullighan CG, Marshall SE, Welsh KI. Mannose-binding lectin polymorphisms are associated with early age of disease onset and autoimmunity in common variable immunodeficiency. *Scand J Immunol* 2000; **51**: 111–22.

Classical and atypical *HFE* hemochromatosis

Hemochromatosis and *HFE* mutations

The "classical" type of familial hemochromatosis that is transmitted as an autosomal recessive disorder is usually due to homozygosity for the C282Y mutation of the *HFE* gene. It is expected that mutations of *HFE* cause the great majority of the cases of heritable iron overload in humans. There are at least 37 known mutations of the *HFE* gene (Table 8.1) (Chapter 4). Some individuals who are homozygous for any of the known mutations may develop heavy iron overload. At least six mutations are associated with mild iron accumulation; and at least six mutations were discovered in patients who did not have iron overload. There is insufficient reported information in the literature to determine if six of the mutations are sufficiently deleterious to result in iron overload. Approximately 1500 mutations of the cystic fibrosis gene (*CF*) are known, and the gene encodes a 1480 amino acid protein. In contrast, *HFE* is much smaller than *CF*, and encodes a protein of only 343 amino acids. Thus, it is expected that fewer mutations of *HFE* than mutations of *CF* will be eventually discovered.

Molecular genetics

Although the autosomal recessive inheritance pattern of "classical" hemochromatosis had long been recognized, identification of the responsible gene remained elusive for many years (Table 8.1). An important breakthrough in the search for the gene occurred in 1976 when hemochromatosis was found to be linked closely to the human leukocyte antigen (HLA)-A*03 region of the short arm of chromosome 6.[1] Twenty years later, the affected gene, *HFE*, was identified using a positional cloning technique.[2] A single nucleotide change, resulting in the substitution of tyrosine for cysteine at amino acid 282 of the unprocessed protein (p.C282Y), was identified in nearly all patients with HLA-linked hemochromatosis.[2] A second common mutation in *HFE* was also identified; this results in the substitution

of aspartate for histidine at amino acid 63 (p.H63D).[2] Proof that *HFE* is the gene defective in "classical" hemochromatosis was provided when knockout of the mouse *Hfe* gene and knockin of the C282Y mutation resulted in iron overload.[3,4]

HFE gene and protein

The *HFE* gene is located on chromosome 6p21.3 and contains 7 exons spanning 12 kb.[2] It was clear from the predicted structure of HFE protein that it was unlikely to be a metal transporter.[2] Rather, the *HFE* gene encodes a protein of 343 amino acids that is structurally similar to major histocompatibility (MHC) class I proteins. These include a 22 amino-acid signal peptide, a large extracellular domain consisting of three loops ($\alpha 1$ to $\alpha 3$), a single transmembrane domain, and a short cytoplasmic tail.[2] HFE protein, like other MHC class I molecules, is physically associated with β_2-microglobulin via its $\alpha 3$ loop.[5] The C282Y mutation leads to disruption of the disulfide bond needed to form this loop, and consequential loss of the interaction of mutant HFE protein with β_2-microglobulin.[5,6] As a result, the C282Y mutant protein is retained in the endoplasmic reticulum and middle Golgi compartments, and fails to undergo late Golgi processing.[6] This leads to accelerated degradation of the mutant protein and reduced expression on the cell surface.[6] The hemochromatosis-like phenotype of β_2-microglobulin knockout mice provides independent evidence of the importance of the association between β_2-microglobulin and HFE protein for normal HFE function.[7] Although HFE is structurally similar to other MHC class I proteins, it is not capable of antigen presentation.[8]

HFE mutations

The *HFE* mutation found in the majority of "classical" hemochromatosis patients is the substitution of tyrosine for cysteine at amino acid 282 of the unprocessed

Table 8.1. *HFE* mutations

Type of mutation	Designation (amino acid change)	Mutation (nucleotide change)	Prevalence	Effect on iron homeostasis
Missense	V53M	G157A	Rare	Unknown
	V59M	G175A	Rare	Unknown
	H63D	C187G	~0.16	Modest
	S65C	A193T	~0.016	Weak
	G93R	G277C	Rare	Probable
	I105T	T314C	Rare	Probable
	Q127H	A381C	Rare	Unknown
	E168Q	G502T	Rare	Modest
	V272L	G815T	Rare	Unknown
	E277K	G829A	Rare	Unknown
	C282S	G845C	Rare	Marked
	C282Y	G845A	~0.08	Marked
	Q283P	A848C	Rare	Marked
	R330M	G989T	Rare	Unknown
Nonsense	R74X	C211T	Rare	Marked
	E168X	G502A	Rare	Marked
	W169X	G506A	Rare	Marked
Splice site	IVS3+1 G/T	IVS3+1 G/T	Rare	Marked
	IVS5+1 G/A	IVS5+1 G/A	Rare	Marked
Frameshift	G93fs	c.del277	Rare	Marked
	A158fs	c.del471	Rare	Marked
Deletion		370del 22	Rare	Modest

protein (C282Y).[2] Approximately 80%–90% of Caucasian subjects of northern European ancestry with hemochromatosis diagnosed in medical care are homozygous for C282Y.[9] In other ethnic populations, the C282Y mutation is less common. Population studies suggest that the C282Y mutation occurred on an ancestral (possibly Celtic) haplotype approximately 2000 years ago.[10] It has been speculated that the C282Y mutation, by causing increased iron absorption and augmenting body iron stores, provided a selective advantage to a population whose dietary iron availability was limited (Chapter 4).

The frequency of the C282Y mutation in western European Caucasian populations is quite high (~10% heterozygotes or "carriers").[9] Nonetheless, the results of many population studies demonstrate that many C282Y homozygotes do not develop clinically significant iron overload,[11] indicating that there is incomplete penetrance of the C282Y mutation. Factors such as blood loss (e.g. menstruation, blood donation) and diet may contribute to the lack of phenotypic expression of C282Y homozygosity, but these factors cannot explain most cases of non-expression. It seems most likely that incomplete penetrance of the C282Y mutation is due in part to genetic modifiers, with potential candidates that include other genes involved in iron homeostasis. For example, it has been proposed that mutations in the *HAMP* gene that encodes hepcidin (Chapter 14) may act as modifiers in some cases.[12]

HFE H63D is more common than C282Y and is found in 15%–40% of Caucasians.[13] Unlike C282Y, this mutation appears to have arisen multiple times in different ethnic populations.[10] Homozygosity for H63D slightly increases serum iron measures (transferrin saturation, ferritin), but does not result in clinically significant iron overload.[14] Compound heterozygosity for the H63D mutation with C282Y is found with greater frequency in patients with iron overload than occurs in the general population.[13] Although the risk for iron loading in C282Y/H63D compound heterozygotes is increased, it is estimated to be nearly 200-fold lower than in C282Y homozygotes.

Rare patients with hemochromatosis phenotypes have *HFE* mutations other than C282Y or H63D[15-18] (Table 8.1). The Human Gene Mutation Database at the Institute of Medical Genetics in Cardiff lists more that 30 *HFE* mutations.[19] These include missense mutations (e.g. G93R, I105T, Q127H, S65C), splice site mutations (e.g. IVS3+1 G/T, IVS5+1 G/A), frameshift mutations (e.g. G93fs, A158fs), and deletions and nonsense mutations (e.g. E168X, R74X, W169X). Each symptomatic patient reported to date with one of the missense mutations also has either C282Y or H63D mutation as his/her second allele. The two identified splice site mutations cause altered mRNA splicing and exon skipping, resulting in abnormal variants of HFE protein. The frameshift and nonsense mutations result in the production of truncated forms of HFE protein. The relative contribution of mutations other than C282Y or H63D to the overall incidence of *HFE* hemochromatosis is small.

HFE expression

The *HFE* gene is expressed at relatively low mRNA levels in most human tissues.[2] In the liver, HFE is expressed in hepatocytes, and also in Kupffer cells and bile duct epithelial cells.[8,20] Other identified sites of HFE protein expression include duodenal crypt enterocytes, placental syncytiotrophoblasts, tissue macrophages, and circulating monocytes and granulocytes.[8,20] It has been proposed that HFE protein in hepatocytes may play a key role in sensing body iron status, and thereby influencing the expression of hepcidin, the master iron-regulatory hormone.[20-22]

HFE regulation

Little is known about the regulation of *HFE* gene expression. In contrast to other MHC molecules, *HFE* expression is not induced by various cytokines in cultured cells. The effect of iron on *HFE* expression appears to be minimal.[20] Little change in intestinal expression of *Hfe* has been identified in mice in response to iron loading or depletion.[20] No sequences homologous to iron-responsive elements have been identified in either the 5′- or 3′-untranslated region of *HFE* mRNA. Although the promoter region of the *HFE* gene contains sequences homologous to several binding sites for known transcription factors, functional characterization is incomplete. The predominant *HFE* mRNA is 4.2 kb in length, although additional minor transcripts, both longer and shorter, have been reported.[8,20] Some of the smaller transcripts are attributable to alternative splicing events and differential use of polyadenylation signals. The levels of translated protein from the *HFE* splice-variant transcripts and their physiological significance are unknown.

Mouse models of *HFE* hereditary hemochromatosis

Transgenic methodology has provided important information about the functional consequences of *HFE* gene disruption in the whole animal. *Hfe* knockout mice and mice homozygous for the C282Y mutation manifest greater hepatic iron levels, transferrin saturation, and intestinal iron absorption than wild-type mice.[6-8] Like patients with *HFE* hemochromatosis, these mice have low hepcidin expression in the liver.[23] Mice with targeted knockout of *Hfe* in hepatocytes also have low hepcidin and iron overload, indicating that Hfe protein within hepatocytes plays a key role in hepcidin regulation.[24] Strain differences determine the severity of iron accumulation in *Hfe* knockout mice, supporting the concept that there are genetic modifiers of the *HFE* hemochromatosis phenotype in humans.[20]

Effect of HFE protein on iron metabolism

Despite intensive investigation, the molecular mechanism by which HFE protein influences iron metabolism remains unclear.[20-22] Both patients with C282Y homozygosity and *Hfe* knockout mice have inappropriately low levels of expression of hepcidin in the liver, suggesting that normal HFE protein plays an important role in the iron-sensing pathway that regulates hepcidin.[21,22] HFE protein binds to both transferrin receptors 1 and 2.[21,22] One hypothesis proposes

Table 8.2. Prevalence (%) of *HFE* genotypes in Americans from ten studies

Population	Subjects (n)	C282Y/C282Y	C282Y/wt	C282Y/H63D	H63D/H63D	H63D/wt	wt/wt	References
Whites								
Alabama	176	0	13.10	6.80	3.40	15.4	60.3	104
Alabama	142	0.70	10.60	3.50	2.80	19.7	62.7	15
California	193	0	15.00	1.00	3.60	24.3	58.0	105
Connecticut	100	1.00	8.00	0	4.00	24.0	63.0	106
Kaiser	30 418	0.44	9.80	1.80	2.40	23.3	62.4	11
Maine	1001	0.70	9.70	2.20	1.70	24.6	61.1	107
Missouri	1450	0.40	8.90	2.40	3.50	23.9	61.0	108
New Mexico	287	0	9.80	2.40	2.40	19.9	65.5	109
NHANES III	2016	0.30	9.50	2.40	2.20	23.6	62.1	13
Total	35 783	0–1.00	8.00–13.10	0–6.80	1.70–4.00	15.4–24.6	58.0–65.0	
Blacks								
Connecticut	56	0	2.00	0	0	3.5	94.5	106
Kaiser	1462	0	3.50	0.30	0.20	8.4	87.5	11
Michigan	172	0	3.00	0	0	3.0	94.0	110
NHANES III	1600	0.06	2.30	0.06	0.32	5.6	91.7	13
Total	3290	0–0.06	2.00–3.50	0–0.30	0–0.32	3.0–8.4	87.5–95.0	
Mexican Americans								
Connecticut	100	0	3.00	1.00	1.00	15.0	82.0	106
Kaiser	4049	0.22	3.50	0.84	1.40	20.6	73.4	11
NHANES III	1555	0.03	2.75	0.19	1.10	19.7	76.3	13
Total	5704	0–0.22	2.80–3.50	0.19–1.00	1.00–1.40	15.0–21.0	73.0–82.0	

that diferric transferrin competitively displaces HFE protein from transferrin receptor 1, and thereby makes more HFE available to bind to transferrin receptor 2.[21,22] The complex of HFE and transferrin receptor 2 may be involved in stimulating a signaling pathway that increases hepcidin gene expression in hepatocytes.[21,22]

Prevalence and population genetics of *HFE* mutations

The prevalence of common *HFE* genotypes has been determined in many populations. The results from ten surveys of *HFE* genotypes in the US are displayed in Table 8.2. The results of studies of at least 1000 people revealed that the prevalence of *HFE* C282Y homozygosity among US Caucasians is about 3–7 per 1000 (population prevalence estimate of 0.3–0.7 percent) (Table 8.2). Studies that included at least 1000 Mexican Americans showed that 0.3–2.2 per 1000 were *HFE* C282Y homozygotes (prevalence estimate of 0.03–0.22 percent) (Table 8.2). Studies that included at least 1000 US blacks showed that 0–0.6 per 1000 were *HFE* C282Y homozygotes (prevalence estimate 0–0.06 percent) (Table 8.2). Iron overload is relatively common among African-Americans, but it is not typically due to mutations of the *HFE* gene (Chapter 18).

Table 8.3. Prevalence (%) of *HFE* C282Y and H63D genotypes in hemochromatosis patients in 16 countries[a]

Country	Subjects (n)	C282Y/ C282Y	C282Y/ wt	C282Y/ H63D	H63D/ H63D	H63D/ wt	wt/wt	References
United Kingdom	277	90.0–100.0	0–1.7	0–5.5	0–0.9	0	0–4.3	111–115
Australia	184	88.8–100.0	0–5.6	0–1.4	0	0	0–4.0	116,117
Canada	128	95.3	0	0	0	1.6	3.1	118
Denmark	58	95	0	1.7	0	0	3.4	119
Germany	288	72.0–94.6	1.1–2.0	0–8.3	2.8	0–6.0	0–5.3	120–123
Belgium	49	93.9	0	4.1	0	2.0	0	124
Spain	259	57.0–92.8	0–6.0	0–11.0	0–4.5	0–11.0	3.2–13.6	125–131
France	1097	67.2–92.4	0.9–4.4	2.3–7.1	1.1–8.2	1.5–4.9	0–9.8	10,132–136
Sweden	125	89.0–92.0	1.1	3.4	1.1	1.1	1.1	137,138
U.S.	818	59.4–88.6	0.6–26.7	4.5–20.3	0–7.0	0–8.1	0.6–12.0	2,15,95,106, 139–141
Norway	258	88.4	3.9	5.4	0	1.1	1.2	142
Portugal	25	88.0	6.2	1.5	0	0	4.6	143
Austria	40	77.5	0	7.5	2.5	2.5	10.0	144
Italy	263	33.3–69.0	2.7–6.3	4.4–10.0	1.3–3.3	4.0–13.3	11.3–36.7	145,146
Brazil	15	53.3	6.6	0	0	6.6	33.5	147
Greece	10	50.0	0	0	0	0	50.0	93
Total	3894	33.0–100.0	0–6.6	0–11.0	0–8.2	0–13.0	0–50.0	

Note: [a]wt = wild-type or normal *HFE* allele.

Worldwide prevalence of *HFE* mutations in hemochromatosis patients

Populations whose ancestry is northern, central, and western European or Scandinavian have a relatively high prevalence of hemochromatosis. In other populations, the prevalence of hemochromatosis and of *HFE* mutations is very low. The frequency of the two most common mutations of *HFE* and the prevalence of different *HFE* genotypes in 42 studies from 16 countries are displayed in Table 8.3.

HEIRS Study

The largest study ever performed to determine the prevalence of mutations of the *HFE* gene in a general population is the HEIRS Study, which was performed in the US and Canada at multiple field centers. Results of the HEIRS Study, including the *HFE* genotypes in different areas and populations of the US and Canada, are displayed in Table 8.4.

Mechanisms of iron absorption and deposition

Iron absorption

The uptake of inorganic iron by absorptive enterocytes differs between C282Y homozygotes and control subjects in some respects. DCYTB (duodenal cytochrome b reductase 1) mRNA levels are not increased in untreated hemochromatosis patients.[25] Untreated C282Y homozygotes have inappropriate upregulation of DMT1 (divalent metal transporter-1) mRNA expression for a given level of serum ferritin concentration, although the absolute level of expression of this iron transport gene does not differ significantly from that of normal subjects.[25] In addition to iron,

Table 8.4. Prevalence of *HFE* C282Y and H63D genotypes in 99 711 HEIRS Study participants[a]

Race/ethnicity (n)	C282Y/C282Y	C282Y/H63D	H63D/H63D	C282Y/wt	H63D/wt	wt/wt
White (44 082)	0.44	2.0	2.4	10	24	61
Native American (648)	0.11	0.77	1.3	5.7	20	72
Hispanic (12 459)	0.027	0.33	1.1	2.9	18	78
Black (27 124)	0.014	0.071	0.089	2.3	5.7	92
Pacific Islander (698)	0.012	0.096	0.20	2.0	8.4	89
Asian (12 772)	0.000039	0.0055	0.20	0.012	8.4	91
Multiple/unknown (1928)	0.0031	0.0010	0.011	0.058	0.16	76

Note: [a]Adapted from Adams *et al.*[93] This includes observations on all participants for whom there were complete phenotype and genotype screening data, except 1457 subjects who heard about the study from a participating family member. Within the five single race/ethnicity groups, prevalence rates were derived using Hardy–Weinberg proportions and data from non-C282Y homozygotes. wt = wild-type or normal *HFE* allele.

DMT1 probably transports non-ferrous divalent metal cations in *HFE* hemochromatosis (Chapters 4, 8). Absorption of heme iron by persons with hemochromatosis is also increased in proportion to their serum ferritin levels.[26,27]

Ferroportin mRNA is inappropriately increased for a given level of serum ferritin concentration in untreated hemochromatosis patients, although the absolute level of expression does not differ significantly from that of control subjects.[25] Hephaestin mRNA levels are not upregulated in hemochromatosis.[25] Phlebotomy therapy increases expression of DMT1 and ferroportin mRNA in C282Y homozygotes, a consequence of phlebotomy-induced erythropoiesis. Enterocytes express transferrin and transferrin receptors on their basolateral membranes.[28] Mucosal transferrin is significantly lower in hemochromatosis subjects than in controls, presumably due to a decrease in mucosal transferrin receptors.[29] The interaction of transferrin, transferrin receptor, and HFE protein at this location is incompletely understood.[30,31] Nonetheless, HFE appears to play a minor role in the regulation of iron absorption by duodenal enterocytes.[32]

Iron transport

Absorbed and recycled iron is transported in plasma bound to transferrin. In hemochromatosis homozygotes, transferrin is normal by electrophoresis and its affinity for iron is similar to that of control subjects.[33–35] Serum transferrin levels in most hemochromatosis homozygotes are normal or slightly decreased.

In some C282Y homozygotes, transferrin in plasma or serum is always saturated to an abnormally great degree with iron.[36] This occurs long before iron overload develops and is attributed to increased iron export by macrophages. Additional iron may be transported in the plasma of C282Y homozygotes as non-transferrin-bound iron (NBTI). Serum ceruloplasmin and serum ferroxidase concentrations are lower in untreated C282Y homozygotes than in normal control subjects,[37,38] but return to normal levels after phlebotomy therapy.[38]

Iron in plasma, either bound to transferrin or as NTBI, reaches hepatocytes via radicles of the hepatic artery and portal vein. In hemochromatosis, primary hepatic transferrin receptors (TFR1) are down-regulated in accordance with the severity of iron overload.[39,40] Hepatocytes have a low-affinity, transferrin-mediated pathway that accounts for most of their iron uptake.[41,42] TFR2 protein is expressed on the basolateral surface of hepatocytes[43] and is thought to modulate the signaling pathway that controls hepcidin expression.[42,44] Of all organs, expression of HFE is greatest in the liver. TFR2 binds to membrane-anchored HFE,[21] although the physiologic significance of this interaction has not been defined. HFE protein does not appear to alter the unloading of iron from transferrin in the endosome.[44]

Iron deposition in target organs

NTBI is rapidly removed by hepatocytes as it passes through hepatic sinusoids by a process that is linear, concentration-dependent, and saturable (Chapter 2). This mechanism is important in *HFE* hemochromatosis because transferrin saturation with iron is often markedly elevated.[36] Plasma membrane expression of DMT1 is upregulated in the livers of hemochromatosis patients, and thus facilitative transport of Fe^{2+} via DMT1 could account for the uptake of plasma NTBI characteristic of *HFE* hemochromatosis.[45] It is probable that a gradient of iron in the hepatic sinusoids is produced by transferrin receptor- and DMT1-mediated iron transport into hepatocytes from plasma, such that portal areas of hepatic acini are exposed to higher iron concentrations and central areas are exposed to lower iron levels. These features are consistent with the anatomical distribution of hepatic iron seen in hemochromatosis, i.e. predominance of hepatocellular iron loading with a portal to central gradient. The prompt removal of NTBI from the hepatic circulation also accounts for the fact that hepatic iron loading precedes the accumulation of iron in other organs in hemochromatosis. Concentrations of certain non-ferrous divalent metals such as zinc and manganese are increased in the livers of patients with hemochromatosis; their transport into hepatocytes may be another consequence of transferrin or DMT1 pathways.

Diabetes mellitus occurs in ~15% of patients with hemochromatosis and C282Y homozygosity (Chapter 5). Pancreatic iron overload causes or contributes to this complication in some cases. There is predominance of iron overload of the exocrine tissue of the pancreas; iron levels in the pancreatic islets are quite variable.[46] Electron microscopy of islet cells reveals that iron deposits are restricted to B cells and are associated with loss of their endocrine granules.[46] In severe transfusion iron overload, hemosiderin is also selectively deposited in B cells of the islet.[47] Fibrosis of the pancreatic exocrine glands and islets can occur if iron overload is severe.[48]

The anterior pituitary gland is a target organ of iron overload, and impaired function of the gonadotrophs with consequent hypogonadism is the most commonly encountered non-diabetes endocrinopathy in *HFE* hemochromatosis (Chapter 5). Iron in the anterior pituitary gland is predominantly deposited in gonadotroph cells and, to a lesser degree, in other secretory cells.[49,50] Gonadotrophin-secreting cells express more surface transferrin receptors than other hormone-producing cells in the anterior pituitary gland,[51] and thus may have a greater requirement for iron than other pituitary cell types.[52] This could underlie the reason why gonadotroph cells are especially susceptible to iron loading. In two cases of hemochromatosis, reduction of pituitary gonadotroph numbers was also implicated in the genesis of hypogonadism.[50] Fibrosis of the anterior pituitary occurs in some cases.[48] Most hemochromatosis patients with C282Y homozygosity and hypogonadotrophic hypogonadism also have severe hepatic iron overload.[53]

Iron and erythrocytes

Values of mean hemoglobin and mean corpuscular volume (but not erythrocyte count) are significantly greater in subjects with C282Y homozygosity and hemochromatosis phenotypes than in control subjects.[54–56] HFE is not expressed in erythroid colonies with a normal *HFE* genotype.[57] Therefore, it is unlikely that *HFE* mutations alter erythroid iron handling directly, but increase the supply of iron to developing erythroid tissues via highly-saturated transferrin.[54,58,57] It can be inferred from studies of blood erythrocytes that hemoglobin synthesis by immature erythroid cells in hemochromatosis is increased.[54,56] There is also a putative locus for mean corpuscular volume on chromosome 6q24 (near the *HFE* locus at chromosome 6p21.3).[58] An early report suggested that hemochromatosis patients have megaloblastic erythropoiesis.[59] *HFE* C282Y homozygotes have increased plasma iron turnover and increased erythropoiesis.[57] The slightly increased erythropoiesis in C282Y homozygotes may be due to ineffective erythropoiesis.[57] Heme-mediated erythroblast toxicity such as that characteristic of hereditary deficiency of FLVCR, a heme exporter[60,61] could explain ineffective erythropoiesis in hemochromatosis, although this is unproven.

Control of iron absorption

Hepcidin is produced by hepatocytes under conditions of iron availability (Chapter 2). Hepcidin mRNA expression is inappropriately decreased in *HFE* hemochromatosis.[62] *HFE* C282Y homozygotes have a blunted urine hepcidin response to an oral iron challenge.[63] HFE protein may exert its iron-regulatory activity principally in hepatocytes by modulating the production of hepcidin.[64] The increased plasma iron turnover and the slightly increased erythropoiesis that occur in *HFE* hemochromatosis could also act as an "erythropoiesis regulator" and contribute to the relative deficiency of hepcidin. Growth/differentiation factor 15 (GDF15), a member of the transforming growth factor-beta superfamily, may be such a "regulator" in beta-thalassemia patients with severe iron overload.[65] In contrast, volunteer blood superdonors have markedly decreased serum hepcidin levels, but most have normal GDF15 expression. This indicates that GDF15 over expression arising from the expanded erythroid pool necessary to replace donated red cells is not the biochemical mechanism for their decreased serum hepcidin levels.[66] To date, there are no reports of GDF15 expression in hemochromatosis.

Penetrance of hemochromatosis

Expressivity of iron phenotypes in C282Y homozygotes (and other persons with hemochromatosis-associated *HFE* genotypes) is highly variable. Only a small proportion of C282Y homozygotes develop severe iron overload and consequential multi-organ damage. Thus, C282Y homozygosity is necessary but not sufficient for the development of deleterious iron overload, although it is an important and determinable risk factor. It is plausible that mutations in other known iron-related genes account for much of this variability. Nonetheless, pathogenic alleles in numerous pertinent genes have not been detected in most C282Y homozygotes,[67–72] regardless of the degree of their iron overload. The concordance of iron phenotypes in hemochromatosis probands with C282Y homozygosity and their haploidentical sibs is not great.[73] Disparate frequencies of human leukocyte antigen (HLA) haplotypes occur in men and women with C282Y homozygosity, and common HLA haplotypes are not independent variables associated with iron overload severity.[74] These observations suggest that a combination of presently undefined heritable traits, sex-related characteristics, dietary or other environmental factors, non-physiologic mechanisms, or the complex interplay of various known (and undescribed) modulators of iron homeostasis largely account for phenotype differences among C282Y homozygotes.

Absorption and metabolism of non-ferrous metals

The absorption or retention of some non-ferrous metals is increased in persons with hemochromatosis and other iron overload disorders. Many non-ferrous metals are normal dietary constituents; others are environmental contaminants or occupational hazards.

Absorption

Divalent metal transporter-1 (DMT1), expressed on the luminal surfaces of absorptive enterocytes, is the major Fe^{2+} transporter that mediates cellular iron uptake in mammals. DMT1 is upregulated in *HFE* hemochromatosis, in iron deficiency, and after phlebotomy. DMT1 has an unusually broad substrate range that includes Fe^{2+}, Zn^{2+}, Mn^{2+}, Co^{2+}, Cd^{2+}, Cu^{2+}, Ni^{2+}, and Pb^{2+}. This could account for the increased absorption of Co^{2+}, Cd^{2+}, and Pb^{2+} in persons with hemochromatosis.[75–77] Intestinal absorption of inorganic iron, cobalt, and lead in hemochromatosis homozygotes diagnosed in medical care is 1.5–3 times greater than that observed in normal control subjects, is increased in men and women, and is not significantly affected by the presence or absence of iron overload, hepatic cirrhosis, or diabetes mellitus.[77] Increased absorption of lead also occurs in hemochromatosis heterozygotes.[77] In homozygotes, hepatic concentrations of zinc, manganese, and copper are several-fold greater than normal, and are unassociated with the presence or absence of hepatic cirrhosis.[78] Levels of copper are increased in some tissues, especially the choroid plexus and thyroid. This implies that increased quantities of Zn^{2+}, Mn^{2+}, and Cu^{2+} are also absorbed by persons with hemochromatosis, possibly via DMT1 binding. Physiologic concentrations of Ca^{2+} inhibit DMT1, consistent with impaired mucosal uptake and absorption of iron, cobalt, iron, zinc, lead, and plutonium in the presence of calcium.[78]

Enterocyte transferrin receptors occur only at the basolateral membranes. mRNA for duodenal transferrin receptors is inappropriately increased in hemochromatosis.[79] The C282Y *HFE* protein, associated with most "classical" cases of hemochromatosis, binds transferrin receptor poorly[80] but, like normal HFE, is not itself a metal-binding protein. These circumstances could facilitate the transport of non-ferrous metals from enterocytes into the circulation in persons with hemochromatosis. Some divalent cations, especially Zn^{2+}, Cd^{2+}, Cu^{2+}, and Pb^{2+} are exported via mechanisms apparently uninvolved with iron absorption. It is also possible that some non-ferrous metals that bind DMT1 are exported from enterocytes via ferroportin, although this is unproven.

Transport in blood

The affinity of unsaturated transferrin appears to be greatest for iron, but transferrin binds many other metals in a competitive (or non-competitive) manner in vitro and in vivo, including Al, V, Cr, Mn, Co, Ni, Cu, Zn, Ga, Ru, Cd, In, Hf, Pb, Bi, Ac, Gd, Th, Pa, U, Np, Pu, Am, Cm, and Cf.[78] Thus, transferrin may be a physiologic transporter for these metals. Physico-chemical characteristics of transferrin in hemochromatosis are normal,[78] and mutations in the transferrin gene or its regulatory elements have not been identified in patients with hemochromatosis or iron overload. Like iron, non-ferrous metals can alter transferrin synthesis by modulating regulatory sequences or altering post-translational production. In untreated and treated persons with hemochromatosis, plasma transferrin saturation is usually elevated and therefore few binding sites on transferrin may be available for non-ferrous metals. Regardless, many non-ferrous metals are largely transported by albumin (e.g. zinc) or more specific binders (e.g. ceruloplasmin).

Cellular uptake

The cellular uptake some non-ferrous metals, e.g. Co^{2+} or Ga^{2+}, occurs via transferrin receptors. Transferrin receptor function and regulation appear to be appropriate for the degree of iron overload in *HFE* hemochromatosis. Transferrin receptor gene structure is also normal, except in rare cases of hemochromatosis due to mutations in the alternate transferrin receptor gene *TFR2*. The uptake of many non-ferrous metals probably occurs via non-transferrin-associated mechanisms. Hepatocyte uptake of NTB iron is much more efficient than that of transferrin-bound iron, and this could account for the predominantly hepatocellular iron loading with a portal to central gradient observed in hemochromatosis.[78] Non-transferrin mechanisms could also account for the relatively selective hepatic deposition of manganese and zinc in hemochromatosis.[81,82]

Organ distribution and storage

Blood zinc concentrations are often normal in hemochromatosis homozygotes[83] and thus do not reflect increased hepatic zinc retention characteristic of hemochromatosis.[82] Liver concentrations of manganese are significantly increased in hemochromatosis.[81] Ferritin, the primary iron storage protein, can also bind non-ferrous metals in vivo and in vitro, including Be, Al, Cu, Zn, Ga, Cd, Pb, and Bi.[78] Absorbed cobalt is not incorporated into ferritin.[79] Body retention of intravenously administered radiochromium

is depressed in hemochromatosis.[84] Aluminum concentrations in the livers of hemochromatosis patients are subnormal,[78] and cobalt was almost undetectable in multiple tissues obtained at autopsy from patients with hemochromatosis.[78] In African iron overload patients from South Africa, significantly increased concentrations of lead were detected in liver, pancreas, jejunum, heart, and spleen. This suggests that lead absorption is increased in such persons.[78]

Excretion

The renal excretion of absorbed inorganic cobalt is rapid and quantitative in persons with hemochromatosis.[75] Whole-body zinc excretion in hemochromatosis homozygotes is normal or increased.[85] The urinary excretion of intravenously administered chromium is normal or increased in hemochromatosis,[84] and urinary excretion of lead is probably normal.[77] Taken together, these observations suggest that the overall function of excretory mechanisms for non-ferrous metals in hemochromatosis is not impaired.

Implications for management

Many non-prescription nutritional supplements contain chromium, manganese, copper, or zinc, in addition to iron. It is prudent for known hemochromatosis homozygotes or heterozygotes to limit their use of non-ferrous metal supplements to the treatment of specific nutritional deficiencies.[86] Zinc absorption and retention are increased in hemochromatosis, yet serum zinc concentrations are usually normal.[83] Persons with avocational or occupational exposure to toxic metals, especially cadmium, lead, and the actinides need appropriate testing on a regular basis. The excess retention of zinc, manganese, and lead in persons with hemochromatosis is probably not decreased significantly by therapeutic phlebotomy, because concentrations of these metals in the blood are low.[77,83] There are no reported investigations of possible synergy of excess iron and zinc, manganese, or lead in the livers or other tissues of persons with hemochromatosis. In unusual patients with hemochromatosis and Wilson disease, there was no evidence of severe hepatic injury despite significant accumulations of iron and copper in the liver.[87,88]

Reports of non-ferrous metal toxicity in persons with hemochromatosis are rare.[78] In hemochromatosis patients whose mean blood lead concentrations were greater than normal (including some subjects with occupational or avocational lead exposure), no evidence of plumbism was observed.[77] The scale of undue exposure to and absorption and retention of non-ferrous metals in persons with *HFE* mutations is potentially great.[89] Patients with hemochromatosis should not be treated with chelation therapy for non-ferrous metal retention unless they have manifestations of metal toxicity.

Variable expression of iron overload associated with *HFE* mutations

Phenotype heterogeneity

The amount of body iron stores is a major determinant of clinical outcome in patients with hemochromatosis. Patients with greater iron overload, as assessed by hepatic iron concentration and/or the amount of total iron removed by phlebotomy, have an increased prevalence of cirrhosis, diabetes mellitus, cardiomyopathy, and hypogonadism and an increased risk of mortality. Hepatic iron concentration greater than 400–500 µmol/g is an important risk factor for hepatic fibrosis and cirrhosis. In contrast, arthropathy is unrelated to iron stores and, unlike other clinical manifestations, is not significantly improved by phlebotomy therapy. It is generally accepted that the liver is the first site of iron deposition in persons with hemochromatosis, and that other organs are involved later. Previous studies have suggested that there may be a threshold in the liver for iron accumulation. Increments of hepatic iron concentration are progressively smaller in patients with hemochromatosis until values of hepatic iron concentration reach a plateau at ∼350 µmol/g. Thereafter, iron accumulation progresses in extrahepatic sites as shown by the increase of both serum ferritin concentration and iron removed by phlebotomy, and by the higher prevalence of clinical extrahepatic manifestations other than arthropathy.[90] Iron stores accumulate progressively in many individuals with hemochromatosis[90] but not in others.[11] The organ distribution of excessive iron may differ depending on pathophysiology. In persons with transfusion iron overload, for example, iron may be deposited preferentially in extra-hepatic organs such as the heart when total body iron levels are relatively low.[91]

A genotypic definition of hemochromatosis became possible after the discovery of the *HFE* gene in 1996 and the subsequent description of mutations in other genes related to iron metabolism (Chapter 4).

Hemochromatosis in most Caucasians is associated with homozygosity for *HFE* C282Y. A small proportion of Caucasians with iron overload have compound heterozygosity for C282Y and another *HFE* mutation such as H63D or S65C. Heterogeneity in body iron measures in persons with *HFE* hemochromatosis-associated genotypes is great.[92]

Definition of penetrance

The term *penetrance* refers to the proportion of people with a specified genotype who have an abnormal phenotype due to that genotype. The most prevalent biochemical abnormality found in individuals with *HFE* hemochromatosis-associated genotypes is increased saturation of plasma transferrin with iron. If iron stores are increased, the plasma ferritin level is also elevated. Thus, serum transferrin saturation and ferritin levels are commonly used as biochemical markers of penetrance, although these attributes alone do not increase risks for morbidity or mortality. Further, these measures are elevated in many persons with a variety of non-hemochromatosis conditions, and are normal (or even subnormal) in some patients with *HFE* hemochromatosis-associated genotypes.

Iron overload is deemed by some to have clinical penetrance only when it can be demonstrated that there is a change in organ function that is unambiguously related to an increase in body iron, and that there is consequential morbidity or premature mortality. The prevalence of some symptoms often associated with hemochromatosis and iron overload, e.g. arthralgias and fatigue, is great in persons with *HFE* C282Y homozygosity identified by screening. These observations have led some investigators to conclude that the clinical penetrance of hemochromatosis for these manifestations is moderately high. Regardless, analyses of observations in large screening programs reveals that the prevalence of these and most other symptoms does not differ significantly between C282Y homozygotes and age- and sex-matched non-C282Y homozygotes.[11,93] In some persons diagnosed to have hemochromatosis in medical care, however, these manifestations sometimes improve or resolve after iron depletion is achieved with phlebotomy, indicating that excess iron may contribute to their development.

Hepatic cirrhosis is generally regarded as a consequence of severe iron overload in subjects in whom there are no other known causes of liver disease.

In the past, cirrhosis was an almost universal attribute of persons diagnosed to have hemochromatosis, because occurrence of the triad of skin bronzing, diabetes mellitus, and cirrhosis was the essence of diagnosis. Since the publication of phenotype screening of blood bank donors in 1988[95] and the discovery of *HFE* in 1996,[2] it has become widely accepted that the spectrum of phenotypes in C282Y homozygotes is very heterogeneous.

Today, the prevalence of cirrhosis in C282Y homozygotes diagnosed in medical care and family studies remains relatively great, but is low in C282Y homozygotes identified in screening.[11,95] Organ dysfunction other than cirrhosis due to elevated tissue iron deposits (e.g. diabetes mellitus and hypogonadism) occurs in a high proportion of persons with hemochromatosis diagnosed in medical care,[91] but in a very small percentage of persons found to have hemochromatosis in family or screening studies.[95] The ultimate measure of penetrance is the presence of organ dysfunction with associated reduction of life expectancy. The proportion of persons with *HFE* hemochromatosis in whom longevity is reduced due to iron overload is small. Taken together, screening populations for hemochromatosis with serum iron measures or *HFE* mutation analyses identifies many C282Y homozygotes whose iron and symptom phenotypes are quite different from older "textbook" descriptions of hemochromatosis, because very few of the C282Y homozygotes detected by screening have (or will develop) life-threatening manifestations of hemochromatosis.[11,96]

Variability in penetrance

Several population screening studies have defined the prevalence of the common *HFE* mutations and the penetrance of the *HFE* C282Y/C282Y genotype. The biochemical penetrance of homozygosity for C282Y differs across reports. A compilation of data from cross-sectional general population screening studies reveals that at least 75% of male *HFE* C282Y homozygotes had elevated transferrin saturation levels, and that 58–76% had elevated serum ferritin levels.[97] The prevalence of elevated serum iron measures is more variable among female than male homozygotes. The proportion of adult female C282Y homozygotes with normal serum iron measures is as high as 50%, and some have iron deficiency. Among *HFE* C282Y homozygotes identified by population

genetic screening, 38% of those undergoing further evaluation met criteria for iron overload, 25% had hepatic fibrosis, and 6% had cirrhosis. The occurrence of significant organ dysfunction that can be reliably attributed to iron overload is low in most studies. Overall, definitions of penetrance often vary and many screening studies lack an appropriate control population. Studies designed to identify potential mechanisms that mediate differences in hemochromatosis penetrance are the critical next step in the development of better management models.

Genotypic factors that affect penetrance

Nature of the *HFE* mutation

The majority of patients with clinically defined "classical" hemochromatosis are homozygous for the *HFE* C282Y mutation. A significant minority are compound heterozygotes with *HFE* genotypes C282Y/H63D or C282Y/S65C; a much smaller proportion have other *HFE* genotypes (Chapter 4). C282Y homozygotes have significantly higher serum iron measures than C282Y/H63D or C282Y/S65C compound heterozygotes or patients heterozygous or homozygous for H63D or S65C. This difference in disease penetrance is consistent with the laboratory observation that the C282Y mutation abrogates the ability of cells to express surface HFE protein, whereas the H63D and S65C mutations lead to the surface expression of an abnormal protein with reduced function.

Ancestral haplotype

Univariate analyses of observations of *HFE* C282Y homozygotes diagnosed in medical care indicated that the presence of the ancestral haplotype minimally defined by HLA-A*03, B*07 was associated with a more severe phenotype than in subjects lacking HLA-A*03, B*07.[98–100] Multivariate analyses in a large patient series of C282Y homozygotes diagnosed in medical care suggest that the ancestral haplotype is not associated with penetrance (measured as iron removed by phlebotomy to achieve iron depletion) in *HFE* C282Y homozygotes.[101] Whether another 6p-linked gene(s) accounts for the association between the ancestral haplotype and more severe iron overload remains to be defined (Chapter 4).

Other genetic determinants of penetrance

The concordance of the severity of iron overload in affected siblings provide strong evidence that the phenotypic expression of this disorder is influenced by genetic factors. The iron phenotypes of different strains of laboratory mice with the homologs of human C282Y homozygosity also differ significantly. Scattered reports have attributed variability in penetrance to the co-inheritance of mutations in other iron-associated genes (e.g. *HAMP, TFR2, HJV, HP*), tumor necrosis factor-alpha promoter alleles, manganese superoxide dismutase alleles, and mitochondrial DNA mutations. Genome-wide screening studies may identify genetic co-factors that influence penetrance. To date, a single "modifier gene" that explains most of the observed variability in penetrance (if it exists) remains unreported. It is possible that penetrance is determined by multiple co-inherited genetic factors and environmental or dietary factors.

Non-genetic variables

Age

The accumulation of iron in hemochromatosis homozygotes is age-dependent. Thus, the risk of most clinical complications of hemochromatosis increases with age and with body iron stores. Based on these observations, an age-related index, e.g. the hepatic iron index (hepatic iron concentration/age in years) has been used to differentiate hemochromatosis homozygotes diagnosed in medical care from heterozygotes and patients with alcohol-dependent hepatic iron excess (Chapters 4, 8, 9). Recently, the relationship between hepatic iron concentration and age has been questioned. A positive correlation of hepatic iron concentration with age exists in younger homozygotes who develop iron loading. In older homozygotes with iron overload, however, the hepatic iron concentration may not rise as rapidly as it does in younger patients. Hepcidin dysregulation could explain the apparent self-limiting nature of iron overload in hemochromatosis.

These observations suggest that the rate of iron accumulation rate is not constant throughout the lives of hemochromatosis patients because the rate of intestinal iron absorption decreases with progressive iron accumulation. These observations also indicate that the rate of iron accumulation rate varies among hemochromatosis patients. For example, the iron accumulation rate ranged from 110–880 mg Fe/y in 47 Italian male patients, as assessed by the ratio of iron removed by phlebotomy adjusted by age (Fe, mg/age, y). The second hypothesis does not exclude the former, and is supported by the presence of interfamilial heterogeneity and intrafamilial homogeneity of phenotype expression. That the rate of iron accumulation varies widely among hemochromatosis patients explains the highly variable rate of increase of serum ferritin concentration after iron depletion is achieved. These data can only be explained by iron accumulation rates that differ markedly in hemochromatosis patients, although it is not clear whether these observations are due to genetic attributes, acquired factors, or both.

Sex

This variable has the greatest known influence on penetrance of iron overload in hemochromatosis homozygotes. Clinical manifestations of iron overload predominate in male hemochromatosis homozygotes. Among hemochromatosis probands, there is a higher proportion of men than women in all populations studied, ranging from 2:1 to 8:1, whereas the ratio of men to women approaches 1:1 in cases discovered through family studies or screening. The accumulation rate of iron is fourfold greater in men than in women. Thus, the difference in clinical expression of the condition between men and women has been attributed, in large part, to the lower magnitude of iron stores and levels of iron absorption in female than in male probands. Among affected siblings discordant for sex, the hepatic iron concentration was lower in women than their male siblings. Similarly, in affected siblings of different sex, the total iron removed by phlebotomy was markedly lower in women than in men, unless amenorrhea was present. Menses doubles or triples daily iron losses; the average total iron requirement for a normal singleton pregnancy is ~800 mg (range 500–1400 mg). Because some hemochromatosis subjects accumulate 300–500 mg iron per year, the iron balance in menstruating women who are hemochromatosis homozygotes may be slightly positive or neutral. Approximately 6% of menstruating women with hemochromatosis diagnosed in medical care or family studies have normal serum iron measures. Nonetheless, some women with hemochromatosis develop severe iron overload.

Dietary iron content

Excess iron cannot be absorbed unless the diet provides more available iron than is required. It is required for growth, pregnancy, and lactation, than is sufficient to replace unavoidable losses. The assumption that the amount of dietary iron influences the phenotypic expression of hemochromatosis is based on the evidence that heme iron is readily absorbed and promotes the absorption of non-heme iron, whereas non-heme iron has a low bioavailability and its absorption is influenced by other dietary ingredients (Chapter 2). It has been proposed that the great *per capita* consumption of meat, for example, would explain the high prevalence and relative early age of presentation of iron overload disease in hemochromatosis patients in Australia. Nonetheless, a study of 41 hemochromatosis homozygotes in Australia revealed that meat consumption or alcohol intake did not account for phenotype variability. Further, another study concluded that diet, and especially meat consumption, significantly influenced serum ferritin levels in women but not men in a large, healthy Australian population. There are no other reports of studies designed specifically to evaluate the role of dietary iron in determining the phenotypic variability of hemochromatosis.

Other factors

Blood donation status has the second greatest influence on serum ferritin concentration. Regular blood donations and pathological blood loss (e.g. peptic ulcer, hookworm infestation, and inflammatory bowel disease) may delay the appearance of iron overload or reduce its ultimate severity in hemochromatosis homozygotes. It is prudent to suspect iron malabsorption or pathologic blood loss in men with hemochromatosis who do not have iron overload or who do not reaccumulate iron after achieving iron depletion with phlebotomy. Use of proton pump inhibitors, regular consumption of calcium as antacids or as nutritional supplements, celiac disease, or bariatric surgery may reduce iron absorption in some subjects with hemochromatosis. Regular tea drinking reduces iron absorption; tannins in tea bind inorganic iron and inhibit its absorption.

Heavy alcohol intake is common in patients with hemochromatosis, although great differences exist in different hemochromatosis populations. Whether alcohol ingestion significantly increases iron absorption in humans with or without hemochromatosis is controversial. Even in South African blacks who ingest large amounts of iron in traditional beer brewed in iron pots, the development of iron overload requires the additional presence of a putative iron-loading gene (Chapter 18). There is no direct evidence that heavy alcohol intake increases iron overload in hemochromatosis homozygotes. Nonetheless, chronic heavy alcohol intake accelerates organ damage, increasing storage of iron in extrahepatic sites, and increases the risk of hepatocellular carcinoma in patients with hemochromatosis. Similarly, chronic hepatitis B or C infections favor the development of hepatic cirrhosis and hepatocellular carcinoma, but do not increase total body iron. Some persons who have heritable types of anemia develop iron overload. Hemochromatosis has been reported to occur in some persons who have hereditary spherocytosis, although if is not clear that this type of hemolytic anemia enhances iron absorption. Many persons with erythrocyte pyruvate kinase deficiency, congenital dyserythropoietic anemia, or thalassemia major develop iron overload. Some of them co-inherit common *HFE* mutations, but the development of iron overload is due predominantly to ineffective erythropoiesis (mediated by growth/differentiation factor 15; GDF15) and chronic transfusion (Chapters 21–25, 27). Some investigators have suggested that patients with beta-thalassemia minor who were hemochromatosis homozygotes had unusually severe iron overload, although other investigators have reported that iron overload phenotypes in patients with hemochromatosis with and without beta-thalassemia minor are similar.

Despite major advances in the comprehension of the genetic basis of hemochromatosis and iron overload, several questions remain unresolved. The discovery of a single major mutation (C282Y) in the *HFE* gene does not explain the variability of iron overload among C282Y homozygotes. The concordance of disease expression between siblings, in addition to the association between disease severity and the presence of the ancestral haplotype, suggest that other genetic factors are involved in the regulation of iron metabolism and that they interact with or modulate the expression of common *HFE* mutations, if not also expression of the wild-type or normal *HFE* allele. The elucidation of the mechanisms of regulation of iron absorption by the *HFE* protein will provide new insights into the comprehension of genotype–phenotype correlations in hemochromatosis.

Basis of diagnosis
Early definitions of hemochromatosis

The definition of hemochromatosis has undergone a great metamorphosis from the initial description of "bronze diabetes" in 1865 to the identification of the

HFE gene in 1996. The original definition was descriptive and syndromic: skin pigmentation and diabetes mellitus. Six years later, the definition was modified to include iron deposition in a cirrhotic liver. In 1889, von Recklinghausen advanced the definition to emphasize the presumed pathophysiologic abnormality: iron from circulating blood accumulated in and caused pigmentation of the liver.

During most of the twentieth century, hemochromatosis was considered to be an idiopathic disorder. Some authors included in the definition a statement about possible causes of iron overload, such as an unidentified environmental effect, disordered copper metabolism, or alcohol abuse. Sheldon considered the possibility that hemochromatosis is an inborn error of metabolism.[48] Before 1949, hemochromatosis was regarded as untreatable, because there was no known reliable therapy for iron overload or its complications. The first reports of phlebotomy therapy for hemochromatosis appeared at mid-century. By 1955, hemochromatosis was believed to be a rare idiopathic disorder of iron metabolism, primarily of middle-aged men, that caused heavy iron overload. Signs and symptoms included gray skin pigmentation, hepatomegaly, splenomegaly, ascites, diabetes mellitus, hypogonadism, heart failure, hepatic cirrhosis, and hepatocellular carcinoma. Most reports described only patients who had end-stage organ damage due to iron overload. Because hemochromatosis was not generally acknowledged to be a heritable disorder, family members of probands were not routinely evaluated for iron overload or its complications. Thus, there are few descriptions from this era of young individuals who had no organ damage. Most patients described were men approximately 50 years of age; few women were diagnosed. The apparent gender bias added confusion about the nature of the disorder. It is now understood that affected women are granted some reprieve from iron accumulation due to their losses of iron during menstruation, pregnancy, and childbirth, although it is clear that this easily-understood explanation for phenotype differences between men and women is not wholly adequate.

Changing definition based on segregation analysis and HLA type

In the 1970s, a major advancement occurred: the hypothesis that hemochromatosis is an inherited disorder.[102] The mode of genetic transmission, however, was obscured because penetrance of hemochromatosis is incomplete, and because iron overload is more severe in men than women. Nonetheless, the heritable nature of hemochromatosis was accepted due to three observations. First, hemochromatosis occurs with greater frequency than expected among siblings of affected individuals and among the offspring of consanguineous marriages. Second, segregation analysis of informative pedigrees revealed that hemochromatosis is transmitted as an autosomal recessive trait. Third, the results of segregation analysis also demonstrated that diabetes mellitus and hemochromatosis segregate independently as genetic traits. These findings resulted in a change of the definition of hemochromatosis to indicate that it is an autosomal recessive disorder that causes iron overload.

In the mid 1970s, the observation that hemochromatosis is associated with the human leukocyte antigen (HLA) serotype A3 changed thinking about the disorder for two main reasons. First, confirmation of the tight genetic linkage of hemochromatosis to the major histocompatibility complex, and physical mapping of the HLA class I region to 6p21.3 raised the possibility of identifying the hemochromatosis gene. Second, the hypothesis of a founder mutation for hemochromatosis provided the single most important piece of information that later contributed to cloning of the hemochromatosis gene (Chapter 4).

Further understanding of the phenotypic expression of hemochromatosis was achieved in the 1980s. Incremental understanding of iron balance in affected individuals and postulates about the natural history of the disorder contributed to an evolving definition. The phenotypic expression of hemochromatosis, including the iron phenotypes of homozygotes and heterozygotes, was characterized. Among heterozygotes, 10%–25% have an elevated transferrin saturation value or serum ferritin concentration, but most do not develop heavy iron overload or its complications unless they have an additional condition that contributes to increased iron absorption.

A large screening study for hemochromatosis among healthy volunteer blood donors was performed in Utah in 1988.[94] The results demonstrated that it is possible to identify young, asymptomatic homozygotes before the onset of illness caused by iron overload. In fact, most of the homozygotes who were identified by a transferrin saturation value >60% were not iron-loaded. Evaluation of the first-degree relatives of the probands (by HLA typing and measurement of serum transferrin saturation and ferritin levels) resulted in the identification of additional, asymptomatic homozygotes. The Utah blood bank screening study confirmed previous estimates of the frequency of homozygosity for hemochromatosis among Caucasians of European ancestry (5 per 1000). These results and those of many other population and family screening studies added evidence to support a revised definition of hemochromatosis: an autosomal recessive trait that can be identified prior to the development of iron overload and organ damage.

Definition after identification of the hemochromatosis gene

A hemochromatosis-associated gene (*HFE*) was isolated in 1996.[2] The existence of a founder mutation enabled researchers to localize the candidate region by analyzing conserved haplotypes on chromosomes bearing a hemochromatosis gene. Initial genetic analysis suggested that the hemochromatosis locus was within one centimorgan of HLA-A. Subsequent studies revealed that this estimate was low due to reduced recombination in this region. Positional cloning based on borders defined by conserved regions identified a sequence having a mutation common in hemochromatosis chromosomes. Homozygosity for a mutation resulting in a c.845G→A change (cysteine to tyrosine at residue 282; p.C282Y) was present in a majority, but not all, patients with hemochromatosis. In four reports, the frequency of homozygosity for the *HFE* C282Y mutation among hemochromatosis homozygotes varied from 82%–90%. In a study restricted to pedigrees having two or more affected individuals, the C282Y mutation was detected in 100% of cases.

The etiology of iron overload in the 11%–18% of individuals with hemochromatosis phenotypes who are not homozygous for the C282Y mutation may be due to other mutations that occur in the *HFE* gene, or to other genes are involved in the regulation of iron absorption. A second common mutation in *HFE* (c.187C→G; H63D) was also identified in 1996. This polymorphism also contributes to iron loading. Other non-synonymous exon mutations in *HFE* have also been described in individuals with iron overload, especially S65C, although many of these persons have a copy of C282Y or H63D. Therefore, hemochromatosis can now be defined as a disorder of iron metabolism that is inherited as an autosomal recessive trait due to two mutant *HFE* alleles.[103]

It is understood that such genotypes may increase the susceptibility to develop iron overload, although this genetic definition does not require the presence of symptoms or signs of illness, or the development of iron overload.

Non-*HFE* inherited hemochromatosis

Hereditary forms of hemochromatosis can occur that are associated with mutations in genes other than *HFE*.[103] Some of these familial syndromes have clinical characteristics that differ from those of "classical" *HFE* hemochromatosis (Chapters 12–16). A modern genotypic definition of hemochromatosis should include these disorders as distinct entities.

The Online Mendelian Inheritance in Man (OMIM) database

This currently recognizes four forms of heritable hemochromatosis. The classification has limited utility because it is not descriptive, and because mutations in two different genes account for "type II" hemochromatosis.

Type I

"Classical" autosomal recessive hemochromatosis associated with mutations of *HFE* (HFE gene) on chromosome 6p21.3 (OMIM No. +235200) (Chapters 4, 8).

Type II

"Juvenile" or early age-of-onset autosomal recessive hemochromatosis due to mutations in either *HJV* (hemojuvelin gene) on chromosome 1q (type IIA, OMIM # 602930), or the *HAMP* (hepcidin gene) (type IIB, OMIM #606464) (Chapters 13, 14).

Type III

Transferrin receptor-2 autosomal recessive hemochromatosis (OMIM #604250) due to mutations in *TFR2* (transferrin receptor-2 gene) on chromosome 7 (Chapter 15).

Type IV

Autosomal dominant hemochromatosis linked to *SLC40A1* (ferroportin gene) mutations on chromosome 2q32 (OMIM # 606069). Two fundamental phenotypes depend on the specific *SLC40A1* mutations (Chapter 12).

Other rare disorders associated with multi-organ iron overload include atransferrinemia (Chapter 19), aceruloplasminemia (Chapter 28), ferritin heavy-chain ("Japanese") iron overload (Chapter 16), DMT1 iron overload (Chapter 20), glutaredoxin deficiency (Chapter 25), and some other types of heritable anemia (Chapters 21–25). Other syndromes of inherited iron overload are likely to be described in the future.

Problems with a genetic definition

The result of diverse genetically defined iron-related disorders is that they cause progressive increase in body iron that may eventually cause organ dysfunction. From the viewpoint of the clinician, it is often more important to recognize the early phenotypic manifestations of disease than to seek genetic definitions in every patient with possible iron overload. The predominant genetic profile underlying hemochromatosis in individuals of northern European descent is *HFE* C282Y homozygosity. Although the prevalence of this genotype is high, its penetrance, particularly that defined as the chance of developing organ dysfunction due to iron overload, is relatively low. Thus, persons defined as having *HFE* hemochromatosis because they have *HFE* C282Y homozygosity will include a large proportion of individuals who may never develop significant iron overload. This definition is therefore less relevant to the clinician than criteria to identify persons whose risk of developing deleterious iron overload is high and thus need treatment. Accordingly, it is important to consider a definition of hemochromatosis that describes a clinically significant phenotype in a standard manner, regardless of genotype.

Phenotypic definition of hemochromatosis

Most phenotypic definitions include three basic components. First, the specific exclusion of "secondary" forms of iron overload such as those related to ineffective erythropoiesis or chronic erythrocyte transfusions is important because the clinical approach to patients with iron overload differs according to the presence or absence of heritable anemia. Second, the syndrome of iron overload should be familial and seemingly inherited. Third, the presence of significant iron overload should be demonstrated.

Assessment of body iron stores is described in Chapter 4. The normal adult has about 1000 mg of storage iron; in general, the level is higher in men than women (Chapter 2). Although definitions of excess body iron vary, it is generally accepted that individuals with 4–5 g or more of excess body iron have iron overload. Greater quantities are probably needed to cause iron overload disease. The clinical significance of more modest degrees excess body iron (2–4 g) is unknown.

Practical approach for clinicians

Clinicians should have a high awareness of the early phenotypic manifestations of iron overload and evaluate patients for hemochromatosis. In most patients with potentially injurious iron overload, the serum transferrin saturation is usually elevated. Some persons with ferroportin hemochromatosis have normal or low transferrin saturation levels. All persons with increased body iron stores have elevated serum ferritin levels (Chapter 4). If the serum iron measures suggest that diagnosis of hemochromatosis or iron overload, *HFE* mutation analysis is commercially available and can help to confirm the diagnosis of *HFE* hemochromatosis typical of western European Caucasians. If the *HFE* genotype is not one that is typically associated with iron overload, performing a liver biopsy to document hepatic iron overload may be indicated, especially if the serum ferritin level is greater than 1000 μg/L. Otherwise, a carefully monitored trial of quantitative phlebotomy that serves both as diagnosis and treatment is indicated (Chapter 36).

The demonstration of iron overload in patients without *HFE* hemochromatosis-associated genotypes indicates that a search for less common hemochromatosis alleles may be warranted. Identification of the causative genetic abnormality supports diagnosis of the proband. Further, this augments phenotype screening of family members that is important for early diagnosis and prevention of iron overload and associated organ dysfunction. Biochemical (phenotype) testing alone should be used in families whose proband has no demonstrable iron-related mutation.

References

1. Simon M, Bourel M, Fauchet R, Genetet B. Association of HLA-A3 and HLA-B14 antigens with idiopathic haemochromatosis. *Gut* 1976; **17**: 332–4.

2. Feder JN, Gnirke A, Thomas W, *et al.* A novel MHC class I-like gene is mutated in patients with hereditary haemochromatosis. *Nat Genet* 1996; **13**: 399–408.

3. Zhou XY, Tomatsu S, Fleming RE, *et al*. *HFE* gene knockout produces mouse model of hereditary hemochromatosis. *Proc Natl Acad Sci USA* 1998; **95**: 2492–7.

4. Levy JE, Montross LK, Cohen DE, Fleming MD, Andrews NC. The C282Y mutation causing hereditary hemochromatosis does not produce a null allele. *Blood* 1999; **94**: 9–11.

5. Feder JN, Tsuchihashi Z, Irrinki A, *et al*. The hemochromatosis founder mutation in *HLA-H* disrupts beta2-microglobulin interaction and cell surface expression. *J Biol Chem* 1997; **272**: 14025–8.

6. Waheed A, Parkkila S, Zhou XY, *et al*. Hereditary hemochromatosis: effects of C282Y and H63D mutations on association with beta2-microglobulin, intracellular processing, and cell surface expression of the HFE protein in COS-7 cells. *Proc Natl Acad Sci USA* 1997; **94**: 12384–9.

7. Santos M, Schilham MW, Rademakers LH, Marx JJ, de Sousa M, Clevers H. Defective iron homeostasis in beta2-microglobulin knockout mice recapitulates hereditary hemochromatosis in man. *J Exp Med* 1996; **184**: 1975–85.

8. Fleming RE, Britton RS, Waheed A, Sly WS, Bacon BR. Pathogenesis of hereditary hemochromatosis. *Clin Liver Dis* 2004; **8**: 755–73, vii.

9. Beckman LE, Saha N, Spitsyn V, Van Landeghem G, Beckman L. Ethnic differences in the *HFE* codon 282 (Cys/Tyr) polymorphism. *Hum Hered* 1997; **47**: 263–7.

10. Rochette J, Pointon JJ, Fisher CA, *et al*. Multicentric origin of hemochromatosis gene (*HFE*) mutations. *Am J Hum Genet* 1999; **64**: 1056–62.

11. Beutler E, Felitti VJ, Koziol JA, Ho NJ, Gelbart T. Penetrance of 845G-> A (C282Y) *HFE* hereditary haemochromatosis mutation in the USA. *Lancet* 2002; **359**: 211–18.

12. Jacolot S, Le Gac G, Scotet V, Quere I, Mura C, Ferec C. *HAMP* as a modifier gene that increases the phenotypic expression of the *HFE* pC282Y homozygous genotype. *Blood* 2004; **103**: 2835–40.

13. Steinberg KK, Cogswell ME, Chang JC, *et al*. Prevalence of C282Y and H63D mutations in the hemochromatosis (*HFE*) gene in the United States. *JAMA* 2001; **285**: 2216–22.

14. Gochee PA, Powell LW, Cullen DJ, Du SD, Rossi E, Olynyk JK. A population-based study of the biochemical and clinical expression of the H63D hemochromatosis mutation. *Gastroenterology* 2002; **122**: 646–51.

15. Barton JC, Shih WW, Sawada-Hirai R, *et al*. Genetic and clinical description of hemochromatosis probands and heterozygotes: evidence that multiple genes linked to the major histocompatibility complex are responsible for hemochromatosis. *Blood Cells Mol Dis* 1997; **23**: 135–45.

16. Pointon JJ, Wallace D, Merryweather-Clarke AT, Robson KJ. Uncommon mutations and polymorphisms in the hemochromatosis gene. *Genet Test* 2000; **4**: 151–61.

17. Beutler E, Griffin MJ, Gelbart T, West C. A previously undescribed nonsense mutation of the *HFE* gene. *Clin Genet* 2002; **61**: 40–2.

18. Barton JC, West C, Lee PL, Beutler E. A previously undescribed frameshift deletion mutation of *HFE* (c.del277; G93fs) associated with hemochromatosis and iron overload in a C282Y heterozygote. *Clin Genet* 2004; **66**: 214–16.

19. Human Gene Mutation Database at the Institute of Medical Genetics in Cardiff. 01–23–2010.

20. Fleming RE, Britton RS. Iron Imports. VI. *HFE* and regulation of intestinal iron absorption. *Am J Physiol Gastrointest Liver Physiol* 2006; **290**: G590–4.

21. Goswami T, Andrews NC. Hereditary hemochromatosis protein, HFE, interaction with transferrin receptor 2 suggests a molecular mechanism for mammalian iron sensing. *J Biol Chem* 2006; **281**: 28 494–8.

22. Schmidt PJ, Toran PT, Giannetti AM, Bjorkman PJ, Andrews NC. The transferrin receptor modulates Hfe-dependent regulation of hepcidin expression. *Cell Metab* 2008; **7**: 205–14.

23. Bridle KR, Frazer DM, Wilkins SJ, *et al*. Disrupted hepcidin regulation in *HFE*-associated haemochromatosis and the liver as a regulator of body iron homoeostasis. *Lancet* 2003; **361**: 669–73.

24. Vujic Spasic M, Kiss J, Herrmann T, *et al*. Hfe acts in hepatocytes to prevent hemochromatosis. *Cell Metab* 2008; **7**: 173–8.

25. Stuart KA, Anderson GJ, Frazer DM, *et al*. Duodenal expression of iron transport molecules in untreated haemochromatosis subjects. *Gut* 2003; **52**: 953–9.

26. Bezwoda WR, Disler PB, Lynch SR, *et al*. Patterns of food iron absorption in iron-deficient white and Indian subjects and in venesected haemochromatotic patients. *Br J Haematol* 1976; **33**: 425–36.

27. Lynch SR, Skikne BS, Cook JD. Food iron absorption in idiopathic hemochromatosis. *Blood* 1989; **74**: 2187–93.

28. Parmley RT, Barton JC, Conrad ME. Ultrastructural localization of transferrin, transferrin receptor, and iron-binding sites on human placental and duodenal microvilli. *Br J Haematol* 1985; **60**: 81–9.

29. Whittaker P, Skikne BS, Covell AM, *et al*. Duodenal iron proteins in idiopathic hemochromatosis. *J Clin Invest* 1989; **83**: 261–7.

30. Feder JN, Penny DM, Irrinki A, *et al.* The hemochromatosis gene product complexes with the transferrin receptor and lowers its affinity for ligand binding. *Proc Natl Acad Sci USA* 1998; **95**: 1472–7.

31. Lebron JA, Bennett MJ, Vaughn DE, *et al.* Crystal structure of the hemochromatosis protein HFE and characterization of its interaction with transferrin receptor. *Cell* 1998; **93**: 111–23.

32. Kelleher T, Ryan E, Barrett S, *et al.* Increased *DMT1* but not *IREG1* or *HFE* mRNA following iron depletion therapy in hereditary haemochromatosis. *Gut* 2004; **53**: 1174–9.

33. Turnbull A, Giblett ER. The binding and transport of iron by transferrin variants. *J Lab Clin Med* 1961; **57**: 450–9.

34. Bothwell TH, Jacobs P, Torrance JD. Studies on the behavior of transferrin in idiopathic haemochromatosis. *S Afr J Med Sci* 1962; **27**: 35–9.

35. Wheby MS, Balcerzak SP, Anderson P, Crosby WH. Clearance of iron from hemochromatotic and normal transferin in vivo. *Blood* 1964; **24**: 765–9.

36. Batey RG, Lai Chung FP, Shamir S, Sherlock S. A non-transferrin-bound serum iron in idiopathic hemochromatosis. *Dig Dis Sci* 1980; **25**: 340–6.

37. Cairo G, Conte D, Bianchi L, Fraquelli M, Recalcati S. Reduced serum ceruloplasmin levels in hereditary haemochromatosis. *Br J Haematol* 2001; **114**: 226–9.

38. Laine F, Ropert M, Lan CL, *et al.* Serum ceruloplasmin and ferroxidase activity are decreased in *HFE* C282Y homozygote male iron overloaded patients. *J Hepatol* 2002; **36**: 60–5.

39. Sciot R, Paterson AC, Van den Oord JJ, Desmet VJ. Lack of hepatic transferrin receptor expression in hemochromatosis. *Hepatology* 1987; **7**: 831–7.

40. Lombard M, Bomford A, Hynes M, *et al.* Regulation of the hepatic transferrin receptor in hereditary hemochromatosis. *Hepatology* 1989; **9**: 1–5.

41. Kawabata H, Yang R, Hirama T, *et al.* Molecular cloning of transferrin receptor 2. A new member of the transferrin receptor-like family. *J Biol Chem* 1999; **274**: 20826–32.

42. Chua ACG, Delima RD, Morgan EH, *et al.* Iron uptake from plasma transferrin by a transferrin receptor 2 mutant mouse model of haemachromatosis, *J Hepatol* (in press).

43. Merle U, Theilig F, Fein E, *et al.* Localization of the iron-regulatory proteins hemojuvelin and transferrin receptor 2 to the basolateral membrane domain of hepatocytes. *Histochem Cell Biol* 2007; **127**: 221–6.

44. Davies PS, Zhang AS, Anderson EL, *et al.* Evidence for the interaction of the hereditary haemochromatosis protein, HFE, with the transferrin receptor in endocytic compartments. *Biochem J* 2003; **373**: 145–53.

45. Mackenzie B, Ujwal ML, Chang MH, Romero MF, Hediger MA. Divalent metal-ion transporter DMT1 mediates both H+ coupled Fe2+ transport and uncoupled fluxes. *Pflugers Arch* 2006; **451**: 544–58.

46. Rahier J, Loozen S, Goebbels RM, Abrahem M. The haemochromatotic human pancreas: a quantitative immunohistochemical and ultrastructural study. *Diabetologia* 1987; **30**: 5–12.

47. Lu JP, Hayashi K. Selective iron deposition in pancreatic islet B cells of transfusional iron overloaded autopsy cases. *Pathol Int* 1994; **44**: 194–9.

48. Sheldon JH. *Haemochromatosis.* London, Oxford University Press, 1935.

49. Peillon F, Racadot J. [Histopathological modification in the hypophysis in 6 cases of hemochromatosis.] *Ann Endocrinol (Paris)* 1969; **30**: 800–7.

50. Bergeron C, Kovacs K. Pituitary siderosis. A histologic, immunocytologic, and ultrastructural study. *Am J Pathol* 1978; **93**: 295–309.

51. Atkin SL, Burnett HE, Green VL, White MC, Lombard M. Expression of the transferrin receptor in human anterior pituitary adenomas is confined to gonadotrophinomas. *Clin Endocrinol (Oxf)* 1996; **44**: 467–71.

52. Tampanaru-Sarmesiu A, Stefaneanu L, Thapar K, Kontogeorgos G, Sumi T, Kovacs K. Transferrin and transferrin receptor in human hypophysis and pituitary adenomas. *Am J Pathol* 1998; **152**: 413–22.

53. McDermott JH, Walsh CH. Hypogonadism in hereditary hemochromatosis. *J Clin Endocrinol Metab* 2005; **90**: 2451–5.

54. Barton JC, Bertoli LF, Rothenberg BE. Peripheral blood erythrocyte parameters in hemochromatosis: evidence for increased erythrocyte hemoglobin content. *J Lab Clin Med* 2000; **135**: 96–104.

55. Beutler E, Felitti V, Gelbart T, Ho N. The effect of *HFE* genotypes on measurements of iron overload in patients attending a health appraisal clinic. *Ann Intern Med* 2000; **133**: 329–37.

56. McLaren CE, Barton JC, Gordeuk VR, *et al.* Determinants and characteristics of mean corpuscular volume and hemoglobin concentration in white *HFE* C282Y homozygotes in the hemochromatosis and iron overload screening study. *Am J Hematol* 2007; **82**: 898–905.

57. Feeney GP, Carter K, Masters GS, Jackson HA, Cavil I, Worwood M. Changes in erythropoiesis in hereditary hemochromatosis are not mediated by HFE expression in nucleated red cells. *Haematologica* 2005; **90**: 180–7.

58. Lin JP, O'Donnell CJ, Jin L, Fox C, Yang Q, Cupples LA. Evidence for linkage of red blood cell size and count: genome-wide scans in the Framingham Heart Study. *Am J Hematol* 2007; **82**: 605–10.

59. Kozewski BJ. The occurrence of megaloblastic erythropoiesis in patients with hemochromatosis. *Blood* 1952; **7**: 1182–95.

60. Quigley JG, Yang Z, Worthington MT, *et al.* Identification of a human heme exporter that is essential for erythropoiesis. *Cell* 2004; **118**: 757–66.

61. Keel SB, Doty RT, Yang Z, *et al.* A heme export protein is required for red blood cell differentiation and iron homeostasis. *Science* 2008; **319**: 825–8.

62. Gehrke SG, Kulaksiz H, Herrmann T, *et al.* Expression of hepcidin in hereditary hemochromatosis: evidence for a regulation in response to the serum transferrin saturation and to non-transferrin-bound iron. *Blood* 2003; **102**: 371–6.

63. Piperno A, Girelli D, Nemeth E, *et al.* Blunted hepcidin response to oral iron challenge in *HFE*-related hemochromatosis. *Blood* 2007; **110**: 4096–100.

64. Ganz T. Iron homeostasis: fitting the puzzle pieces together. *Cell Metab* 2008; **7**: 288–90.

65. Tanno T, Bhanu NV, Oneal PA, *et al.* High levels of GDF15 in thalassemia suppress expression of the iron regulatory protein hepcidin. *Nat Med* 2007; **13**: 1096–101.

66. Mast AE, Foster TM, Pinder HL, *et al.* Behavioral, biochemical, and genetic analysis of iron metabolism in high-intensity blood donors. *Transfusion* 2008; **48**: 2197–204.

67. Lee PL, Gelbart T, West C, Halloran C, Felitti V, Beutler E. A study of genes that may modulate the expression of hereditary hemochromatosis: transferrin receptor-1, ferroportin, ceruloplasmin, ferritin light and heavy chains, iron regulatory proteins (IRP)-1 and -2, and hepcidin. *Blood Cells Mol Dis* 2001; **27**: 783–802.

68. Hofmann WK, Tong XJ, Ajioka RS, Kushner JP, Koeffler HP. Mutation analysis of transferrin-receptor 2 in patients with atypical hemochromatosis. *Blood* 2002; **100**: 1099–100.

69. Lee P, Gelbart T, West C, Halloran C, Beutler E. Seeking candidate mutations that affect iron homeostasis. *Blood Cells Mol Dis* 2002; **29**: 471–87.

70. Kelleher T, Ryan E, Barrett S, O'Keane C, Crowe J. *DMT1* genetic variability is not responsible for phenotype variability in hereditary hemochromatosis. *Blood Cells Mol Dis* 2004; **33**: 35–9.

71. Lee PL, Barton JC, Brandhagen D, Beutler E. Hemojuvelin (*HJV*) mutations in persons of European, African-American and Asian ancestry with adult onset haemochromatosis. *Br J Haematol* 2004; **127**: 224–9.

72. Le Gac G, Scotet V, Ka C, *et al.* The recently identified type 2A juvenile haemochromatosis gene (*HJV*), a second candidate modifier of the C282Y homozygous phenotype. *Hum Mol Genet* 2004; **13**: 1913–18.

73. Mura C, Le Gac G, Scotet V, Raguenes O, Mercier AY, Ferec C. Variation of iron loading expression in C282Y homozygous haemochromatosis probands and sib pairs. *J Med Genet* 2001; **38**: 632–6.

74. Barton JC, Wiener HW, Acton RT, Go RC. HLA haplotype A*03-B*07 in hemochromatosis probands with *HFE* C282Y homozygosity: frequency disparity in men and women and lack of association with severity of iron overload. *Blood Cells Mol Dis* 2005; **34**: 38–47.

75. Olatunbosun D, Corbett WE, Ludwig J, Valberg LS. Alteration of cobalt absorption in portal cirrhosis and idiopathic hemochromatosis. *J Lab Clin Med* 1970; **75**: 754–62.

76. Akesson A, Stal P, Vahter M. Phlebotomy increases cadmium uptake in hemochromatosis. *Environ Health Perspect* 2000; **108**: 289–91.

77. Barton JC, Patton MA, Edwards CQ, *et al.* Blood lead concentrations in hereditary hemochromatosis. *J Lab Clin Med* 1994; **124**: 193–8.

78. Barton JC. The absorption and metabolism of non-ferrous metals in hemochromatosis. In: Barton JC, Edwards CQ, eds. *Hemochromatosis: Genetics, Pathophysiology, Diagnosis and Treatment.* Cambridge, Cambridge University Press. 2000; 131–44.

79. Pietrangelo A, Rocchi E, Casalgrandi G, *et al.* Regulation of transferrin, transferrin receptor, and ferritin genes in human duodenum. *Gastroenterology* 1992; **102**: 802–9.

80. Feder JN, Penny DM, Irrinki A, *et al.* The hemochromatosis gene product complexes with the transferrin receptor and lowers its affinity for ligand binding. *Proc Natl Acad Sci USA* 1998; **95**: 1472–7.

81. Altstatt LB, Pollack S, Feldman MH, Reba RC, Crosby WH. Liver manganese in hemochromatosis. *Proc Soc Exp Biol Med* 1967; **124**: 353–5.

82. Adams PC, Bradley C, Frei JV. Hepatic zinc in hemochromatosis. *Clin Invest Med* 1991; **14**: 16–20.

83. Brissot P, Le Treut A, Dien G, Cottencin M, Simon M, Bourel M. Hypovitaminemia A in idiopathic hemochromatosis and hepatic cirrhosis. Role of retinol-binding protein and zinc. *Digestion* 1978; **17**: 469–78.

84. Sargent T, 3rd, Lim TH, Jenson RL. Reduced chromium retention in patients with hemochromatosis, a possible basis of hemochromatotic diabetes. *Metabolism* 1979; **28**: 70–9.

85. Spencer H, Sontag SJ, Derler J, Osis D. Intestinal absorption of iron in patients with hemochromatosis.

In: Weintraub LR, Edwards CQ, Krikker M, eds. *Hemochromatosis. Proceedings of the First International Conference.* New York, The New York Academy of Sciences. 1988; 336–8.

86. Barton JC, Bertoli LF. Zinc gluconate lozenges for treating the common cold. *Ann Intern Med* 1997; **126**: 738–9.

87. Walshe JM, Cox DW. Effect of treatment of Wilson's disease on natural history of haemochromatosis. *Lancet* 1998; **352**: 112–13.

88. Dib N, Valsesia E, Malinge MC, Mauras Y, Misrahi M, Cales P. Late onset of Wilson's disease in a family with genetic haemochromatosis. *Eur J Gastroenterol Hepatol* 2006; **18**: 43–7.

89. Onalaja AO, Claudio L. Genetic susceptibility to lead poisoning. *Environ Health Perspect* 2000; **108** Suppl 1: 23–8.

90. Mandelli C, Cesarini L, Piperno A, et al. Saturability of hepatic iron deposits in genetic hemochromatosis. *Hepatology* 1992; **16**: 956–9.

91. Niederau C, Fischer R, Sonnenberg A, Stremmel W, Trampisch HJ, Strohmeyer G. Survival and causes of death in cirrhotic and in non-cirrhotic patients with primary hemochromatosis. *N Engl J Med* 1985; **313**: 1256–62.

92. Wood MJ, Powell LW, Ramm GA. Environmental and genetic modifiers of the progression to fibrosis and cirrhosis in hemochromatosis. *Blood* 2008; **111**: 4456–62.

93. Adams PC, Reboussin DM, Barton JC, et al. Hemochromatosis and iron overload screening in a racially diverse population. *N Engl J Med* 2005; **352**: 1769–78.

94. Edwards CQ, Griffen LM, Goldgar D, Drummond C, Skolnick MH, Kushner JP. Prevalence of hemochromatosis among 11 065 presumably healthy blood donors. *N Engl J Med* 1988; **318**: 1355–62.

95. Bulaj ZJ, Ajioka RS, Phillips JD, et al. Disease-related conditions in relatives of patients with hemochromatosis. *N Engl J Med* 2000; **343**: 1529–35.

96. McLaren GD, McLaren CE, Adams PC, et al. Clinical manifestations of hemochromatosis in *HFE* C282Y homozygotes identified by screening. *Can J Gastroenterol* 2008; **22**: 923–30.

97. Adams PC. Non-expressing homozygotes for C282Y hemochromatosis: minority or majority of cases? *Mol Genet Metab* 2000; **71**: 81–6.

98. Barton JC, Harmon L, Rivers C, Acton RT. Hemochromatosis: association of severity of iron overload with genetic markers. *Blood Cells Mol Dis* 1996; **22**: 195–204.

99. Pratiwi R, Fletcher LM, Pyper WR, et al. Linkage disequilibrium analysis in Australian haemochromatosis patients indicates bipartite association with clinical expression. *J Hepatol* 1999; **31**: 39–46.

100. Piperno A, Arosio C, Fargion S, et al. The ancestral hemochromatosis haplotype is associated with a severe phenotype expression in Italian patients. *Hepatology* 1996; **24**: 43–6.

101. Barton JC, Wiener HW, Acton RT, Go RC. HLA haplotype A*03-B*07 in hemochromatosis probands with *HFE* C282Y homozygosity: frequency disparity in men and women and lack of association with severity of iron overload. *Blood Cells Mol Dis* 2005; **34**: 38–47.

102. Cartwright GE, Edwards CQ, Kravitz K, et al. Hereditary hemochromatosis. Phenotypic expression of the disease. *N Engl J Med* 1979; **301**: 175–9.

103. Pietrangelo A. Hereditary hemochromatosis—a new look at an old disease. *N Engl J Med* 2004; **350**: 2383–97.

104. Barton JC, Sawada-Hirai R, Rothenberg BE, Acton RT. Two novel missense mutations of the *HFE* gene (I105T and G93R) and identification of the S65C mutation in Alabama hemochromatosis probands. *Blood Cells Mol Dis* 1999; **25**: 147–55.

105. Beutler E, Gelbart T, West C, et al. Mutation analysis in hereditary hemochromatosis. *Blood Cells Mol Dis* 1996; **22**: 187–94.

106. Marshall DS, Linfert DR, Tsongalis GJ. Prevalence of the C282Y and H63D polymorphisms in a multi-ethnic control population. *Int J Mol Med* 1999; **4**: 389–93.

107. Bradley LA, Johnson DD, Palomaki GE, Haddow JE, Robertson NH, Ferrie RM. Hereditary haemochromatosis mutation frequencies in the general population. *J Med Screen* 1998; **5**: 34–6.

108. McDonnell SM, Hover A, Gloe D, Ou CY, Cogswell ME, Grummer-Strawn L. Population-based screening for hemochromatosis using phenotypic and DNA testing among employees of health maintenance organizations in Springfield, Missouri. *Am J Med* 1999; **107**: 30–7.

109. Garry PJ, Montoya GD, Baumgartner RN, Liang HC, Williams TM, Brodie SG. Impact of *HLA-H* mutations on iron stores in healthy elderly men and women. *Blood Cells Mol Dis* 1997; **23**: 277–87.

110. Monaghan KG, Rybicki BA, Shurafa M, Feldman GL. Mutation analysis of the *HFE* gene associated with hereditary hemochromatosis in African-American(s). *Am J Hematol* 1998; **58**: 213–17.

111. A simple genetic test identifies 90% of UK patients with haemochromatosis. The UK Haemochromatosis Consortium. *Gut* 1997; 41: 841–4.

112. Willis G, Jennings BA, Goodman E, Fellows IW, Wimperis JZ. A high prevalence of *HLA-H* 845A mutations in hemochromatosis patients and the

normal population in eastern England. *Blood Cells Mol Dis* 1997; **23**: 288–91.

113. Murphy S, Curran MD, McDougall N, Callender ME, O'Brien CJ, Middleton D. High incidence of the Cys282Tyr mutation in the *HFE* gene in the Irish population—implications for haemochromatosis. *Tissue Antigens* 1998; **52**: 484–8.

114. Ryan E, O'Keane C, Crowe J. Hemochromatosis in Ireland and *HFE*. *Blood Cells Mol Dis* 1998; **24**: 428–32.

115. Miedzybrodzka Z, Loughlin S, Baty D, *et al.* Haemochromatosis mutations in northeast Scotland. *Br J Haematol* 1999; **106**: 385–7.

116. Jazwinska EC, Cullen LM, Busfield F, *et al.* Haemochromatosis and *HLA-H. Nat Genet* 1996; **14**: 249–51.

117. Rossi E, Henderson S, Chin CY, *et al.* Genotyping as a diagnostic aid in genetic haemochromatosis. *J Gastroenterol Hepatol* 1999; **14**: 427–30.

118. Adams PC, Chakrabarti S. Genotypic/phenotypic correlations in genetic hemochromatosis: evolution of diagnostic criteria. *Gastroenterology* 1998; **114**: 319–23.

119. Milman N, Koefoed P, Pedersen P, Nielsen FC, Eiberg H. Frequency of the *HFE* C282Y and H63D mutations in Danish patients with clinical haemochromatosis initially diagnosed by phenotypic methods. *Eur J Haematol* 2003; **71**: 403–7.

120. Erhardt A, Niederau C, Osman Y, Hassan M, Haussinger D. [Demonstration of *HFE* polymorphism in German patients with hereditary haemochromatosis.] *Dtsch Med Wochenschr* 1999; **124**: 1448–52.

121. Gottschalk R, Seidl C, Schilling S, *et al.* Iron overload and genotypic expression of *HFE* mutations H63D/C282Y and transferrin receptor Hin6I and BanI polymorphism in German patients with hereditary haemochromatosis. *Eur J Immunogenet* 2000; **27**: 129–34.

122. Hellerbrand C, Bosserhoff AK, Seegers S, *et al.* Mutation analysis of the *HFE* gene in German hemochromatosis patients and controls using automated SSCP-based capillary electrophoresis and a new PCR-ELISA technique. *Scand J Gastroenterol* 2001; **36**: 1211–16.

123. Nielsen P, Carpinteiro S, Fischer R, Cabeda JM, Porto G, Gabbe EE. Prevalence of the C282Y and H63D mutations in the *HFE* gene in patients with hereditary haemochromatosis and in control subjects from northern Germany. *Br J Haematol* 1998; **103**: 842–5.

124. Van Vlierberghe H, Messiaen L, Hautekeete M, De Paepe A, Elewaut A. Prevalence of the Cys282Tyr and His63Asp mutation in Flemish patients with hereditary haemochromatosis. *Acta Gastroenterol Belg* 2000; **63**: 250–3.

125. de Juan D, Reta A, Castiella A, Pozueta J, Prada A, Cuadrado E. *HFE* gene mutations analysis in Basque hereditary haemochromatosis patients and controls. *Eur J Hum Genet* 2001; **9**: 961–4.

126. Guix P, Picornell A, Parera M, *et al.* Prevalence of the C282Y mutation for haemochromatosis on the Island of Majorca. *Clin Genet* 2000; **58**: 123–8.

127. Sanchez M, Bruguera M, Quintero E, *et al.* Hereditary hemochromatosis in Spain. *Genet Test* 2000; **4**: 171–6.

128. Fabrega E, Castro B, Sanchez-Castro L, Benito A, Fernandez-Luna JL, Pons-Romero F. [The prevalence of the Cys282Tyr mutation in the hemochromatosis gene in Cantabria in patients diagnosed with hereditary hemochromatosis.] *Med Clin (Barc)* 1999; **112**: 451–3.

129. Sanchez M, Bruguera M, Bosch J, Rodes J, Ballesta F, Oliva R. Prevalence of the Cys282Tyr and His63Asp *HFE* gene mutations in Spanish patients with hereditary hemochromatosis and in controls. *J Hepatol* 1998; **29**: 725–8.

130. Moreno L, Vallcorba P, Boixeda D, Cabello P, Bermejo F, San Roman C. [The usefulness of the detection of Cys282Tyr and His63Asp mutations in the diagnosis of hereditary hemochromatosis.] *Rev Clin Esp* 1999; **199**: 632–6.

131. Jorquera F, Dominguez A, Diaz-Golpe V, *et al.* C282Y and H63D mutations of the haemochromatosis gene in patients with iron overload. *Rev Esp Enferm Dig* 2001; **93**: 293–302.

132. Jouanolle AM, Fergelot P, Gandon G, Yaouanq J, Le Gall JY, David V. A candidate gene for hemochromatosis: frequency of the C282Y and H63D mutations. *Hum Genet* 1997; **100**: 544–7.

133. Mura C, Raguenes O, Ferec C. *HFE* mutations analysis in 711 hemochromatosis probands: evidence for S65C implication in mild form of hemochromatosis. *Blood* 1999; **93**: 2502–5.

134. Aguilar-Martinez P, Biron C, Blanc F, *et al.* Compound heterozygotes for hemochromatosis gene mutations: may they help to understand the pathophysiology of the disease? *Blood Cells Mol Dis* 1997; **23**: 269–76.

135. Borot N, Roth M, Malfroy L, *et al.* Mutations in the MHC class I-like candidate gene for hemochromatosis in French patients. *Immunogenetics* 1997; **45**: 320–4.

136. Mercier G, Burckel A, Bathelier C, Boillat E, Lucotte G. Mutation analysis of the *HLA-H* gene in French hemochromatosis patients, and genetic counseling in families. *Genet Couns* 1998; **9**: 181–6.

137. Cardoso EM, Stal P, Hagen K, *et al. HFE* mutations in patients with hereditary haemochromatosis in Sweden. *J Intern Med* 1998; **243**: 203–8.

138. Olsson KS, Ritter B, Sandberg L, Raha-Chowdhury R, Gruen J, Worwood M. The ancestral haplotype in patients with genetic hemochromatosis from central and western Sweden. 1997. St. Malo, International Symposium on Iron in Biology and Medicine.

139. Calandro L, Thorsen T, Barcellos L, Griggs J, Baer D, Sensabaugh GF. Mutation analysis in hereditary hemochromatosis. *Blood Cells Mol Dis* 1996; **22**: 194A–4B.

140. Sham RL, Ou CY, Cappuccio J, Braggins C, Dunnigan K, Phatak PD. Correlation between genotype and phenotype in hereditary hemochromatosis: analysis of 61 cases. *Blood Cells Mol Dis* 1997; **23**: 314–20.

141. Brandhagen DJ, Fairbanks VF, Baldus WP, *et al.* Prevalence and clinical significance of *HFE* gene mutations in patients with iron overload. *Am J Gastroenterol* 2000; **95**: 2910–14.

142. Asberg A, Hveem K, Thorstensen K, *et al.* Screening for hemochromatosis: high prevalence and low morbidity in an unselected population of 65 238 persons. *Scand J Gastroenterol* 2001; **36**: 1108–15.

143. Porto G, de Sousa M. Variation of hemochromatosis prevalence and genotype in national groups. In: Barton JC, Edwards CQ, eds. *Hewmochromatosis; Genetics, Pathophysiology, Diagnosis and Treatment.* Cambridge, Cambridge University Press. 2000; 51–62.

144. Datz C, Lalloz MR, Vogel W, *et al.* Predominance of the *HLA-H* Cys282Tyr mutation in Austrian patients with genetic haemochromatosis. *J Hepatol* 1997; **27**: 773–9.

145. Carella M, D'Ambrosio L, Totaro A, *et al.* Mutation analysis of the *HLA-H* gene in Italian hemochromatosis patients. *Am J Hum Genet* 1997; **60**: 828–32.

146. Piperno A, Sampietro M, Pietrangelo A, *et al.* Heterogeneity of hemochromatosis in Italy. *Gastroenterology* 1998; **114**: 996–1002.

147. Papanikolaou G, Politou M, Roetto A, *et al.* Linkage to chromosome 1q in Greek families with juvenile hemochromatosis. *Blood Cells Mol Dis* 2001; **27**: 744–9.

Heterozygosity for *HFE* C282Y

The C282Y polymorphism of the *HFE* gene on chromosome 6p21.3 is the most common known human mutation that has a marked effect on iron absorption and homeostasis. Approximately 12% of Caucasians of northern or western European descent living in Europe or in derivative countries such as the US, Canada, Australia, or New Zealand are simple heterozygotes for C282Y, and they outnumber C282Y homozygotes in these populations by approximately 25:1. In the US alone, approximately 20 million whites are C282Y heterozygotes. If iron-related organ injury or another deleterious allele on C282Y-bearing chromosome 6p haplotypes were to occur in C282Y heterozygotes, the number of individuals at potential risk is great. This has led to an interest in defining: (a) the iron phenotype and any related iron or liver morbidity of C282Y heterozygotes and their management; (b) the optimal means to identify C282Y heterozygotes and to estimate their prevalence in populations; and (c) the association of C282Y with various non-iron-related disorders.

History

The *HFE* C282Y mutation arose in northwestern Europe, perhaps in the Neolithic Age.[1–3] The original C282Y mutation probably occurred on a chromosome 6 haplotype characterized by human leukocyte antigens (HLA)-A*03, B*07, and by the marker allele D6S105(8). C282Y spread with various population movements, especially Viking migrations.[1–4] Many C282Y homozygotes alive today have one or two copies of the ancestral haplotype. Likewise, all C282Y heterozygotes have inherited a common *HFE* polymorphism, but also much or all of an ancestral chromosome with its other component genes and alleles, the effects of which must be considered in understanding fully the effects of C282Y heterozygosity. Although C282Y and HLA-A

and -B loci are tightly linked, other C282Y-bearing haplotypes have appeared over the centuries due to recombination events. Thus, many C282Y haplotypes occur in western European whites, some of which are common and typify certain geographic areas or ethnic groups.

It is presumed that C282Y heterozygosity conferred an evolutionary advantage, although the basis of this presumption is poorly understood. *HFE* is a non-classical, class I HLA gene that influences iron absorption and metabolism.[5] Other HLA genes and alleles influence disease resistance and mate selection.[6] It has been hypothesized that C282Y was a beneficial trait for the transformation of Neolithic Europeans to an agrarian existence in which dietary iron was less plentiful and absorbable than in a meat-based diet typical of hunters.[2,3] A popular conjecture contends that women with C282Y heterozygosity may have once had a reproductive advantage because they could absorb more iron than other women, although the mechanism(s) of this putative advantage is unclear. The evidence that iron deficiency in present day white women with C282Y heterozygosity is lower than that in white women without C282Y is conflicting.[7,8] The risk of ovulatory infertility may be lower in women who consume iron supplements and non-heme iron from other sources, although *HFE* genotypes were not determined in these subjects.[9] In two studies, the mean number of children that hemochromatosis or C282Y heterozygotes had did not differ significantly from that of control subjects.[10,11] C282Y heterozygotes may have a increased resistance to certain infections[12] such as plague that were common in Europe for centuries. Contrariwise, mildly elevated plasma levels of iron typical of persons with *HFE* C282Y may increase their susceptibility to cosmopolitan siderophilic bacteria such as *Escherichia coli* or *Vibrio vulnificus*.[13]

Clinical aspects
Definition of heterozygosity

Hemochromatosis is tightly linked to the HLA class I region on chromosome 6p. Before the discovery of *HFE* in 1996, hemochromatosis homozygotes were diagnosed by iron phenotyping and evaluated further with human leukocyte antigen (HLA)-A and -B testing. It is therefore possible to assign a *HFE* hemochromatosis genotype within a pedigree based on HLA-A and -B types and haplotypes shared with the proband. Because *HFE* hemochromatosis is transmitted as an autosomal recessive disorder, parents and offspring of a proband are, at least, obligate heterozygotes for a hemochromatosis gene. In this manner, presumed hemochromatosis heterozygotes can be identified among the first-degree relatives of presumed homozygotes. In early studies, persons who shared a single HLA haplotype with a first-degree relative diagnosed to have hemochromatosis were defined to be heterozygotes.[14,15] (Chapters 4, 8).

Based on these ascertainment criteria, it was estimated that approximately 12% of white Caucasians in the US were hemochromatosis heterozygotes.[16] Similar population frequency estimates of presumed heterozygotes were derived mathematically by mixture modeling of transferrin saturation and ferritin values in large numbers of whites from the general population.[17] After the discovery of *HFE*, it became possible to detect C282Y heterozygotes by mutation analysis. Therefore, *HFE* genotyping is now routinely used to identify C282Y heterozygotes among family members of hemochromatosis probands or in large-scale general population screening programs.

Symptoms, signs, and physical examination

Most C282Y heterozygotes have no symptoms, signs, or physical characteristics that distinguish them from persons of the same sex and age in the general population. This is due to the fact that most C282Y heterozygotes do not develop harmful degrees of iron overload in the absence of other conditions that also augment iron absorption. In exceptional cases, C282Y heterozygotes come to clinical attention because they have skin lesions due to porphyria cutanea tarda (Chapters 5, 10). Other persons are discovered to have C282Y heterozygosity because they have heritable forms of anemia such as spherocytosis that may act in concert with C282Y heterozygosity to enhance iron absorption and therefore cause or exacerbate iron overload. In such cases, it may be possible to demonstrate that certain symptoms, signs, or abnormalities on physical examination correspond to iron overload-related morbidity.

Laboratory studies
Serum iron measures

An early study performed analyzed the effects of age, sex, heterozygosity, and homozygosity for hemochromatosis on the expected results of tests of iron metabolism; the results were compared to those of normal subjects. Presumed heterozygosity was associated with a modest increase in serum iron concentration, transferrin saturation, serum ferritin concentration, and the grade of stainable iron in hepatocytes. Heterozygosity was associated with a modest decrement in the total iron-binding capacity, presumably the response of normally-functioning hepatocytes to the presence of adequate supplies of transferrin-bound iron.[15]

Utah investigators investigated the iron phenotypes of 1058 hemochromatosis heterozygotes in 202 pedigrees and of 321 normal control subjects.[14] Individuals were classified as heterozygotes based on half-HLA identity to a homozygous proband. Heterozygotes and control subjects were divided by sex into age groups of 1–30 years, 31–60 years, and 61–90 years. A comparison of the results of serum iron measures between the heterozygotes and the control subjects is displayed in Table 9.1. When compared by age and sex, heterozygotes had significantly higher serum iron concentration values than control subjects, consistent with earlier results.[15] The mean transferrin saturation was significantly higher among all groups of male and female heterozygotes than that of the age- and sex-matched control subjects (Table 9.1). Heterozygotes had transferrin saturation values about 22% higher than the age- and sex-matched normal individuals. Male heterozygotes had transferrin saturation values about 20% higher than female heterozygotes. The mean transferrin saturation remained constant across all respective groups of heterozygotes and control subjects.

Using a threshold value of 60% for transferrin saturation and 325 µg/L for serum ferritin for males (50% and 125 µg/L, respectively, for females), only 1% of males and 0.4% of female hemochromatosis heterozygotes had an elevation of both transferrin

Table 9.1 Effects of *HFE* C282Y heterozygosity on iron measures

Test	Expected normal value	Heterozygous effect on test result (+/−)
Serum iron concentration, μg/dL	87 (144)	+17 (238)
Total iron-binding capacity, μg/dL	356 (144)	−31 (238)
Transferrin saturation, %	24 (144)	+9 (238)
Serum ferritin concentration, μg/L	104 (135)	+6 (228)
HPCSI,[a] grade 0–4	0.2 (39)	+0.9 (29)

Note: [a]Hepatic parenchymal cell stainable iron.
Adapted from refs.[14,15]
Serum iron concentration, total iron-binding capacity, transferrin saturation, serum ferritin concentration, and hepatic parenchymal cell stainable iron, expressed as an increment or decrement in expected arithmetic mean values in normal subjects:[14,15] results of multivariate linear analysis. The number of subjects tested appears in parentheses beside the test result.

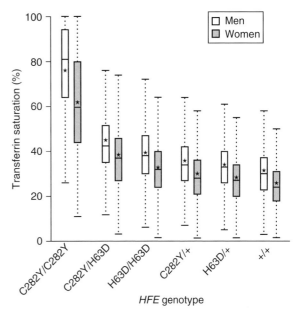

Fig. 9.1. Non-fasting serum transferrin saturation in men and women according to genotype. An elevated transferrin saturation was defined as higher than 45% in women and higher than 50% in men. Data are presented as box plots. The box stretches from the 25th to the 75th percentile. The median is shown with a line across the box, and the mean with an asterisk. The whiskers indicate 1.5 times the interquartile range above the third and below the first quartiles, or the upper or lower extreme values, whichever is closer. Participants who joined the study only because they heard about it from a participating family member or who reported a previous diagnosis of hemochromatosis or iron overload were excluded. Adapted from Adams *et al.* 2005[34] with permission.

saturation and serum ferritin values.[14,15] These results demonstrate that heterozygotes rarely have marked elevation of blood tests of iron metabolism. The serum iron measures in C282Y heterozygotes in screening studies are similar to those reported before the discovery of *HFE* (Figs. 9.1, 9.2). *HFE* C282Y-heterozygotes did not absorb dietary iron more efficiently, even when foods were highly fortified with iron from ferrous sulfate and ascorbic acid, than did control subjects.[18]

Hepatic iron content

Hepatic iron levels in 39 hemochromatosis heterozygotes (22 men, 17 women; age 8–71 years) in a Utah study were measured using atomic absorption spectrophotometry and estimated microscopically by grading the stainable iron in hepatocytes.[14] Iron loading in heterozygotes was uncommon, and massive hepatic iron loading was not detected in any heterozygote (Table 9.2).[14] These results are consistent with those of earlier studies.[15,19] In family or population screening programs or in clinical practice, liver biopsy is not usually indicated or performed in C282Y heterozygotes, unless iron measures are extremely high or there is evidence of a liver disorder

that cannot be diagnosed otherwise. Among 181 patients with hemochromatosis phenotypes who underwent *HFE* genotyping and percutaneous liver biopsy, C282Y heterozygotes comprised less than 1% and none had cirrhosis.[20] Nonetheless, C282Y heterozygosity cannot be inferred from measures of hepatic iron content alone.

Decreased serum ferritin concentration

A serum ferritin value <12 μg/L was detected in 21% of female heterozygotes of reproductive age (12–50 years), and in 32% of age-matched control female subjects. A serum ferritin value <12 μg/L was present in 2% of male heterozygotes age 19 years or greater, and in 4% of age-matched control male subjects.[14,15] In screening studies in southern California and Australia, the prevalence of iron deficiency was slightly lower in women with C282Y heterozygosity than in women without C282Y.[8,21,23]

Table 9.2. Measures of hepatic iron in 39 hemochromatosis heterozygotes[14]

Iron measure	All heterozygotes (*n* = 39)	Heterozygotes with elevated liver iron (*n* = 11)	Reference range
Mean hepatic iron, µg Fe/g dry liver (µmol/g)	1449 µg Fe/g (26 µmol Fe/g)	2411 µg Fe/g (43 µmol Fe/g)	<1400 µg Fe/g (<25 µmol Fe/g)
Hepatocyte iron grade	grade 2 (*n* = 8); grade 3 (*n* = 3)	grades 2–4	grade 0–1

Notes: *Hepatic iron stores were measured by atomic absorption spectrophotometry and microscopically by grading the stainable iron in hepatocytes (grades 0–4). The upper reference limit for hepatic iron concentration is 1400 µg Fe/g dry weight of liver (25 µmol Fe/g dry liver). The reference range for stainable hepatocyte iron is grade 0–1. There were 22 males and 17 females (ages 8–71 years).[14]

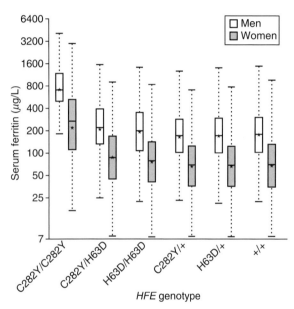

Fig. 9.2. Serum ferritin levels in men and women according to genotype. An elevated serum ferritin level was defined as a level greater than 200 µg/L in women and greater than 300 µg/L in men. Data are presented as box plots. The box stretches from the 25th to 75th percentile. The median is shown with a line across the box, and the mean, which is a geometric mean, with an asterisk. The whiskers indicate 1.5 times the interquartile range above the third and below the first quartiles, or the upper or lower extreme values, whichever is closer. Participants who joined the study only because they heard about it from a participating family member or who reported a previous diagnosis of hemochromatosis or iron overload were excluded. Adapted from Adams *et al.* 2005[34] with permission.

Serum concentrations of hepatic enzymes

Mean serum levels of aspartate aminotransferase did not differ significantly in *HFE* C282Y homozygotes not previously treated with phlebotomy and in *HFE* wt/wt controls in a large screening program.[23] Therefore, it is assumed that C282Y heterozygotes have, on average, serum levels of hepatic enzymes that are similar to those of other persons of the same age and sex. In contrast, some patients who undergo evaluation of elevated serum concentrations of hepatic enzymes or other evidence of liver disease are discovered to have C282Y heterozygosity. Some of these persons have iron overload of varying degrees, usually associated with the co-inheritance of *HFE* H63D, or with porphyria cutanea tarda, some heritable types of anemia, or a novel *HFE* missense mutation. Others have a liver disorder not caused by iron overload alone, such as excessive alcohol consumption, viral hepatitis, or non-alcoholic hepatic steatosis. Hepatic iron levels may be somewhat higher in the latter group of patients than would be expected in persons who have C282Y heterozygosity alone associated with a liver disorder.[8,21,22]

Erythrocyte measures

Erythrocyte measures are influenced by *HFE* alleles, other genetic factors, and various acquired conditions. Hemoglobin and mean corpuscular volume (MCV) are influenced by iron availability and its delivery to developing erythroid cells. *HFE* C282Y homozygotes typically have significantly higher mean values of hemoglobin and MCV than *HFE* wt/wt control subjects.[24–26] Mean values of MCV in C282Y heterozygotes are between those of C282Y homozygotes and control subjects.[8,21,24] Transferrin saturation and serum ferritin levels are somewhat greater in persons with C282Y. This partly explains the greater mean MCV in C282Y heterozygotes (and homozygotes).[26–30]

Hemoglobin and MCV levels are also influenced by other genetic traits. Linkage analyses have identified loci for hemoglobin on chromosomes 6q23 and 9q,[31,32] fetal hemoglobin on 6q23,[33] and MCV on chromosomes 7q, 11p15, and 6q24.[31,32] Hematocrit, derived from erythrocyte and MCV values, has been linked to loci on chromosomes 6q23–24 and 9q.[31,32] In Caucasian adults analyzed by ethnicity, mean hemoglobin and MCV were significantly lower in those who reported southern than northern European ancestry, but participants with C282Y nonetheless had higher mean hemoglobin than other participants in both ethnic groups.[25] Regardless, it is unlikely that *HFE* alleles (6p21.3) are closely linked to putative hemoglobin and MCV loci on the long arm of chromosome 6, although this is unproven.

Hemoglobin and MCV values cannot be used as sensitive or specific indicators C282Y heterozygosity. Some C282Y heterozygotes have hemoglobin or MCV levels greater than the respective upper reference limits because they have unrelated conditions that cause erythrocytosis or macrocytosis. In the general white population, the most common cause of subnormal hemoglobin or MCV values is iron deficiency, although screening programs have identified some C282Y heterozygotes (and homozygotes) who have evidence of iron depletion.[34] In some geographic regions, persons with C282Y may also have thalassemia, a common cause of anemia and microcytosis.

C282Y heterozygosity, hepcidin, and non-*HFE* hemochromatosis phenotypes

Hepcidin plays a central role in iron homeostasis (Chapter 2). Serum concentrations of prohepcidin (a hepcidin precursor) and iron absorption were measured in healthy men, and its relationship with iron status in men carrying *HFE* mutations, hemochromatosis patients, and pregnant women was evaluated. Iron absorption was determined in 30 healthy men (15 *HFE* wt/wt, 15 C282Y heterozygotes) using a stable isotope, erythrocyte incorporation technique.[35] Iron status was measured in 138 healthy men (91 *HFE* wt/wt, 47 C282Y heterozygotes), 6 C282Y homozygotes with a hemochromatosis phenotype, and 13 pregnant women. Mean serum prohepcidin concentrations were 208 ± 118 (S.D.) ng/mL in *HFE* wt/wt subjects and 225 ± 109 ng/mL in C282Y heterozygotes, 177 ± 36 ng/mL in hemochromatosis patients, and 159 ± 59 ng/mL in pregnant women. There was no relationship between serum prohepcidin concentration and serum ferritin in any subject group, nor was the prohepcidin concentration

associated with efficiency of iron absorption. This suggests that hepcidin expression in healthy C282Y heterozygotes does not differ significantly from that in healthy subjects.[35] This agrees with observations that C282Y heterozygosity (or inheritance of other common *HFE* alleles) probably does not act as a "modifier" of non-*HFE* hemochromatosis.[36] Patients with C282Y heterozygosity who have an iron overload phenotype should be evaluated for novel *HFE* mutations, non-*HFE* iron overload disorders, or other conditions that also augment iron absorption.

DNA analyses

DNA analysis to detect *HFE* C282Y can be performed using a variety of techniques (Chapter 4). Genomic DNA derived from blood buffy coat (leukocytes) is the usual source, although DNA suitable for analysis can also be obtained from saliva, buccal swabs, fresh tissue specimens or, in some cases, from paraffin embedded tissues.

Population genetics

The prevalence of *HFE* C282Y is greatest in white persons who reside in or whose ancestors arose from the British Isles, the western and northwestern coastal areas of France, Iceland, and southwestern Scandinavia.[4,37–39] Even in these regions, there may be significant local, regional, or ethnic differences in the prevalence of C282Y.[4,37–40] Lower frequencies of C282Y occur in middle and eastern Europe and in central and south America. In the absence of admixture with whites, C282Y does not appear to occur in Natives of the Americas, Natives of sub-Saharan Africa, Asians, or Pacific Islanders.[37] C282Y occurs in African-Americans, Hispanics, and Native Americans, but its prevalence in these groups is low.[23,34] It has been postulated that C282Y arose as an independent mutation in Sri Lanka.[37]

Predisposition of *HFE* C282Y heterozygotes to various conditions

Many studies have been performed to evaluate a possible relationship of diverse conditions with C282Y heterozygosity, and many have design or methodologic limitations. The usual approach is to perform C282Y mutation analysis in persons who have been previously diagnosed to have the condition of interest. Thus, these retrospective studies do

Table 9.3. Iron-related and liver conditions with increased prevalence of *HFE* C282Y heterozygosity

Condition	Study population	Reference
Porphyria cutanea tarda	Many populations of European descent[a]	51–61
Iron overload in hereditary spherocytosis	Swiss, Spanish families	62,63
Iron overload in hepatitis C	Italy	64
Iron overload and hepatocellular carcinoma in non-cirrhotic livers	France	65
Myelodysplasia with ringed sideroblasts	Hungary; Ohio	66,67
Venous leg ulceration[b]	Italy	45
Increased blood lead concentration[c]	Alabama and Utah	41
Hepatic fibrosis in nonalcoholic steatohepatitis[d]	North America	68
Hepatitis B in patients with cirrhosis	Italy	46
Early onset of liver decompensation in hepatitis C	Czech Republic	47
Hepatocellular carcinoma in alcoholic cirrhosis	France	48,49

Notes: [a]An association of hemochromatosis alleles with porphyria cutanea tarda was first reported in kinships studied with HLA typing.[69] A study of patients with porphyria cutanea tarda in Bulgaria did not report increased prevalence of C282Y heterozygosity.[70]
[b]This condition was included because chronic venous disease leads to local iron overload in the affected legs.[45]
[c]These subjects were studied before the discovery of *HFE* in 1996, and therefore they did not undergo *HFE* genotyping. They were identified according to iron phenotype and HLA haplotypes. Increased absorption of several non-ferrous metals in hemochromatosis homozygotes and heterozygotes may be mediated by increased expression of divalent metal transporter-1 (Chapters 2, 4).
[d]This conclusion was not confirmed in two other studies.[71,72]

not provide a direct indication of the relative risk of the condition of interest among persons with various *HFE* genotypes. A few studies have identified persons of defined haplotype or genotype and then evaluated for a condition of interest.[41] Studies performed in cohorts or populations in which the prevalence of C282Y is relatively high have a greater statistical likelihood of demonstrating altered risk in persons with C282Y than studies of cohorts or populations in which the background prevalence of C282Y is relatively low. Accordingly, the conclusions about the same condition of interest may differ greatly according to the geographic or ethnic composition of the respective study cohorts. Almost uniformly, C282Y disease association studies performed in geographic areas or racial/ethnic groups in which the overall population frequency of C282Y is low (e.g. Asia, African-Americans) are unable to detect increased (or reduced) risk in C282Y heterozygotes for the condition of interest. Many studies have used univariate comparisons only, although some employed multivariable analyses. Some datasets have little statistical power, because the numbers of study subjects evaluated were suboptimal. One early study

made disease association estimates solely on the basis of responses to a questionnaire.[42] Altogether, it is prudent to interpret "positive" association studies carefully.

After the discovery of *HFE*, cohorts of patients with iron-related and liver conditions were evaluated to determine whether they had a higher prevalence of C282Y. Relatively few significant results have been reported (Table 9.3). Several large studies of patients with intermediate and severe forms of thalassemia have been performed, but have revealed no significant differences in iron phenotypes in person and those without C282Y. Many studies in various European and derivative populations have reported that myocardial infarction, stroke, carotid atherosclerosis, and diabetes mellitus (type 2) are not significantly associated with C282Y heterozygosity. A spectrum of neurologic disorders, including Alzheimer disease, multiple sclerosis, and amyotrophic lateral sclerosis, do not appear to be associated with C282Y heterozygosity. In many populations, cohorts of patients with common forms of cancer and leukemia have undergone *HFE* genotyping, revealing few positive (or negative) associations with C282Y heterozygosity

Table 9.4. Conditions for which risk may be altered in *HFE* C282Y heterozygotes

Condition	Study population	Risk	Reference
Breast cancer, women	Tennessee	Increased	73
Colon cancer	North Carolina	Increased	74
Acute lymphoblastic leukemia, childhood	British Isles	Increased[a]	75,76
Parkinson disease	Portugal	Increased	77
Diabetes mellitus, type 2[b]	Ontario; Poland	Increased	78,79
Gestational diabetes mellitus	North and central Europe	Increased	80
Early age of onset, presence of nephropathy in diabetes mellitus, type 2	Spain	Increased	44
Elevated low-density lipoproteins	US	Decreased	81,82

Notes: [a]The investigators concluded that this risk may be due to a gene linked to C282Y.
[b]Other studies of European cohorts have reported no significant increase in the prevalence of C282Y heterozygotes or homozygotes among patients with diabetes mellitus.

(Table 9.4). Altogether, these results are consistent with observations that C282Y heterozygotes identified in population screening do not have decreased longevity.[43]

There appear to be several underlying explanations for disease associations with C282Y heterozygosity. Among iron-related and liver disorders, the relatively mild effect of C282Y heterozygosity on inorganic iron absorption or serum iron measures probably contributes directly to the occurrence or aggravation of the some conditions (Table 9.3). In other disorders (Table 9.4), it is probable that any causal relationship is unrelated to iron, the *HFE* locus, or the C282Y allele, but to other deleterious or disease-associated alleles that are in linkage disequilibrium with *HFE*. In some studies, it is reported that the condition of interest occurs at different rates in males than females. In population screening studies, however, the prevalence of C282Y is the same in men and women. Taken together, these observations imply that C282Y or linked genes may be expressed differentially in males and females, or that these putative genes may influence the expression of potentially deleterious genetic determinants on chromosomes other than 6p.

Prevention and treatment

Persons of European descent who have certain iron overload or iron-related disorders other than typical *HFE* hemochromatosis (Table 9.3) should undergo mutation analysis to determine whether they have C282Y (or other common *HFE* missense alleles). Results sometimes help to understand the pathophysiology of iron overload, and may aid investigation of at-risk family members. Sequencing or denaturing high-pressure liquid chromatography of *HFE* in some patients with iron phenotypes typical of hemochromatosis who appear to have simple C282Y heterozygosity on initial testing can identify novel *HFE* mutations (Chapters 4, 8). In general, it is not appropriate test children for C282Y. Routine *HFE* mutation analysis for patients with other at-risk disorders (Table 9.4) is not indicated outside research protocols. However, the available data suggest that demonstrating C282Y heterozygosity may have some prognostic implications in persons with diabetes mellitus, type 2,[44] venous leg ulceration,[45] or hepatitis B, hepatitis C, or alcoholic cirrhosis.[46–49] Some heterozygotes benefit from considerate genetic counseling (Chapter 38).

Iron overload in *HFE* C282Y heterozygotes is managed with therapeutic phlebotomy in a manner similar to that described for C282Y homozygotes[50] (Chapter 36). It has been suggested that iron fortification of foods should not pose a health risk to *HFE* C282Y heterozygotes.[18] C282Y heterozygotes should avoid routine ingestion of certain mineral supplements unless a corresponding deficiency has been demonstrated, and should avoid excessive vocational or hobby exposure to non-ferrous metals that share absorptive pathways with iron.

References

1. Lucotte G, Dieterlen F. A European allele map of the C282Y mutation of hemochromatosis: Celtic versus Viking origin of the mutation? *Blood Cells Mol Dis* 2003; **31**: 262–7.

2. Distante S, Robson KJ, Graham-Campbell J, Arnaiz-Villena A, Brissot P, Worwood M. The origin and spread of the *HFE*-C282Y haemochromatosis mutation. *Hum Genet* 2004; **115**: 269–79.

3. Naugler C. Hemochromatosis: a Neolithic adaptation to cereal grain diets. *Med Hypotheses* 2008; **70**: 691–2.

4. Fairbanks VF. Hemochromatosis: population genetics. In: Barton JC, Edwards CQ, eds. *Hemochromatosis: Genetics, Pathophysiology, Diagnosis and Treatment.* Cambridge, Cambridge University Press. 2000; 42–50.

5. Feder JN, Gnirke A, Thomas W, *et al.* A novel MHC class I-like gene is mutated in patients with hereditary haemochromatosis. *Nat Genet* 1996; **13**: 399–408.

6. Gruen JR, Weissman SM. Evolving views of the major histocompatibility complex. *Blood* 1997; **90**: 4252–65.

7. Datz C, Haas T, Rinner H, Sandhofer F, Patsch W, Paulweber B. Heterozygosity for the C282Y mutation in the hemochromatosis gene is associated with increased serum iron, transferrin saturation, and hemoglobin in young women: a protective role against iron deficiency? *Clin Chem* 1998; **44**: 2429–32.

8. Rossi E, Olynyk JK, Cullen DJ, *et al.* Compound heterozygous hemochromatosis genotype predicts increased iron and erythrocyte indices in women. *Clin Chem* 2000; **46**: 162–6.

9. Chavarro JE, Rich-Edwards JW, Rosner BA, Willett WC. Iron intake and risk of ovulatory infertility. *Obstet Gynecol* 2006; **108**: 1145–52.

10. De Braekeleer M. A prevalence and fertility study of haemochromatosis in Saguenay-Lac-Saint-Jean. *Ann Hum Biol* 1993; **20**: 501–5.

11. Nelson RL, Persky V, Davis F, Becker E. Is hereditary hemochromatosis a balanced polymorphism: an analysis of family size among hemochromatosis heterozygotes. *Hepatogastroenterology* 2001; **48**: 523–6.

12. Rochette J, Pointon JJ, Fisher CA, *et al.* Multicentric origin of hemochromatosis gene (*HFE*) mutations. *Am J Hum Genet* 1999; **64**: 1056–62.

13. Bullen JJ. Bacterial infections in hemochromatosis. In: Barton JC, Edwards CQ, eds. *Hemochromatosis: Genetics, Pathophysiology, Diagnosis, and Treatment.* Cambridge, Cambridge University Press. 2000; 381–6.

14. Bulaj ZJ, Griffen LM, Jorde LB, Edwards CQ, Kushner JP. Clinical and biochemical abnormalities in people heterozygous for hemochromatosis. *N Engl J Med* 1996; **335**: 1799–805.

15. Edwards CQ, Griffen LM, Bulaj ZJ, Ajioka RS, Kushner JP. The iron phenotype of hemochromatosis heterozygotes. In: Barton JC, Edwards CQ, eds. *Hemochromatosis: Genetics, Pathophysiology, Diagnosis and Treatment.* Cambridge, Cambridge University Press. 2000; 411–18.

16. Edwards CQ, Griffen LM, Goldgar D, Drummond C, Skolnick MH, Kushner JP. Prevalence of hemochromatosis among 11 065 presumably healthy blood donors. *N Engl J Med* 1988; **318**: 1355–62.

17. McLaren CE, Gordeuk VR, Looker AC, *et al.* Prevalence of heterozygotes for hemochromatosis in the white population of the United States. *Blood* 1995; **86**: 2021–7.

18. Hunt JR, Zeng H. Iron absorption by heterozygous carriers of the *HFE* C282Y mutation associated with hemochromatosis. *Am J Clin Nutr* 2004; **80**: 924–31.

19. Bassett ML, Halliday JW, Powell LW. HLA typing in idiopathic hemochromatosis: distinction between homozygotes and heterozygotes with biochemical expression. *Hepatology* 1981; **1**: 120–6.

20. Morrison ED, Brandhagen DJ, Phatak PD, *et al.* Serum ferritin level predicts advanced hepatic fibrosis among US patients with phenotypic hemochromatosis. *Ann Intern Med* 2003; **138**: 627–33.

21. Rossi E, Bulsara MK, Olynyk JK, Cullen DJ, Summerville L, Powell LW. Effect of hemochromatosis genotype and lifestyle factors on iron and red cell indices in a community population. *Clin Chem* 2001; **47**: 202–8.

22. George DK, Goldwurm S, MacDonald GA, *et al.* Increased hepatic iron concentration in non-alcoholic steatohepatitis is associated with increased fibrosis. *Gastroenterology* 1998; **114**: 311–18.

23. Beutler E, Felitti V, Gelbart T, Ho N. The effect of *HFE* genotypes on measurements of iron overload in patients attending a health appraisal clinic. *Ann Intern Med* 2000; **133**: 329–37.

24. Barton JC, Bertoli LF, Rothenberg BE. Peripheral blood erythrocyte parameters in hemochromatosis: evidence for increased erythrocyte hemoglobin content. *J Lab Clin Med* 2000; **135**: 96–104.

25. Beutler E, Felitti V, Gelbart T, Waalen J. Haematological effects of the C282Y *HFE* mutation in homozygous and heterozygous states among subjects of northern and southern European ancestry. *Br J Haematol* 2003; **120**: 887–93.

26. McLaren CE, Barton JC, Gordeuk VR, *et al.* Determinants and characteristics of mean corpuscular volume and hemoglobin concentration in white *HFE* C282Y homozygotes in the hemochromatosis and iron overload screening study. *Am J Hematol* 2007; **82**: 898–905.

27. Jacobs P, Finch CA. Iron for erythropoiesis [abstract]. *Blood* 1971; **37**: 220.

28. Cazzola M, Huebers HA, Sayers MH, MacPhail AP, Eng M, Finch CA. Transferrin saturation, plasma iron turnover, and transferrin uptake in normal humans. *Blood* 1985; **66**: 935–9.

29. Feeney GP, Carter K, Masters GS, Jackson HA, Cavil I, Worwood M. Changes in erythropoiesis in hereditary hemochromatosis are not mediated by HFE expression in nucleated red cells. *Haematologica* 2005; **90**: 180–7.

30. Goodnough LT. Erythropoietin and iron-restricted erythropoiesis. *Exp Hematol* 2007; **35**: 167–72.

31. Iliadou A, Evans DM, Zhu G, *et al*. Genome-wide scans of red cell indices suggest linkage on chromosome 6q23. *J Med Genet* 2007; **44**: 24–30.

32. Lin JP, O'Donnell CJ, Levy D, Cupples LA. Evidence for a gene influencing haematocrit on chromosome 6q23–24: genome-wide scan in the Framingham Heart Study. *J Med Genet* 2005; **42**: 75–9.

33. Garner C, Mitchell J, Hatzis T, Reittie J, Farrall M, Thein SL. Haplotype mapping of a major quantitative-trait locus for fetal hemoglobin production, on chromosome 6q23. *Am J Hum Genet* 1998; **62**: 1468–74.

34. Adams PC, Reboussin DM, Barton JC, *et al*. Hemochromatosis and iron-overload screening in a racially diverse population. *N Engl J Med* 2005; **352**: 1769–78.

35. Roe MA, Spinks C, Heath AL, *et al*. Serum prohepcidin concentration: no association with iron absorption in healthy men; and no relationship with iron status in men carrying *HFE* mutations, hereditary haemochromatosis patients undergoing phlebotomy treatment, or pregnant women. *Br J Nutr* 2007; **97**: 544–9.

36. Rivard SR, Mura C, Simard H, *et al*. Clinical and molecular aspects of juvenile hemochromatosis in Saguenay-Lac-Saint-Jean (Quebec, Canada). *Blood Cells Mol Dis* 2000; **26**: 10–14.

37. Merryweather-Clarke AT, Pointon JJ, Jouanolle AM, Rochette J, Robson KJ. Geography of *HFE* C282Y and H63D mutations. *Genet Test* 2000; **4**: 183–98.

38. Mortimore M, Merryweather-Clarke AT, Robson KJ, Powell LW. The haemochromatosis gene: a global perspective and implications for the Asia-Pacific region. *J Gastroenterol Hepatol* 1999; **14**: 838–43.

39. Porto G, de Sousa M. Variation of hemochromatosis prevalence and genotype in national groups. In: Barton JC, Edwards CQ, eds. *Hemochromatosis: Genetics, Pathophysiology, Diagnosis and Treatment*. Cambridge, Cambridge University Press. 2000; 51–62.

40. Acton RT, Barton JC, Snively BM, *et al*. Geographic and racial/ethnic differences in *HFE* mutation frequencies in the Hemochromatosis and Iron Overload Screening (HEIRS) Study. *Ethn Dis* 2006; **16**: 815–21.

41. Barton JC, Patton MA, Edwards CQ, *et al*. Blood lead concentrations in hereditary hemochromatosis. *J Lab Clin Med* 1994; **124**: 193–8.

42. Nelson RL, Davis FG, Persky V, Becker E. Risk of neoplastic and other diseases among people with heterozygosity for hereditary hemochromatosis. *Cancer* 1995; **76**: 875–9.

43. Waalen J, Beutler E. No age-related decrease in frequency of heterozygotes for the *HFE* C282Y haemochromatosis mutation. *J Hepatol* 2004; **40**: 1044–5.

44. Oliva R, Novials A, Sanchez M, *et al*. The *HFE* gene is associated to an earlier age of onset and to the presence of diabetic nephropathy in diabetes mellitus type 2. *Endocrine* 2004; **24**: 111–14.

45. Zamboni P, Tognazzo S, Izzo M, *et al*. Hemochromatosis C282Y gene mutation increases the risk of venous leg ulceration. *J Vasc Surg* 2005; **42**: 309–14.

46. Fracanzani AL, Fargion S, Stazi MA, *et al*. Association between heterozygosity for *HFE* gene mutations and hepatitis viruses in hepatocellular carcinoma. *Blood Cells Mol Dis* 2005; **35**: 27–32.

47. Pacal L, Husa P, Znojil V, Kankova K. *HFE* C282Y gene variant is a risk factor for the progression to decompensated liver disease in chronic viral hepatitis C subjects in the Czech population. *Hepatol Res* 2007; **37**: 740–7.

48. Nahon P, Sutton A, Rufat P, *et al*. Liver iron, *HFE* gene mutations, and hepatocellular carcinoma occurrence in patients with cirrhosis. *Gastroenterology* 2008; **134**: 102–10.

49. Lauret E, Rodriguez M, Gonzalez S, *et al*. *HFE* gene mutations in alcoholic and virus-related cirrhotic patients with hepatocellular carcinoma. *Am J Gastroenterol* 2002; **97**: 1016–21.

50. Barton JC, McDonnell SM, Adams PC, *et al*. Management of hemochromatosis. Hemochromatosis Management Working Group. *Ann Intern Med* 1998; **129**: 932–9.

51. Bonkovsky HL, Poh-Fitzpatrick M, Pimstone N, *et al*. Porphyria cutanea tarda, hepatitis C, and *HFE* gene mutations in north America. *Hepatology* 1998; **27**: 1661–9.

52. Stuart KA, Busfield F, Jazwinska EC, *et al*. The C282Y mutation in the haemochromatosis gene (*HFE*) and

hepatitis C virus infection are independent cofactors for porphyria cutanea tarda in Australian patients. *J Hepatol* 1998; **28**: 404–9.

53. Martinelli AL, Zago MA, Roselino AM, *et al.* Porphyria cutanea tarda in Brazilian patients: association with hemochromatosis C282Y mutation and hepatitis C virus infection. *Am J Gastroenterol* 2000; **95**: 3516–21.

54. Tannapfel A, Stolzel U, Kostler E, *et al.* C282Y and H63D mutation of the hemochromatosis gene in German porphyria cutanea tarda patients. *Virchows Arch* 2001; **439**: 1–5.

55. Egger NG, Goeger DE, Payne DA, Miskovsky EP, Weinman SA, Anderson KE. Porphyria cutanea tarda: multiplicity of risk factors including *HFE* mutations, hepatitis C, and inherited uroporphyrinogen decarboxylase deficiency. *Dig Dis Sci* 2002; **47**: 419–26.

56. Hift RJ, Corrigall AV, Hancock V, Kannemeyer J, Kirsch RE, Meissner PN. Porphyria cutanea tarda: the etiological importance of mutations in the *HFE* gene and viral infection is population-dependent. *Cell Mol Biol (Noisy-le-grand)* 2002; **48**: 853–9.

57. Lamoril J, Andant C, Gouya L, *et al.* Hemochromatosis (*HFE*) and transferrin receptor-1 (*TFRC1*) genes in sporadic porphyria cutanea tarda (sPCT). *Cell Mol Biol (Noisy-le-grand)* 2002; **48**: 33–41.

58. Chiaverini C, Halimi G, Ouzan D, Halfon P, Ortonne JP, Lacour JP. Porphyria cutanea tarda, C282Y, H63D and S65C *HFE* gene mutations and hepatitis C infection: a study from southern France. *Dermatology* 2003; **206**: 212–16.

59. Nagy Z, Koszo F, Par A, *et al.* Hemochromatosis (*HFE*) gene mutations and hepatitis C virus infection as risk factors for porphyria cutanea tarda in Hungarian patients. *Liver Int* 2004; **24**: 16–20.

60. Toll A, Celis R, Ozalla MD, Bruguera M, Herrero C, Ercilla MG. The prevalence of *HFE* C282Y gene mutation is increased in Spanish patients with porphyria cutanea tarda without hepatitis C virus infection. *J Eur Acad Dermatol Venereol* 2006; **20**: 1201–6.

61. Kratka K, Dostalikova-Cimburova M, Michalikova H, Stransky J, Vranova J, Horak J. High prevalence of *HFE* gene mutations in patients with porphyria cutanea tarda in the Czech Republic. *Br J Dermatol* 2008; **159**: 585–90.

62. Brandenberg JB, Demarmels BF, Lutz HU, Wuillemin WA. Hereditary spherocytosis and hemochromatosis. *Ann Hematol* 2002; **81**: 202–9.

63. Montes-Cano MA, Rodriguez-Munoz F, Franco-Osorio R, Nunez-Roldan A, Gonzalez-Escribano MF. Hereditary spherocytosis associated with mutations in *HFE* gene. *Ann Hematol* 2003; **82**: 769–72.

64. Valenti L, Pulixi EA, Arosio P, *et al.* Relative contribution of iron genes, dysmetabolism and hepatitis C virus (HCV) in the pathogenesis of altered iron regulation in HCV chronic hepatitis. *Haematologica* 2007; **92**: 1037–42.

65. Blanc JF, De Ledinghen V, Bernard PH, *et al.* Increased incidence of *HFE* C282Y mutations in patients with iron overload and hepatocellular carcinoma developed in non-cirrhotic liver. *J Hepatol* 2000; **32**: 805–11.

66. Varkonyi J, Tarkovacs G, Karadi I, *et al.* High incidence of hemochromatosis gene mutations in the myelodysplastic syndrome: the Budapest Study on 50 patients. *Acta Haematol* 2003; **109**: 64–7.

67. Nearman ZP, Szpurka H, Serio B, *et al.* Hemochromatosis-associated gene mutations in patients with myelodysplastic syndromes with refractory anemia with ringed sideroblasts. *Am J Hematol* 2007; **82**: 1076–9.

68. Nelson JE, Bhattacharya R, Lindor KD, *et al. HFE* C282Y mutations are associated with advanced hepatic fibrosis in Caucasians with non-alcoholic steatohepatitis. *Hepatology* 2007; **46**: 723–9.

69. Kushner JP, Edwards CQ, Dadone MM, Skolnick MH. Heterozygosity for HLA-linked hemochromatosis as a likely cause of the hepatic siderosis associated with sporadic porphyria cutanea tarda. *Gastroenterology* 1985; **88**: 1232–8.

70. Ivanova A, von Ahsen N, Adjarov D, Krastev Z, Oellerich M, Wieland E. C282Y and H63D mutations in the *HFE* gene are not associated with porphyria cutanea tarda in Bulgaria. *Hepatology* 1999; **30**: 1531–2.

71. Chitturi S, Weltman M, Farrell GC, *et al. HFE* mutations, hepatic iron, and fibrosis: ethnic-specific association of NASH with C282Y but not with fibrotic severity. *Hepatology* 2002; **36**: 142–9.

72. Bugianesi E, Manzini P, D'Antico S, *et al.* Relative contribution of iron burden, *HFE* mutations, and insulin resistance to fibrosis in non-alcoholic fatty liver. *Hepatology* 2004; **39**: 179–87.

73. Kallianpur AR, Hall LD, Yadav M, *et al.* Increased prevalence of the *HFE* C282Y hemochromatosis allele in women with breast cancer. *Cancer Epidemiol Biomarkers Prev* 2004; **13**: 205–12.

74. Shaheen NJ, Silverman LM, Keku T, *et al.* Association between hemochromatosis (*HFE*) gene mutation carrier status and the risk of colon cancer. *J Natl Cancer Inst* 2003; **95**: 154–9.

75. Dorak MT, Burnett AK, Worwood M. Hemochromatosis gene in leukemia and lymphoma. *Leuk Lymphoma* 2002; **43**: 467–77.

76. Dorak MT, Burnett AK, Worwood M, Sproul AM, Gibson BE. The C282Y mutation of *HFE* is

another male-specific risk factor for childhood acute lymphoblastic leukemia. *Blood* 1999; **94**: 3957.

77. Guerreiro RJ, Bras JM, Santana I, *et al.* Association of *HFE* common mutations with Parkinson's disease, Alzheimer's disease, and mild cognitive impairment in a Portuguese cohort. *BMC Neurol* 2006; **6**: 24.

78. Kwan T, Leber B, Ahuja S, Carter R, Gerstein HC. Patients with type 2 diabetes have a high frequency of the C282Y mutation of the hemochromatosis gene. *Clin Invest Med* 1998; **21**: 251–7.

79. Moczulski DK, Grzeszczak W, Gawlik B. Role of hemochromatosis C282Y and H63D mutations in *HFE* gene in development of type 2 diabetes and diabetic nephropathy. *Diabetes Care* 2001; **24**: 1187–91.

80. Cauza E, Hanusch-Enserer U, Bischof M, *et al.* Increased C282Y heterozygosity in gestational diabetes. *Fetal Diagn Ther* 2005; **20**: 349–54.

81. Rasmussen ML, Folsom AR, Catellier DJ, Tsai MY, Garg U, Eckfeldt JH. A prospective study of coronary heart disease and the hemochromatosis gene (*HFE*) C282Y mutation: the Atherosclerosis Risk in Communities (ARIC) Study. *Atherosclerosis* 2001; **154**: 739–46.

82. Pankow JS, Boerwinkle E, Adams PC, *et al. HFE* C282Y homozygotes have reduced low-density lipoprotein cholesterol: the Atherosclerosis Risk in Communities (ARIC) Study. *Transl Res* 2008; **152**: 3–10.

Chapter 10

Porphyria cutanea tarda

Porphyrias are disorders caused by heritable or acquired deficiency of an enzyme that is required for the normal synthesis of heme. A ring structure, heme is formed by the insertion of an iron atom into protoporphyrin in the final step of the porphyrin synthesis pathway. The usual presenting symptoms and signs of porphyrias are either skin photosensitivity or neurovisceral symptoms and signs. Three types of porphyria are characterized by a predominance of photosensitivity (porphyria cutanea tarda (PCT), congenital erythropoietic porphyria, and erythropoietic protoporphyria). Two types of porphyria are characterized mainly by neurovisceral symptoms and signs (acute intermittent porphyria and aminolevulinate dehydratase deficiency). The two remaining types of porphyria are characterized by both photosensitivity and neurovisceral symptoms and signs (hereditary coproporphyria and variegate porphyria). The seven main types of porphyria, the associated enzyme deficiency, the mode of inheritance, and the major presenting symptoms and signs are displayed in Table 10.1. The only type of porphyria discussed here is PCT, the most common of all porphyrias.

Porphyria cutanea tarda (PCT)

PCT is estimated to occur in about 1 per 5000 to 25 000 individuals in the general population.[1] PCT is caused by decreased specific activity of the uroporphyrinogen decarboxylase enzyme, the fifth enzyme in the heme synthesis pathway. Three types of PCT can be identified on the basis of decreased activity of the uroporphyrinogen decarboxylase enzyme (URO-D) in liver cells or in erythrocytes.

Sporadic or type I PCT

The total amount of the URO-D is normal in both liver cells and in red blood cells, but URO-D activity is about 50% of normal in liver cells. URO-D activity in

red blood cells is normal. Other family members have normal URO-D activity in liver cells and in red blood cells. Sporadic or type I PCT accounts for about 75% of patients who have PCT, and it is the most common type of porphyria. Sporadic type I PCT usually occurs in adults who have increased liver iron stores, drink excessive alcohol, take oral contraceptives or estrogen replacement therapy, have viral hepatitis C, or have accidental exposure to polyhalogenated chemicals such as polychlorinated biphenyls. There is no mutation of the URO-D gene in this subtype of PCT. In typical families, only the index patient is affected, and no other family members are predicted to develop the photosensitive bullous dermatosis typical of this type of PCT.

Familial or type II PCT

The activity of the URO-D is about 50% of normal in liver cells and in red blood cells. This subtype of PCT is transmitted as an autosomal dominant trait, and thus more than one person in the family may have decreased URO-D activity and experience episodes of cutaneous photosensitivity. Nonetheless, only one person is affected in many families. Type II PCT accounts for about 25% of patients who have PCT.

Rare individuals who inherit a URO-D gene mutation from each parent develop an autosomal recessive disorder called hepatoerythropoietic porphyria; this disorder usually appears in childhood. The URO-D activity in liver cells and red blood cells of patients with hepatoerythropoietic porphyria is about 15% of normal, whereas the activity of URO-D in the usual familial type II PCT is about 50% of normal.

Type III PCT

URO-D activity in liver cells is decreased, similar to sporadic type I PCT. In type III PCT, however, other family members may have decreased URO-D activity

Table 10.1. Characteristics of porphyrias

Acute porphyrias	Deficient enzyme	Heritability (autosomal)	Presenting symptoms/signs
Acute intermittent	Porphobilinogen deaminase	Dominant	Neurovisceral
Hereditary coproporphyria	Coproporphyrinogen oxidase	Dominant	Neurovisceral, photosensitivity
Variegate	Protoporphyrinogen oxidase	Dominant	Neurovisceral, photosensitivity
Aminolevulinate dehydratase deficiency	Aminolevulinate dehydratase	Recessive	Neurovisceral
Other porphyrias	**Deficient enzyme**	**Heritability**	**Presenting symptoms/signs**
Porphyria cutanea tarda	Uroporphyrinogen decarboxylase	Sporadic or dominant	Photosensitivity
Congenital erythropoietic	Uroporphyrinogen III cosynthase	Recessive	Photosensitivity
Erythropoietic protoporphyria	Ferrochelatase	Recessive or dominant?	Photosensitivity

in liver cells and may develop photosensitivity dermatosis. This subtype of PCT usually occurs during childhood.

Outbreaks or clusters of PCT

Outbreaks of PCT have been reported in association with accidental ingestion of, or accidental exposure to, industrial chemical compounds by relatively large numbers of persons. The largest known clustering of patients with PCT occurred in about 4000 patients in Turkey 50 years ago following the ingestion of wheat contaminated with hexachlorobenzene ("porphyria turcica"). PCT has occurred in smaller clusters of patients who were accidentally exposed to other polyhalogenated aromatic hydrocarbons, including herbicides and polychlorinated biphenyls. All of these compounds caused PCT by inhibiting the activity of URO-D, resulting in the accumulation of excessive amounts of uroporphyrin. This, in turn, caused photosensitivity dermatosis.

Clinical manifestations

The most common reason for patients with PCT to seek medical attention is for evaluation and treatment of a skin rash. Patients often state that their skin problem started with small blisters or vesicles (4–10 mm diameter) that contained a small amount of clear fluid; many report unusual degrees of skin fragility, especially in areas not covered by clothing. The blisters may enlarge to cover a diameter of a few centimeters. Patients also comment that minor bumps, scratches, or scrapes that used to cause no injury, recently started causing large areas of skin to peel off, leaving tender or painful open sores that heal very slowly, followed by scarring. This history is characteristic of the photosensitive bullous dermatosis of porphyria cutanea tarda that occurs in skin that is exposed to sunlight. Some patients volunteer that they recently developed increased amounts of facial hair, especially lateral to the eyes in the temporal areas and in the skin below the eyes, high over the cheekbones. The scalp, face, nose, neck, arms, and the back of the hands are the most commonly affected areas. The chest, abdomen, and legs may be affected in people whose clothing doesn't cover these areas.

Physical examination findings

Active skin lesions reveal small vesicles that rupture with minimal pressure, skin fragility, painful superficial ulcers at the sites of ruptured vesicles, thin scars over healed areas, increased amounts of hair over the temporal and malar areas, and milia in some areas of the face and over the dorsum of hands and fingers. Milia are tiny, raised, palpable areas of skin.

Some patients develop full-thickness skin ulcerations over the dorsa of the hands or fingers that expose tendons and predispose to severe infections.

Skin fluorescence

The skin of patients who have active porphyric dermatitis fluoresces neon pink or purple color under a Wood's lamp (that emits light of a long wavelength ~ 410 nm). Some urine and liver biopsy samples of affected persons also fluoresce when held under a Wood's lamp. The fluorescence is caused by the presence of markedly increased amounts of uroporphyrin I in the skin and in the liver, and occurs in many but not in all patients who have PCT.

Pathology

Liver biopsy specimens from PCT patients show increased amounts of iron within hepatocytes. The amount of iron in the liver cells varies according to the presence of other precipitating factors such as the presence of one or two copies of *HFE* C282Y. For example, PCT patients who are C282Y homozygotes typically have heavy iron-loading of liver cells. Patients who are heterozygous for C282Y usually have mildly or moderately increased iron stores. Under high microscopic magnification, porphyrin crystals are visible in hepatocytes in some cases. The liver biopsy specimen may fluoresce a "hot" pink or purple color under Wood's light. Liver disease in PCT patients can progress to fibrosis or cirrhosis. Some PCT patients with cirrhosis develop hepatocellular carcinoma.

The livers of patients whose expression of PCT is triggered by viral hepatitis C typically have a prominent infiltration of inflammatory cells, especially in the portal areas. Liver injury in PCT patients with viral hepatitis C can progress to include fibrosis or cirrhosis. In some cases, there is no identified precipitating factor. Even in these individuals, the liver has increased amounts of storage iron. Patients with PCT, viral hepatitis C of long duration, and hepatic cirrhosis can develop hepatocellular carcinoma. Hepatitis C is a common cause of cirrhosis and liver failure that results in liver transplantation in the US.

Genetics

Type I or sporadic PCT is an acquired disorder. First-degree relatives typically have normal URO-D enzyme activity in hepatocytes and erythrocytes, and do not develop the photosensitive dermatosis of PCT. Type II PCT is transmitted as an autosomal dominant trait. About half of the first-degree relatives of an affected individual have decreased activity of the URO-D enzyme, but some of them do not develop photosensitive bullous dermatosis. This means that there is incomplete expression of the URO-D mutations. Individuals with type III PCT have decreased activity of the URO-D enzyme in liver cells, similar to patients with sporadic type I. The difference between type III and sporadic type I PCT is that relatives of patients with type III also have decreased URO-D enzyme activity and may experience a photosensitive bullous dermatosis.

Genetic abnormality

The gene that codes for the uroporphyrinogen decarboxylase gene *UROD* is situated on the chromosome 1p34. More than 60 mutations of *UROD* have been identified. *UROD* mutations are usually missense mutations and induce substitution of an abnormal amino acid. The activity of the abnormal URO-D enzyme is usually about 50% of normal, even though the total amount of the enzyme protein produced may be normal.

Function of URO-D

Uroporphyrinogen decarboxylase catalyzes the fifth step in the heme synthesis pathway, which involves the removal of one carboxyl (-COOH) group from uroporphyrinogen I or III to produce coproporphyrinogen I or III. Normally, coproporphyrinogen III is converted to protoporphyrin IX, which can then receive an iron atom to form heme. When URO-D does not function properly, uroporphyrinogen is not converted to coproporphyrin, and uroporphyrin accumulates in skin, liver, and other organs.

Pathophysiology

In sporadic type I PCT, modest amounts of iron decrease the activity of URO-D enzyme. This inhibition of URO-D activity is caused by the production of uroporphomethene, a uroporphyrinogen ring (referred to as a macrocycle) that has an oxidized carbon in the bridge between porphobilinogen molecules.[2] Iron is involved in the generation of the uroporphomethene inhibitor of URO-D activity.

When the activity of URO-D is decreased, uroporphyrinogen accumulates in skin, liver, and other organs. When long wavelength light of about 410 nm contacts exposed skin that has increased amounts of uroporphyrinogen, vacuoles develop in the superficial dermis. Reactive oxygen species then contribute to the development of vacuoles or blisters in the skin. These blisters cause markedly increased fragility of the skin. Large areas of skin can be scraped off as a result of trivial contact with some object. Flare-ups of the bullous dermatosis of PCT can be triggered in some patients by iron, ethanol, viral hepatitis C, or estrogens in oral contraceptives or postmenopausal estrogen hormone replacement therapy. In familial type II PCT, modest amounts of iron decrease the activity of the URO-D enzyme. When the activity of the URO-D enzyme is decreased, uroporphyrinogen accumulates in skin, liver, and other organs.

Laboratory findings
Urinary excretion of porphyrins

The most characteristic laboratory abnormality during a flare-up of PCT is the presence of increased amounts of urinary uroporphyrins. In normal individuals, the total amount of porphyrin that is excreted in the urine in 24 hours is less than 200 μg, and 24-hour urinary excretion of uroporphyrin is about 50 μg. The major porphyrin that is excreted in the urine of normal people is coproporphyrin. In a report of 77 patients with a flare-up of sporadic type I PCT, the 24-hour total urinary excretion of porphyrins averaged 4932 μg (range 730–26 921 μg). The average 24-hour total urinary excretion of porphyrins in 29 patients with familial type II PCT was also markedly increased at 4061 μg (range 749–9376 μg).[3]

In both sporadic type I and familial type II PCT, the types of porphyrins that are excreted are the same–increased amounts of uroporphyrin I and 7-carboxyl porphyrins. The explanation for this similarity in excreted porphyrins is that the same URO-D enzyme is involved in each of these types of PCT. The urine color in PCT patients is usually a normal yellow hue. Uncommonly, patients with PCT report that their urine seems to have a faint pink color. During a flare-up of PCT, the urine typically fluoresces a faint neon pink or a "hot" purple color when it is held under a Wood's light.

Viral hepatitis C and elevated liver enzymes

Another common laboratory abnormality in people who have a flare-up of PCT is elevated serum concentrations of aspartate and alanine aminotransferases. Elevated serum levels of hepatic transaminases, a non-specific abnormality, are common in patients who have either sporadic type I or familial type II PCT. In a report of seropositivity for hepatitis C in persons with sporadic or familial PCT, 80% of men and 23% of women with PCT were positive for hepatitis C.[3] Many studies demonstrate that hepatitis C virus infection is common in patients with PCT [4–8]. Nonetheless, the presence of viral hepatitis C is not sufficient for the expression of PCT, because many PCT patients do not have hepatitis C. Additional factors are involved in triggering and expression of PCT.

Blood tests of iron stores

In a report of 99 patients with either sporadic type I PCT or familial type II PCT, the average serum ferritin concentration was 472 μg/L in men and 498 μg/L in women. In 99 normal control subjects, the mean serum ferritin concentration was 88 μg/L in men and 49 μg/L in women. These differences in serum ferritin were very significant.[3] The results of serum iron concentration, transferrin saturation, and serum ferritin concentration in 99 PCT patients and 99 normal control subjects are displayed in Table 10.2. Some PCT patients have normal serum iron measures.

HFE C282Y mutations in PCT patients

Iron is a common underlying element that results in decreased activity of the URO-D enzyme in PCT patients. There is much variation in the prevalence of the *HFE* mutations C282Y and H63D among persons who have PCT. The results of a study of *HFE* genotyping of 87 American patients with either type of PCT revealed that 19% were homozygous and 15% were heterozygous for the C282Y mutation.[3] Similar results have been published by investigators in some other areas of the world.[4–7,9–12] In some other countries, especially those in which the population frequency of C282Y is relatively low, there is no increased prevalence of the C282Y mutation among PCT patients.[10,13,14]

The presence of *HFE* C282Y or H63D is not sufficient for the expression of PCT, because many PCT patients do not have these mutations. Additional contributing factors are involved in the triggering and expression of PCT. The results of testing for the C282Y and H63D mutations in PCT patients in 28 studies from 16 countries are displayed in Table 10.3.[3,5–7,9,10,12–33]

Table 10.2. Iron phenotypes of porphyria cutanea tarda patients and normal controls[a]

	Men (n = 65)			Women (n = 34)		
Iron Measure	PCT	Control[a]	P value	PCT	Control[a]	P value
Serum iron, µmol/L	26.0 ± 1.8	19.3 ± 0.72	0.0030	23.3 ± 1.8	16.5 ± 1.25	0.0046
Transferrin saturation, %	44 ± 3	30 ± 1	0.0003	46 ± 4	26 ± 2	0.0010
Serum ferritin, µg/L	472 ± 42	88 ± 8	0.0001	498 ± 107	49 ± 9	0.0001

Note: [a]Adapted from Bulaj *et al.*[3]; used with permission. PCT = porphyria cutanea tarda. Controls (65 men, 34 women) were matched by sex and age (± 5 y) with PCT patients. Controls were members of hemochromatosis pedigrees who shared no HLA alloantigen with the hemochromatosis homozygote pedigree proband. *P* values (two-tailed) were calculated with the paired two-sample Wilcoxon signed rank test. Values are expressed as the mean ± SEM.[3]

Table 10.3. Percentages of *HFE* genotypes in porphyria cutanea tarda (PCT) patients

Country	Author year	No. PCT patients[a]	C282Y/C282Y	C282Y/wt	C282Y/H63D	H63D/H63D	H63D/wt
USA	Bonkovsky 1998[6]	26 s	15	23	0	8	23
	Bulaj 2000[3]	87 f+s	19	15	7	7	15
	Egger 2002[15]	34 f+s	9	9	12	9	26
	Mehrany 2004[16]	6	50	17	17	0	17
Denmark	Christiansen 1999[17]	57 f+s	16	18	0	5	23
United Kingdom	Roberts 1997[38]	41 s	17	25	7	—	—
	Brady 2000[18]	65 s, 19 f	23 s, 26 f	19 s, 16 f	5 s, 21 f	2 s	25 s
Spain	de Salamanca 1999[13]	69 s, 19 f	4 s, 0 f	6 s, 5 f	7 s, 11 f	15 s, 0 f	29 s, 21 f
	Gonzalez-Hevilla 2005[20]	63 s	3	13	8	10	40
	Toll 2006[19]	99 s	0	16	7	10	43
France	Dereure 2001[23]	36 f+s	0	19	3	14	19
	Skowron 2001[22]	56	0	16	14	7	
	Lamoril 2002[5]	65 s	6	8	5	8	40
	Chiaverini 2003[21]	33 s	0	15	3	6	48
Italy	D'Amato 1998[10]	50 f+s	2	8	4	2	20

Table 10.3. *(cont.)*

Country	Author year	No. PCT patients[a]	C282Y/C282Y	C282Y/wt	C282Y/H63D	H63D/H63D	H63D/wt
	Sampietro 1998[24]	68 s	0	3	1	7	43
Germany	Tannapfel 2001[26]	196 s	12	28	9	2	43
	Stolzel 2003[9]	62 f+s	5	15	13	0	29
	Frank 2006[25]	51	8	16	2	4	35
Hungary	Nagy 2004[27]	50	6	8	2	2	32
Czech Republic	Malina 2000[28]	65 s, 6 f	4	17	—	—	—
Bulgaria	Ivanova 1999[29]	48 f+s	0	0	2	0	19
Japan	Furuyama 1999[14]	20	0	0	0	0	5
Australia	Stuart 1998[7]	27	11	33	0	7	37
Chile	Wolff 2006[30]	20 f+s	0	10	5	5	25
Argentina	Mendez 2005[31]	10 s, 20 f	0	0	0	10	60
			0	0	5	10	30
Brazil	Martinelli 2000[32]	23	0	13	4	4	22
South Africa	Hift 2002[33]	57	5	11	0	0	32

Note: [a]s = sporadic PCT; f = familial PCT. Patients without s or f designations were not classified by respective authors. Percentages of subjects with wild-type *HFE* genotype are not displayed.

Treatment

Phlebotomy

The best treatment for patients who experience a flare of the bullous dermatosis of sporadic type I or familial type II porphyria cutanea tarda is depletion of excessive iron stores. The most reliable way to deplete iron stores is to perform phlebotomy therapy, repeated removal of 500 mL units of whole blood. Each mL of centrifuged red blood cells contains 1 mg of iron. In a person whose hematocrit is 40 mL/dL, each 500 mL phlebotomy contains 200 mL of red blood cells. The result is that each 500 mL whole blood phlebotomy removes 200 mg of iron. Normal men usually have adequate storage iron to allow removal of 4–5 units of whole blood (800–1000 mg Fe) before they become iron deficient. Normal pre-menopausal women usually have adequate storage iron to allow removal of 1–2 units of whole blood (200–400 mg Fe)

before they become iron deficient. Because they have modestly or moderately increased iron stores, many men and women with PCT need to undergo 6–14 units of phlebotomy therapy (1200–2800 mg Fe) to deplete their iron stores, and to induce a remission of the photosensitive bullous dermatosis. Individuals who have PCT and are homozygous for the C282Y mutation of the *HFE* gene typically have to undergo 20–40 units of phlebotomy therapy (4000–8000 mg Fe), similar to many hemochromatosis homozygotes who do not have PCT. The diagnosis of iron deficiency is established when the patient develops anemia (hematocrit of 34–36 mL/dL) and mean corpuscular volume ~75 fL. Iron deficiency can be proved by measurement of a transferrin saturation value ~5% and a serum ferritin concentration ~10 μg/L. Some blood centers charge patients with PCT who need to undergo phlebotomy therapy. Phlebotomy is less convenient than an oral medication.

Phlebotomy therapy usually is tolerated well by people who have PCT. Phlebotomy therapy eliminates the adverse effects of medications.

Oral iron chelation

Deferoxamine, deferiprone, or deferasirox could be used to deplete excess storage iron in patients who have PCT plus either anemia or cardiac angina, which could preclude phlebotomy therapy. Of these medications, deferoxamine must be given parenterally, either as a subcutaneous infusion, or intramuscularly, or by intravenous infusion. Deferiprone and deferasirox can be taken by mouth. Deferiprone is not available in the US, but it used in some other countries. It is more convenient to take an oral medication than to arrange for repeated phlebotomies in a blood center.

Chloroquine therapy

Chloroquine has been used for at least 32 years to treat patients during flare-ups of PCT. Chloroquine causes a decrease in blood tests of iron stores, decreased excretion of urinary porphyrins, and remission of the bullous dermatosis of PCT. A recent study was performed to determine the effectiveness of chloroquine therapy in 74 PCT patients according to their *HFE* genotypes. PCT patients who were heterozygous for the C282Y mutation, or were compound heterozygotes for the *HFE* C282Y/H63D mutations of the *HFE* gene responded well to chloroquine therapy; their blood tests of iron stores improved and their bullous dermatosis improved. Individuals who were homozygous for the C282Y mutation did not experience improvement in their blood tests of iron stores and did not experience remission of the flare-up of PCT. The authors concluded that the iron stores of C282Y homozygotes were too high for chloroquine to deplete the iron stores and recommended that PCT patients who were C282Y homozygotes should not be treated with chloroquine.[9]

Transdermal estrogen replacement

In a study of seven postmenopausal women with inactive PCT and 19 postmenopausal women without PCT, the 7 PCT patients applied an estrogen skin patch twice each week for 1 year. Of the 19 normal women, 10 applied an estrogen skin patch twice each week and 9 took oral estrogen daily for 1 year.

All of the women underwent evaluation by a physician at time 0 and every 2 months therafter during the study. None of the PCT patients and none of the normal control women experienced a rise in urinary porphyrin excretion, and none of the PCT patients experienced a flare of PCT. The results of this year-long study suggested that postmenopausal women whose iron stores and urinary porphyrin excretion were normalized by phlebotomy therapy could be treated safely with an estrogen skin patch.[34]

The Women's Health Initiative randomized controlled trial demonstrated that estrogen–progestin replacement for an average of 5.2 years caused health risks that exceeded potential benefits in postmenopausal women, and that estrogen and progestin replacement should not be started or continued for primary prevention of coronary heart disease. All cause mortality did not increase, but there were greater rates of coronary heart disease events, strokes, pulmonary emboli, and invasive breast cancers in the group of women who were treated with estrogen–progestin replacement than in women who did not receive hormone replacement.[35]

Anastrazole therapy

Some women have both PCT and another serious health disorder including need for estrogen replacement or treatment of breast cancer. In two cases, anastrazole therapy resulted in remission of the bullous dermatosis of sporadic type I PCT. Anastrazole is an inhibitor of aromatase, an enzyme involved in the conversion of androgens to estrogens. It is thought that the remission of PCT in these women was caused by inhibition of aromatase, and by an anti-estrogenic effect of anastrazole.[36,37]

References

1. Elder GH. Molecular genetics of disorders of haem biosynthesis. *J Clin Pathol* 1993; **46**: 977–81.

2. Phillips JD, Bergonia HA, Reilly CA, Franklin MR, Kushner JP. A porphomethene inhibitor of uroporphyrinogen decarboxylase causes porphyria cutanea tarda. *Proc Natl Acad Sci USA* 2007; **104**: 5079–84.

3. Bulaj ZJ, Phillips JD, Ajioka RS, *et al.* Hemochromatosis genes and other factors contributing to the pathogenesis of porphyria cutanea tarda. *Blood* 2000; **95**: 1565–71.

4. Lambrecht RW, Thapar M, Bonkovsky HL. Genetic aspects of porphyria cutanea tarda. *Semin Liver Dis* 2007; **27**: 99–108.

5. Lamoril J, Andant C, Gouya L, *et al*. Hemochromatosis (*HFE*) and transferrin receptor-1 (*TFRC1*) genes in sporadic porphyria cutanea tarda (sPCT). *Cell Mol Biol (Noisy-le-grand)* 2002; **48**: 33–41.

6. Bonkovsky HL, Poh-Fitzpatrick M, Pimstone N, *et al*. Porphyria cutanea tarda, hepatitis C, and *HFE* gene mutations in north America. *Hepatology* 1998; **27**: 1661–9.

7. Stuart KA, Busfield F, Jazwinska EC, *et al*. The C282Y mutation in the haemochromatosis gene (*HFE*) and hepatitis C virus infection are independent cofactors for porphyria cutanea tarda in Australian patients. *J Hepatol* 1998; **28**: 404–9.

8. Fargion S, Piperno A, Cappellini MD, *et al*. Hepatitis C virus and porphyria cutanea tarda: evidence of a strong association. *Hepatology* 1992; **16**: 1322–6.

9. Stolzel U, Kostler E, Schuppan D, *et al*. Hemochromatosis (*HFE*) gene mutations and response to chloroquine in porphyria cutanea tarda. *Arch Dermatol* 2003; **139**: 309–13.

10. D'Amato M, Macri A, Griso D, Biolcati G, Ameglio F. Are His63Asp or Cys282Tyr *HFE* mutations associated with porphyria cutanea tarda? Data of patients from central and southern Italy. *J Invest Dermatol* 1998; **111**: 1241–2.

11. Santos M, Clevers HC, Marx JJ. Mutations of the hereditary hemochromatosis candidate gene *HLA-H* in porphyria cutanea tarda. *N Engl J Med* 1997; **336**: 1327–8.

12. Roberts AG, Whatley SD, Morgan RR, Worwood M, Elder GH. Increased frequency of the haemochromatosis Cys282Tyr mutation in sporadic porphyria cutanea tarda. *Lancet* 1997; **349**: 321–3.

13. de Salamanca RE, Morales P, Castro MJ, Rojo R, Gonzalez M, Arnaiz-Villena A. The most frequent *HFE* allele linked to porphyria cutanea tarda in Mediterraneans is His63Asp. *Hepatology* 1999; **30**: 819–20.

14. Furuyama K, Kondo M, Hirata K, Fujita H, Sassa S. Extremely rare association of *HFE* mutations with porphyria cutanea tarda in Japanese patients. *Hepatology* 1999; **30**: 1532–3.

15. Egger NG, Goeger DE, Payne DA, Miskovsky EP, Weinman SA, Anderson KE. Porphyria cutanea tarda: multiplicity of risk factors including *HFE* mutations, hepatitis C, and inherited uroporphyrinogen decarboxylase deficiency. *Dig Dis Sci* 2002; **47**: 419–26.

16. Mehrany K, Drage LA, Brandhagen DJ, Pittelkow MR. Association of porphyria cutanea tarda with hereditary hemochromatosis. *J Am Acad Dermatol* 2004; **51**: 205–11.

17. Christiansen L, Bygum A, Thomsen K, Brandrup F, Horder M, Petersen NE. Denaturing gradient gel electrophoresis analysis of the hemochromatosis (*HFE*) gene: impact of *HFE* gene mutations on the manifestation of porphyria cutanea tarda. *Clin Chem* 1999; **45**: 2025–6.

18. Brady JJ, Jackson HA, Roberts AG, *et al*. Co-inheritance of mutations in the uroporphyrinogen decarboxylase and hemochromatosis genes accelerates the onset of porphyria cutanea tarda. *J Invest Dermatol* 2000; **115**: 868–74.

19. Toll A, Celis R, Ozalla MD, Bruguera M, Herrero C, Ercilla MG. The prevalence of *HFE* C282Y gene mutation is increased in Spanish patients with porphyria cutanea tarda without hepatitis C virus infection. *J Eur Acad Dermatol Venereol* 2006; **20**: 1201–6.

20. Gonzalez-Hevilla M, de Salamanca RE, Morales P, *et al*. Human leukocyte antigen haplotypes and *HFE* mutations in Spanish hereditary hemochromatosis and sporadic porphyria cutanea tarda. *J Gastroenterol Hepatol* 2005; **20**: 456–62.

21. Chiaverini C, Halimi G, Ouzan D, Halfon P, Ortonne JP, Lacour JP. Porphyria cutanea tarda, C282Y, H63D, and S65C *HFE* gene mutations and hepatitis C infection: a study from southern France. *Dermatology* 2003; **206**: 212–16.

22. Skowron F, Berard F, Grezard P, Wolf F, Morel Y, Perrot H. [Role of the hemochromatosis gene in prophyria cutanea tarda. Prospective study of 56 cases.] *Ann Dermatol Venereol* 2001; **128**: 600–4.

23. Dereure O, Aguilar-Martinez P, Bessis D, *et al*. *HFE* mutations and transferrin receptor polymorphism analysis in porphyria cutanea tarda: a prospective study of 36 cases from southern France. *Br J Dermatol* 2001; **144**: 533–9.

24. Sampietro M, Piperno A, Lupica L, *et al*. High prevalence of the His63Asp *HFE* mutation in Italian patients with porphyria cutanea tarda. *Hepatology* 1998; **27**: 181–4.

25. Frank J, Poblete-Gutierrez P, Weiskirchen R, Gressner O, Merk HF, Lammert F. Hemochromatosis gene sequence deviations in German patients with porphyria cutanea tarda. *Physiol Res* 2006; **55** Suppl 2: S75–83.

26. Tannapfel A, Stolzel U, Kostler E, *et al*. C282Y and H63D mutation of the hemochromatosis gene in German porphyria cutanea tarda patients. *Virchows Arch* 2001; **439**: 1–5.

27. Nagy Z, Koszo F, Par A, *et al.* Hemochromatosis (*HFE*) gene mutations and hepatitis C virus infection as risk factors for porphyria cutanea tarda in Hungarian patients. *Liver Int* 2004; **24**: 16–20.

28. Malina L, Zd'arsky E, Dandova S, Michalikova H, Cerna M, Cimburova M. [Significance and prevalence of the C282Y gene mutation of primary hemochromatosis in the pathogenesis of pophyria cutanea tarda.] *Cas Lek Cesk* 2000; **139**: 728–30.

29. Ivanova A, von Ahsen N, Adjarov D, Krastev Z, Oellerich M, Wieland E. C282Y and H63D mutations in the *HFE* gene are not associated with porphyria cutanea tarda in Bulgaria. *Hepatology* 1999; **30**: 1531–2.

30. Wolff CF, Armas RM, Frank J, Poblete PG. [Mutations of hemochromatosis gene in volunteer blood donors and Chilean porphyria cutanea tarda patients.] *Medicina (B Aires)* 2006; **66**: 421–6.

31. Mendez M, Rossetti MV, Del C Battle AM, Parera VE. The role of inherited and acquired factors in the development of porphyria cutanea tarda in the Argentinean population. *J Am Acad Dermatol* 2005; **52**: 417–24.

32. Martinelli AL, Zago MA, Roselino AM, *et al.* Porphyria cutanea tarda in Brazilian patients: association with hemochromatosis C282Y mutation and hepatitis C virus infection. *Am J Gastroenterol* 2000; **95**: 3516–21.

33. Hift RJ, Corrigall AV, Hancock V, Kannemeyer J, Kirsch RE, Meissner PN. Porphyria cutanea tarda: the etiological importance of mutations in the *HFE* gene and viral infection is population-dependent. *Cell Mol Biol (Noisy-le-grand)* 2002; **48**: 853–9.

34. Bulaj ZJ, Franklin MR, Phillips JD, *et al.* Transdermal estrogen replacement therapy in postmenopausal women previously treated for porphyria cutanea tarda. *J Lab Clin Med* 2000; **136**: 482–8.

35. Rossouw JE, Anderson GL, Prentice RL, *et al.* Risks and benefits of estrogen plus progestin in healthy postmenopausal women: principal results from the Women's Health Initiative randomized controlled trial. *JAMA* 2002; **288**: 321–33.

36. Bertoli LF, Barton JC. Remission of porphyria cutanea tarda after anastrozole treatment of breast cancer. *Clin Breast Cancer* 2007; **7**: 716–18.

37. Roche M, Daly P, Crowley V, Darby C, Barnes L. A case of porphyria cutanea tarda resulting in digital amputation and improved by anastrazole. *Clin Exp Dermatol* 2007; **32**: 327–8.

38. Roberts AG, Whatley SD, Nicklin S, *et al.* The frequency of hemochromatosis-associated alleles is increased in British patients with sporadic porphyria cutanea tarda. *Hepatology* 1997; **25**: 159–61.

Mitochondrial mutations as modifiers of hemochromatosis

In health, mitochondria are crucial organelles for iron metabolism and heme synthesis,[1] and contain a specific iron importer known as mitoferrin.[2] In disease, mutations in *ALAS2* or *ABCB7* result in impaired heme synthesis with the consequent accumulation of iron in mitochondria. In a zebrafish mutant, *frascati*, there is profound hypochromic anemia and erythroid maturation arrest due to defective mitochondrial iron uptake,[2] although a human counterpart of this zebrafish mutant has not been described to date. Heteroplasmic point mutations of mitochondrial DNA (mtDNA) affecting subunit I of cytochrome c oxidase have been identified in patients with acquired idiopathic sideroblastic anemia.[3] Mitochondria, especially those of hepatocytes, may be injured by iron overload through diverse mechanisms.[4]

Heteroplasmy in certain regions of mtDNA, including that of the non-coding mitochondrial polymorphism at nt 16189, seems to be inherited and is not the result of somatic age-related accumulation.[5] In several populations, the mtDNA 16189 variant is associated with type 2 diabetes mellitus, dilated cardiomyopathy, and low body fat at birth.[6–11] The 16189 variant lies close to conserved sequences that control replication and transcription of mitochondrial DNA, and it has been proposed that this variant may induce replication slippage.[10,11] Thus, the 16189 polymorphism has been investigated as a possible heritable factor or "modifier" that could influence the severity of iron overload in *HFE* hemochromatosis or in other conditions.

The prevalence of the 16189 mtDNA variant was significantly greater in British, French, and Australian adults with iron overload phenotypes and *HFE* C282Y homozygosity (14.1%) than in population control subjects (3.1%) and "asymptomatic" C282Y homozygotes without iron overload (8.4%).[12] In a study of American C282Y homozygotes, there was no significant relationship between the occurrence of the 16189 polymorphism and serum ferritin levels at diagnosis.[13] In a study of

Spanish subjects, the prevalence of the 16189 mtDNA variant in persons with hemochromatosis phenotypes and hemochromatosis-associated *HFE* genotypes did not differ significantly from that in control subjects.[14] In the same study, the prevalence of the 16189 mtDNA variant was similar in patients with beta-thalassemia and in those without. Taken together, the available evidence suggests that it is unlikely that the mtDNA 16189 variant is either a "modifier" or a surrogate marker of a factor that influences the severity of iron overload in C282Y homozygotes or beta-thalassemia. Nonetheless, studies that compare the prevalence of the 16189 mtDNA variant in persons with iron overload with and without diabetes mellitus or other specific complications may renew interest in this common genetic variant as a "modifier" of iron overload.

References

1. Bottomley SS. Iron overload in sideroblastic and other non-thalassemic anemias. In: Barton JC, Edwards CQ, eds. *Hemochromatosis: Genetics, Pathophysiology, Diagnosis and Treatment*. Cambridge, Cambridge University Press. 2000; 435–41.

2. Shaw GC, Cope JJ, Li L, *et al.* Mitoferrin is essential for erythroid iron assimilation. *Nature* 2006; **440**: 96–100.

3. Gattermann N, Retzlaff S, Wang YL, *et al.* Heteroplasmic point mutations of mitochondrial DNA affecting subunit I of cytochrome c oxidase in two patients with acquired idiopathic sideroblastic anemia. *Blood* 1997; **90**: 4961–72.

4. Britton RS. Mechanisms of iron toxicity. In: Barton JC, Edwards CQ, eds. *Hemochromatosis: Genetics, Pathophysiology, Diagnosis and Treatment*. Cambridge, Cambridge University Press. 2000; 229–38.

5. Lagerstrom-Fermer M, Olsson C, Forsgren L, Syvanen AC. Heteroplasmy of the human mtDNA control region remains constant during life. *Am J Hum Genet* 2001; **68**: 1299–301.

6. Kim JH, Park KS, Cho YM, *et al.* The prevalence of the mitochondrial DNA 16189 variant in non-diabetic

Korean adults and its association with higher fasting glucose and body mass index. *Diabet Med* 2002; **19**: 681–4.

7. Lin TK, Chen SD, Wang PW, *et al.* Increased oxidative damage with altered antioxidative status in type 2 diabetic patients harboring the 16189 T to C variant of mitochondrial DNA. *Ann N Y Acad Sci* 2005; **1042**: 64–9.

8. Park KS, Chan JC, Chuang LM, *et al.* A mitochondrial DNA variant at position 16189 is associated with type 2 diabetes mellitus in Asians. *Diabetologia* 2008; **51**: 602–8.

9. Poulton J, Brown MS, Cooper A, Marchington DR, Phillips DI. A common mitochondrial DNA variant is associated with insulin resistance in adult life. *Diabetologia* 1998; **41**: 54–8.

10. Poulton J, Marchington DR, Scott-Brown M, Phillips DI, Hagelberg E. Does a common mitochondrial DNA polymorphism underlie susceptibility to diabetes and the thrifty genotype? *Trends Genet* 1998; **14**: 387–9.

11. Poulton J, Luan J, Macaulay V, Hennings S, Mitchell J, Wareham NJ. Type 2 diabetes is associated with a common mitochondrial variant: evidence from a population-based case-control study. *Hum Mol Genet* 2002; **11**: 1581–3.

12. Livesey KJ, Wimhurst VL, Carter K, *et al.* The 16189 variant of mitochondrial DNA occurs more frequently in C282Y homozygotes with haemochromatosis than those without iron loading. *J Med Genet* 2004; **41**: 6–10.

13. Beutler E, Beutler L, Lee PL, Barton JC. The mitochondrial nt 16189 polymorphism and hereditary hemochromatosis. *Blood Cells Mol Dis* 2004; **33**: 344–5.

14. Salvador M, Villegas A, Llorente L, Ropero P, Gonzalez FA, Bustamante L. 16189 Mitochondrial variant and iron overload. *Ann Hematol* 2007; **86**: 463–4.

Mutations in the *SLC40A1* (*FPN1*) gene that encodes ferroportin (OMIM *604653) cause an uncommon, heterogeneous group of iron overload disorders characterized by an autosomal dominant pattern of inheritance (OMIM #606069). Ferroportin hemochromatosis has been described worldwide in a variety of race/ethnicity groups. *SLC40A1* mutations cause two major iron overload phenotype patterns, each depending on the particular mutation and its effect on the function of the transcribed ferroportin protein. In many ferroportin hemochromatosis kinships, serum iron measures and complications of iron overload typical of other types of hemochromatosis are relatively uncommon. The collective term "ferroportin disease" or "hemochromatosis type 4" is sometimes used to describe the clinical manifestations of ferroportin mutations.

History

In 1990, an autosomal dominant form of hemochromatosis was reported in a Melanesian pedigree from the Solomon Islands. All affected individuals had serum iron measures and a pattern of liver iron staining similar to those of *HFE* hemochromatosis, although linkage of this disorder to chromosome 6p was excluded.[1] In 1999, Pietrangelo and colleagues reported a large Italian family that included persons with an iron overload condition that occurred in pattern consistent with autosomal dominant inheritance. Based on microsatellite marker analyses, this disorder was also not linked to chromosome 6p.[2] In 2001, Njajou and colleagues identified the *SLC40A1* mutation N144H associated with autosomal dominant hemochromatosis in a large multi-generation family from the Netherlands.[3] In the same year, Montosi *et al.* mapped the autosomal dominant iron overload in the large Italian kinship to chromosome 2q32, and demonstrated the missense mutation *SLC40A1* A77D in affected family members.[4] In 2003, Arden and colleagues identified the *SLC40A1* mutation N144T in a

Solomon Islander with iron overload.[5] although it remains unproven whether this mutation accounts for the large Melanesian kinship with autosomal dominant hemochromatosis previously reported.[1]

Clinical description

Many patients report no distinctive symptoms and have no significant physical abnormalities attributable to iron overload. Chronic fatigue, hepatomegaly, or stigmata of chronic liver disease and cirrhosis occur in some patients, especially those with severe iron overload. In a large Dutch kindred, the main and most common symptoms were arthralgias and premature signs of degenerative arthropathy.[6] In unusual cases, cirrhosis, heart disease, or hormonal disorders including diabetes mellitus and hypogonadotrophic hypogonadism occur.

Genetics

An autosomal dominant pattern of inheritance is characteristic of ferroportin hemochromatosis (Fig. 12.1). In affected families, adults in two or more successive generations typically have hemochromatosis or iron overload phenotypes, although the occurrence of iron overload in children in some kinships has been reported.[2,7] Provisional diagnosis of ferroportin hemochromatosis depends critically on the preparation of an accurate pedigree and iron phenotyping of multiple family members.

Most reported ferroportin mutations are restricted to single families ("private" mutations), and are relatively uncommon (Table 12.1). Although the geographic extent of the various reported mutations is worldwide, only a few specific mutations have been identified in diverse populations. The most prevalent of these is characterized by the deletion of one of a group of three valine residues (V162del). This mutation has been reported in kinships from Australia,

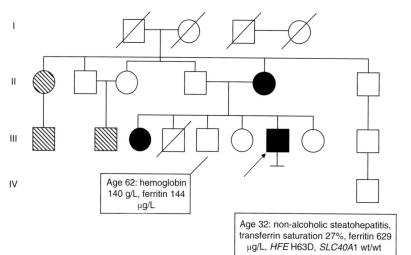

Fig. 12.1. Pedigree of iron phenotypes and *SLC40A1* c.1402G→A heterozygosity. Family members with c.1402G→A are shown as black figures (arrow = proband); phenotype data were not available for the proband's sister or mother. Family members reported to have hemochromatosis treated with phlebotomy are shown as shaded figures. Adapted from Lee *et al*.[57]

Age 62: hemoglobin 140 g/L, ferritin 144 μg/L

Age 32: non-alcoholic steatohepatitis, transferrin saturation 27%, ferritin 629 μg/L, *HFE* H63D, *SLC40A1* wt/wt

Table 12.1. Geographic distribution and race/ethnicity of persons with ferroportin gene (*SLC40A1*) mutations[a]

Exon	Protein alteration	cDNA alteration	Location or Race/Ethnicity	Reference(s)
—	—	−59–45del	French	40
—	—	−188A→G	Japanese	41
3	Y64N	190T→C	Japanese	42
3	V72F	214G→T	Italian	43
3	A77D	230C→A	Italian; Indian; Australia	4,15,16
3	G80S	238G→A	Italian	44,45
3	G80V	239G→T	Italian	46
3	R88G	262A→G	French	40
3	R88T	263G→C	Spanish	47
5	N144H	430A→C	Dutch	3
5	N144D	430A→G	Australian	48
5	N144T	431A→C	Solomon Islander	5
5	I152F	"758A→T"	Italian	49
5	D157G	"744A→G"	French	50
5	D157N	469G→A	Italian	43
5	V162del	484–486delGTT	Australia; UK; Italy; Greece; Sri Lanka; Austria	8–13
6	N174I	521A→T	Italian	44,45
6	R178G	532C→A	Greek	51
6	I180T	539T→C	Spanish	47
6	D181V	"846A→T"	Italian	46
6	Q182H	546G→T	French	50

Table 12.1. (*cont.*)

Exon	Protein alteration	cDNA alteration	Location or Race/Ethnicity	Reference(s)
6	R178Q	533G→A	French	40
6	N185D	553A→G	Scandinavian	52
6	L233P	698T→C	Italian	49
7	G267D	"1104G→A"	Chinese	46
7	D270V	809A→T	Black South African	53
7	G323V	968G→T	French	50
7	C326S	977G→C	USA	7
7	C326Y	977G→A	Thailand	54,55
7	S338R	1014T→G	New Zealand	56
7	G468S[b]	1402G→A	Scottish-Irish (USA)[a]	57
8	R489K	1466G→A	English	58
8	R489S	1467A→C	Japanese	42
8	G490S[c]	1468G→A	French	40
8	G490D[c]	1468G→A	Caucasian-Asian	59
8	Y501C	1502A→G	Italian	60

Notes: [a]*SLC40A1* Q248H (c.744G→T) occurs as a polymorphism in Native Africans and in African-Americans; persons with this allele may have slightly higher serum ferritin levels than those without Q248H.[17–19] *SLC40A1* G339D (c.1016G→A), L384M (c.1148T→A), and L384B (c.1149T→G) are also common in African-Americans, but have no defined association with abnormal iron measures.[18] *SLC40A1* L384M (c.1149T→A) and L384V (c.1149T→G) were detected in Italian blood donors at frequencies of 10% and 5%, respectively.[61] Pathogenicity, if any, of *SLC40A1* F405S (c.1214T→C) (ENSEMBL database), and M432V (c.1294A→G), P443L (c.1328C→T), and R561G (c.1681A→G) (NCBI SNP database) is unreported.
[b]This allele, a splice site mutation, caused premature truncation of ferroportin transcription at amino acid 330, and thus is the functional equivalent of G330X.[57]
[c]Identical cDNA alterations were reported for these different protein alterations.

UK, Italy, Greece, Sri Lanka, and Austria.[8–13] It has been proposed that this mutation has occurred independently, several times, due to slippage mispairing in a repeat sequence.[14] The A77D mutation has been described in iron overloaded patients from Italy, Australia, and India.[4,15,16] The common Q248H allele occurs as a polymorphism in persons who reside in diverse areas of sub-Saharan Africa and in African-Americans (Table 12.1).[17–21]

Pathophysiology

Ferroportin, the receptor for hepcidin,[22] occurs as a multimer on the surfaces of cells responsible for gathering and recycling iron: enterocytes (basolateral surfaces), macrophages, hepatocytes, and placental syncytiotrophoblasts.[22–25] The hepcidin-binding site on ferroportin is evolutionarily conserved.[26] The binding of cell surface ferroportin by hepcidin results in ferroportin tyrosine phosphorylation at the plasma membrane, and subsequent ferroportin internalization, dephosphorylation, and degradation by ubiquitination. Hepcidin-induced internalization of ferroportin requires binding and co-operative interaction with Janus Kinase 2 (JAK2).[27] Thus, hepcidin participates in regulation of plasma iron levels and tissue distribution of iron by post-translational regulation of ferroportin.[22–25] Hepcidin regulation is normal in ferroportin hemochromatosis, whereas dysregulation of hepcidin underlies the pathophysiology in some types of hemochromatosis, such as those associated with mutations in *HFE*, *HJV*, or *TFR2*.

In patients with a pathogenic *SLC40A1* mutation, ferroportin multimers consist of both normal and abnormal molecules. Human ferroportin mutations introduced into mice generate proteins that either are defective in cell surface localization or have a decreased ability to be internalized and degraded in response to hepcidin.[28] The *flatiron (ffe)* mouse has a missense mutation (H32R) in the first putative transmembrane segment of ferroportin. The H32R mutant form of ferroportin inhibits the function of normal ferroportin protein, acting as a "dominant negative."[29,30] Accordingly, the dominant inheritance of iron overload due to ferroportin mutations has been attributed to a dominant negative effect of the mutant *SLC40A1* allele that prevents the normal function of wild-type (normal) ferroportin, not to haploinsufficiency.[31]

Ferrokinetic consequences of the "dominant negative" effect account for the two different iron overload phenotypes that occur in persons with ferroportin hemochromatosis. *SLC40A1* mutations that encode ferroportin that either is not presented normally to the cell surface or has defective iron export activity ("abnormal ferroportin trafficking") are associated with "loss-of-function," normal or low transferrin saturation, and predominance of iron retention in macrophages. The overall effect of such mutations is to decrease iron absorption from the intestine and inhibit iron egress from macrophages (Fig. 12.2).

Mutations that encode ferroportin that cannot bind hepcidin normally or be internalized after hepcidin binding ("hepcidin resistance") are associated with "gain-of-function," and cause elevated transferrin saturation and iron deposition in hepatocytes (Fig. 12.2). The overall effect of such mutations is to increase iron absorption from enterocytes (Fig. 12.2) and stimulate iron export from macrophages, both of which promote iron loading of hepatocytes and other parenchymal tissues. The *SLC40A1* mutations involving N144, Y64N, and C326 residues cause autosomal dominant parenchymal iron overload.[32] Human ferroportin constructs bearing these pathogenic mutations localized to cell surfaces and exported iron normally, but were partially or completely resistant to hepcidin-mediated internalization and continued to export iron despite the presence of hepcidin.[33] The primary defect with C326 substitutions was the loss of hepcidin binding, which resulted in the most severe phenotype. The thiol form of C326 was essential for interaction with hepcidin, suggesting that C326-SH homology is located in or near the binding site of hepcidin. In contrast, N144 and Y64 residues were not required for hepcidin binding, but their mutations impaired the subsequent internalization of the ligand-receptor complex.[33]

Ferroportin also interacts with hephaestin, an X-linked iron transporter, to transport iron out of enterocytes.[34,35] This could account for sex-associated differences in the function of normal or abnormal ferroportin as an iron exporter.

Laboratory evaluation

Persons with "loss-of-function" ferroportin hemochromatosis typically have normal or low plasma transferrin saturation, elevated serum ferritin concentration, and a predominance of iron deposition in Kupffer cells and other macrophage populations such as those in the bone marrow, spleen, and lymph nodes (Table 12.2).[2,36] Some patients with "loss-of-function" mutations present with isolated hyperferritinemia, especially those with *SLC40A1* N174I, Q182H, or G323V. The differential diagnosis of this phenotype therefore includes common liver disorders such as hepatic steatosis, alcohol-related liver disease, and viral hepatitis; chronic infection or inflammation; malignancy; and hereditary hyperferritinemia-cataract syndrome (Chapter 17). Some patients with "loss-of-function" mutations also have hemoglobin levels that are at the lower reference range or have mild anemia. In kinships with "gain-of-function" ferroportin mutations, affected persons have high transferrin saturation, elevated serum ferritin level, and preferential iron loading of hepatocytes and other parenchymal cells. In some "gain-of-function" kinships, early age-of-onset iron overload occurs (Table 12.2).[7] In some ferroportin hemochromatosis kinships, there is moderate phenotype heterogeneity among affected family members.

Liver specimens obtained by biopsy are usually needed to ascertain that iron overload is present, and to distinguish ferroportin hemochromatosis from other causes of hyperferritinemia. Predominance of iron deposition in Kupffer cells suggests a "loss-of-function" mutation. Iron deposits that appear predominantly in hepatocytes suggest a "gain-of-function" mutation. Some patients have increased iron deposition in both cell populations. The liver biopsy should be evaluated for the presence of fibrosis, cirrhosis, or other histologic abnormalities, and its iron concentration and the patient's hepatic iron index should be quantified. An elevated hepatic iron index is observed in some cases. Because the hepatic iron index was originally devised to assess patients with *HFE* hemochromatosis, it may not be as useful in

(a)

**Effects of abnormal ferroportins:
enterocytes**

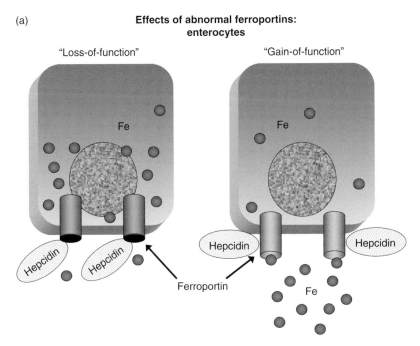

"Loss-of-function"   "Gain-of-function"

(b)

**Effects of abnormal ferroportins:
macrophages**

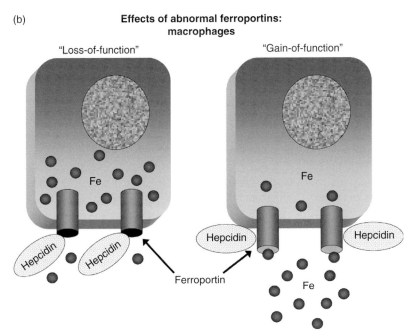

"Loss-of-function"   "Gain-of-function"

Fig. 12.2. *SLC40A1* mutations that encode ferroportin that either is not presented normally to the cell surface or has defective iron export activity are associated with "loss-of-function," normal or low transferrin saturation, and predominance of iron retention in macrophages. Such mutations decrease iron absorption from the intestine (a) and inhibit iron egress from macrophages (b). *SLC40A1* mutations that encode ferroportin that cannot bind hepcidin normally or be internalized after hepcidin binding ("hepcidin resistance") are associated with "gain-of-function," and cause elevated transferrin saturation and iron deposition in hepatocytes. The effect of such mutations is to increase iron absorption from enterocytes (a) and stimulate iron export from macrophages (b), both of which promote iron loading of hepatocytes and other parenchymal tissues.

patients with ferroportin hemochromatosis. Hepatic fibrosis and micronodular hepatic cirrhosis is present in some patients; primary liver cancer has been reported.[37] Magnetic resonance imaging (MRI) can be used to estimate liver iron content and provide information about iron deposition in other organs and tissues (Chapter 4).[38] Pietrangelo and colleagues used MRI to evaluate 22 patients from four different pedigrees with different ferroportin mutations (A77D, N144H, G80S, and Val 162del). In treated patients with "lack-of-function" ferroportin hemochromatosis (A77D, G80S, and Val 162del), MRI revealed that the spleen and the spine had iron accumulation even when serum ferritin was normal and

Table 12.2. Characteristics of two major hemochromatosis phenotypes due to altered ferroportin protein activity

Characteristic	"Loss-of-function"	"Gain-of-function"
Representative mutations	A77D, V162del, G490D	Y64N, C326Y, N144D, N144H
Mechanism of action of abnormal ferroportin	Abnormal ferroportin trafficking	Hepcidin resistance
Location of altered portion of ferroportin[a]	Mostly intracellular	Mostly extracellular
Hepcidin levels	Elevated	Normal but disproportionately low for degree of iron loading
Iron absorption	Secondarily increased	Increased due resistance of ferroportin to hepcidin binding
Transferrin saturation	Normal or mildly subnormal	Elevated
Serum ferritin level	Normal to very elevated	Elevated
Iron-limited erythropoiesis	In some cases	No
Predominant sites of iron retention or deposition	Macrophages	Hepatocytes, other parenchymal cells

Note: [a] The mutation *SLC40A1* A77D affects a transmembrane portion of the ferroportin molecule, and is associated with a "mixed" phenotype. Other *SLC40A1* mutations reported to be associated with "mixed" or both iron phenotypes ("gain-of-function" and "loss-of-function") include R88T, N144H, N174I, R178G, N185D, R489S, G490S, and G490D.

liver iron content was low.[38] Patients with severe hepatic iron overload should be evaluated for heart disease, diabetes mellitus, and hypogonadism. In some cases, heart disease, diabetes mellitus, or arthropathy appear to be unrelated to iron overload.

The ferroportin allele Q248H occurs as a polymorphism in sub-Saharan Native Africans and in African-Americans with and without iron overload phenotypes.[17,18] Q248H has not been reported in other race or ethnicity groups. Aggregate Q248H frequencies in African-Americans and Native Africans differ significantly (0.0525 vs. 0.0946, respectively). Q248H has been weakly associated with hyperferritinemia.[17–21] The odds ratios estimates of iron overload in African-Americans and Native Africans with Q248H who lack *HFE* C282Y are not significantly greater than unity, suggesting that the role of Q248H in the causation of iron overload is minimal, if any.[20] This is consistent with observations that the amino acid encoded at the 248 position of ferroportin protein is not highly conserved across species, and that the mutation does not affect a portion of the ferroportin molecule critical to hepcidin binding or iron transport.[20,39] (Fig. 12.3)

SLC40A1 mutation analysis by direct sequencing or denaturing high-performance liquid chromatography is often used to evaluate the DNA of index patients suspected to have autosomal dominant hemochromatosis and iron overload (Fig. 12.3). After a specific *SLC40A1* mutation is identified, other family members can be evaluated using the same or other analysis techniques. Because mutation analysis to identify ferroportin gene mutations is usually not available commercially or in screening programs, it may be necessary to refer patients with autosomal dominant hemochromatosis to a research investigator to obtain a molecular diagnosis.

HFE mutation analysis sometimes reveals C282Y or H63D heterozygosity in persons with ferroportin hemochromatosis, but such results are usually incidental findings and do not explain the phenotype or pattern of inheritance of hemochromatosis associated with *SLC40A1* mutations. In some kinships, hemochromatosis associated with *HFE* homozygosity sometimes occurs in a pseudo-dominant pattern of inheritance due to the relatively high prevalence of C282Y in some populations, but is readily distinguished from ferroportin hemochromatosis by *HFE* mutation analysis.

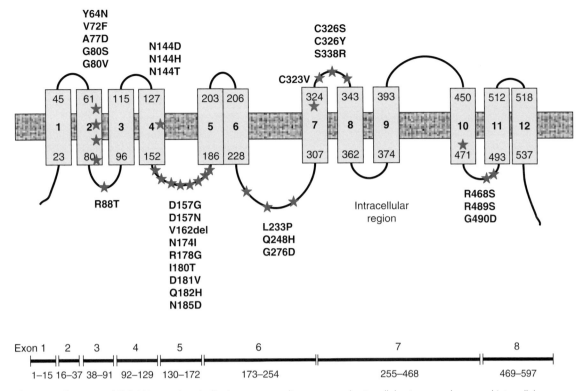

Fig. 12.3. Summary of *SLC40A1* mutations, indicating corresponding exons, and extracellular, transmembrane, and intracellular domains of ferroportin. Adapted from E. Beutler and P. Lee.

Treatment

Therapeutic phlebotomy is the treatment of choice for persons who have autosomal dominant iron overload, even if a pathogenic ferroportin mutation has not been demonstrated. Some patients with a "loss-of-function" mutation have mild anemia and may experience slow recovery of hemoglobin concentrations after phlebotomy sessions due to a decreased rate of export of storage iron from macrophages. Therefore, it may be desirable or necessary to reduce the volume of phlebotomy to less than would be prescribed for patients with other types of hemochromatosis, and phlebotomy sessions may need to be spaced several weeks apart. Nonetheless, administration of erythropoietin is usually unnecessary. Patients with "gain-of-function" mutations usually tolerate phlebotomy well, and can be treated in the same manner as patients with "classical" *HFE* hemochromatosis. At present, there are no reports of erythrocytapheresis or iron chelation therapy in persons with ferroportin hemochromatosis.

Once iron depletion is achieved, phlebotomy therapy to maintain low iron stores should be performed, especially in those with "gain-of-function" mutations. Other patients re-accumulate iron slowly or not at all. A diet with a low iron content is not indicated in most cases, although no patient should consume supplemental iron. Hepatic cirrhosis, diabetes mellitus, other endocrinopathy, cardiomyopathy, and arthropathy should be managed in a manner that is similar to that appropriate for patients without hemochromatosis.

References

1. Eason RJ, Adams PC, Aston CE, Searle J. Familial iron overload with possible autosomal dominant inheritance. *Aust N Z J Med* 1990; **20**: 226–30.

2. Pietrangelo A, Montosi G, Totaro A, *et al.* Hereditary hemochromatosis in adults without pathogenic mutations in the hemochromatosis gene. *N Engl J Med* 1999; **341**: 725–32.

3. Njajou OT, Vaessen N, Joosse M, *et al.* A mutation in *SLC11A3* is associated with autosomal dominant hemochromatosis. *Nat Genet* 2001; **28**: 213–14.

4. Montosi G, Donovan A, Totaro A, *et al.* Autosomal-dominant hemochromatosis is associated with a

mutation in the ferroportin (*SLC11A3*) gene. *J Clin Invest* 2001; **108**: 619–23.

5. Arden KE, Wallace DF, Dixon JL, *et al.* A novel mutation in ferroportin 1 is associated with haemochromatosis in a Solomon Islands patient. *Gut* 2003; **52**: 1215–17.

6. Njajou OT, de Jong G, Berghuis B, *et al.* Dominant hemochromatosis due to N144H mutation of *SLC11A3*: clinical and biological characteristics. *Blood Cells Mol Dis* 2002; **29**: 439–43.

7. Sham RL, Phatak PD, West C, Lee P, Andrews C, Beutler E. Autosomal dominant hereditary hemochromatosis associated with a novel ferroportin mutation and unique clinical features. *Blood Cells Mol Dis* 2005; **34**: 157–61.

8. Cazzola M, Cremonesi L, Papaioannou M, *et al.* Genetic hyperferritinaemia and reticuloendothelial iron overload associated with a three base pair deletion in the coding region of the ferroportin gene (*SLC11A3*). *Br J Haematol* 2002; **119**: 539–46.

9. Devalia V, Carter K, Walker AP, *et al.* Autosomal dominant reticuloendothelial iron overload associated with a 3-base pair deletion in the ferroportin 1 gene (*SLC11A3*). *Blood* 2002; **100**: 695–7.

10. Roetto A, Merryweather-Clarke AT, Daraio F, *et al.* A valine deletion of ferroportin 1: a common mutation in hemochromastosis type 4. *Blood* 2002; **100**: 733–4.

11. Wallace DF, Pedersen P, Dixon JL, *et al.* Novel mutation in ferroportin1 is associated with autosomal dominant hemochromatosis. *Blood* 2002; **100**: 692–4.

12. Wallace DF, Browett P, Wong P, Kua H, Ameratunga R, Subramaniam VN. Identification of ferroportin disease in the Indian subcontinent. *Gut* 2005; **54**: 567–8.

13. Zoller H, McFarlane I, Theurl I, *et al.* Primary iron overload with inappropriate hepcidin expression in V162del ferroportin disease. *Hepatology* 2005; **42**: 466–72.

14. Wallace DF, Subramaniam VN. Non-*HFE* haemochromatosis. *World J Gastroenterol* 2007; **13**: 4690–8.

15. Subramaniam VN, Wallace DF, Dixon JL, Fletcher LM, Crawford DHG. Ferroportin disease due to the A77D mutation in Australia. *Gut* 2005; **54**: 1048–9.

16. Agarwal S, Sankar VH, Tewari D, Pradhan M. Ferroportin (*SLC40A1*) gene in thalassemic patients of Indian descent. *Clin Genet* 2006; **70**: 86–7.

17. Barton JC, Acton RT, Rivers CA, *et al.* Genotypic and phenotypic heterogeneity of African-Americans with primary iron overload. *Blood Cells Mol Dis* 2003; **31**: 310–19.

18. Beutler E, Barton JC, Felitti VJ, *et al.* Ferroportin 1 (*SCL40A1*) variant associated with iron overload in African-Americans. *Blood Cells Mol Dis* 2003; **31**: 305–9.

19. Gordeuk VR, Caleffi A, Corradini E, *et al.* Iron overload in Africans and African-Americans and a common mutation in the *SCL40A1* (ferroportin 1) gene. *Blood Cells Mol Dis* 2003; **31**: 299–304.

20. Barton JC, Acton RT, Lee PL, West C. *SLC40A1* Q248H allele frequencies and Q248H-associated risk of non-*HFE* iron overload in persons of sub-Saharan African descent. *Blood Cells Mol Dis* 2007; **39**: 206–11.

21. Rivers CA, Barton JC, Gordeuk VR, *et al.* Association of ferroportin Q248H polymorphism with elevated levels of serum ferritin in African-Americans in the Hemochromatosis and Iron Overload Screening (HEIRS) Study. *Blood Cells Mol Dis* 2007; **38**: 247–52.

22. Nemeth E, Tuttle MS, Powelson J, *et al.* Hepcidin regulates cellular iron efflux by binding to ferroportin and inducing its internalization. *Science* 2004; **306**: 2090–3.

23. Donovan A, Brownlie A, Zhou Y, *et al.* Positional cloning of zebrafish ferroportin 1 identifies a conserved vertebrate iron exporter. *Nature* 2000; **403**: 776–81.

24. Donovan A, Lima CA, Pinkus JL, *et al.* The iron exporter ferroportin/Slc40a1 is essential for iron homeostasis. *Cell Metab* 2005; **1**: 191–200.

25. McKie AT, Marciani P, Rolfs A, *et al.* A novel duodenal iron-regulated transporter, IREG1, implicated in the basolateral transfer of iron to the circulation. *Mol Cell* 2000; **5**: 299–309.

26. De Domenico I, Nemeth E, Nelson JM, *et al.* The hepcidin-binding site on ferroportin is evolutionarily conserved. *Cell Metab* 2008; **8**: 146–56.

27. De Domenico I, Lo E, Ward DM, Kaplan J. Hepcidin-induced internalization of ferroportin requires binding and co-operative interaction with Jak2. *Proc Natl Acad Sci USA* 2009; **106**: 3800–5.

28. De Domenico I, Ward DM, Nemeth E, *et al.* The molecular basis of ferroportin-linked hemochromatosis. *Proc Natl Acad Sci USA* 2005; **102**: 8955–60.

29. Andrews NC. Of mice and iron: ferroportin disease. *Blood* 2007; **109**: 4115.

30. Zohn IE, De Domenico I, Pollock A, *et al.* The flatiron mutation in mouse ferroportin acts as a dominant negative to cause ferroportin disease. *Blood* 2007; **109**: 4174–80.

31. De Domenico I, Ward DM, Musci G, Kaplan J. Iron overload due to mutations in ferroportin. *Haematologica* 2006; **91**: 92–5.

32. Sham RL, Phatak PD, Nemeth E, Ganz T. Hereditary hemochromatosis due to resistance to hepcidin: high hepcidin concentrations in a family with C326S ferroportin mutation. *Blood* 2009; **114**: 493–4.

33. Fernandes A, Preza GC, Phung Y, *et al*. The molecular basis of hepcidin-resistant hereditary hemochromatosis. *Blood* 2009; **114**: 437–43.

34. Aisen P, Enns C, Wessling-Resnick M. Chemistry and biology of eukaryotic iron metabolism. *Int J Biochem Cell Biol* 2001; **33**: 940–59.

35. Syed BA, Beaumont NJ, Patel A, *et al*. Analysis of the human hephaestin gene and protein: comparative modeling of the N-terminus ecto-domain based upon ceruloplasmin. *Protein Eng* 2002; **15**: 205–14.

36. Pietrangelo A. The ferroportin disease. *Blood Cells Mol Dis* 2004; **32**: 131–8.

37. Corradini E, Ferrara F, Pollicino T, *et al*. Disease progression and liver cancer in the ferroportin disease. *Gut* 2007; **56**: 1030–2.

38. Pietrangelo A, Corradini E, Ferrara F, *et al*. Magnetic resonance imaging to identify classic and non-classic forms of ferroportin disease. *Blood Cells Mol Dis* 2006; **37**: 192–6.

39. Drakesmith H, Schimanski LM, Ormerod E, *et al*. Resistance to hepcidin is conferred by hemochromatosis-associated mutations of ferroportin. *Blood* 2005; **106**: 1092–7.

40. Cunat S, Giansily-Blaizot M, Bismuth M, *et al*. Global sequencing approach for characterizing the molecular background of hereditary iron disorders. *Clin Chem* 2007; **53**: 2060–9.

41. Liu W, Shimomura S, Imanishi H, *et al*. Hemochromatosis with mutation of the ferroportin 1 (*IREG1*) gene. *Intern Med* 2005; **44**: 285–9.

42. Koyama C, Wakusawa S, Hayashi H, *et al*. A Japanese family with ferroportin disease caused by a novel mutation of *SLC40A1* gene: hyperferritinemia associated with a relatively low transferrin saturation of iron. *Intern Med* 2005; **44**: 990–3.

43. Pelucchi S, Mariani R, Salvioni A, *et al*. Novel mutations of the ferroportin gene (*SLC40A1*): analysis of 56 consecutive patients with unexplained iron overload. *Clin Genet* 2008; **73**: 171–8.

44. Corradini E, Montosi G, Ferrara F, *et al*. Lack of enterocyte iron accumulation in the ferroportin disease. *Blood Cells Mol Dis* 2005; **35**: 315–18.

45. De Domenico I, McVey WD, Nemeth E, *et al*. Molecular and clinical correlates in iron overload associated with mutations in ferroportin. *Haematologica* 2006; **91**: 1092–5.

46. Cremonesi L, Forni GL, Soriani N, *et al*. Genetic and clinical heterogeneity of ferroportin disease. *Br J Haematol* 2005; **131**: 663–70.

47. Bach V, Remacha A, Altes A, Barcelo MJ, Molina MA, Baiget M. Autosomal dominant hereditary hemochromatosis associated with two novel Ferroportin 1 mutations in Spain. *Blood Cells Mol Dis* 2006; **36**: 41–5.

48. Wallace DF, Clark RM, Harley HA, Subramaniam VN. Autosomal dominant iron overload due to a novel mutation of ferroportin1 associated with parenchymal iron loading and cirrhosis. *J Hepatol* 2004; **40**: 710–13.

49. Girelli D, De Domenico I, Bozzini C, *et al*. Clinical, pathological, and molecular correlates in ferroportin disease: a study of two novel mutations. *J Hepatol* 2008; **49**: 664–71.

50. Hetet G, Devaux I, Soufir N, Grandchamp B, Beaumont C. Molecular analyses of patients with hyperferritinemia and normal serum iron values reveal both L ferritin IRE and 3 new ferroportin (*slc11A3*) mutations. *Blood* 2003; **102**: 1904–10.

51. Speletas M, Kioumi A, Loules G, *et al*. Analysis of *SLC40A1* gene at the mRNA level reveals rapidly the causative mutations in patients with hereditary hemochromatosis type IV. *Blood Cells Mol Dis* 2008; **40**: 353–9.

52. Morris TJ, Litvinova MM, Ralston D, Mattman A, Holmes D, Lockitch G. A novel ferroportin mutation in a Canadian family with autosomal dominant hemochromatosis. *Blood Cells Mol Dis* 2005; **35**: 309–14.

53. Zaahl MG, Merryweather-Clarke AT, Kotze MJ, van der Merwe S, Warnich L, Robson KJ. Analysis of genes implicated in iron regulation in individuals presenting with primary iron overload. *Hum Genet* 2004; **115**: 409–17.

54. Robson KJ, Merryweather-Clarke AT, Cadet E, *et al*. Recent advances in understanding haemochromatosis: a transition state. *J Med Genet* 2004; **41**: 721–30.

55. Lok CY, Merryweather-Clarke AT, Viprakasit V, *et al*. Iron overload in the Asian community. *Blood* 2009; **114**: 20–5.

56. Wallace DF, Dixon JL, Ramm GA, Anderson GJ, Powell LW, Subramaniam VN. A novel mutation in ferroportin implicated in iron overload. *J Hepatol* 2007; **46**: 921–6.

57. Lee PL, Gelbart T, West C, Barton JC. *SLC40A1* c.1402G→A results in aberrant splicing, ferroportin truncation after glycine 330, and an autosomal dominant hemochromatosis phenotype. *Acta Haematol* 2007; **118**: 237–41.

58. Griffiths WJ, Mayr R, McFarlane I, *et al*. Clinical presentation and molecular pathophysiology of

179

autosomal dominant hemochromatosis caused by a novel ferroportin mutation. *Hepatology* 2009, Oct 19. [Epub ahead of print]

59. Jouanolle AM, Douabin-Gicquel V, Halimi C, *et al.* Novel mutation in ferroportin 1 gene is associated with autosomal dominant iron overload. *J Hepatol* 2003; **39**: 286–9.

60. Letocart E, Le Gac G, Majore S, *et al.* A novel missense mutation in *SLC40A1* results in resistance to hepcidin

and confirms the existence of two ferroportin-associated iron overload diseases. *Br J Haematol* 2009; **147**: 379–85.

61. Duca L, Delbini P, Nava I, Vaja V, Fiorelli G, Cappellini MD. Mutation analysis of hepcidin and ferroportin genes in Italian prospective blood donors with iron overload. *Am J Hematol* 2009; **84**: 592–3.

Hemochromatosis associated with hemojuvelin gene (*HJV*) mutations

The term "juvenile hemochromatosis" (JH) (OMIM #602390) is used to describe rare forms of hereditary hemochromatosis characterized by severe iron overload, heart failure, and hypogonadotrophic hypogonadism in children, adolescents, or adults less than 30 years of age.[1–3] The average daily rate of iron absorption in young persons with JH is much greater than that of adults with *HFE* hemochromatosis. Although the pattern of parenchymal iron deposition in these two disorders is similar, cardiac damage and hypogonadotrophic hypogonadism occur much earlier in life and are more prevalent in JH than in adult-onset *HFE* hemochromatosis. Testicular atrophy or amenorrhea are the most common presenting symptoms of JH. Heart failure and arrhythmia due to cardiomyopathy are the predominant causes of death. JH is associated with an autosomal recessive pattern of inheritance in most kinships. Most persons with JH have two mutations of the hemojuvelin gene (*HJV*) on chromosome 1q (OMIM *608374). A major pathophysiologic attribute of JH hemochromatosis is dysregulation of hepcidin. Animal studies confirm that hemojuvelin is critical for the regulation of iron homeostasis and the induction of hepcidin synthesis. JH is sometimes designated as "type 2" hemochromatosis to distinguish it from *HFE* hemochromatosis.

Other persons with JH phenotypes have autosomal recessive iron overload associated with mutations in the hepcidin gene (*HAMP*) (Chapter 14) or in the transferrin receptor-2 gene (*TFR2*) (Chapter 15). In rare cases, JH phenotypes may appear in young persons who have autosomal dominant hemochromatosis due to "gain-of-function" ferroportin gene (*SLC40A1*) mutations.[4,5] (Chapter 12). JH is unrelated to neonatal hemochromatosis that occurs in late fetal life or in neonates (Chapter 33).

History

The clinical syndrome now known as JH was first described by French authors in the early 1930s as "le syndrome endocrine-hepato-cardiaque."[1–3] The rarity of hemochromatosis phenotypes in young persons was recognized by Sheldon in 1930.[6] In a review of hemochromatosis cases published in 1955 by Finch and Finch, only 3.5% of 787 patients were younger than age 30 years.[7] Series of young persons with JH phenotypes were reported during the interval 1979–2000.[8–10] The genetic basis of JH was described in 1999–2004,[11,12] and in 2004 the name hemojuvelin was proposed for the protein encoded by *HJV*.[12]

Clinical description

Some patients report the insidious onset of unexplained weight loss, weakness, lassitude, dyspnea on exertion, or joint discomfort. Failure of normal sexual development at adolescence, erectile dysfunction, or amenorrhea are common but non-specific signs of JH. Inadequate sexual maturation or loss of secondary sexual characteristics after puberty leads to poor breast development, testicular atrophy, or decreased or absent axillary and pubic hair. Patients with advanced iron overload may present with signs of congestive heart failure or cirrhosis. A high proportion of patients with JH have bone and joint disease, especially pain and swelling in metacarpophalangeal joints.[13] Some JH patients are somewhat taller than their siblings without iron overload. Some younger patients, especially pre-adolescents, have only mild hepatomegaly, and others have no symptoms or physical abnormalities attributable to iron overload.

Patients with *HJV* hemochromatosis are significantly younger than patients with *HFE* hemochromatosis, and are more likely to have hypogonadism, cardiomyopathy, and impaired glucose tolerance than patients with *HFE* hemochromatosis (Table 13.1). Cirrhosis and arthropathy are also common in *HJV* hemochromatosis, but the prevalence of these conditions is similar to that in patients diagnosed to have *HFE* hemochromatosis in medical care (Table 13.1).

Table 13.1. Comparison of *HFE* and *HJV* hemochromatosis[a]

Characteristic	*HFE* Hemochromatosis	*HJV* Hemochromatosis
Age at diagnosis, years[b]	45 ± 11	23 ± 6
Male: female ratio	Male predominance	Equal proportions of males and females
Iron absorption	Increased in some cases, especially males	Markedly increased
Transferrin saturation, %	88 ± 12	89 ± 10
Serum ferritin, g/L	2,830 ± 2,239	3,146 ± 1,270
Hypogonadism[b]	18%	96%
Cardiomyopathy[b]	7%	35%
Reduced glucose tolerance[b]	27%	58%
Cirrhosis	52%	42%
Arthropathy	12%	27%
Iron removed, g	14 ± 9	14 ± 5
Iron removed, g/year of age[b]	0.32 ± 0.20	0.65 ± 0.30

Notes: [a]Data adapted in part from de Gobbi et al.[30] These subjects were diagnosed in medical care. Characteristics are displayed as mean ± 1 SD or percentage of subjects, as indicated.
[b]These characteristics differ significantly between *HFE* and *HJV* hemochromatosis.

Genetics and pathophysiology

In 1999, Roetto and colleagues performed a genome-wide search to map the JH locus in nine Italian families, of which six were consanguineous and three had multiple affected patients.[11] This early age-of-onset phenotype mapped to the centromeric region of chromosome 1q. In 2004, Papanikolaou and colleagues reported using a positional cloning technique to identify a previously unknown gene on chromosome 1q as the cause of JH in French, Greek, and Italian patients.[12] All affected individuals had mutations in each copy of a gene subsequently named hemojuvelin (*HJV*). The most common of these mutations is G320V; this allele accounted for two-thirds of *HJV* mutations in French, Greek, and Italian JH patients and their families,[12] and has been reported in many other populations. Other pathogenic *HJV* alleles have been reported (Fig. 13.1).

Most JH cases have been described in whites from European populations,[10–12,14,15] but few patients in different kinships appear to be closely related by geography or ethnicity. It is unknown whether *HJV* mutations are more common in European whites than in other racial/ethnic groups, or whether research efforts to discover such cases to date have been greater in European countries and derivative nations. A few *HJV* mutations have been detected in more than one population, especially G320V.[10–12,14,16] *HJV* mutations and JH phenotypes have also been described in families of sub-Saharan African descent,[17,18] in Japanese kinships,[19] and in other Asian populations.[20] Many *HJV* mutations other than G320V are "private" and have been detected only in single families. Many persons with JH phenotypes occur in consanguineous marriages, or reside in isolated communities or populations in which the prospect of marriages among distant relatives is relatively great. JH has been described in identical twins.[10] Some patients with JH phenotypes are homozygous for a pathogenic *HJV* allele, especially those in consanguineous kinships. Other patients are compound heterozygotes for two different pathogenic mutations. In some extended kinships, three or more *HJV* mutations are sometimes discovered.

Hemojuvelin is homologous to the repulsive guidance (RGD) molecule family of proteins. Hemojuvelin is highly expressed in heart, liver, and skeletal muscle. The glycosylphosphatidylinositol-linked membrane protein hemojuvelin (GPI-hemojuvelin) is an essential upstream regulator of hepcidin, a polypeptide

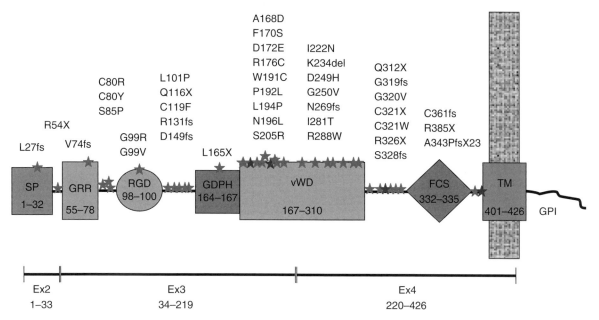

Fig. 13.1. Schematic diagram of reported pathogenic mutations in hemojuvelin (*HJV*) hemochromatosis. SP: signal peptide (not in mature protein); RGD: tri-amino acid adhesion motif; GRR: glycine-rich region; GDPH: tetra-amino acid conserved proteolytic cleavage site; vWD: partial von Willebrand type D domain; FCS: furin proteolytic cleavage site; TM: transmembrane domain (not in mature protein); and GPI: glycosylphosphatidyl inositol membrane anchor. The mutations mainly retained in the endoplasmic reticulum include F170S, W191C, G320V, and R385X.[22] Adapted from E. Beutler and P. Lee.

synthesized by hepatocytes that controls iron absorption. Hemojuvelin is transcribed in several isoforms; five alternative splicing variants have been identified. The major isoform is predicted to encode a 426-amino acid protein characterized by a RGD motif and a von Willebrand type D domain (Fig. 13.1). A soluble form of hemojuvelin (s-hemojuvelin) exists in blood and acts as antagonist of GPI-hemojuvelin (membrane-bound or m-hemojuvelin) to downregulate hepcidin expression. The release of s-hemojuvelin is negatively regulated by both transferrin-bound iron and non-transferrin-bound iron, indicating that s-hemojuvelin could be one of the mediators of hepcidin regulation by iron.[21] s-Hemojuvelin is released by a proprotein convertase through the cleavage at a conserved polybasic RNRR site.[21] The loss of hemojuvelin membrane export is central to the pathogenesis of JH, and hemojuvelin cleavage is essential for the export. These and other observations support the postulate that there is a dual function for s- and m-hemojuvelin proteins in iron deficiency and overload, respectively.[22] *HJV* may regulate hepcidin synthesis through signaling pathways that involve bone morphogenetic proteins and their subsequent effects on SMAD 1/5/8.[23] All *HJV* mutations discovered in

patients with iron overload phenotypes encode ineffective forms of mutant hemojuvelin ("loss-of-function mutations"). Urinary hepcidin levels are depressed or undetectable in individuals with JH due to *HJV* mutations.[12,24] The increased cellular export of iron from macrophages by ferroportin is almost unopposed due to the near-absence of hepcidin. This also accounts for the high levels of transferrin saturation usually observed in *HJV* hemochromatosis (Table 13.1).

Iron absorption is markedly increased in many persons with *HJV* hemochromatosis. This accounts for their severe parenchymal iron overload that occurs at an early age. For example, one untreated patient absorbed 100% of an oral test-dose of 0.5 mg of radioactive iron (normal range for adult men $28 \pm 9\%$); another male patient retained 60% (20.4 mg) of an orally administered dose of 35 mg of iron.[10] The estimated daily iron absorption in three siblings with JH due to *HJV* mutations was 2.3, 3.1, and 1.7 mg, respectively (normal ~ 1.0 mg daily).[14] Altogether, many types of mutant hemojuvelin are associated with severe hepcidin deficiency, and thus permit iron absorption to a far greater extent than do mutant HFE proteins. Other persons who inherit two *HJV* missense mutations are diagnosed to have hemochromatosis relatively late in life.[12] It is presumed that iron overload in these cases is less severe in part because their specific *HJV* mutation(s) are less effective in down-regulating hepcidin expression than certain other *HJV* mutation(s).

Laboratory evaluation

Most persons with JH phenotypes and *HJV* hemochromatosis have markedly elevated serum iron levels and transferrin saturation values. Elevated serum ferritin concentrations are present in most patients from an early age, and even higher values are observed in many teenagers or young adults (Table 13.1). Patients with hypogonadism have low normal or subnormal levels of luteinizing and follicle-stimulating hormones, subnormal age-adjusted levels of testosterone or estradiol, and anterior pituitary density by magnetic resonance imaging consistent with iron deposition. Mild elevation of serum concentrations of hepatic transaminases occurs in many patients due to iron deposition in hepatocytes.

Echocardiography often reveals a low left ventricular ejection fraction and an infiltrative pattern in the myocardium. Ventricular dilatation occurs in many patients with overt cardiomyopathy.[25] Endomyocardial biopsy specimens reveal heavy iron deposition in cardiac myocytes and fibrosis of the myocardium, although obtaining such biopsy specimens is not essential to diagnosis in most cases. Liver specimens obtained by biopsy reveal heavy iron deposition in hepatocytes, although iron may also be deposited in Kupffer cells and bile ductular cells. Micronodular cirrhosis develops in some patients. Bone and joint imaging studies may reveal osteoporosis, arthropathic changes similar to those of degenerative arthritis,[13] and sometimes delayed closure of epiphyses associated with hypogonadism.

HJV mutations reported to be associated with iron overload phenotypes are displayed in Fig. 13.1. *HJV* mutation analysis is not usually commercially available, although some research physicians and scientists will perform appropriate genetic testing. Study of parents and siblings of JH index patients is often needed to ensure that mutations that are discovered are, in fact, pathogenic and have caused the JH syndrome. Clinicians must often establish the diagnosis of JH on clinical grounds and manage patients and their families, as indicated, in the absence of *HJV*

mutation analyses. After the discovery of *HFE* in 1996, some patients with JH phenotypes were discovered to have common *HFE* mutations such as C282Y, H63D, or S65C. The JH phenotype does not segregate with *HFE* mutations in JH kinships, nor does the inheritance of *HFE* C282Y, H63D, or S65C in heterozygous configurations appear to alter the phenotype of JH hemochromatosis significantly.[26,27] Heterozygosity for certain *HJV* mutations has been discovered in some persons without iron overload who participated in population screening studies or who were control subjects (Table 13.2). Some of these mutations are probably pathogenic, and may eventually be discovered in persons with iron overload; such persons would be expected to have a second *HJV* mutation.

Heterozygosity for a *HJV* missense mutation (e.g. S105L, E302K, N372D, R335Q, L101P, and G320V) was associated with increased severity of iron overload in 9 of 310 French patients with hemochromatosis and *HFE* C282Y homozygosity.[28] In 48 white US hemochromatosis patients with *HFE* C282Y homozygosity studied with similar technique, no *HJV* coding region mutation was detected.[17] Aggregate *HJV* coding region mutation frequencies in C282Y homozygotes with a hemochromatosis phenotype in France and the US were similar (0.0148 vs. 0, respectively; $P = 0.2716$).[16] The aggregate frequency of *HJV* coding region mutations was also similar in French hemochromatosis patients with *HFE* C282Y homozygosity and in French control subjects (0.0145 vs. 0.0045, respectively; $P = 0.0564$).[16,28] Double heterozygosity for *HJV* I222N and *HFE* C282Y was not associated with evidence of increased iron absorption in a 29-year-old woman.[16] Various iron measures were similar in multiple family members with and without *HJV* L165X when stratified by *HFE* genotypes that included C282Y homozygosity and heterozygosity, indicating the absence of a clinically relevant modifying effect on the *HFE* genotypes.[29] Altogether, it remains unclear that heterozygosity for *HJV* mutations is a modifier of iron overload phenotypes in *HFE* C282Y homozygotes or heterozygotes.

Family screening

In typical JH kinships, each parent of a patient with a JH phenotype is heterozygous for a *HJV* mutation, and thus approximately 25% of all children of these parents will have JH. Transferrin saturation and

Table 13.2. Some *HJV* mutations detected in persons without iron overload[a]

Exon	Amino acid substitution	Comments
1	Q6H	Signal peptide mutation HJV Q6H (18G→C) occurred in *cis* with C321X, a premature termination mutation (962G→A and 963C→A). Unknown if Q6H itself is functional. Glutamine at this position is not conserved in rat hemojuvelin.[41]
—	IVS2 + 395C→G	Reported in patient with hyperferritinemia. Could affect splicing, but simple heterzygosity for this mutation alone would not explain an iron overload phenotype.[15]
3	G69-G70	Reported in African-American with hyperferritinemia; mutation caused glycine insertion (insG).[42]
3	S105L	
4	E275E	
4	R288Y	Associated phenotype not reported.[43] HJV R288W is associated with an iron overload phenotype.[44]
4	E302K	
4	A310G	Polymorphism without known effect on iron phenotypes.
4	R335Q	
4	N372D	Reported in heterozygous configuration in persons with hemochromatosis and homozygosity for *HFE* C282Y.[28] Asparagine at residue 372 is highly conserved.[28]

Note: [a]Compiled in part from data displayed in Beutler and Beutler[42] and Wallace and Subramaniam.[43] These *HJV* mutations, usually in heterozygous configuration, have been reported predominantly in persons without iron overload who participated in population screening studies or who were control subjects, or in persons without proven iron overload. Some mutations are probably pathogenic, and may eventually be discovered in persons with iron overload. Such persons would be expected to have a second pathogenic *HJV* mutation.

ferritin measurements should be performed in all children in JH kinships promptly after JH is discovered in the index case. If possible, each sibling should undergo *HJV* genotyping. In this manner, JH is sometimes identified in very young family members before manifestations of iron overload disease occur (Fig. 13.2). Such persons should be treated to achieve and maintain iron depletion with therapeutic phlebotomy, because early diagnosis and treatment can prevent complications of iron overload that would otherwise develop. Simple heterozygosity for a *HJV* mutation is typical of parents and some siblings of JH patients. Heterozygotes for pathogenic *HJV* mutations usually have normal iron phenotypes and do not develop iron overload.[14,30]

Treatment

Cardiomyopathy due to iron overload in patients with JH must be treated aggressively and promptly (Chapters 5, 36). Cardiomyopathy can be immediately life-threatening, and life expectancy after diagnosis without effective treatment is brief (days to a few years). Heart failure and arrhythmia should be treated in the same manner as in patients with similar cardiac complications unassociated with iron overload. Therapeutic phlebotomy is the mainstay of treatment of iron overload in patients with cardiomyopathy due to myocardial siderosis, and phlebotomy removes more iron in a shorter interval than other treatments (Chapter 36). Nonetheless, the addition of deferoxamine infusions or administration of an oral iron chelator such as deferiprone or deferasirox may promote a greater rate of net iron loss than can be achieved with phlebotomy alone (Chapter 36).[31,32] Combination chelation therapy may be advantageous in some cases.[33] Nonetheless, oral iron chelators are incapable of removing iron specifically from the myocardium. Treatment with phlebotomy and iron chelation drugs should be continued until iron depletion indicated by low normal serum ferritin concentration is achieved. Heart or liver transplantation should be considered in patients whose major organ failure cannot be managed satisfactorily by iron depletion and other routine ancillary measures.[34]

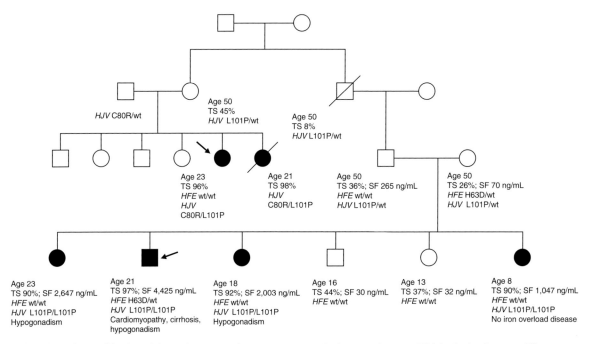

Fig. 13.2. Pedigree of family with hemochromatosis due to mutations in the hemojuvelin gene (*HJV*). In this kinship, two different pathogenic *HJV* alleles caused juvenile hemochromatosis phenotypes in two successive generations. Persons with hemochromatosis phenotypes are indicated by solid figures. Index cases of each generation are indicated by arrows. TS = transferrin saturation; SF = serum ferritin. Absence of missense *HFE* or *HJV* mutation is denoted wt. Genotypes displayed in parentheses were deduced. Adapted from Lee *et al.*[40]

In patients without cardiomyopathy, performing therapeutic phlebotomy once or twice weekly until iron depletion is achieved is recommended. Most patients tolerate this treatment very well. Administration of erythropoietin to support erythropoiesis is usually unnecessary, but may permit more aggressive phlebotomy in patients who also have thalassemia.[35] Phlebotomy therapy to maintain low iron stores should be performed in all patients. Daily consumption of green tea may decrease the rate of iron absorption,[10,36] but does not promote iron excretion. A diet of low iron content is not indicated, although JH patients should not consume supplemental iron.

Hypogonadism, diabetes mellitus, and osteoporosis should be managed by an endocrinologist. In many cases, lifelong replacement treatment with sex hormones and insulin is needed. Reversal of hypogonadism after iron depletion improves testicular function or helps achieve pregnancy and childbearing in some patients with JH phenotypes.[37–39] The treatment of arthropathy is similar to that in patients with other forms of degenerative joint disease. The arthritis usually progresses despite phlebotomy therapy.[13] Although unreported to date, patients with JH who

also have cirrhosis probably have an increased risk to develop primary liver cancer. The low prevalence of JH and the high rate of mortality due to cardiomyopathy in persons with cirrhosis and JH phenotypes could account for the apparent rarity of primary liver cancer.

References

1. Bezançon F, de Gennes L, DeLarue J, Oumensky V. *Cirrhose pigmentaire avec infantilisme et insuffisance cardiaque et aplasie endocriniennes multiples. Bull Mém Soc Méd Hôp Paris* 1932; **48**: 967–74.

2. de Gennes L, DeLarue J, de Vericourt R. *Sur un nouveau cas de cirrhose pigmentaire avec infantilisme et myocarde. Le syndrome endocrine-hepato-cardiaque. Bull Mém Soc Méd Hôp Paris* 1935; **51**: 1228.

3. de Vericourt R. *Le syndrome endocrino-hepato-myocardiaque (sur an aspect des cirrhoses pigmentaires).* Paris, 1935.

4. Pietrangelo A, Caleffi A, Henrion J, *et al.* Juvenile hemochromatosis associated with pathogenic mutations of adult hemochromatosis genes. *Gastroenterology* 2005; **128**: 470–9.

5. Sham RL, Phatak PD, West C, Lee P, Andrews C, Beutler E. Autosomal dominant hereditary

hemochromatosis associated with a novel ferroportin mutation and unique clinical features. *Blood Cells Mol Dis* 2005; **34**: 157–61.

6. Sheldon JH. *Haemochromatosis*. London, Oxford University Press, 1935; 381.

7. Finch SC, Finch CL. Idiopathic hemochromatosis, an iron storage disease. A. Iron metabolism in hemochromatosis. *Medicine* 1955; **34**: 381–430.

8. Goossens JP. Idiopathic haemochromatosis: Juvenile and familial type—endocrine aspects. *Neth J Med* 1975; **18**: 161–9.

9. Lamon JM, Marynick SP, Roseblatt R, Donnelly S. Idiopathic hemochromatosis in a young female. A case study and review of the syndrome in young people. *Gastroenterology* 1979; **76**: 178–83.

10. Kaltwasser JP. Juvenile hemochromatosis. In: Barton JC, Edward CQ, eds. *Hemochromatosis: Genetics, Pathogenesis, Diagnosis and Treatment*. Cambridge, Cambridge University Press. 2000; 318–25.

11. Roetto A, Totaro A, Cazzola M, *et al.* Juvenile hemochromatosis locus maps to chromosome 1q. *Am J Hum Genet* 1999; **64**: 1388–93.

12. Papanikolaou G, Samuels ME, Ludwig EH, *et al.* Mutations in *HFE2* cause iron overload in chromosome 1q-linked juvenile hemochromatosis. *Nat Genet* 2004; **36**: 77–82.

13. Vaiopoulos G, Papanikolaou G, Politou M, Jibreel I, Sakellaropoulos N, Loukopoulos D. Arthropathy in juvenile hemochromatosis. *Arthritis Rheum* 2003; **48**: 227–30.

14. Barton JC, Rao SV, Pereira NM, *et al.* Juvenile hemochromatosis in the southeastern United States: a report of seven cases in two kinships. *Blood Cells Mol Dis* 2002; **29**: 104–15.

15. Mendes AI, Ferro A, Martins R, *et al.* Non-classical hereditary hemochromatosis in Portugal: novel mutations identified in iron metabolism-related genes. *Ann Hematol* 2009; **88**: 229–34.

16. Barton JC, Rivers CA, Niyongere S, Bohannon SB, Acton RT. Allele frequencies of hemojuvelin gene (*HJV*) I222N and G320V missense mutations in white and African-American subjects from the general Alabama population. *BMC Med Genet* 2004; **5**: 29.

17. Lee PL, Barton JC, Brandhagen D, Beutler E. Hemojuvelin (*HJV*) mutations in persons of European, African-American and Asian ancestry with adult onset haemochromatosis. *Br J Haematol* 2004; **127**: 224–9.

18. Murugan RC, Lee PL, Kalavar, MR, Barton JC. Early age-of-onset iron overload and homozygosity for the novel hemojuvelin mutation *HJV* R54X (exon 3; c.160>T) in an African-American male of West Indies descent. *Clin Genet* 2008; **74**: 88–92.

19. Koyama C, Hayashi H, Wakusawa S, *et al.* Three patients with middle-age-onset hemochromatosis caused by novel mutations in the hemojuvelin gene. *J Hepatol* 2005; **43**: 740–2.

20. Lok CY, Merryweather-Clarke AT, Viprakasit V, *et al.* Iron overload in the Asian community. *Blood* 2009; **114**: 20–5.

21. Lin L, Nemeth E, Goodnough JB, Thapa DR, Gabayan V, Ganz T. Soluble hemojuvelin is released by proprotein convertase-mediated cleavage at a conserved polybasic RNRR site. *Blood Cells Mol Dis* 2008; **40**: 122–31.

22. Silvestri L, Pagani A, Fazi C, *et al.* Defective targeting of hemojuvelin to plasma membrane is a common pathogenetic mechanism in juvenile hemochromatosis. *Blood* 2007; **109**: 4503–10.

23. Truksa J, Peng H, Lee P, Beutler E. Bone morphogenetic proteins 2, 4, and 9 stimulate murine hepcidin 1 expression independently of Hfe, transferrin receptor-2 (Tfr2), and IL-6. *Proc Natl Acad Sci USA* 2006; **103**: 10289–93.

24. Zhang AS, Anderson SA, Meyers KR, Hernandez C, Eisenstein RS, Enns CA. Evidence that inhibition of hemojuvelin shedding in response to iron is mediated through neogenin. *J Biol Chem* 2007; **282**: 12547–56.

25. Muhlestein JB. Cardiac abnormalities in hemochromatosis. In: Barton JC, Edwards CQ, eds. *Hemochromatosis: Genetics, Pathophysiology, Diagnosis and Treatment*. Cambridge, Cambridge University Press. 2000; 297–311.

26. Rivard SR, Mura C, Simard H, *et al.* Mutation analysis in the *HFE* gene in patients with hereditary haemochromatosis in Saguenay-Lac-Saint-Jean (Quebec, Canada). *Br J Haematol* 2000; **108**: 854–8.

27. Rivard SR, Mura C, Simard H, *et al.* Clinical and molecular aspects of juvenile hemochromatosis in Saguenay-Lac-Saint-Jean (Quebec, Canada). *Blood Cells Mol Dis* 2000; **26**: 10–14.

28. Le Gac G, Scotet V, Ka C, *et al.* The recently identified type 2A juvenile haemochromatosis gene (*HJV*), a second candidate modifier of the C282Y homozygous phenotype. *Hum Mol Genet* 2004; **13**: 1913–18.

29. van Dijk BA, Kemna EH, Tjalsma H, *et al.* Effect of the new *HJV*-L165X mutation on penetrance of *HFE*. *Blood* 2007; **109**: 5525–6.

30. de Gobbi M, Roetto A, Piperno A, *et al.* Natural history of juvenile haemochromatosis. *Br J Haematol* 2002; **117**: 973–9.

31. Kelly AL, Rhodes DA, Roland JM, Schofield P, Cox TM. Hereditary juvenile haemochromatosis: a genetically heterogeneous life-threatening iron-storage disease. *QJM* 1998; **91**: 607–18.

32. Fabio G, Minonzio F, Delbini P, Bianchi A, Cappellini MD. Reversal of cardiac complications by deferiprone and deferoxamine combination therapy in a patient affected by a severe type of juvenile hemochromatosis (JH). *Blood* 2007; **109**: 362–4.

33. Barton JC. Chelation therapy for iron overload. *Curr Gastroenterol Rep* 2007; **9**: 74–82.

34. Jensen PD, Bagger JP, Jensen FT, Baandrup U, Christensen T, Ellegaard J. Heart transplantation in a case of juvenile hereditary haemochromatosis followed up by MRI and endomyocardial biopsies. *Eur J Haematol* 1993; **51**: 199–205.

35. De Gobbi M, Pasquero P, Brunello F, Paccotti P, Mazza U, Camaschella C. Juvenile hemochromatosis associated with B-thalassemia treated by phlebotomy and recombinant human erythropoietin. *Haematologica* 2000; **85**: 865–7.

36. Kaltwasser JP, Werner E, Schalk K, Hansen C, Gottschalk R, Seidl C. Clinical trial on the effect of regular tea drinking on iron accumulation in genetic haemochromatosis. *Gut* 1998; **43**: 699–704.

37. Cazzola M, Ascari E, Barosi G, et al. Juvenile idiopathic haemochromatosis: a life-threatening disorder presenting as hypogonadotropic hypogonadism. *Hum Genet* 1983; **65**: 149–54.

38. Kelly TM, Edwards CQ, Meikle AW, Kushner JP. Hypogonadism in hemochromatosis: reversal with iron depletion. *Ann Intern Med* 1984; **101**: 629–32.

39. Farina G, Pedrotti C, Cerani P, et al. Successful pregnancy following gonadotropin therapy in a young female with juvenile idiopathic hemochromatosis and secondary hypogonadotropic hypogonadism. *Haematologica* 1995; **80**: 335–7.

40. Lee PL, Beutler E, Rao SV, Barton JC. Genetic abnormalities and juvenile hemochromatosis: mutations of the *HJV* gene encoding hemojuvelin. *Blood* 2004; **103**: 4669–71.

41. Huang FW, Rubio-Aliaga I, Kushner JP, Andrews NC, Fleming MD. Identification of a novel mutation (C321X) in *HJV*. *Blood* 2004; **104**: 2176–7.

42. Beutler L, Beutler E. Hematologically important mutations: iron storage diseases. *Blood Cells Mol Dis* 2004; **33**: 40–4.

43. Wallace DF, Subramaniam VN. Non-*HFE* haemochromatosis. *World J Gastroenterol* 2007; **13**: 4690–8.

44. Filali M, Le Jeunne C, Durand E, et al. Juvenile hemochromatosis *HJV*-related revealed by cardiogenic shock. *Blood Cells Mol Dis* 2004; **33**: 120–4.

14 Hemochromatosis associated with hepcidin gene (*HAMP*) mutations

Hepcidin, an antimicrobial peptide produced by hepatocytes, is a central negative regulator of iron absorption that is encoded by the *HAMP* gene on chromosome 19q13 (Chapter 2). In humans, *HAMP* mutations account for a rare subtype of juvenile-onset hemochromatosis (OMIM #602390). Some patients have an autosomal recessive disorder associated with homozygosity for rare pathogenic *HAMP* mutations. Others have hemochromatosis phenotypes due to heterozygosity for a pathogenic *HAMP* mutation and co-inheritance of heterozygosity or homozygosity for *HFE* C282Y.

The precursor of hepcidin comprises 84 amino acids, from which 3 active peptides of 25, 22, and 20 amino acids, respectively, are produced by protease cleavage.[1,2] The 25 and 20 amino acid peptides represent the major forms.[1] Active forms of hepcidin contain numerous cysteines.[3] Eight highly-conserved cysteine residues form four disulfide bonds, the critical basis of a rigid structure of the final peptide.[4] The *HAMP* promoter contains consensus sequences for the transcription factor CCAAT/enhancer binding protein-α (CEBP/α) that confers liver tissue specificity.[5] The *HAMP* promoter also responds to interleukin-6 (IL-6), and has a bone morphogenetic protein-responsive element (BMP-RE) that binds SMAD 1/5/8/4 protein complex.[6–9] Hepcidin expression is decreased in *HFE*, "gain-of-function" *SLC40A1*, and *TFR2* hemochromatosis, and increased in "loss-of-function" *SLC40A1* hemochromatosis in the absence of *HAMP* mutations[3,10–14] (Chapters 8, 12, 15). In experimental animals, hepcidin synthesis is increased by iron loading and inflammation and is inhibited by iron deficiency anemia and hypoxia.[15–17]

Clinical and laboratory features

Patients who are homozygous for deleterious *HAMP* mutations have clinical phenotypes similar to those of patients with *HJV* hemochromatosis.[18] (Chapter 13) In general, index patients are relatively young, and have elevated transferrin saturation and moderate or severe hyperferritinemia.[18–21] In patients homozygous for *HAMP* −25G→A, urinary hepcidin was absent in one case[20] and present in an unrelated patient.[22] Hepcidin was not appropriately induced by an iron challenge test.[22] A 21-year-old Pakistani man homozygous for *HAMP* R42Sfs also had hypogonadism and gynecomastia.[21] A 29-year-old Portuguese man with *HAMP* −25G→A homozygosity also had insulin-dependent diabetes mellitus, severe heart failure, skin hyperpigmentation, hepatosplenomegaly, and hypogonadism.[20] Younger homozygotes in some kinships may be asymptomatic. Heterozygotes for deleterious *HAMP* mutations in these kinships had normal iron phenotypes, consistent with observations in population screening studies.[23] Patients with digenic hemochromatosis associated with co-inheritance of a pathogenic *HAMP* mutation and one or two copies of *HFE* C282Y also have relatively severe, early-onset hemochromatosis phenotypes.[7,24] Many subjects with *HAMP* hemochromatosis have elevated serum levels of hepatic transaminases. Liver biopsy specimens reveal marked iron overload that is localized predominantly in periportal hepatocytes, with or without cirrhosis. Two *HAMP* −72C→T heterozygotes also had beta-thalassemia trait and hepatitis C.[25]

Genetics

HAMP hemochromatosis occurs in at least two defined patterns of inheritance. The first pattern is an autosomal recessive disorder. These deleterious *HAMP* mutations are rare and have been reported as private mutations in consanguineous kinships.[18–21,26] (Table 14.1) *HAMP* −25G→A has been reported in apparently unrelated Portuguese kinships.[20,22] In a consanguineous Australian kinship, both a father and his daughter were *HAMP* C78T homozygotes, resulting in a pseudo-dominant pattern of inheritance.[19]

Table 14.1. Pathogenic mutations of the hepcidin gene (*HAMP*)

cDNA	Exon	Amino acid substitution	Genotypes with high iron phenotypes	Region/ethnicity	Reference(s)
c.−153C→T	—	—	Digenic with C282Y	French; US Hispanic	7,29
−72C→T	—	—	Digenic with C282Y[a]	Italian; US whites	23,33
−25G→A (+14G→A, 5′ UTR)[b]	—	—	Homozygosity	Portuguese	20,22
93delG[c]	1	G32fs (T31fsX180)	Homozygosity	Italian/Greek	18
148–IVS2(+1) delATGG[d]	2	M50fs	Digenic with C282Y	English	24
126–127delAG	2	R42Sfs	Homozygosity	Pakistani	21
166C→T[e]	3	R56X	Homozygosity; digenic with C282Y	Italian/Greek	18,27
175C→G	3	R59G	Digenic with C282Y	French, US white	23,27
208T→C	3	C70R	Homozygosity; digenic with C282Y	Italian	26,34
212G→A	3	G71D	Digenic with C282Y	English, Italian, US Hispanic	23,24,33
233G→A	3	C78T	Homozygosity	Australian	19

Notes: [a]Two Italian subjects with this mutation also had beta-thalassemia trait, hepatitis C, and iron overload.[25]
[b]This mutation creates a new initiation codon at position +14 of the 5′ UTR, which induces a shift of the reading frame and the generation of an abnormal protein. In one patient, this protein was probably unstable or otherwise degraded, because it was not found on bidirectional protein gel electrophoresis.[20,31] In another patient, there was detectable hepcidin, suggesting that the start of translation was maintained at the original ATG with some normal protein production.[22]
[c]This deletion resulted in a frameshift, and, if mutated RNA achieved translation, generated an abnormal elongated (179 residues) prohepcidin peptide, in contrast to the normal hepcidin propeptide of 84 amino acids.[18]
[d]This four-nucleotide ATGG deletion (last codon of exon 2 (met50) and first base of the splice donor site of intron 2 (IVS+1(-G)); this causes a 4-bp *HAMP* frameshift. The mutation was predicted to result in retention of the splice consensus site, but altered the reading frame, extending it beyond the end of the normal transcript.[24]
[e]This mutation affects a propeptide cleavage site.

The second pattern of inheritance is digenic hemochromatosis associated with co-inheritance of a pathogenic *HAMP* mutation and *HFE* C282Y. Such configurations have been detected in groups of *HFE* C282Y homozygotes who were tested for *HAMP* alleles. In a cohort of 392 French *HFE* homozygotes with hemochromatosis phenotypes, Jacolot and colleagues found that five were also heterozygous for a *HAMP* mutation (R59G, G71D, or R56X).[27] Biasiotto *et al.* tested 136 C282Y homozygous, 43 heterozygous, and 42 C282Y/H63D compound heterozygous, and 62 control Italian subjects for *HAMP* mutations using denaturing high-performance liquid chromatography (DHPLC). Abnormally high indices of iron status were found in a C282Y/H63D heterozygote who also had *HAMP* −72C→T; the iron phenotype of another

C282Y/H63D compound heterozygote who also had *HAMP* G71D was normal.[28] In the HEIRS Study, DHPLC analysis of 191 C282Y homozygotes identified in screening was performed; two were heterozygous for *HAMP* mutations. One had the *HAMP* promoter mutation −72C→T and the other had *HAMP* R59G; both study participants had high transferrin saturation and serum ferritin values.[29] In the same study, *HAMP* −153C→T was not detected in any of 191 *HFE* C282Y homozygotes.[29] *HAMP* mutations that would account for iron overload were not detected in a group of white, Asian, and African-American subjects with and without iron overload.[30]

HAMP G71D was detected in the general English population at an allele frequency of 0.3%.[24] In the HEIRS Study, the allele frequencies of *HAMP* R59G in white controls and *HAMP* G71D in Hispanic controls were 0.7% and 0.6%, respectively. *HAMP* −153C→T was not detected in 100 French subjects with normal serum iron and hemoglobin measures.[7] In the HEIRS Study, *HAMP* −153C→T occurred in a single Hispanic participant, but was not detected in large cohorts of white, African-American, or Asian study participants.[29] Taken together, these observations indicate *HAMP* mutations are uncommon in general populations, and account for little of the iron phenotype heterogeneity in persons with or without *HFE* C282Y.[23]

Genotype-phenotype correlations

Two missense *HAMP* mutations (C70R, C78T) directly affect highly-conserved cysteine residues that form disulfide bonds crucial for normal structure and function of mature hepcidin (Table 14.1). Other coding region mutations result in premature truncation of the protein (Table 14.1). Thus, homozygosity for *HAMP* R42Sfs or C78T, for example, abrogates production of normally functional hepcidin.[19] *HAMP* −25G→A creates a new initiation codon at position +14 of the 5′ UTR[20,31] (Table 14.1). One *HAMP* −25G→A homozygote had detectable hepcidin, suggesting that the start of translation was maintained at the original ATG with some normal protein production.[22]

In vitro, *HAMP* −153C→T decreased transcriptional activity of the promoter, altered its IL-6 responsiveness, and prevented binding of SMAD 1/5/8/4 protein complex to the BMP responsive element (RE) of *HAMP* (Table 14.1). Thus, −153C→T could decrease hepcidin levels and contribute to iron overload.[7] Two highly conserved and sequence-identical BMP-RE at positions −84/−79 and −2255/−2250 of the *HAMP* promoter are critical for basal hepcidin mRNA expression and hepcidin response to BMP-2 and BMP-6.[32] The former BMP-RE is proximal to a STAT-binding site important for hepcidin response to IL-6.[32] *HAMP* promoter mutations in areas outside BMP-REs or the STAT-binding site may also contribute to the development of iron overload. For example, two Italian patients with beta-thalassemia trait, hepatitis C, and iron overload were *HAMP* −72C→T heterozygotes[25] (Table 14.1).

Prevention and treatment

All first-degree relatives of probands with *HAMP* hemochromatosis should undergo iron phenotyping

and analysis to identify *HAMP* and *HFE* mutations. Thus, asymptomatic subjects with pathogenic genotypes (especially young persons and women) can be treated before they develop target organ injury due to iron overload.

Therapy for iron overload due to *HAMP* hemochromatosis is similar to that for *HJV* hemochromatosis. Therapeutic phlebotomy alleviates iron overload in persons homozygous for *HAMP* mutations and is tolerated well.[18–21] Subjects with evidence of iron-induced cardiomyopathy may benefit from combined phlebotomy and iron chelation therapy (Chapters 5, 36). Similarly, persons with C282Y homozygosity or heterozygosity who have iron overload phenotypes should be treated with phlebotomy (Chapters 5, 36). Hypogonadism, arthropathy, and diabetes mellitus should be managed as described in Chapter 5.

References

1. Park CH, Valore EV, Waring AJ, Ganz T. Hepcidin, a urinary antimicrobial peptide synthesized in the liver. *J Biol Chem* 2001; **276**: 7806–10.

2. Krause A, Neitz S, Magert HJ, *et al.* LEAP-1, a novel highly disulfide-bonded human peptide, exhibits antimicrobial activity. *FEBS Lett* 2000; **480**: 147–50.

3. Gehrke SG, Kulaksiz H, Herrmann T, *et al.* Expression of hepcidin in hereditary hemochromatosis: evidence for a regulation in response to the serum transferrin saturation and to non-transferrin-bound iron. *Blood* 2003; **102**: 371–6.

4. Hunter HN, Fulton DB, Ganz T, Vogel HJ. The solution structure of human hepcidin, a peptide hormone with antimicrobial activity that is involved in iron uptake and hereditary hemochromatosis. *J Biol Chem* 2002; **277**: 37 597–603.

5. Courselaud B, Pigeon C, Inoue Y, *et al.* C/EBPalpha regulates hepatic transcription of hepcidin, an antimicrobial peptide and regulator of iron metabolism. Cross-talk between C/EBP pathway and iron metabolism. *J Biol Chem* 2002; **277**: 41163–70.

6. Truksa J, Peng H, Lee P, Beutler E. Different regulatory elements are required for response of hepcidin to interleukin-6 and bone morphogenetic proteins 4 and 9. *Br J Haematol* 2007; **139**: 138–47.

7. Island ML, Jouanolle AM, Mosser A, *et al.* A new mutation in the hepcidin promoter impairs its BMP response and contributes to a severe phenotype in *HFE*-related hemochromatosis. *Haematologica* 2009; **94**: 720–4.

8. Lee PL, Beutler E. Regulation of hepcidin and iron overload disease. *Annu Rev Pathol* 2009; **4**: 489–515.

191

9. Truksa J, Lee P, Beutler E. Two BMP responsive elements, STAT, and bZIP/HNF4/COUP motifs of the hepcidin promoter are critical for BMP, SMAD1, and HJV responsiveness. *Blood* 2009; **113**: 688–95.

10. Nemeth E, Roetto A, Garozzo G, Ganz T, Camaschella C. Hepcidin is decreased in *TFR2* hemochromatosis. *Blood* 2005; **105**: 1803–6.

11. Zoller H, McFarlane I, Theurl I, *et al.* Primary iron overload with inappropriate hepcidin expression in V162del ferroportin disease. *Hepatology* 2005; **42**: 466–72.

12. Ganz T, Nemeth E. Regulation of iron acquisition and iron distribution in mammals. *Biochim Biophys Acta* 2006; **1763**: 690–9.

13. Origa R, Galanello R, Ganz T, *et al.* Liver iron concentrations and urinary hepcidin in beta-thalassemia. *Haematologica* 2007; **92**: 583–8.

14. Piperno A, Girelli D, Nemeth E, *et al.* Blunted hepcidin response to oral iron challenge in *HFE*-related hemochromatosis. *Blood* 2007; **110**: 4096–100.

15. Nicolas G, Chauvet C, Viatte L, *et al.* The gene encoding the iron regulatory peptide hepcidin is regulated by anemia, hypoxia, and inflammation. *J Clin Invest* 2002; **110**: 1037–44.

16. Nicolas G, Bennoun M, Porteu A, *et al.* Severe iron deficiency anemia in transgenic mice expressing liver hepcidin. *Proc Natl Acad Sci USA* 2002; **99**: 4596–601.

17. Ganz T. Hepcidin, a key regulator of iron metabolism and mediator of anemia of inflammation. *Blood* 2003; **102**: 783–8.

18. Roetto A, Papanikolaou G, Politou M, *et al.* Mutant antimicrobial peptide hepcidin is associated with severe juvenile hemochromatosis. *Nat Genet* 2003; **33**: 21–2.

19. Delatycki MB, Allen KJ, Gow P, *et al.* A homozygous *HAMP* mutation in a multiply consanguineous family with pseudo-dominant juvenile hemochromatosis. *Clin Genet* 2004; **65**: 378–83.

20. Matthes T, Aguilar-Martinez P, Pizzi-Bosman L, *et al.* Severe hemochromatosis in a Portuguese family associated with a new mutation in the 5'-UTR of the *HAMP* gene. *Blood* 2004; **104**: 2181–3.

21. Lok CY, Merryweather-Clarke AT, Viprakasit V, *et al.* Iron overload in the Asian community. *Blood* 2009; **114**: 20–5.

22. Porto G, Roetto A, Daraio F, *et al.* A Portuguese patient homozygous for the -25G>A mutation of the *HAMP* promoter shows evidence of steady-state transcription but fails to up-regulate hepcidin levels by iron. *Blood* 2005; **106**: 2922–3.

23. Barton JC, LaFreniere S, Leiendecker-Foster C, *et al. HFE, SLC40A1, HAMP, HJV, TFR2,* and *FTL* mutations detected by denaturing high-performance liquid chromatography after iron phenotyping and *HFE* C282Y and H63D genotyping in 785 HEIRS Study participants. *Am J Hematol* 2009; **84**: 710–14.

24. Merryweather-Clarke AT, Cadet E, Bomford A, *et al.* Digenic inheritance of mutations in *HAMP* and *HFE* results in different types of haemochromatosis. *Hum Mol Genet* 2003; **12**: 2241–7.

25. Valenti L, Pulixi EA, Arosio P, *et al.* Relative contribution of iron genes, dysmetabolism and hepatitis C virus (HCV) in the pathogenesis of altered iron regulation in HCV chronic hepatitis. *Haematologica* 2007; **92**: 1037–42.

26. Roetto A, Daraio F, Porporato P, *et al.* Screening hepcidin for mutations in juvenile hemochromatosis: identification of a new mutation (C70R). *Blood* 2004; **103**: 2407–9.

27. Jacolot S, Le Gac G, Scotet V, Quere I, Mura C, Ferec C. *HAMP* as a modifier gene that increases the phenotypic expression of the *HFE* pC282Y homozygous genotype. *Blood* 2004; **103**: 2835–40.

28. Biasiotto G, Belloli S, Ruggeri G, *et al.* Identification of new mutations of the *HFE*, hepcidin, and transferrin receptor-2 genes by denaturing HPLC analysis of individuals with biochemical indications of iron overload. *Clin Chem* 2003; **49**: 1981–8.

29. Barton JC, LaFreniere S, Leiendecker-Foster C, *et al. HAMP* promoter mutation nc.−153C>T in 785 HEIRS Study participants. *Haematologica* 2009; **94**: 1465.

30. Lee PL, Gelbart T, West C, Halloran C, Felitti V, Beutler E. A study of genes that may modulate the expression of hereditary hemochromatosis: transferrin receptor-1, ferroportin, ceruloplasmin, ferritin light and heavy chains, iron regulatory proteins (IRP)-1 and -2, and hepcidin. *Blood Cells Mol Dis* 2001; **27**: 783–802.

31. Rideau A, Mangeat B, Matthes T, Trono D, Beris P. Molecular mechanism of hepcidin deficiency in a patient with juvenile hemochromatosis. *Haematologica* 2007; **92**: 127–8.

32. Casanovas G, Mleczko-Sanecka K, Altamura S, Hentze MW, Muckenthaler MU. Bone morphogenetic protein (BMP)-responsive elements located in the proximal and distal hepcidin promoter are critical for its response to HJV/BMP/SMAD. *J Mol Med* 2009; **87**: 471–80.

33. Biasiotto G, Roetto A, Daraio F, *et al.* Identification of new mutations of hepcidin and hemojuvelin in patients with *HFE* C282Y allele. *Blood Cells Mol Dis* 2004; **33**: 338–43.

34. Majore S, Binni F, Pennese A, De Santis A, Crisi A, Grammatico P. *HAMP* gene mutation c.208T>C (p.C70R) identified in an Italian patient with severe hereditary hemochromatosis. *Hum Mutat* 2004; **23**: 400.

Hemochromatosis associated with transferrin receptor-2 gene (*TFR2*) mutations

TFR2 hemochromatosis (OMIM #604250) is a rare autosomal recessive disorder characterized by elevated serum iron measures, parenchymal iron deposition, and complications of iron overload. In some kinships, severe iron overload occurs in children or young adults. In individual cases, the *TFR2* hemochromatosis phenotype may resemble that of *HFE* hemochromatosis or *HJV* hemochromatosis (Chapter 8).

History

In 1999, Kawabata and colleagues cloned and sequenced a human gene homologous to the *TFR* gene that encodes classical transferrin receptor (TFR1). They named the newly discovered gene *TFR2* (OMIM *604720), and mapped it to chromosome 7q22.[1] Two transcripts (alpha and beta) are expressed from this gene; the alpha transcript is expressed predominantly in the liver. TFR2-alpha is a second transferrin receptor that mediates cellular iron transport in vitro.[1] In normal subjects, most iron uptake by the liver is transferrin mediated. Expression of TFR1 in hepatocytes, as in other non-reticuloendothelial cell types, is downregulated in response to increased intracellular iron. Consequently, hepatocyte TFR1 is undetectable in patients with *HFE* hemochromatosis and hepatic iron loading. Nonetheless, hepatic iron loading in *HFE* hemochromatosis is progressive. Experiments in mice demonstrate that TFR2 makes only a minor contribution to the uptake of transferrin-bound iron by the liver, but rather TFR2 is thought to modulate the signaling pathway that controls hepcidin expression.[2] In 2000, Camaschella and colleagues described persons with hemochromatosis phenotypes in two unrelated Sicilian families who had mutations in *TFR2*.[3]

Clinical characteristics

The age of onset and severity of iron overload varies moderately in patients with *TFR2* hemochromatosis.[4–6] Some patients have early-onset iron overload typical of "juvenile" hemochromatosis due to *HJV* or *HAMP* mutations (Chapters 13, 14).[4,5,7,8] In early-onset cases, fatigue, loss of libido, amenorrhea, or cardiomyopathy can occur as consequences of iron overload.[8–10] Weight loss, hepatomegaly, stigmata of cirrhosis, arthralgias, arthropathy, diabetes mellitus, and bronze discoloration of the skin have been described in adolescents and adults with *TFR2* hemochromatosis.[11] Overall, these manifestations are similar to those in *HJV* or *HFE* hemochromatosis. In *HFE* C282Y homozygotes, however, the development of severe iron overload before age 30 years is unusual, and iron overload is typically less severe than in persons of similar age with *TFR2* hemochromatosis.

Laboratory findings

TFR2 hemochromatosis is associated with elevated transferrin saturation, hyperferritinemia, and multiorgan iron overload, especially hepatocytes.[3,4,9] Serum activities of hepatic transaminases may be elevated. It is recommended that liver biopsy be performed in patients with serum ferritin >1000 µg/L, hepatomegaly, or suspected presence of a liver disorder in addition to iron overload. Patients with cardiac symptoms or signs should be evaluated with electrocardiography and echocardiography. Serum levels of estradiol (women) and testosterone (men) are decreased in patients with evidence of hypogonadism. Thus, serum levels of luteinizing and follicle-stimulating hormones are also subnormal in most such cases, implicating failure of pituitary gonadotroph cells due to iron overload as the cause of hypogonadism (hypogonadotrophic hypogonadism). A gonadotrophin-releasing hormone test may be informative in some patients. Biochemical manifestations of diabetes mellitus are similar to those in patients without hemochromatosis. Radiographs of abnormal joints should be performed and evaluated. Untreated patients have levels of hepcidin (measured in urine) that are disproportionately low in comparison with the degree of iron overload.[12] One patient had thrombocytopenia.[10]

Magnetic resonance imaging (MRI) scans reveal decreased T2-weighted signal intensity over liver, spleen, pancreas, and pituitary gland in patients with advanced iron overload. Specimens of liver obtained by biopsy from untreated patients and prepared with Perls' technique show marked deposition of iron, predominantly in hepatocytes.[8,13,14] There is a decreasing gradient of iron, predominantly in hepatocytes, from portal to centrilobular areas. Various degrees of hepatocellular necrosis, hepatic fibrosis, and cirrhosis may be present.[8,13,14] The hepatic iron index is markedly elevated. Hepatic cirrhosis is common in individuals whose hepatic iron concentration is $>20\,000\,\mu g$ ($\sim400\,\mu mol$) Fe/g liver dry weight. Hepatocellular carcinoma has not been reported.[11] Urinary hepcidin was low or undetectable in eight of ten patients with homozygosity for deleterious *TFR2* alleles, irrespective of the previous phlebotomy treatments.[12] Two patients with normal hepcidin values had concomitant inflammatory conditions.[12] Altogether, the clinical laboratory phenotypes of individuals with *TFR2* hemochromatosis

cannot be reliably distinguished from those of patients with *HFE* or *HJV* hemochromatosis.

DNA-based testing should only be performed in subjects in whom a diagnosis of iron overload is proven by serum iron measures and liver biopsy, and in whom there is no explanatory *HFE* genotype or other known cause of iron overload. Specific *TFR2* mutations can be detected by one of several strategies; mutation analysis may be available as a clinical or commercial test in some regions. Nonetheless, there is no predominant mutation among patients with *TFR2* hemochromatosis, and thus mutation-specific analysis may not demonstrate causative alleles. Mutation scanning for pathologic mutations has a very high detection rate, but is usually available only as a research technique. Most persons who are heterozygous for *TFR2* mutations have normal iron phenotypes.

Genetics

The TFR2-alpha transcript contains 18 exons, including a cytosolic domain, a transmembrane domain, a protease-associated domain, and a transferrin receptor-like dimerization region (Fig. 15.1). Pathogenic,

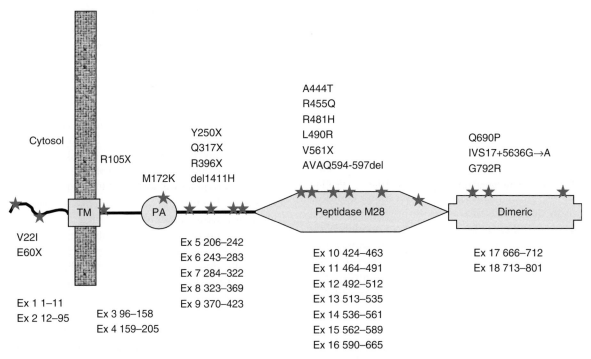

Fig. 15.1. Summary of pathogenic *TFR2* mutations, corresponding exons, and TFR2 protein structure. TM: transmembrane domain, PA: protease-associated domain, Dimeric: transferrin receptor-like dimerization region. See Table 15.1. Adapted from E. Beutler and P. Lee.

Table 15.1. Pathogenic mutations of the transferrin receptor-2 gene *TFR2*[a]

Exon or intervening sequence	Amino acid substitution	Race/ethnicity, other comments	Reference(s)
2	V22I	Italian subject with "altered iron status"	19
2	E60X[b]	Italian, including one with beta-thalassemia trait	9,24
3	R105X	North French	4
4	M172K	Italian	5,9
6	Y250X	several Sicilian, Italian families	3,7
7	Q317X	Italian	8
7	R396X	Scotch-Irish American; in *cis* with G792R	15
9	del411H	Italian	6
10	A444T	Italian	6
10	R455Q	Scotch-Irish American	15
11	R481H	Taiwanese	14
11	L490R	Japanese	28
14	V561X (P555fsX561; S556AfsX6)	Japanese	28
16	AVAQ594–597del[c]	Italian; Japanese	13,29
17	Q690P	Portuguese	10
IVS17 + 5636G→A	—	Italian	6
18	G792R	Scotch-Irish American, in *cis* with R396X; French, not in *cis* with another mutation	15,30

Notes: [a]All mutations were reported to cause iron overload phenotypes as homozygosity or compound heterozygosity with other deleterious *TFR2* alleles.
[b]There are reports of two corresponding mutations: c.ins88C (p.R30PfsX31);[9] and c.313C→T (p.R105X).[4] The former was subsequently reported by Wallace and Subramaniam as R30fsX60.[31]
[c]Identified by Beutler and Beutler as A621-Q624;[32] and by Camaschella and Roetto as 1902–1213del (AVAQ621–624del).[11]

"gain-of-function" mutations that occur in each of these regions have been described (Fig. 15.1; Table 15.1). The beta transcript lacks exons 1 through 3 and has an additional 142 bases at the 5′ end of exon 4.

TFR2 hemochromatosis has been reported in subjects of European and Asian ancestry (Table 15.1). The typical pattern of genetic transmission is autosomal recessive with moderate or complete penetrance (Fig. 15.2). Many pathogenic mutations are "private." Some have been detected in consanguineous kinships. Some pathogenic mutations, especially *TFR2* Y250X and R455Q, have appeared in individuals or kindreds who were not closely related (Table 15.1), suggesting that these mutations may have arisen more than once or may occur at low frequency in some populations. In one man, *TFR2* R396X and G792R probably occurred on the same haplotype.[15]

TFR2 Y250X was not identified in large samples of persons of various race/ethnicity (including African-Americans), with or without iron overload and related conditions.[16–18] *TFR2* AVAQ594–597del was not detected in 100 healthy Italian controls.[13] Other population testing programs have detected few pathologic or other *TFR2* alleles.[19–21] Sequencing *TFR2* in persons who reported having, or were proven to have, hemochromatosis or iron overload confirms that pathologic *TFR2* mutations are rare.[18,22,23]

TFR2 I238M is a polymorphism detected in an Asian population sample at a frequency of ∼0.0192. The prevalence of *TFR2* I238M in Asian subjects with

Table 15.2. *TFR2* mutations unproven to cause iron overload

Exon or intervening sequence	Amino acid substitution	Race/ethnicity, other comments	Reference(s)
2	H33N	Italian; not expected to be pathologic	6
2	A75V	Italian	19
IVS3 + 49C→A	—	Italian; polymorphism	6
4	D189N	Native American/white reported having hemochromatosis; also had *HAMP* promoter mutation −443C→T	23
5	I238M[a]	White, Chinese, Japanese subjects with, without iron overload; polymorphism	18,28,33,34
6	F280L	Portuguese	34
IVS − 9T→A	—	Portuguese	34
10	I449V	Heterozygosity in white American without iron overload	35
10	R455G	Heterozygosity in American with *HFE* C282Y homozygosity	22
15	V583I	Heterozygosity in white American without iron overload	36
16	D590D[b]	White American	18
16	A617A[c]	White American; Italian	18,37
17	R678P	French	30
18	M705HfsX87	French	30

Notes: [a]Polymorphism in Asian population at a frequency of 0.0192; not associated with increased transferrin saturation or ferritin levels in heterozygotes or an I238M homozygote.[18]
[b]Polymorphism in white American population at a frequency of 0.037; not associated with increased transferrin saturation or ferritin levels in heterozygotes.[18]
[c]Polymorphism in Asian population (allele frequency 0.33); not associated with increased transferrin saturation or ferritin levels in heterozygotes.[18] In Italian subjects, allele frequencies were 0.11 in controls and 0.14 in hemochromatosis patients.[37]

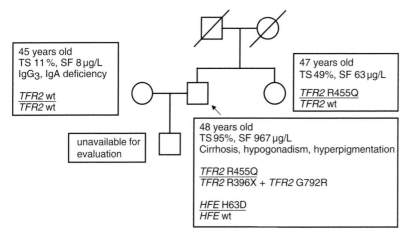

45 years old
TS 11 %, SF 8 μg/L
IgG₃, IgA deficiency

TFR2 wt
TFR2 wt

unavailable for evaluation

47 years old
TS 49%, SF 63 μg/L

TFR2 R455Q
TFR2 wt

48 years old
TS 95%, SF 967 μg/L
Cirrhosis, hypogonadism, hyperpigmentation

TFR2 R455Q
TFR2 R396X + *TFR2* G792R

HFE H63D
HFE wt

Fig. 15.2. Pedigree of a family of Scottish descent in which *TFR2* hemochromatosis occurred in a middle-aged male proband with a severe iron overload phenotype (arrow). The novel *TFR2* premature stop-codon mutation R396X mutation occurred in *cis* with another missense mutation (G792R). Because it was predicted that R396X would prevent transcription of a TFR2 polypeptide bearing the G792R amino acid substitution, it was not possible to determine whether or not G792R is a pathogenic mutation. The *TFR2* R455Q mutation has been described in another *TFR2* hemochromatosis kinship.[15]

and without iron overload phenotypes is similar, and simple heterozygosity for I238M was not associated with an increase in transferrin saturation or ferritin levels in control subjects.[18] Some other *TFR2* mutations are also unassociated with a hemochromatosis or iron overload phenotype (Table 15.2).

Hofmann and colleagues evaluated relatives with atypical hemochromatosis to determine whether differences in penetrance of the *HFE* C282Y mutation were associated with mutations in the *TFR2* gene.[22] They reported two brothers, each of whom were C282Y homozygotes; only the brother with liver fibrosis had *TFR2* R455Q. This suggested that R455Q functions as a "modifier" of the hemochromatosis phenotype when it is co-inherited with C282Y homozygosity. In two other brothers in the same kinship, the brother who co-inherited *TFR2* Q317 homozygosity and *HFE* C282Y/H63D had more severe iron loading than his sibling who had *TFR2* Q317 homozygosity alone.[8] In a young Italian patient with homozygosity for *TFR2* E60X and beta-thalassemia trait, iron overload was relatively severe at an early age.[24] Overall, known pathogenic *TFR2* mutations are so uncommon that they cannot be considered as common "modifiers" of the expression of *HFE* or other types of non-*TFR2* hemochromatosis or iron overload.

Prevention and treatment

TFR2 hemochromatosis is rare, even among patients with hemochromatosis unassociated with *HFE* C282Y.[10] A north American screening study used both iron phenotyping and DNA sequencing to detect deleterious *TFR2* mutations in participants under the age of 30 years who gave previous reports of hemochromatosis or iron overload, and in young participants who were discovered to have iron overload phenotypes in screening. No participant had two pathogenic *TFR2* mutations.[23,25] There is no reason to suspect that healthy persons in the general population have *TFR2* hemochromatosis, nor to perform general population or clinic screening for *TFR2* mutations outside a research protocol.

A high proportion of persons with *TFR2* hemochromatosis develop signs and symptoms of iron overload at a relatively early age. In kinships in which the diagnosis of *TFR2* hemochromatosis has been proven in an index case, *TFR2* testing should be performed in other at-risk family members to identify pathogenic *TFR2* genotypes. Penetrance of *TFR2* genotypes is less than 100%. In one family, for example, a middle-aged female homozygous for *TFR2* E60X had no evidence of clinical disease; a second female with the same *TFR2* genotype had iron deficiency.[3] Even untreated, iron overload may not be progressive.[9,13] Nonetheless, it is recommended that subjects with iron overload undergo iron depletion

treatment before they develop irreversible organ injury occurs. Treatment of iron overload should not be deferred in a patient with iron overload because his/her *TFR2* genotype has not been defined.

Phlebotomy is the treatment of choice for iron overload due to *TFR2* hemochromatosis (Chapter 36). Patients with cardiac symptoms or signs should be investigated promptly and thoroughly (Chapter 4). If cardiomyopathy due to myocardial siderosis is detected, aggressive combination treatment with phlebotomy and iron chelation drugs to reduce iron burdens should be initiated (Chapters 5, 36). Subcutaneous infusions of deferoxamine alone were ineffective in alleviating iron overload in one patient.[14] In a patient who also had beta-thalassemia trait and anemia, 26 grams of iron were removed with deferoxamine therapy.[24]

After iron depletion is achieved, serum transferrin saturation may remain elevated, but ferritin and hepatic transaminase levels usually return to their respective reference ranges. Repeat liver biopsy specimens reveal little or no iron deposition. Hyperpigmentation resolves after iron depletion. Hypogonadism is often irreversible. Cardiac arrhythmia, complications of cirrhosis or other liver disease, diabetes mellitus, hypogonadism, and arthropathy should be managed in a manner similar to that of patients without hemochromatosis or iron overload.[11] Like persons with *HFE* hemochromatosis,[26,27] it is presumed that patients with *TFR2* hemochromatosis should avoid consumption of medicinal iron, mineral supplements, excess vitamin C, and uncooked shellfish. Patients with liver disease should restrict alcohol intake that could exacerbate hepatocellular injury.[11] Maintenance phlebotomy should be used to sustain iron depletion.[14,15]

References

1. Kawabata H, Yang R, Hirama T, *et al.* Molecular cloning of transferrin receptor-2. A new member of the transferrin receptor-like family. *J Biol Chem* 1999; **274**: 20826–32.

2. Chua ACG, Delima RD, Morgan EH, *et al.* Iron uptake from plasma transferin by a transform receptor-2 mutant mouse model of haemochromatosis. *J Hepatiol* 2010; **52**: 425–31.

3. Camaschella C, Roetto A, Cali A, *et al.* The gene *TFR2* is mutated in a new type of haemochromatosis mapping to 7q22. *Nat Genet* 2000; **25**: 14–15.

4. Le Gac G, Mons F, Jacolot S, Scotet V, Ferec C, Frebourg T. Early onset hereditary hemochromatosis

resulting from a novel *TFR2* gene nonsense mutation (R105X) in two siblings of north French descent. *Br J Haematol* 2004; **125**: 674–8.

5. Majore S, Milano F, Binni F, *et al*. Homozygous p.M172K mutation of the *TFR2* gene in an Italian family with type 3 hereditary hemochromatosis and early onset iron overload. *Haematologica* 2006; **91**: ECR33.

6. Biasiotto G, Camaschella C, Forni GL, Polotti A, Zecchina G, Arosio P. New *TFR2* mutations in young Italian patients with hemochromatosis. *Haematologica* 2008; **93**: 309–10.

7. Piperno A, Roetto A, Mariani R, *et al*. Homozygosity for transferrin receptor-2 Y250X mutation induces early iron overload. *Haematologica* 2004; **89**: 359–60.

8. Pietrangelo A, Caleffi A, Henrion J, *et al*. Juvenile hemochromatosis associated with pathogenic mutations of adult hemochromatosis genes. *Gastroenterology* 2005; **128**: 470–9.

9. Roetto A, Totaro A, Piperno A, *et al*. New mutations inactivating transferrin receptor-2 in hemochromatosis type 3. *Blood* 2001; **97**: 2555–60.

10. Mattman A, Huntsman D, Lockitch G, *et al*. Transferrin receptor-2 (*TfR2*) and *HFE* mutational analysis in non-C282Y iron overload: identification of a novel *TfR2* mutation. *Blood* 2002; **100**: 1075–7.

11. Camaschella C, Roetto A. *TFR2*-related hereditary hemochromatosis [Type 3 hereditary hemochromatosis.] In: Pagon RA, ed. *GeneReviews*. Seattle, University of Washington. 2006.

12. Nemeth E, Roetto A, Garozzo G, Ganz T, Camaschella C. Hepcidin is decreased in *TFR2* hemochromatosis. *Blood* 2005; **105**: 1803–6.

13. Girelli D, Bozzini C, Roetto A, *et al*. Clinical and pathologic findings in hemochromatosis type 3 due to a novel mutation in transferrin receptor-2 gene. *Gastroenterology* 2002; **122**: 1295–302.

14. Hsiao PJ, Tsai KB, Shin SJ, *et al*. A novel mutation of transferrin receptor-2 in a Taiwanese woman with type 3 hemochromatosis. *J Hepatol* 2007; **47**: 303–6.

15. Lee PL, Barton JC. Hemochromatosis and severe iron overload associated with compound heterozygosity for *TFR2* R455Q and two novel mutations *TFR2* R396X and G792R. *Acta Haematol* 2006; **115**: 102–5.

16. Barton EH, West PA, Rivers CA, Barton JC, Acton RT. Transferrin receptor-2 (*TFR2*) mutation Y250X in Alabama Caucasian and African-American subjects with and without primary iron overload. *Blood Cells Mol Dis* 2001; **27**: 279–84.

17. Dereure O, Esculier C, Aguilar-Martinez P, Dessis D, Guillot B, Guilhou JJ. No evidence of Y250X transferrin receptor type 2 mutation in patients with porphyria cutanea tarda. A study of 38 cases. *Dermatology* 2002; **204**: 158–9.

18. Lee PL, Halloran C, West C, Beutler E. Mutation analysis of the transferrin receptor-2 gene in patients with iron overload. *Blood Cells Mol Dis* 2001; **27**: 285–9.

19. Biasiotto G, Belloli S, Ruggeri G, *et al*. Identification of new mutations of the *HFE*, hepcidin, and transferrin receptor-2 genes by denaturing HPLC analysis of individuals with biochemical indications of iron overload. *Clin Chem* 2003; **49**: 1981–8.

20. De Gobbi M, Daraio F, Oberkanins C, *et al*. Analysis of *HFE* and *TFR2* mutations in selected blood donors with biochemical parameters of iron overload. *Haematologica* 2003; **88**: 396–401.

21. Mariani R, Salvioni A, Corengia C, *et al*. Prevalence of *HFE* mutations in upper northern Italy: study of 1132 unrelated blood donors. *Dig Liver Dis* 2003; **35**: 479–81.

22. Hofmann WK, Tong XJ, Ajioka RS, Kushner JP, Koeffler HP. Mutation analysis of transferrin receptor-2 in patients with atypical hemochromatosis. *Blood* 2002; **100**: 1099–100.

23. Barton JC, Acton RT, Leiendecker-Foster C, *et al*. Characteristics of participants with self-reported hemochromatosis or iron overload at HEIRS Study initial screening. *Am J Hematol* 2008; **83**: 126–32.

24. Riva A, Mariani R, Bovo G, *et al*. Type 3 hemochromatosis and beta-thalassemia trait. *Eur J Haematol* 2004; **72**: 370–4.

25. Barton JC, Acton RT, Leiendecker-Foster C, *et al*. HFE C282Y homozygotes aged 25–29 years at HEIRS Study initial screening. *Genet Test* 2007; **11**: 269–75.

26. Witte DL, Crosby WH, Edwards CQ, Fairbanks VF, Mitros F. A Practice guideline development task force of the College of American Pathologists. Hereditary hemochromatosis. *Clin Chim Acta* 1996; **245**: 139–200.

27. Barton JC, McDonnell SM, Adams PC, *et al*. Management of hemochromatosis. Hemochromatosis Management Working Group. *Ann Intern Med* 1998; **129**: 932–9.

28. Koyama C, Wakusawa S, Hayashi H, *et al*. Two novel mutations, L490R and V561X, of the transferrin receptor-2 gene in Japanese patients with hemochromatosis. *Haematologica* 2005; **90**: 302–7.

29. Hattori A, Wakusawa S, Hayashi H, *et al*. AVAQ 594–597 deletion of the *TfR2* gene in a Japanese family with hemochromatosis. *Hepatol Res* 2003; **26**: 154–6.

30. Jouanolle AM, Mosser A, David V, *et al*. Early onset iron overload in two patients presenting with new mutations in *TFR2* [abstract]. *The Second Congress of the International BioIron Society* 2007; 72.

31. Wallace DF, Subramaniam VN. Non-*HFE* haemochromatosis. *World J Gastroenterol* 2007; **13**: 4690–8.

32. Beutler L, Beutler E. Hematologically important mutations: iron storage diseases. *Blood Cells Mol Dis* 2004; **33**: 40–4.

33. Chan V, Wong MS, Ooi C, *et al*. Can defects in transferrin receptor-2 and hereditary hemochromatosis genes account for iron overload in HbH disease? *Blood Cells Mol Dis* 2003; **30**: 107–11.

34. Mendes AI, Ferro A, Martins R, *et al*. Non-classical hereditary hemochromatosis in Portugal: novel mutations identified in iron metabolism-related genes. *Ann Hematol* 2009; **88**: 229–34.

35. Barton JC, Lee PL. Disparate phenotypic expression of *ALAS2* R452H (nt 1407 G>A) in two brothers, one with severe sideroblastic anemia and iron overload, hepatic cirrhosis, and hepatocellular carcinoma. *Blood Cells Mol Dis* 2006; **36**: 342–6.

36. Barton JC, Lee PL, West C, Bottomley SS. Iron overload and prolonged ingestion of iron supplements: clinical features and mutation analysis of hemochromatosis-associated genes in four cases. *Am J Hematol* 2006; **81**: 760–7.

37. Meregalli M, Pellagatti A, Bissolotti E, Fracanzani AL, Fargion S, Sampietro M. Molecular analysis of the *TFR2* gene: report of a novel polymorphism (1878C>T). *Hum Mutat* 2000; **16**: 532.

Iron overload associated with IRE mutation of ferritin heavy-chain gene (*FTH1*)

Ferritin H- and L-chains form a shell of 24 subunits that stores iron. Each type of chain has a distinct role in iron storage.[1] The H-chain is encoded by the *FTH1* gene (chromosome 11q12–q13) and the L-chain by the *FTL* gene (chromosome 19q13.13–13.4).[2,3] A common cytosolic protein, iron regulatory protein (IRP), binds to the iron-responsive element (IRE) of the 5′ untranslated regions (UTRs) of the H- and L-subunit RNAs, and thus controls the synthesis of both proteins.[4–8] Heterogeneous mutations in the IRE of L-ferritin reduce the binding affinity of IRE to IRPs and thereby diminish the negative control of L-ferritin (but not H-ferritin) synthesis. This leads to the constitutive upregulation of ferritin L-chain synthesis characteristic of the autosomal dominant disorder known as hereditary hyperferritinemia-cataract syndrome (HHCS) (Chapter 17). In 2001, Kato and colleagues described a unique Japanese family in which a mutation in the H-ferritin IRE (A49U) caused hyperferritinemia and autosomal dominant iron overload (OMIM +134770).[9]

Clinical description

The proband, a 56-year-old woman, was discovered to have a markedly increased liver density on computerized tomography scanning. A T2-weighted magnetic resonance imaging study also showed markedly decreased signal intensity in the liver; signal intensity in the heart and bone marrow was similar to that of the liver. These results were interpreted as iron overload; this was confirmed by her serum ferritin level of 1654 μg/L. She had elevated serum iron and transferrin saturation measures and normal total iron-binding capacity.[9] A liver biopsy specimen revealed heavy iron deposition in hepatocytes, and some stainable iron in Kupffer cells. The pattern of iron staining in hepatic lobules was similar to that of *HFE* hemochromatosis. Splenectomy was performed as part of a treatment protocol for gastric cancer that was discovered incidentally. There was also heavy iron staining of splenic macrophages.[9]

The three family members with an iron overload phenotype and the A49U mutation (proband, a brother, and a sister) were 56–65 years old at diagnosis. These subjects gave no history of thalassemia, blood transfusion or donation, abnormal dietary iron intake, alcohol abuse, or pathological iron loss.[9] There was no report of cirrhosis, diabetes mellitus, other endocrinopathy, or arthropathy. Liver and spleen sizes or other physical attributes were not described for any of the iron overload subjects.[9] MRI evaluation of a brother of the proband yielded results similar to those in the proband.

Genetics

Total RNA was extracted from the liver biopsy specimen of the proband and reverse transcribed using an oligo-dT primer. The entire cDNA sequence of the L- and H-ferritin subunits was amplified and sequenced. This revealed heterozygosity for a single A→U conversion at position 49 (A49U) in the second residue of the five-base IRE loop sequence (CAGUG) of the H-ferritin subunit (Fig. 16.1).[9] This mutation was detected in a heterozygous configuration in the genomic DNA of the three family members (proband and two siblings) who had an iron overload phenotype defined by elevated serum iron measures and imaging evidence of excessive iron deposition in liver and bone marrow, and in the 28-year-old daughter of the proband. The segregation of A49U and iron overload in the family members is consistent with an autosomal dominant pattern of inheritance. This mutation was not detected in the genomic DNA of 42 unrelated control subjects.[9]

Pathophysiology

Under physiological conditions, regulation of ferritin synthesis is finely controlled at the translational level by iron availability. Ferritin H-subunits generate ferroxidase activity essential for incorporation of iron into the

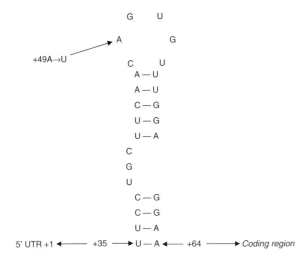

Fig. 16.1. Predicted secondary structure of H-ferritin subunit iron-responsive element (IRE) mRNA and the mutation identified in a unique Japanese family described by Kato and colleagues.[9] Numbering starts at the first transcripted nucleotide.[14] The ferritin heavy-chain gene (*FTH1*) on chromosome 11q12–q13 encodes this IRE.

protein shell, whereas L-subunits facilitate iron core formation.[1] Regulation is achieved by the high-affinity interaction of non-coding stem-loop structures located in the 5′ UTR of L- and H-ferritin mRNAs (IREs) with cytoplasmic mRNA-binding IRPs.[2,4–6,10] A single noncoding IRE is located on the 5′ UTR of the genes that encode L- and H-ferritin. Binding of IRPs to IREs normally represses translation of their corresponding *cis* genes.[2] Four persons in a Japanese kinship with autosomal dominant iron overload had the same point mutation (A49U) in the IRE motif of H-ferritin.[9]

In vitro studies revealed that the mutated IRE had a higher binding affinity to IRP than did the wild-type probe.[11] When mutated H-ferritin subunit was overexpressed in a cell line in vitro, there was suppression of H-subunit synthesis, decreased radioiron incorporation into ferritin, and increased iron uptake. This suggested that the decrease in H-ferritin subunit impaired iron uptake into the ferritin molecule, and caused iron accumulation in the cytosol, possibly due to decreased ferroxidase activity.[9] In an H-ferritin gene knockout mouse model, affected mice die *in utero* due to massive iron overload.[12] These observations demonstrate that the physiologic role of H-ferritin subunits in the incorporation of iron into the ferritin protein shell is essential, and suggest that the novel A49U mutation accounts for hereditary iron overload, presumably related to impairment of the ferroxidase activity generated by the H-ferritin subunit. It is

probable that other families will eventually be identified who have autosomal dominant iron overload caused by the same or other IRE mutations of *FTH1*.

Laboratory evaluation

The three family members with iron overload and the *FTH1* A49U mutation had serum ferritin levels of 742–1657 µg/L and serum transferrin concentrations of 212–231 mg/dL. Transferrin saturation was increased in each subject. None had anemia. Microscopic evaluation of bone marrow was not reported. The 28-year-old daughter of the proband was also heterozygous for A49U, but had serum ferritin 98 µg/L. The absence of iron overload in this young woman was attributed to her relatively young age, recent childbirth, and lactation.[9] Family members had normal levels of ceruloplasmin and serum copper. They did not have *HFE* C282Y or H63D, or *TFR2* Y250X.[9]

Iron overload transmitted as an autosomal dominant trait is typically associated with mutations of the *SLC40A1* gene that encodes ferroportin. In kinships with "loss-of-function" mutations, normal or reduced transferrin saturation and mild anemia are often present. In kinships with "gain-of-function" *SLC40A1* mutations, transferrin saturation is usually increased and anemia is absent, similar to the clinical picture of members of the Japanese family who had the A49U mutation of H-ferritin IRE.[9] Deposition of iron in macrophages in the liver, spleen, and bone marrow are features common to both ferroportin and H-ferritin IRE iron overload. Kawanaka and colleagues described three siblings with non-*HFE* autosomal dominant iron overload in another Japanese kinship.[11] This disorder was associated with homozygosity for the AVAQ 594–597 deletion of *TFR2*.[13] *HFE* hemochromatosis assumes a pseudo-dominant pattern of inheritance in some kinships. HHCS is associated with an autosomal dominant pattern of inheritance and with cataract development at various ages. In contrast to persons with *FTH1* autosomal dominant iron overload, persons with HHCS have normal transferrin saturation values. They have no evidence of excessive iron deposition demonstrable by imaging studies, in liver or bone marrow biopsy specimens, or by therapeutic trials of phlebotomy to quantify iron burdens. Regardless of the clinical features, the molecular basis of autosomal dominant hyperferritinemia or iron overload in most kinships must be ascertained by DNA mutation analysis.

Therapy

Kato and colleagues did not report the results of therapy to induce iron depletion in members of this unusual family.[9] It is presumed that iron overload in these cases could be treated with phlebotomy, and that such treatment would prevent or reduce iron-related organ injury.

References

1. Harrison PM, Arosio P. The ferritins: molecular properties, iron storage function and cellular regulation. *Biochim Biophys Acta* 1996; **1275**: 161–203.

2. Hentze MW, Rouault TA, Caughman SW, Dancis A, Harford JB, Klausner RD. A cis-acting element is necessary and sufficient for translational regulation of human ferritin expression in response to iron. *Proc Natl Acad Sci USA* 1987; **84**: 6730–4.

3. McGill JR, Naylor SL, Sakaguchi AY, *et al.* Human ferritin H and L sequences lie on ten different chromosomes. *Hum Genet* 1987; **76**: 66–72.

4. Eisenstein RS. Iron regulatory proteins and the molecular control of mammalian iron metabolism. *Annu Rev Nutr* 2000; **20**: 627–62.

5. Hentze MW, Caughman SW, Rouault TA, *et al.* Identification of the iron-responsive element for the translational regulation of human ferritin mRNA. *Science* 1987; **238**: 1570–3.

6. Leibold EA, Munro HN. Cytoplasmic protein binds in vitro to a highly conserved sequence in the 5′ untranslated region of ferritin heavy- and light-subunit mRNAs. *Proc Natl Acad Sci USA* 1988; **85**: 2171–5.

7. Theil EC. Ferritin: structure, gene regulation, and cellular function in animals, plants, and microorganisms. *Annu Rev Biochem* 1987; **56**: 289–315.

8. Thomson AM, Rogers JT, Leedman PJ. Iron-regulatory proteins, iron-responsive elements and ferritin mRNA translation. *Int J Biochem Cell Biol* 1999; **31**: 1139–52.

9. Kato J, Fujikawa K, Kanda M, *et al.* A mutation, in the iron-responsive element of H ferritin mRNA, causing autosomal dominant iron overload. *Am J Hum Genet* 2001; **69**: 191–7.

10. Caughman SW, Hentze MW, Rouault TA, Harford JB, Klausner RD. The iron-responsive element is the single element responsible for iron-dependent translational regulation of ferritin biosynthesis. Evidence for function as the binding site for a translational repressor. *J Biol Chem* 1988; **263**: 19 048–52.

11. Kawanaka M, Kinoyama S, Niiyama G, *et al.* [A case of idiopathic hemochromatosis which occurred in three siblings with high level of serum CA 19-9.] *Nippon Shokakibyo Gakkai Zasshi* 1998; **95**: 910–15.

12. Ferreira C, Bucchini D, Martin ME, *et al.* Early embryonic lethality of H ferritin gene deletion in mice. *J Biol Chem* 2000; **275**: 3021–4.

13. Hattori A, Wakusawa S, Hayashi H, *et al.* AVAQ 594–597 deletion of the *TfR2* gene in a Japanese family with hemochromatosis. *Hepatol Res* 2003; **26**: 154–6.

14. Hentze MW, Keim S, Papadopoulos P, *et al.* Cloning, characterization, expression, and chromosomal localization of a human ferritin heavy-chain gene. *Proc Natl Acad Sci USA* 1986; **83**: 7226–30.

Hereditary hyperferritinemia-cataract syndrome: IRE mutations of ferritin light-chain gene (*FTL*)

Hereditary hyperferritinemia-cataract syndrome (HHCS) is an autosomal dominant disorder characterized by increased serum L-ferritin levels and bilateral cataracts, in the absence of iron overload (OMIM #600886) (Fig. 17.1). Under physiological conditions, regulation of ferritin synthesis is finely controlled at the translational level by iron availability. This is achieved by the high-affinity interaction of noncoding stem-loop structures located in the untranslated regions (UTRs) of L- and H-ferritin mRNAs known as iron-responsive elements (IREs) with cytoplasmic mRNA-binding proteins. A single noncoding IRE is located on the 5′ UTR of the genes that encode L- and H-ferritin. Binding of IRPs to IREs normally represses translation of their corresponding *cis* genes. Heterogeneous mutations in the IRE of L-ferritin reduce the binding affinity of IRPs to IREs and thereby diminish the negative control of L-ferritin (but not H-ferritin) synthesis. This leads to the constitutive up-regulation of ferritin L-chain synthesis characteristic of HHCS.[1]

History

In 1995, Girelli and colleagues reported two Italian families in which elevated serum ferritin unrelated to iron overload and congenital bilateral nuclear cataract were co-transmitted as an autosomal dominant trait.[2] Affected persons in these kinships had normal or low levels of serum iron, normal transferrin saturation, and absence of iron overload in parenchymal organs, unlike persons with hemochromatosis. In a subsequent report, these investigators coined the descriptive name HHCS to describe the syndrome. By RNA single-strand conformation polymorphism screening of the L-subunit ferritin gene (*FTL*) on chromosome 19q13.13–13.4, they identified a mutation in the 5′ UTR in HHCS subjects. This mutation involved the highly conserved, hexanucleotide sequence [CAGUGU] that

comprises the apical loop of the iron-responsive element (IRE). (Fig. 17.2). This sequence is critical for the post-transcriptional regulation of L-ferritin synthesis by means of IRP.[3] In 1995, Bonneau *et al.* reported co-segregation of severe hyperferritinemia and dominantly inherited cataract with in a three-generation pedigree and suggested two possible explanations: (1) HHCS is a disorder of ferritin metabolism leading to lens opacity; or (2) HHCS is a contiguous gene syndrome involving the L-ferritin gene and the gene encoding lens membrane protein MP19 on chromosome 19q.[4] In 1998, Levi reported that the lens of a HHCS patient contained tenfold more L-ferritin than control lenses; the lens ferritin was fully soluble and had a low iron content.[5]

Pathophysiology
Ferritin metabolism

Hyperferritinemia unrelated to elevated iron stores is a hallmark of HHCS. Serum ferritin in HHCS patients and in normal persons is almost entirely glycosylated L-ferritin.[6] Circulating mononuclear cells from persons with HHCS have normal amounts of immunoreactive H-ferritin, whereas their L-ferritin content is markedly increased.[6] The positive correlation between mononuclear cell L-type ferritin content and serum ferritin concentration is highly significant, suggesting that the excess production of ferritin by mononuclear cells causes or contributes greatly to the increased levels of serum ferritin in persons with HHCS.[6] In HHCS lymphoblastoid cell lines, a large proportion of L-ferritin is non-functional L-chain 24 homopolymers. There is a five- to tenfold expansion of ferritin heteropolymers, with a shift to L-chain-rich isoferritins in the absence of major effects on cellular iron metabolism.[5]

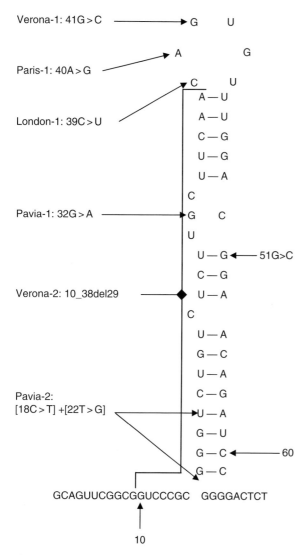

Fig. 17.1. Predicted secondary structure of L-subunit iron-responsive element (IRE) mRNA and selected mutations identified in families with hereditary hyperferritinemia-cataract syndrome. Numbering starts at the first transcribed nucleotide. The ferritin light-chain gene (*FTL*) on chromosome 19q13.13–13.4 encodes this IRE.

Lens

HHCS cataract is due to numerous small opacities, predominantly in the lens cortex, that comprise light-diffracting ferritin crystals.[7] Viewed by slit lamp examination, cataracts in persons with HHCS have been described as "pulverulent," like a "sunflower," and as "breadcrumb-like nuclear and cortical lens opacities."[8] Some reports provide much detail of lens morphology across several HHCS kinships and *FTL*

IRE mutations.[9] By transmission electron microscopy, the lens deposits have a macromolecular crystalline structure consistent with a face-centered cubic crystal with a unit crystal cell size of 17 nm, characteristic of ferritin crystals grown in vitro.[8] The lens ferritin is fully soluble and has a low iron content.[5] Immunohistochemical analysis reveals strong anti-L-ferritin reactivity in the crystalline lens deposits.[8] Ferritin content of a lens in one case was five to tenfold higher that in a cataract from a patient without HHCS,[5] and about 1500-fold higher than in control lenses from two subjects without HHCS of the same kinship.[10] It has been proposed that L-chain accumulation may induce cataract formation by altering the delicate equilibrium between water-soluble proteins (i.e. crystallins) normally found in the ocular lens, or by changing lens antioxidant properties.[5] The human lens L-ferritin sequence is identical to that of human liver L-ferritin.[11]

Clinical description

There appear to be no relevant symptoms associated with HHCS other than impaired vision.[10] Cataract in HHCS has been graded as "severe" when there was a marked loss in visual acuity in the first decades (with some individuals requiring surgery), "mild" when the defect in visual acuity could be corrected with the use of appropriate eyeglasses, and "asymptomatic" when the lens defect did not impair visual acuity.[6] The very early development of cataracts in persons with HHCS has been interpreted as an L-ferritin IRE mutation-specific attribute.[12] The early onset of cataract observed in some HHCS kinships excludes the possibility that the cataracts are due solely to age-related accumulation of ferritin.[13]

Phenotype–genotype correlations in HHCS have yielded heterogeneous results. Cazzola and colleagues observed that mutations of the CAGUGU RNA sequence of the apical loop ("Verona-1," "Paris-1") were associated with marked hyperferritinemia and earlier age of onset and greater severity of cataract (Fig. 17.2). A mutation in the distal stem was associated with milder cataract ("Pavia-1"), and another mutation located lower in the stem ("Pavia-2") was associated with asymptomatic cataract.[6] Other reports corroborate that there is a general relationship of mutation location with severity of hyperferritinemia

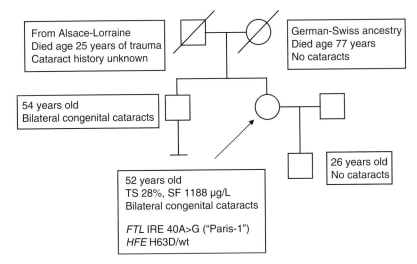

Fig. 17.2. Pedigree of a family with hereditary hyperferritinemia-cataract syndrome. Two siblings had bilateral congenital cataracts. The proband (arrow) was a double heterozygote for the A→G mutation of the CAGUGU motif of the iron-responsive element (IRE) loop of the ferritin L-chain gene (*FTL*) chromosome on 19q13.13–13.4, and for the 187C→G (H63D) mutation of the hemochromatosis-associated *HFE* gene on chromosome 6p21.3. The proband's *FTL* IRE mutation was previously reported as the "Paris-1" mutation (see Fig. 17.2). There is no known interaction between these two iron-associated mutations.[19] Phlebotomy therapy does not lower the serum ferritin value in patients with hereditary hyperferritinemia-cataract syndrome, because their hyperferritinemia is not due to iron overload.

and cataract.[14] Some persons with *FTL* IRE mutations have clinically insignificant cataracts.[10] An Italian subject with a mutation in the ATG start codon of L-ferritin had no hematological or neurological symptoms,[15] whereas hyperferritinemia and cataracts across three generations were associated with a 25 bp deletion encompassing the transcription start site in an Australian kinship.[16]

The in vitro affinity of IRPs to IREs was related to the clinical severity of HHCS in one study.[17] Thermodynamic analysis has revealed that some HHCS mutations lead to changes in the stability and secondary structure of the IRE, whereas others disrupt IRE–IRP recognition with minimal effect on IRE stability.[17] Regardless, there is marked phenotypic variability among subjects sharing the same mutation, whether they belong to the same family or not. In 49 individuals from 7 HHCS kindreds with premature cataract from the United Kingdom, Lachlan *et al.* observed that the severity of the clinical phenotype was variable both within and between kindreds and showed no clear relationship with *FTL* genotype,[18] consistent with the findings in a European case series reported earlier by Girelli *et al.*[10] Thus, it appears that factors other than L-ferritin IRE genotype modulate the severity of lens involvement in patients with HHCS.[1]

Laboratory abnormalities

Serum ferritin levels range from approximately 350 µg/L in some cases to more than 2000 µg/L in others. In individual patients with HHCS and in their affected blood relatives, serum ferritin levels tend to be relatively constant over time. Serum iron concentrations and transferrin saturation values are usually normal in persons with HHCS. Liver biopsy specimens typically reveal normal amounts of stainable iron.[3] Although HHCS mononuclear cells, especially macrophages, produce large quantities of L-ferritin, increased stainable iron is not detected in the bone marrow, because the iron content of the aberrant L-ferritin is low. Some HHCS patients have common *HFE* mutations, especially *HFE* H63D.[19,20]

FTL mutation analysis

Genomic DNA derived from blood buffy coat or other sources can be evaluated using denaturing high-performance liquid chromatography, direct sequencing, DNA scanning, or single mutation-specific technique to detect HHCS *FTL* mutations. Most mutations have been detected using direct sequencing of DNA from persons with high serum ferritin levels without elevated body iron stores. At present, most such testing is performed in research laboratories, and is not available commercially. DNA microchip technology may permit diagnostic testing for HHCS (and other iron-related disorders) on a large scale and at relatively low cost.[21]

More than 35 *FTL* mutations have been identified in HHCS kinships (Table 17.1; Fig. 17.2). Most persons reported to have HHCS have western European ancestry. Most mutations are "private" alleles restricted to single kindreds and are not present in members of the general population, although some

Table 17.1. *FTL* IRE mutations associated with hereditary hyperferritinemia-cataract syndrome[a]

Mutation	Race/ethnicity[b]	References
c.−220_−196del25[c]	Australian	16
10C→G	Italian	31
10_38del29	Italian	32
14G→C	Italian	24
16C→U	Italian	31
18C→T	Italian	21
[18C→T] + [22T→G]	Italian	6
22T→G	Italian	6
22_27del6	Italian	22
29C→G	Italian	33
32G→A	Italian, French, Indian	6,14,34
32G→C	French, Australian	9,12–14
32G→T	French, Canadian, Italian	14,35,36
32G→U	Australian	9
33C→A	French	14
33C→T	American, French, Spanish	7,14,30,37
33C→U	Spanish	38
34T→C	French	14
36C→A	English, French	14,39
36C→G	Italian	31
37A→C	Italian	21
37A→G	Italian	31
37A→T	Spanish	30
38_39delAC	French	14
39C→A	Australian	9
39C→G	French, Greek	40,41
39C→T	Italian, French	14,42
39C→U	English, Italian	39,43
40A→G	French, Basque, American, Australian, Spanish	9,14,19, 44–47
[40A→C] + [41G→C]	Italian	24
41G→C	Italian	3
42_57del16	French	14,48
43G→A	American	49
47G→A	French	14
51G→C	American, Italian	8,20
56A→T	French	21
56del1	Italian	31
90C→U	Italian	31

Notes: [a]Names of mutations are those previously reported in the literature. Numbering is from the first transcribed nucleotide. [b]Mutations are informally denoted by names of cities in which they were first identified and characterized include: 10_38del29, Verona-2; [18C→T] + [22T→G], Pavia-2; 32G→A, Pavia-1; 32G→U, Paris-2; 36C→A, London-2; 37A→T, Zaragoza; 39C→U, London-1; 40A→G, Paris-1; and 41G→C, Verona-1. See Fig. 17.2. [c]This mutation consists of a 25 bp deletion encompassing the transcription start site designated c.−220_−196del25, where nucleotide +1 is the A of the ATG translation initiation start site (Genbank accession NM_000146.3).[16] In contrast, an Italian subject with a mutation in the ATG start codon of L-ferritin had no hematological or neurological symptoms.[15]

mutations have been detected in multiple geographic areas or in persons of diverse race/ethnicity (Table 17.1; Fig. 17.1). Some mutations are informally named for the cities in which they were first identified and characterized (Table 17.1; Figs. 17.1, 17.2). There are no reports of HHCS or *FTL* mutation analysis in most other race/ethnicity groups, and thus it cannot be assumed that HHCS is a disorder that occurs predominantly in European whites. Most reported *FTL* mutations associated with HHCS are single nucleotide substitutions; two double point mutations have been reported. Point mutations or deletions in the CAGUGU RNA sequence of the apical loop greatly decrease binding of the mutant IRE with IRPs. Other deletions have also been identified. One of them, del22–27, is predicted to introduce a novel loop in the upper stem of the IRE structure very close to the lateral bulge that would markedly reduce binding to IRPs.[22] There are clusters of mutations that affect nucleotides 22, 32–33, and 36–42.[21]

Population testing

There are few data from which the prevalence of HHCS in general populations can be deduced. The estimated prevalence of HHCS in southeast Australia is approximately 1/200 000.[9] This estimate is probably conservative, because serum ferritin is not routinely measured by ophthalmologists investigating cataracts (including congenital cataracts), and there may be a low awareness of HHCS among ophthalmologists.[9] In addition, some *FTL* IRE mutations result in mild hyperferritinemia and clinically insignificant cataract.[10] A study in Switzerland evaluated 135 persons whose cataracts required excision and lens implants on or before age 51 years; serum ferritin levels were measured in 15 subjects, and elevated values were detected in two subjects. Neither of the two had *FTL* mutations, implying a very low prevalence of HHCS in this population.[23]

The results of three studies of highly selected subjects also suggest that L-ferritin IRE mutations typical of HHCS are collectively rare. Cremonesi and colleagues developed a rapid DNA scanning technique to detect all mutations in the L-ferritin IRE sequence in a single electrophoretic analysis, and scanned DNA samples from 50 healthy Italian subjects and from 230 Italian subjects with serum ferritin >400 μg/L. A single (previously unreported) mutation was detected.[24] Bozzini and colleagues sequenced the L-ferritin IRE in 51 highly selected, "at-risk" Italian subjects. These comprised: 13 blood donors who had serum ferritin >300 μg/L and lens opacities from a cohort of 3249 blood donors; 15 patients with unexplained cataract from 11 685 patients aged less than 41 years in a cataract surgery registry; and 26 patients aged 41 years or older who had unexplained serum ferritin >300 μg/L from 1231 patients with lens cataract. None of the 51 subjects had L-ferritin IRE mutations.[25] In contrast, Hetet and colleagues sequenced *FTL* exon 1 in 52 DNA samples from French patients referred for molecular diagnosis of HHCS; 24 samples (46%) had a point mutation or deletion in the IRE sequence.[14] A pilot study indicates that it may be feasible to develop a DNA microchip for large-scale analyses in epidemiological studies and screening of mutations associated with iron disorders.[21] Regardless, many *FTL* mutations are "private," suggesting that testing "at-risk" subjects will be much more productive than general population screening.

Differential diagnosis

Ferritin is an important regulator of oxidative stress, a primary factor in the etiology of aging-related cataract. Normal humans have disproportionately high levels of L-ferritin mRNA relative to the amounts of ferritin protein present. Lens ferritin in persons with HHCS is L-ferritin.[5,8,11] Among patients with hyperferritinemia and cataract, the presence of cataract does not permit the unambiguous identification of patients with HHCS, although the existence of a family history of cataract is only encountered in HHCS patients.[14]

The respective prevalences of hyperferritinemia and cataract in general populations are relatively great, and their coincidental association in some patients is expected. Persistent elevation of serum ferritin concentrations occurs in a variety of conditions, including common hepatic disorders (e.g. steatosis, viral hepatitis, alcoholic liver disease), chronic ethanol consumption, chronic inflammation or infection, malignancies, and iron overload of diverse etiologies. More than 2% of 1231 patients aged 41 years or more had unexplained serum ferritin >300 μg/L.[25] Higher mean levels of serum ferritin are typically observed in persons who report Asian, African-American, Native American, or Pacific Islander ancestry than are observed in whites.[26–28] It is plausible that some non-whites have *FTL* IRE mutations with or without susceptibility to develop ocular cataracts, although this possibility is largely unstudied.

Three of 52 DNA samples from French patients referred for molecular diagnosis of HHCS revealed *SLC40A1* mutations.[14] This indicates that ferroportin hemochromatosis (Chapter 12) is a diagnostic possibility in persons with persistent hyperferritinemia and cataract.[14] An autosomal dominant pattern of inheritance is typical of HHCS, ferroportin hemochromatosis, and of iron overload due to H-ferritin mutations (Chapter 16). The pattern of inheritance of *HFE* hemochromatosis is pseudo-dominant in some kinships. In these latter disorders, hyperferritinemia is not linked to the development of cataracts.

Persons heterozygous for the coding region mutation *FTL* T301I have elevated serum levels of glycosylated ferritin, report no specific symptoms, and lack iron overload, ocular cataracts, and neurologic abnormality.[29] It has been postulated that *FTL* T301I increases the efficacy of L-ferritin secretion by increasing the hydrophobicity of the N-terminal "A" alpha helix.[29]

Therapy

HHCS does not cause iron overload. Some HHCS patients have common *HFE* mutations, especially *HFE* H63D,[19,30] and are mistakenly believed to have

HFE hemochromatosis. Others may be erroneously diagnosed to have ferroportin hemochromatosis. When treated with therapeutic phlebotomy, patients with HHCS rapidly develop iron deficiency and anemia.[2,19] Elevated serum ferritin levels are unaffected by phlebotomy in persons with HHCS, due to their iron-insensitive constitutive up-regulation of L-ferritin synthesis. Management of lens abnormalities is similar in persons with or without HHCS. Some patients require observation only, whereas others need corrective lenses to improve vision. Patients with severe lens opacity due to L-ferritin accumulation require cataract excision and implantation of a prosthetic lens.

References

1. Roetto A, Bosio S, Gramaglia E, Barilaro MR, Zecchina G, Camaschella C. Pathogenesis of hyperferritinemia cataract syndrome. *Blood Cells Mol Dis* 2002; **29**: 532–5.

2. Girelli D, Olivieri O, De Franceschi L, Corrocher R, Bergamaschi G, Cazzola M. A linkage between hereditary hyperferritinaemia not related to iron overload and autosomal dominant congenital cataract. *Br J Haematol* 1995; **90**: 931–4.

3. Girelli D, Corrocher R, Bisceglia L, *et al*. Molecular basis for the recently described hereditary hyperferritinemia-cataract syndrome: a mutation in the iron-responsive element of ferritin L-subunit gene (the "Verona mutation"). *Blood* 1995; **86**: 4050–3.

4. Bonneau D, Winter-Fuseau I, Loiseau MN, *et al*. Bilateral cataract and high serum ferritin: a new dominant genetic disorder? *J Med Genet* 1995; **32**: 778–9.

5. Levi S, Girelli D, Perrone F, *et al*. Analysis of ferritins in lymphoblastoid cell lines and in the lens of subjects with hereditary hyperferritinemia-cataract syndrome. *Blood* 1998; **91**: 4180–7.

6. Cazzola M, Bergamaschi G, Tonon L, *et al*. Hereditary hyperferritinemia-cataract syndrome: relationship between phenotypes and specific mutations in the iron-responsive element of ferritin light-chain mRNA. *Blood* 1997; **90**: 814–21.

7. Brooks DG, Manova-Todorova K, Farmer J, *et al*. Ferritin crystal cataracts in hereditary hyperferritinemia cataract syndrome. *Invest Ophthalmol Vis Sci* 2002; **43**: 1121–6.

8. Chang-Godinich A, Ades S, Schenkein D, Brooks D, Stambolian D, Raizman MB. Lens changes in hereditary hyperferritinemia-cataract syndrome. *Am J Ophthalmol* 2001; **132**: 786–8.

9. Craig JE, Clark JB, McLeod JL, *et al*. Hereditary hyperferritinemia-cataract syndrome: prevalence, lens morphology, spectrum of mutations, and clinical presentations. *Arch Ophthalmol* 2003; **121**: 1753–61.

10. Girelli D, Bozzini C, Zecchina G, *et al*. Clinical, biochemical, and molecular findings in a series of families with hereditary hyperferritinaemia-cataract syndrome. *Br J Haematol* 2001; **115**: 334–40.

11. Cheng Q, Gonzalez P, Zigler JS, Jr. High level of ferritin light chain mRNA in lens. *Biochem Biophys Res Commun* 2000; **270**: 349–55.

12. Ismail AR, Lachlan KL, Mumford AD, Temple IK, Hodgkins PR. Hereditary hyperferritinemia-cataract syndrome: ocular, genetic, and biochemical findings. *Eur J Ophthalmol* 2006; **16**: 153–60.

13. Campagnoli MF, Pimazzoni R, Bosio S, *et al*. Onset of cataract in early infancy associated with a 32G→C transition in the iron responsive element of L-ferritin. *Eur J Pediatr* 2002; **161**: 499–502.

14. Hetet G, Devaux I, Soufir N, Grandchamp B, Beaumont C. Molecular analyses of patients with hyperferritinemia and normal serum iron values reveal both L ferritin IRE and 3 new ferroportin (*slc11A3*) mutations. *Blood* 2003; **102**: 1904–10.

15. Cremonesi L, Cozzi A, Girelli D, *et al*. Case report: a subject with a mutation in the ATG start codon of L-ferritin has no haematological or neurological symptoms. *J Med Genet* 2004; **41**: e81.

16. Burdon KP, Sharma S, Chen CS, Dimasi DP, Mackey DA, Craig JE. A novel deletion in the *FTL* gene causes hereditary hyperferritinemia-cataract syndrome (HHCS) by alteration of the transcription start site. *Hum Mutat* 2007; **28**: 742.

17. Allerson CR, Cazzola M, Rouault TA. Clinical severity and thermodynamic effects of iron-responsive element mutations in hereditary hyperferritinemia-cataract syndrome. *J Biol Chem* 1999; **274**: 26 439–47.

18. Lachlan KL, Temple IK, Mumford AD. Clinical features and molecular analysis of seven British kindreds with hereditary hyperferritinaemia-cataract syndrome. *Eur J Hum Genet* 2004; **12**: 790–6.

19. Barton JC, Beutler E, Gelbart T. Coinheritance of alleles associated with hemochromatosis and hereditary hyperferritinemia-cataract syndrome. *Blood* 1998; **92**: 4480.

20. Camaschella C, Zecchina G, Lockitch G, *et al*. A new mutation (G51C) in the iron-responsive element (IRE) of L-ferritin associated with hyperferritinaemia-cataract syndrome decreases the binding affinity of the mutated IRE for iron-regulatory proteins. *Br J Haematol* 2000; **108**: 480–2.

21. Ferrari F, Foglieni B, Arosio P, *et al*. Microelectronic DNA chip for hereditary hyperferritinemia-cataract syndrome, a model for large-scale analysis of disorders of iron metabolism. *Hum Mutat* 2006; **27**: 201–8.

22. Cazzola M, Foglieni B, Bergamaschi G, Levi S, Lazzarino M, Arosio P. A novel deletion of the L-ferritin iron-responsive element responsible for severe hereditary hyperferritinaemia-cataract syndrome. *Br J Haematol* 2002; **116**: 667–70.

23. Rosochova J, Kapetanios A, Pournaras C, Vadas L, Samii K, Beris P. Hereditary hyperferritinaemia-cataract syndrome: does it exist in Switzerland? *Schweiz Med Wochenschr* 2000; **130**: 324–8.

24. Cremonesi L, Fumagalli A, Soriani N, *et al*. Double-gradient denaturing gradient gel electrophoresis assay for identification of L-ferritin iron-responsive element mutations responsible for hereditary hyperferritinemia-cataract syndrome: identification of the new mutation C14G. *Clin Chem* 2001; **47**: 491–7.

25. Bozzini C, Galbiati S, Tinazzi E, Aldigeri R, De Matteis G, Girelli D. Prevalence of hereditary hyperferritinemia-cataract syndrome in blood donors and patients with cataract. *Haematologica* 2003; **88**: 219–20.

26. Barton JC, Acton RT, Dawkins FW, *et al*. Initial screening transferrin saturation values, serum ferritin concentrations, and *HFE* genotypes in whites and blacks in the Hemochromatosis and Iron Overload Screening Study. *Genet Test* 2005; **9**: 231–41.

27. Barton JC, Acton RT, Lovato L, *et al*. Initial screening transferrin saturation values, serum ferritin concentrations, and *HFE* genotypes in Native Americans and whites in the Hemochromatosis and Iron Overload Screening Study. *Clin Genet* 2006; **69**: 48–57.

28. Harris EL, McLaren CE, Reboussin DM, *et al*. Serum ferritin and transferrin saturation in Asians and Pacific Islanders. *Arch Intern Med* 2007; **167**: 722–6.

29. Kannengiesser C, Jouanolle AM, Hetet G, *et al*. A new missense mutation in the L ferritin coding sequence associated with elevated levels of glycosylated ferritin in serum and absence of iron overload. *Haematologica* 2009; **94**: 335–9.

30. Garcia Erce JA, Cortes T, Cremonesi L, Cazzola M, Perez-Lungmus G, Giralt M. [Hyperferritinemia-cataract syndrome associated to the *HFE* gene mutation. Two new Spanish families and a new mutation (A37T: "Zaragoza").] *Med Clin (Barc)* 2006; **127**: 55–8.

31. Cremonesi L, Paroni R, Foglieni B, *et al*. Scanning mutations of the 5′UTR regulatory sequence of L-ferritin by denaturing high-performance liquid chromatography: identification of new mutations. *Br J Haematol* 2003; **121**: 173–9.

32. Girelli D, Corrocher R, Bisceglia L, *et al*. Hereditary hyperferritinemia-cataract syndrome caused by a 29-base pair deletion in the iron responsive element of ferritin L-subunit gene. *Blood* 1997; **90**: 2084–8.

33. Bosio S, Campanella A, Gramaglia E, *et al*. C29G in the iron-responsive element of L-ferritin: a new mutation associated with hyperferritinemia-cataract. *Blood Cells Mol Dis* 2004; **33**: 31–4.

34. Vanita V, Hejtmancik JF, Hennies HC, *et al*. Sutural cataract associated with a mutation in the ferritin light-chain gene (*FTL*) in a family of Indian origin. *Mol Vis* 2006; **12**: 93–9.

35. Wong K, Barbin Y, Chakrabarti S, Adams P. A point mutation in the iron-responsive element of the L-ferritin in a family with hereditary hyperferritinemia-cataract syndrome. *Can J Gastroenterol* 2005; **19**: 253–5.

36. Martin ME, Fargion S, Brissot P, Pellat B, Beaumont C. A point mutation in the bulge of the iron-responsive element of the L ferritin gene in two families with the hereditary hyperferritinemia-cataract syndrome. *Blood* 1998; **91**: 319–23.

37. Ladero JM, Balas A, Garcia-Sanchez F, Vicario JL, Diaz-Rubio M. Hereditary hyperferritinemia-cataract syndrome. Study of a new family in Spain. *Rev Esp Enferm Dig* 2004; **96**: 507–1.

38. Balas A, Aviles MJ, Garcia-Sanchez F, Vicario JL. Description of a new mutation in the L-ferritin iron-responsive element associated with hereditary hyperferritinemia-cataract syndrome in a Spanish family. *Blood* 1999; **93**: 4020–1.

39. Mumford AD, Vulliamy T, Lindsay J, Watson A. Hereditary hyperferritinemia-cataract syndrome: two novel mutations in the L-ferritin iron-responsive element. *Blood* 1998; **91**: 367–8.

40. Garderet L, Hermelin B, Gorin NC, Rosmorduc O. Hereditary hyperferritinemia-cataract syndrome: a novel mutation in the iron-responsive element of the L-ferritin gene in a French family. *Am J Med* 2004; **117**: 138–9.

41. Papanikolaou G, Chandrinou H, Bouzas E, *et al*. Hereditary hyperferritinemia-cataract syndrome in three unrelated families of western Greek origin caused by the C39 > G mutation of L-ferritin IRE. *Blood Cells Mol Dis* 2006; **36**: 33–40.

42. Arosio C, Fossati L, Vigano M, Trombini P, Cazzaniga G, Piperno A. Hereditary hyperferritinemia-cataract syndrome: a de novo mutation in the iron responsive element of the L-ferritin gene. *Haematologica* 1999; **84**: 560–1.

43. Cicilano M, Zecchina G, Roetto A, *et al.* Recurrent mutations in the iron regulatory element of L-ferritin in hereditary hyperferritinemia-cataract syndrome. *Haematologica* 1999; **84**: 489–92.

44. Beaumont C, Leneuve P, Devaux I, *et al.* Mutation in the iron responsive element of the L ferritin mRNA in a family with dominant hyperferritinaemia and cataract. *Nat Genet* 1995; **11**: 444–6.

45. Aguilar-Martinez P, Biron C, Masmejean C, Jeanjean P, Schved JF. A novel mutation in the iron responsive element of ferritin L-subunit gene as a cause for hereditary hyperferritinemia-cataract syndrome. *Blood* 1996; **88**: 1895.

46. Perez dN, Castano L, Martul P, *et al.* Molecular analysis of hereditary hyperferritinemia-cataract

47. Del Castillo RA, Fernandez Ruano ML. [Hereditary hyperferritinemia-cataracts syndrome in a Spanish family caused by the A40G mutation (Paris) in the L-ferritin (*FTL*) gene associated with the mutation H63D in the *HFE* gene.] *Med Clin (Barc)* 2007; **129**: 414–17.

48. Feys J, Nodarian M, Aygalenq P, Cattan D, Bouccara AS, Beaumont C. [Hereditary hyperferritinemia syndrome and cataract.] *J Fr Ophtalmol* 2001; **24**: 847–50.

49. Phillips JD, Warby CA, Kushner JP. Identification of a novel mutation in the L-ferritin IRE leading to hereditary hyperferritinemia-cataract syndrome. *Am J Med Genet A* 2005; **134**: 77–9.

syndrome in a large Basque family. *J Pediatr Endocrinol Metab* 2001; **14**: 295–300.

Iron overload in Native Africans and African-Americans

African iron overload

African iron overload occurs in 14%–18% of Bantu-speaking Natives in at least 15 countries in sub-Saharan Africa. This type of non-transfusion iron overload is due primarily to the ingestion of large quantities of iron contained in traditional beer, although unconfirmed evidence suggests that there is an African iron overload gene (Table 18.1).

History

Iron overload in native sub-Saharan Africans was first described by Strachan in his 1929 thesis on tuberculosis.[1] The disorder was originally attributed to infections, to poisoning due to copper, tin, or zinc, or to malnutrition.[2] In 1953, it was hypothesized that the intake of excessive quantities of iron leached from iron vessels used for food preparation could account for "Bantu siderosis."[3] In 1992, the etiology of African iron overload as a purely dietary disorder was contested with the demonstration that heritable factors may influence the development of this condition.[4]

Clinical description

Patients with early iron overload identified during family or other group testing have no symptoms or signs attributable to iron overload.[5] Symptoms usually do not occur until iron overload is severe; they may develop by late adolescence.[6] Iron overload is progressive in most patients. Weakness and fatigue, abdominal discomfort or pain, or low back or hip pain are common presenting complaints. Iron overload occurs with greater frequency and severity among men than in women.[4,7] Physical examination in subjects with severe iron overload may reveal hyperpigmentation, hepatomegaly, kyphosis, or femoral neck fracture.

Genetics

Segregation analyses of native sub-Saharan African populations indicate that values of serum transferrin saturation and ferritin concentration can be explained by a mixture of three normal distributions.[4,8] This supports the hypotheses that: (1) African iron overload is associated with inheritance of homozygosity for a gene that influences iron absorption or metabolism; (2) some homozygotes for the putative allele may develop iron overload even if they have not consumed traditional beer; and (3) heterozygotes for putative African iron overload gene(s) sometimes develop iron overload of lesser severity than is observed in presumed homozygotes.[4,9,10] Evidence consistent with familial transmission of African iron overload has been reported.[10] Although in vitro functional differences in serum iron measures have been attributed to transferrin polymorphisms in healthy Zimbabweans and those at risk for African iron overload, these differences do not explain increased susceptibility to develop iron overload.[11] To date, no candidate gene(s) that would account for susceptibility to African iron overload has been proposed. The apparent occurrence of African iron overload in multiple family members could be due to their similar inheritance of multiple traits that together may influence iron absorption, or to learned or acquired habits of preparing or drinking traditional beer.

The chromosome and gene implicated in the causation of African iron overload differ from those associated with hemochromatosis in Caucasians. African iron overload is neither a human leukocyte antigen (HLA)-linked disorder nor is it associated with the common pathogenic *HFE* mutation C282Y typical of hemochromatosis in western Caucasians.[4,12–15] *HFE* H63D occurs in a minority of native Africans, but this worldwide polymorphism probably contributes little to the development of iron overload in persons who do not also have *HFE* C282Y. Certain types of hemoglobinopathy,

Table 18.1. Comparison of African and African-American iron overload

Characteristic	African iron overload	African-American iron overload
Affected populations	Sub-Saharan African Natives	African-Americans
Population prevalence[a]	0.14, 0.17, 0.18	0.009, 0.015
Prevalence in liver biopsy specimens[b]	0.15, 0.43, 0.75	0.10
Serum transferrin saturation	Usually elevated	Usually elevated
Serum ferritin concentration	Elevated	Elevated
Target organs[c]	Liver, spleen, bone marrow, pancreas, bone marrow	Liver, spleen, bone marrow
Pattern of iron deposition	Predominantly macrophages; less in parenchymal cells	Predominantly macrophages; less in parenchymal cells; sometimes mixed pattern of iron staining
Complications[d]	Hepatic cirrhosis, primary liver cancer, diabetes mellitus, hyperpigmentation, ascorbic acid (vitamin C) deficiency and osteoporosis, tuberculosis, esophageal cancer	Hepatic cirrhosis, diabetes mellitus, arthropathy, hypogonadotrophic hypogonadism, cardiomyopathy, hyperpigmentation
Pattern of inheritance	Autosomal dominant	Autosomal dominant (non-*HFE* linked); autosomal recessive (*HFE*-, *HJV*-associated); X-linked (*ALAS2*-associated)
Associated genes	Putative African iron overload gene(s)	Putative African iron overload gene(s); *HFE*; *HJV*; *ALAS2*
Prevention or treatment of iron overload	Reduce consumption of traditional beer; phlebotomy	Avoid iron supplements; phlebotomy

Notes: [a]Prevalence estimates were derived from these sources: natives of sub-Saharan Africa[9,22,34] and African-Americans.[41,88]
[b]Frequency estimates of iron overload in liver biopsy specimens were derived from these sources: natives of sub-Saharan Africa[10,32,34] and African-Americans.[40]
[c]Target organs and tissues of iron overload in natives of sub-Saharan Africa also include synovium, duodenum and jejunum, thyroid, adrenal, pituitary, and heart.[6] Clinical findings in African-Americans suggest that other organs, particularly the pancreas, heart, synovium and anterior pituitary (gonadotroph cells) may be target organs and tissues of iron overload.
[d]In natives of sub-Saharan Africa, cardiomyopathy definitely attributable to cardiac siderosis seems unreported although excess iron may occur in the myocardium.[6,25] Vitamin C deficiency and scurvy major contributors to the development of osteoporosis.[6,28,89] Cardiomyopathy was reported in African-Americans with iron overload[41] but there was no demonstration of cardiac siderosis.

thalassemia, and viral hepatitis are common in native sub-Saharan Africans, but there is no report of the influence of such disorders on iron absorption and their association with iron overload in native sub-Saharan Africans.

The ferroportin (*SLC40A1*) allele Q248H occurs as polymorphism in approximately 9% of native sub-Saharan Africans with and without iron overload phenotypes.[16,17] *SLC40A1* Q248H is weakly associated with elevated serum ferritin levels, especially in men.[17,18] It had been anticipated that this polymorphism would explain African iron overload.[19] Odds ratios estimates of iron overload in native Africans with *SLC40A1* Q248H who lack *HFE* C282Y were not significantly greater than unity.[20] Therefore, Q248H was not significantly associated with iron overload in native Africans in this study.

Dietary factors

Dietary iron content is the predominant causative factor of iron overload in native Africans. For many years, it was assumed that iron overload was due solely to excessive quantities of dietary iron consumed in a traditional fermented beverage brewed with various locally-produced grains in steel drums by many African Bantu-speaking natives.[5,6] The iron is ionized and bioavailable.[5,21,22] In one study, traditional beer contained more than 15 mg Fe/dL, approximately one-third of which was ferrous iron.[5] The severity of iron overload is directly proportional to the estimated quantities of traditional beverage consumed.[4,9] It has been hypothesized previously that many of the abnormalities observed in persons with iron overload are due to the effects of alcohol on iron absorption and on the liver.[6] The hepatic iron contents of persons with African iron overload exceed those of persons with alcoholic liver disease, and the histologic changes of alcoholic liver disease are usually absent in Africans with primary iron overload.[5,6] In some native Africans, there may be a nutritional benefit associated with consumption of traditional beer. The prevalences of iron deficiency and iron deficiency anemia were significantly lower in rural women of childbearing age in Zimbabwe and South Africa who drank traditional beer than in those who did not.[23] As expected, evidence of iron overload was detected only among those who drank traditional beer.[23]

Laboratory findings

Affected persons typically have elevated serum iron, transferrin saturation, and serum ferritin levels.[6] Many have elevated serum activities of hepatic enzymes. Serum levels of gamma-glutamyl transpeptidase are elevated in many cases, and are often disproportionately greater than measures of hepatic transaminases. Iron deposits, visualized using Perls' acid ferrocyanide staining technique, are prominent in macrophages in the liver, spleen, bone marrow, synovium, and other organs.[6] Parenchymal iron deposits, especially in hepatocytes, are less prominent than macrophage iron deposits.[5,6] Quantification of liver iron content using atomic absorption spectrometry informs diagnosis. The hepatic iron index (hepatic iron concentration adjusted by age = μmol Fe/g dry weight of liver/y) is elevated in typical, symptomatic African iron overload patients.[24] Complications of African iron overload and associated illnesses demonstrable by routine clinical evaluations include micronodular cirrhosis,[7,25,26] diabetes mellitus,[26] ascorbic acid (vitamin C) deficiency and consequent osteoporosis of the

spine and femoral neck,[27–30] and tuberculosis.[1,9,31] Persons with African iron overload also have increased risks to develop primary liver cancer and esophageal carcinoma.[8,31,32]

Prevalence

African iron overload has been reported in at least 15 countries of southern, central, east, and west Africa.[33] Among men who reported that they drank traditional beer, 17% and 14% in western and central Zimbabwe, respectively, had elevated values of transferrin saturation and serum ferritin concentration.[9,22] In rural Zimbabwe, 18% of hospitalized beer drinkers and 16% of apparently healthy beer drinkers had elevated values of transferrin saturation and serum ferritin concentration.[34] In Swaziland natives, 43% of traditional beer drinkers who underwent diagnostic liver biopsy had hepatic iron overload.[34] In Zimbabwe, 15% of persons who underwent diagnostic liver biopsy had significantly increased quantities of hepatic iron.[10] Twenty percent of South African black men at autopsy had hepatic iron concentrations greater than 5 mg Fe/g dry weight of liver, equivalent to hepatic iron levels in severe hemochromatosis in Caucasians.[7] In autopsy studies from these areas, the prevalence of hepatic iron loading of a degree sufficient to cause hepatic cirrhosis was greater than 10%.[4]

Prevention and treatment

It is generally accepted that native Africans with severe iron overload sustain significant morbidity and excessive mortality, should decrease their iron intake, and should undergo phlebotomy therapy.[24,35] Preliminary data from Tanzania suggest that therapeutic phlebotomy is well tolerated by native Africans with iron overload, and that some experience objective and subjective improvement.[6,36,37] Ascorbic acid therapy has also been administered to affected persons, and may help to mobilize stored iron.[6] Diabetes mellitus is managed in the same manner as it is in persons without iron overload. The extent to which African iron overload is a public health problem is unclear.[35] Decreasing the dietary iron content may be effective in either preventing African iron overload or decreasing its frequency and severity. A decline of approximately 50% in the incidence and severity of iron overload detected at autopsy in South African black men coincided with changes in liquor laws that led to a major switch in drinking habits from traditional brews to conventional, commercially available alcoholic beverages.[6,32]

African-American iron overload

In 1950, Krainin and Kahn reported the case of a black man who had severe non-transfusion iron overload.[38] In 1968, Prasad and colleagues reported the occurrence of increased stainable marrow iron in an African-American man with X-linked sideroblastic anemia.[39] In 1995–1996, case series of African-Americans with non-transfusion iron overload demonstrated that this disorder sometimes occurs in more than one family member, that excess iron deposition in Kupffer cells and other macrophage populations is common, and that HLA phenotypes typical of whites with *HFE* hemochromatosis are unusual.[40,41] African-Americans with non-transfusion iron overload have been reported from several states.[38,40–42] In 2003, the ferroportin gene mutation *SLC40A1* Q248H was identified in African-Americans with and without iron overload.[16,17,19] In 2004, it was reported that two African-American men with iron overload phenotypes had *HFE* genotypes typical of hemochromatosis in whites.[43]

Non-transfusion iron overload in African-Americans comprises a group of disorders characterized by phenotypic and genotypic heterogeneity. The genetic basis of primary iron overload has been identified in some patients, whereas a role for excessive dietary iron in the causation of iron overload has not been demonstrated convincingly in any case. Autopsy and liver biopsy studies suggest that excessive hepatic iron is relatively common in African-Americans, but it is unlikely that all such patients have systemic iron overload due to inherited or acquired causes (Table 18.1).

Clinical description

All patients described to date have been adults; a majority have been men.[33,40,41] Symptoms include weakness and fatigue, joint pain, swelling, and deformity, decreased libido, erectile dysfunction, difficulty controlling diabetes mellitus, and hyperpigmentation.[33,40,41,44] Some patients report no symptoms reasonably attributable to iron overload. Objective clinical findings consistent with hepatic fibrosis or cirrhosis (71%), arthritis (31%), diabetes mellitus (31%), and cardiomyopathy (13%) have been reported in cases collected from the literature.[33] Some patients have no objective findings on physical examination, although some have non-specific heart-related abnormalities, joint deformity, or hepatomegaly. Seven of 19 African-Americans with iron overload had malignancies,[33] although to date there have been no reports of African-Americans with primary iron overload who developed primary liver cancer. The relatively high prevalence of cancer in these cases may be due to ascertainment bias, because most patients reported to date were diagnosed by hematologists or medical oncologists.[40,41,45] Nonetheless, a role for iron overload in increasing the risk for certain types of cancer cannot be excluded.

Genetics

Occurrence of the *HFE* C282Y allele in persons of sub-Saharan African descent is due to racial admixture with European whites,[43] whereas the H63D allele occurs in most populations tested worldwide. Differences in frequencies of common *HFE* mutations in African-Americans vary significantly across regions of the US.[43,46] The inheritance of two common mutations of the *HFE* gene accounts for the development of primary iron overload in some African-Americans.[43,47] Penetrance-adjusted estimates indicate that ~9 African-Americans per 100 000 have a hemochromatosis phenotype and two common *HFE* mutations.[43] In large population screening studies in north America, approximately one African-American in 10 000 was homozygous for *HFE* C282Y,[47,48] consistent with previous estimates.[43] *HFE* C282Y heterozygosity in African-Americans may increase their risk to develop iron overload. Regardless, inheritance of common *HFE* alleles accounts for a small proportion of primary iron overload in African-Americans.[49] Unusual pathogenic *HFE* mutations have not been described in African-Americans with or without iron overload.[50]

Severe, early-onset iron overload in an African-American of West Indies descent was due to homozygosity for *HJV* R54X.[51] Heterozygosity for a hemojuvelin (*HJV*) triplet insert was identified in two African-Americans, one with and one without iron overload.[52] *HJV* mutation analysis in African-Americans from the general population[53] or *HJV* sequencing in African-Americans who participated in a hemochromatosis and iron overload screening program,[54] and reported that they had hemochromatosis or iron overload did not reveal pathogenic *HJV* mutations. Homozygosity or compound heterozygosity

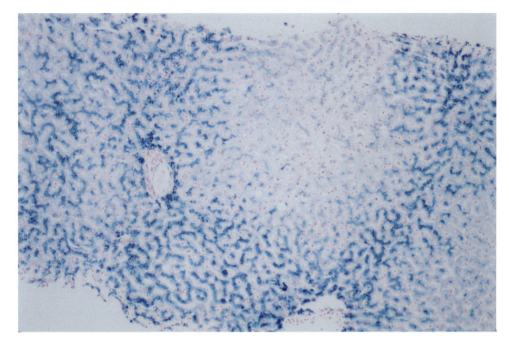

Fig. 4.1. Liver biopsy from a *HFE* C282Y homozygote shows iron deposition predominantly in periportal (zone 1) hepatocytes, with a periportal to pericentral gradient of iron (Perls' Prussian blue stain; hepatic iron concentration 5680 μg/g dry wt).

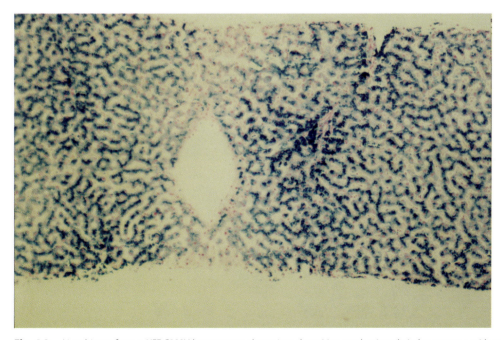

Fig. 4.2. Liver biopsy from a *HFE* C282Y homozygote shows iron deposition predominantly in hepatocytes, with sparing of Kupffer cells (Perls' Prussian blue stain; hepatic iron concentration 8085 μg/g dry wt).

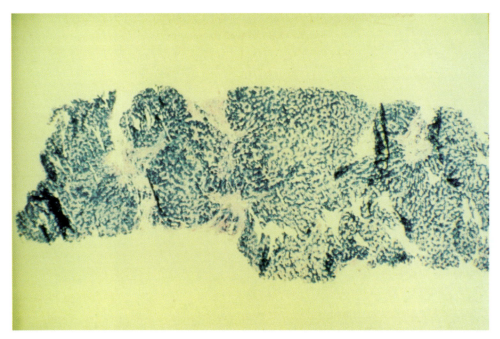

Fig. 4.3a. Panlobular iron deposition and micronodular cirrhosis in patient with hemochromatosis.

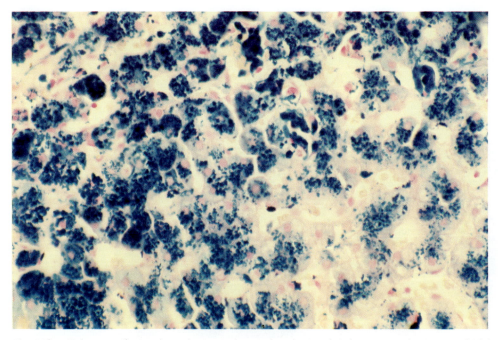

Fig. 4.3b. Higher magnification shows that iron is deposited predominantly in hepatocytes, despite a very high hepatic iron concentration of 40 380 μg/g dry wt (Perls' Prussian blue stain).

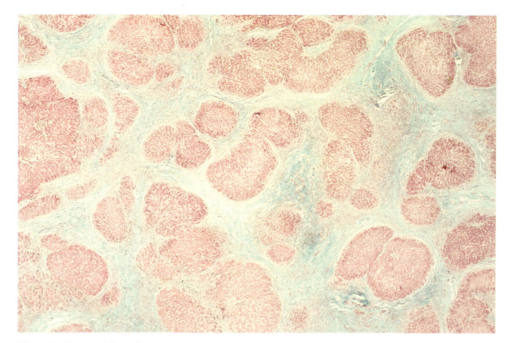

Fig. 4.4. Micronodular cirrhosis in patient with hemochromatosis and *HFE* C282Y homozygosity. The fibrous bands (stained blue) surround islands of hepatocytes (Masson trichrome stain).

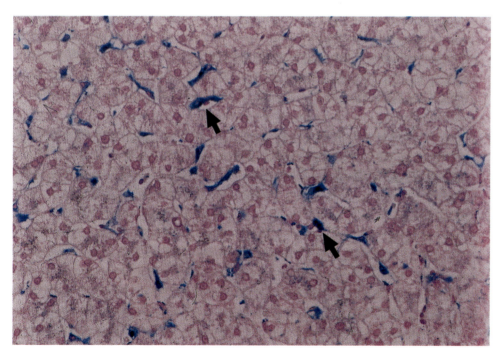

Fig. 4.5. Mild secondary iron overload due to transfusions; iron is located predominantly in Kupffer cells (Perls' Prussian blue stain). Taken from James C. Barton and Corwin Q. Edwards (eds), **Hemochromatosis: Genetics, Pathophysiology, Diagnosis and Treatment**, Cambridge University Press 2000. Reproduced with permission.

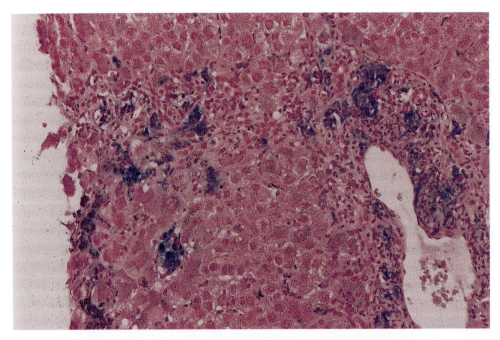

Fig. 4.6. Liver biopsy from a patient with chronic hepatitis C shows iron deposition predominantly in Kupffer cells (Perls' Prussian blue stain). Taken from James C. Barton and Corwin Q. Edwards (eds), **Hemochromatosis: Genetics, Pathophysiology, Diagnosis and Treatment**, Cambridge University Press 2000. Reproduced with permission.

(a)

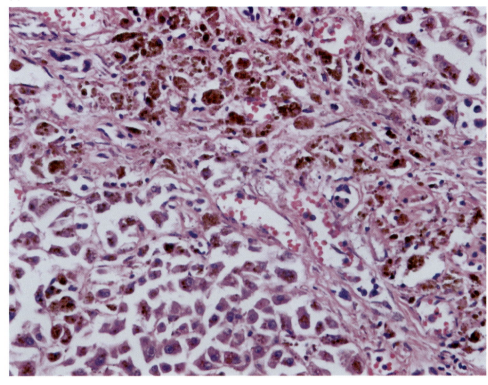

(b)

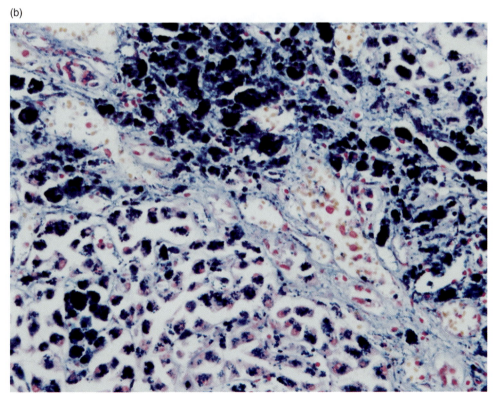

Fig. 5.1. Liver biopsy specimens from woman with pure red cell aplasia treated with numerous transfusions. Hematoxylin and eosin staining reveals brown pigment (hemosiderin) in hepatocytes; an adjacent section stained with Perls' technique reveals grade 4 blue-black intrahepatocytic iron. Original magnification 400×.

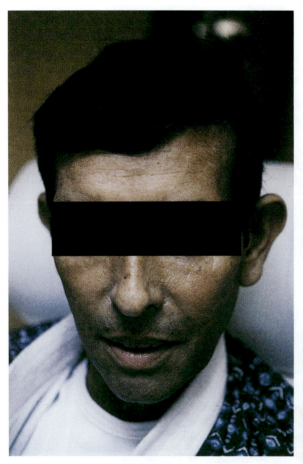
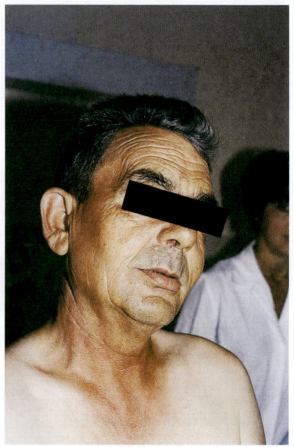

Figs. 5.11 and 5.12. Cutaneous pigmentation in hemochromatosis: (a) grayish hue; (b) brown hue. From Chevrant-Breton.[112] Taken from James C. Barton and Corwin Q. Edwards (eds), **Hemochromatosis: Genetics, Pathophysiology, Diagnosis and Treatment**, Cambridge University Press 2000. Reproduced with permission.

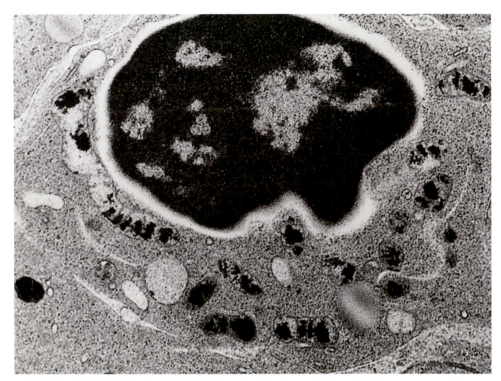

Fig. 25.1a. Features of sideroblastic anemia. Electron micrograph of an erythroblast with iron-laden mitochondria. From S.S. Bottomley.[1] Taken from James C. Barton and Corwin Q. Edwards (eds), **Hemochromatosis: Genetics, Pathophysiology, Diagnosis and Treatment**, Cambridge University Press 2000. Reproduced with permission.

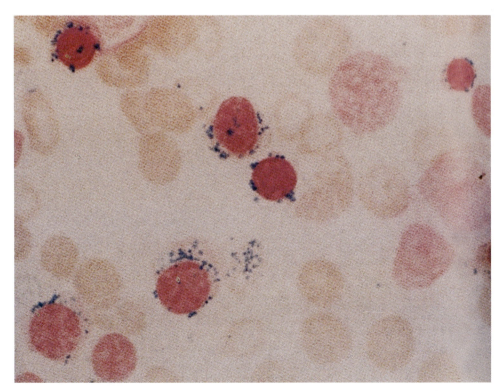

Fig. 25.1b. Bone marrow smear with ringed sideroblasts (Prussian blue stain). From S.S. Bottomley.[1] Taken from James C. Barton and Corwin Q. Edwards (eds), **Hemochromatosis: Genetics, Pathophysiology, Diagnosis and Treatment**, Cambridge University Press 2000. Reproduced with permission.

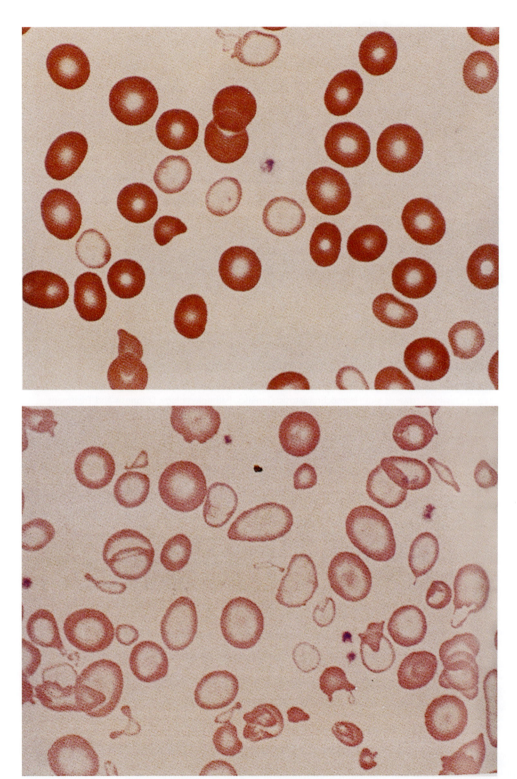

Figs. 25.1c and d. Blood smears of mild and severe sideroblastic anemia, respectively (Wright stain). From S.S. Bottomley.[1] Taken from James C. Barton and Corwin Q. Edwards (eds), **Hemochromatosis: Genetics, Pathophysiology, Diagnosis and Treatment**, Cambridge University Press 2000. Reproduced with permission.

for mutations of the gene that encodes transferrin receptor-2 (*TFR2*) are rare causes of severe hemo-chromatosis phenotypes in Caucasian patients. In African-Americans, *TFR2* mutations were not detected by DNA sequencing,[55] nor was the *TFR2* allele Y250X detected using mutation-specific analysis technique.[56] Likewise, African-Americans with primary iron over-load were not found to have pathogenic mutations of the *HAMP* gene that encodes hepcidin, the ferritin heavy-chain gene (*FTH1*), or the ceruloplasmin gene (*CP*).[50]

The ferroportin (*SLC40A1*) allele Q248H occurs as a polymorphism in native Africans and in African-Americans with and without iron overload pheno-types.[16,17] To date, Q248H has not been reported in other race or ethnicity groups. Aggregate Q248H frequencies in African-Americans and native Africans differ significantly (0.0525 vs. 0.0946, respectively). It is presumed that the lower frequency of Q248H observed in African-Americans than in African natives is due to racial admixture of African-Americans with whites. Because Q248H is weakly associated with elevated serum ferritin levels, especially in men,[17,18] it had been anticipated that this polymorphism could explain iron overload in some African-Americans. Odds ratios estimates of iron overload in African-Americans with *SLC40A1* Q248H who lack *HFE* C282Y are not significantly greater than unity, sug-gesting that the role of Q248H in the causation of iron overload in African-Americans is minimal, if any.[20] The *SLC40A1* allele D270V was identified in a black South African who had iron overload.[57]

Heterozygosity for alpha-thalassemia, beta-thalassemia, or S or C hemoglobinopathy are common among African-Americans in the general population,[40] and in those with iron overload.[16,33,45,58] Some African-Americans have types of thalassemia intermedia or homozygosity for common hemoglobinopathy alleles.[16,59,60] These alleles may act to enhance iron absorption in some cases. A few African-Americans have X-linked sideroblastic anemia and mild iron overload due to mutations in the erythroid-specific aminolevulinate dehydratase gene (*ALAS2*).[39,59,61]

African iron overload often occurs in families.[10,62] A great proportion of the African slaves sold in north America were captured from areas populated by Bantu-speaking people where African iron over-load has been found.[33] Blood relatives of African-American iron overload index patients, including sib-lings and parents, have also been diagnosed to have iron overload.[19,40,41] This implies that a gene or mutation could account for both forms of iron over-load in persons of sub-Saharan African descent. To date, however, no allele has been found in African-Americans that is consistent with a putative African iron overload gene.[4]

Dietary and environmental interactions

Reports of the ingestion of large quantities of dietary or supplemental iron by African-Americans with iron overload are rare,[16] although a role for the quantities of natural dietary or food fortification iron in the penetrance of African-American iron overload cannot be excluded.

Acquired disorders in some African-Americans account for increased hepatic iron deposition. Some patients ingest excessive quantities of alcohol.[40] This could enhance iron absorption[63] and potentiate hepatotoxicity due to oxidative stress, hepatic stellate cell activation, and hepatic fibrogenesis.[64,65] In one autopsy study of African-Americans, however, the prevalence of heavy liver iron staining was similar in subjects with and without histories of chronic alcoholism.[66]

In a study of stainable hepatic iron in African-Americans at coroner autopsy, cirrhosis was not detected in subjects who did not also have inflam-mation and hepatic steatosis.[66] Chronic viral hepatitis C occurs in approximately 1.8% of the overall US population,[67] and the prevalence of chronic hepatitis C is significantly greater in African-Americans than whites.[67,68] A greater proportion of African-Americans than persons of other races respond to chronic hepatitis C infection with an increase in iron stores, after adjustment for age, alcohol intake, gender, menopausal status, education, body mass index, and poverty index.[69] More than half of African-American subjects who had heavy hepatic iron staining also had hepatic inflammation.[66] It is plausible that some of these had viral hepatitis C, although this was not evaluated.[66] More than one-quarter of African-American subjects who had heavy iron staining also had hepatic steatosis. The prevalence of non-alcoholic steatosis and steatohepatitis is lower in African-Americans than in whites,[70,71] although some risk factors for non-alcoholic hepatic steatosis and steato-hepatitis (obesity, insulin resistance, and diabetes mel-litus) are significantly greater in African-Americans than in whites in the US.[71–73] These observations suggest that common liver conditions other than iron overload may augment iron absorption, induce deposition of excessive quantities of iron in the liver, and augment liver injury, even in the absence of systemic iron overload. The development of hepatic fibrosis or cirrhosis in African-Americans who have heavy hepatic iron deposition may require the synergistic effects of inflammation or steatosis. Taken together, these observations could explain the disparity between the relatively high prevalence of elevated measures of hepatic iron content and the paucity of reports of heritable causes of primary iron overload in African-Americans.

Laboratory findings

Mean serum transferrin saturation values are significantly lower and mean serum ferritin levels are significantly higher in African-Americans than in whites.[49] This must be considered in planning a diagnostic approach to African-Americans patients suspected to have iron overload. Some patients present with elevated transferrin saturation; *HFE* mutation analysis should be performed in each case. Other patients have normal or mildly reduced serum iron and transferrin saturation values. Serum ferritin concentrations are increased in all true iron overload cases. Elevated serum levels of hepatic transaminase activities are common. Serum levels of alkaline phosphatase or gamma-glutamyl transpeptidase are often elevated, in contrast to the normal levels of these analytes observed in most whites with hemochromatosis.

In African-American subjects who present with isolated hyperferritinemia, the differential diagnosis must include hemochromatosis due to *SLC40A1* mutations (Chapter 12), common liver disorders such as hepatic steatosis, alcohol-related liver disease, and viral hepatitis; chronic infection or inflammation; malignancy; and hereditary hyperferritinemia-cataract syndrome (Chapter 17). Patients with iron overload and anemia should be evaluated for evidence of iron-loading types of thalassemia or hemoglobinopathy, and for the presence of ringed sideroblasts in the bone marrow.

Liver specimens obtained by biopsy are usually needed to ascertain that iron overload is present, and to distinguish possible iron overload from other causes of hyperferritinemia, especially alcoholism, hepatic steatosis, and hepatitis C. Iron overload is typically characterized by deposition of iron in

macrophages in the liver, spleen, and bone marrow that can be detected by Perls' staining. This pattern of iron deposition resembles that of African iron overload.[6] In other cases, iron deposition occurs predominantly in the parenchymal cells of the liver, spleen, pancreas, and other organs.[40,41] Infrequently, a mixed pattern of hepatocyte-macrophage iron deposition occurs. The iron concentration in liver biopsy specimens should be quantified by atomic absorption spectrometry. The hepatic iron index is often but not invariably elevated.[40] Thus, strict adherence to diagnostic hepatic iron index criteria for *HFE* hemochromatosis in Caucasians (hepatic iron index >1.9) could underestimate the presence of primary iron overload in African-Americans who do not have *HFE* mutations, especially those in whom most excess iron is stored in macrophages. The relationship of iron grades and quantitative liver iron measurements is not well documented in African-American subjects in whom hepatic iron deposition occurs predominantly in macrophages. Hepatic iron concentrations and indices have been used as conservative, surrogate diagnostic criteria for primary iron overload in African-Americans,[40,41,43,74] although there has been no validation of their use in such cases. Further, some African-Americans who had iron overload demonstrated by therapeutic phlebotomy had normal hepatic iron concentrations and indices.[17,40] Elevated hepatic iron indices have also been reported to occur in a variety of other conditions.[75–77]

Hepatic fibrosis and micronodular hepatic cirrhosis are present in some patients, although primary liver cancer has not been reported in African-Americans with iron overload. Magnetic resonance imaging can be used to estimate liver iron content and provide information about iron deposition in other organs and tissues.[78] Patients with severe hepatic iron overload should be evaluated for heart disease, diabetes mellitus, arthropathy, and hypogonadism. These conditions are relatively common, and thus may be unrelated to iron overload in some patients. Hepatitis C is very common in African-Americans with (and without) iron overload. Therefore, it is prudent to evaluate each patient with possible iron overload for this infection.

Prevalence

In a screening program, serum ferritin >200 μg/L in women or >300 μg/L in men who also had transferrin saturation >29% in women or >35% in men was detected in approximately 7% of adult African-American primary care patients.[79] Patients with such iron phenotypes may have increased risk to have or to develop primary iron overload.[79] In liver specimens obtained at autopsy in adult African-Americans, 1.5%–11.0% contained significantly increased quantities of iron by various measures.[41,66,74] Among 249 unselected African-Americans who underwent diagnostic liver biopsy, 10.4% had significantly increased stainable hepatic iron.[80] These observations at first suggest that iron overload is relatively common among African-Americans. In contrast, *HFE* hemochromatosis affects only 9–10 African-Americans per 100 000.[43,47,48] Non-*HFE* mutations that cause hemochromatosis and iron overload in other race/ethnicity groups appear to be rare in African-Americans. Taken together, these observations suggest that elevated serum and liver iron measures in many African-Americans are due to causes other than mutations in genes primarily responsible for iron absorption and homeostasis.

Prevention and treatment

Screening programs have used various phenotype and genotype strategies to identify African-Americans with hemochromatosis or iron overload. The failure to identify many African-Americans with iron overload in one large community-based study was ascribed to the use of transferrin saturation alone as a screening strategy.[81] The combination of an elevated transferrin saturation criterion and *HFE* mutation analysis to identify the common C282Y and H63D alleles was used to screen African-Americans in a health appraisal clinic and in primary care clinics, but the yield of participants with iron overload or *HFE* hemochromatosis genotypes was also very low.[48,49,82] The low prevalence of *HFE* C282Y in African-Americans and the paucity of other iron overload-associated mutations identified to date in African-Americans account for these largely negative outcomes.

Studies of US death certificates reveal that non-whites with a "hemochromatosis" diagnosis at death were reported with increasing frequency over a 14-year interval, were more common in men, and occurred with increasing frequency in older adults.[83] The increasing frequency of "hemochromatosis" diagnoses may be due partly to increasing awareness of hemochromatosis and iron overload, and partly to the erroneous assumption that increased hepatic iron

content constitutes systemic iron overload. In a large hospital autopsy series, the prevalence of severe iron overload in whites and blacks without reports of excessive exogenous iron was similar (0.0019 and 0.0015, respectively).[84] It is presumed that early diagnosis and institution of phlebotomy therapy of African-Americans with primary iron overload before the development of irreversible damage to liver, heart, pancreas, and other organs will reduce the frequency and severity of complications such as hepatic cirrhosis, primary liver cancer, diabetes mellitus, and cardiomyopathy, and extend longevity.

Experience with treatment of African-American patients with primary iron overload mutations is limited but generally favorable.[40,41,43] Therapeutic phlebotomy is the treatment of choice for persons who hemochromatosis-associated *HFE* or *HJV* genotypes. Other patients, especially those with subnormal transferrin saturation or mild anemia, often experience slow recovery of hemoglobin concentrations after phlebotomy sessions. Therefore, their volume of phlebotomy should be less than would be recommended for patients with iron overload of other causes. In addition, it may be necessary to prescribe phlebotomy sessions several weeks apart. In patients with hepatitis C and excessive hepatic iron, phlebotomy therapy to achieve iron depletion decreases hepatic injury.[85,86] The severity of iron overload can be quantified with therapeutic phlebotomy.[33,40,41] At present, there are no reports of parenteral or oral chelation therapy in African-Americans with non-transfusion iron overload.

After iron depletion is achieved, phlebotomy therapy to maintain low iron stores should be prescribed. Some patients re-accumulate iron slowly or not at all. A diet of low iron content is not indicated. Ingestion of excessive or supplemental iron should be avoided in all persons with iron overload.[87] Hepatitis C, alcoholism, hepatic steatosis, cirrhosis, diabetes mellitus, other endocrinopathy, cardiomyopathy, arthropathy, and malignancy should be managed otherwise in a manner that is appropriate for patients without iron overload.

References

1. Strachan AS. Haemosiderosis and haemochromatosis in South African natives with a comment on the etiology of haemochromatosis. MD thesis. University of Glasgow, 1929.

2. Sheldon JH. *Haemochromatosis*. Oxford, Oxford University Press, 1935.

3. Walker ARP, Arvidsson UB. Iron "overload" in the South African Bantu. *Trans Royal Soc Trop Med Hyg* 1964; **47**: 1964.

4. Gordeuk V, Mukiibi J, Hasstedt SJ, *et al*. Iron overload in Africa. Interaction between a gene and dietary iron content. *N Engl J Med* 1992; **326**: 95–100.

5. Pippard MJ. Secondary iron overload. In: Brock JH, Halliday JW, Pippard MJ, Powell LW, eds. *Iron Metabolism in Health and Disease*. London, WB Saunders Company Ltd. 1994; 271–310.

6. Bothwell TH, Charlton RW, Cook JD, Finch CA. Alcohol, iron and liver disease. In: Bothwell TH, Charlton RW, Cook JD, Finch CA, eds. *Iron Metabolism in Man*. Oxford, Oxford University Press. 1979; 156–74.

7. Bothwell TH, Isaacson C. Siderosis in the Bantu. A comparison of incidence in males and females. *Br Med J* 1962; **1**: 522–4.

8. Moyo VM, Makunike R, Gangaidzo IT, *et al*. African iron overload and hepatocellular carcinoma (HA-7-0-080). *Eur J Haematol* 1998; **60**: 28–34.

9. Moyo VM, Gangaidzo IT, Gomo ZA, *et al*. Traditional beer consumption and the iron status of spouse pairs from a rural community in Zimbabwe. *Blood* 1997; **89**: 2159–66.

10. Moyo VM, Mandishona E, Hasstedt SJ, *et al*. Evidence of genetic transmission in African iron overload. *Blood* 1998; **91**: 1076–82.

11. Kasvosve I, Delanghe JR, Gomo ZA, *et al*. Transferrin polymorphism influences iron status in blacks. *Clin Chem* 2000; **46**: 1535–9.

12. McNamara L, MacPhail AP, Gordeuk VR, Hasstedt SJ, Rouault T. Is there a link between African iron overload and the described mutations of the hereditary haemochromatosis gene? *Br J Haematol* 1998; **102**: 1176–8.

13. Roth M, Giraldo P, Hariti G, *et al*. Absence of the hemochromatosis gene Cys282Tyr mutation in three ethnic groups from Algeria (Mzab), Ethiopia, and Senegal. *Immunogenetics* 1997; **46**: 222–5.

14. Gangaidzo IT, Moyo VM, Saungweme T, *et al*. Iron overload in urban Africans in the 1990s. *Gut* 1999; **45**: 278–83.

15. Jeffery S, Crosby A, Plange-Rhule J, *et al*. Evidence from a Ghanaian population of known African descent to support the proposition that hemochromatosis is a Caucasian disorder. *Genet Test* 1999; **3**: 375–7.

16. Barton JC, Acton RT, Rivers CA, *et al*. Genotypic and phenotypic heterogeneity of African-Americans with primary iron overload. *Blood Cells Mol Dis* 2003; **31**: 310–19.

17. Beutler E, Barton JC, Felitti VJ, *et al*. Ferroportin 1 (*SCL40A1*) variant associated with iron overload in African-Americans. *Blood Cells Mol Dis* 2003; **31**: 305–9.

18. Rivers CA, Barton JC, Gordeuk VR, *et al*. Association of ferroportin Q248H polymorphism with elevated levels of serum ferritin in African-Americans in the Hemochromatosis and Iron Overload Screening (HEIRS) Study. *Blood Cells Mol Dis* 2007; **38**: 247–52.

19. Gordeuk VR, Caleffi A, Corradini E, *et al*. Iron overload in Africans and African-Americans and a common mutation in the *SCL40A1* (ferroportin 1) gene. *Blood Cells Mol Dis* 2003; **31**: 299–304.

20. Barton JC, Acton RT, Lee PL, West C. *SLC40A1* Q248H allele frequencies and Q248H-associated risk of non-*HFE* iron overload in persons of sub-Saharan African descent. *Blood Cells Mol Dis* 2007; **39**: 206–11.

21. Bothwell TH, Seftel H, Jacobs P, Torrance JD, Baumslag N. Iron overload in Bantu subjects; studies on the availability of iron in Bantu beer. *Am J Clin Nutr* 1964; **14**: 47–51.

22. Gordeuk VR, Boyd RD, Brittenham GM. Dietary iron overload persists in rural sub-Saharan Africa. *Lancet* 1986; **1**: 1310–13.

23. Mandishona EM, Moyo VM, Gordeuk VR, *et al*. A traditional beverage prevents iron deficiency in African women of childbearing age. *Eur J Clin Nutr* 1999; **53**: 722–5.

24. MacPhail AP, Mandishona EM, Bloom PD, Paterson AC, Rouault TA, Gordeuk VR. Measurements of iron status and survival in African iron overload. *S Afr Med J* 1999; **89**: 966–72.

25. Bothwell TH, Bradlow BA. Siderosis in the Bantu. A combined histopathological and chemical study. *Arch Pathol* 1960; **70**: 279–92.

26. Isaacson C, Seftel HC, Keeley KJ, Bothwell TH. Siderosis in the Bantu: the relationship between iron overload and cirrhosis. *J Lab Clin Med* 1961; **58**: 845–53.

27. Seftel HC, Malkin C, Schmaman A, *et al*. Osteoporosis, scurvy, and siderosis in Johannesburg bantu. *Br Med J* 1966; **1**: 642–6.

28. Lynch SR, Berelowitz I, Seftel HC, *et al*. Osteoporosis in Johannesburg Bantu males. Its relationship to siderosis and ascorbic acid deficiency. *Am J Clin Nutr* 1967; **20**: 799–807.

29. Wapnick AA, Lynch SR, Seftel HC, Charlton RW, Bothwell TH, Jowsey J. The effect of siderosis and ascorbic acid depletion on bone metabolism, with special reference to osteoporosis in the Bantu. *Br J Nutr* 1971; **25**: 367–76.

30. Schnaid E, MacPhail AP, Sweet MB. Fractured neck of femur in black patients: a prospective study. *J Bone Joint Surg Br* 2000; **82**: 872–5.

31. Gordeuk VR, McLaren CE, MacPhail AP, Deichsel G, Bothwell TH. Associations of iron overload in Africa with hepatocellular carcinoma and tuberculosis: Strachan's 1929 thesis revisited. *Blood* 1996; **87**: 3470–6.

32. MacPhail AP, Simon MO, Torrance JD, Charlton RW, Bothwell TH, Isaacson C. Changing patterns of dietary iron overload in black South Africans. *Am J Clin Nutr* 1979; **32**: 1272–8.

33. Bloom PD, Burstein GR, Gordeuk VR. Iron overload in African-Americans. In: Barton JC, Edwards CQ, eds. *Hemochromatosis: Genetics, Pathophysiology, Diagnosis and Treatment*. Cambridge, Cambridge University Press. 2000; 475–83.

34. Friedman BM, Baynes RD, Bothwell TH, *et al.* Dietary iron overload in southern African rural blacks. *S Afr Med J* 1990; **78**: 301–5.

35. Walker AR, Segal I. Iron overload in sub-Saharan Africa: to what extent is it a public health problem? *Br J Nutr* 1999; **81**: 427–34.

36. Speight AN, Cliff J. Iron storage disease of the liver in Dar es Salaam: a preliminary report on venesection therapy. *East Afr Med J* 1974; **51**: 895–902.

37. Cliff JL, Speight AN. Venesection therapy in haemosiderosis. *East Afr Med J* 1976; **53**: 287–91.

38. Krainin P, Kahn BS. Hemochromatosis: report of a case in a Negro; discussion of iron metabolism. *Ann Intern Med* 1950; **33**: 462.

39. Prasad AS, Tranchida L, Konno ET, *et al.* Hereditary sideroblastic anemia and glucose-6-phosphate dehydrogenase deficiency in a Negro family. *J Clin Invest* 1968; **47**: 1415–24.

40. Barton JC, Edwards CQ, Bertoli LF, Shroyer TW, Hudson SL. Iron overload in African-Americans. *Am J Med* 1995; **99**: 616–23.

41. Wurapa RK, Gordeuk VR, Brittenham GM, Khiyami A, Schechter GP, Edwards CQ. Primary iron overload in African-Americans. *Am J Med* 1996; **101**: 9–18.

42. Monaghan KG, Rybicki BA, Shurafa M, Feldman GL. Mutation analysis of the *HFE* gene associated with hereditary hemochromatosis in African-Americans. *Am J Hematol* 1998; **58**: 213–17.

43. Barton JC, Acton RT. Inheritance of two *HFE* mutations in African-Americans: cases with hemochromatosis phenotypes and estimates of hemochromatosis phenotype frequency. *Genet Med* 2001; **3**: 294–300.

44. Rosner IA, Askari AD, McLaren GD, Muir A. Arthropathy, hypouricemia and normal serum iron studies in hereditary hemochromatosis. *Am J Med* 1981; **70**: 870–4.

45. Conrad ME. Sickle cell disease and hemochromatosis. *Am J Hematol* 1991; **38**: 150–2.

46. Acton RT, Barton JC, Snively BM, *et al.* Geographic and racial/ethnic differences in *HFE* mutation frequencies in the Hemochromatosis and Iron Overload Screening (HEIRS) Study. *Ethn Dis* 2006; **16**: 815–21.

47. Adams PC, Reboussin DM, Leiendecker-Foster C, *et al.* Comparison of the unsaturated iron-binding capacity with transferrin saturation as a screening test to detect C282Y homozygotes for hemochromatosis in 101 168 participants in the Hemochromatosis and Iron Overload Screening (HEIRS) Study. *Clin Chem* 2005; **51**: 1048–52.

48. Beutler E, Felitti V, Gelbart T, Ho N. The effect of *HFE* genotypes on measurements of iron overload in patients attending a health appraisal clinic. *Ann Intern Med* 2000; **133**: 329–37.

49. Barton JC, Acton RT, Dawkins FW, *et al.* Initial screening transferrin saturation values, serum ferritin concentrations, and *HFE* genotypes in whites and blacks in the Hemochromatosis and Iron Overload Screening Study. *Genet Test* 2005; **9**: 231–41.

50. Lee PL, Gelbart T, West C, Halloran C, Felitti V, Beutler E. A study of genes that may modulate the expression of hereditary hemochromatosis: transferrin receptor-1, ferroportin, ceruloplasmin, ferritin light and heavy chains, iron regulatory proteins (IRP)-1 and -2, and hepcidin. *Blood Cells Mol Dis* 2001; **27**: 783–802.

51. Murugan RC, Lee PL, Kalavar MR, Barton JC. Early age-of-onset iron overload and homozygosity for the novel hemojuvelin mutation *HJV* R54X (exon 3; c.160>T) in an African-American male of West Indies descent. *Clin Genet* 2008; **74**: 88–92.

52. Lee PL, Barton JC, Brandhagen D, Beutler E. Hemojuvelin (*HJV*) mutations in persons of European, African-American and Asian ancestry with adult onset haemochromatosis. *Br J Haematol* 2004; **127**: 224–9.

53. Barton JC, Rivers CA, Niyongere S, Bohannon SB, Acton RT. Allele frequencies of hemojuvelin gene (*HJV*) I222N and G320V missense mutations in white and African-American subjects from the general Alabama population. *BMC Med Genet* 2004; **5**: 29.

54. Barton JC, Acton RT, Leiendecker-Foster C, *et al.* *HFE* C282Y homozygotes aged 25–29 years at HEIRS Study initial screening. *Genet Test* 2007; **11**: 269–75.

55. Lee PL, Halloran C, West C, Beutler E. Mutation analysis of the transferrin receptor-2 gene in patients with iron overload. *Blood Cells Mol Dis* 2001; **27**: 285–9.

56. Barton EH, West PA, Rivers CA, Barton JC, Acton RT. Transferrin receptor-2 (*TFR2*) mutation Y250X in Alabama Caucasian and African-American subjects with and without primary iron overload. *Blood Cells Mol Dis* 2001; **27**: 279–84.

57. Zaahl MG, Merryweather-Clarke AT, Kotze MJ, van der MS, Warnich L, Robson KJ. Analysis of genes implicated in iron regulation in individuals presenting with primary iron overload. *Hum Genet* 2004; **115**: 409–17.

58. Barton JC, Rothenberg BE, Bertoli LF, Acton RT. Diagnosis of hemochromatosis in family members of probands: a comparison of phenotyping and *HFE* genotyping. *Genet Med* 1999; **1**: 89–93.

59. Barton JC, Lee PL, Bertoli LF, Beutler E. Iron overload in an African-American woman with SS hemoglobinopathy and a promoter mutation in the X-linked erythroid-specific 5-aminolevulinate synthase (*ALAS2*) gene. *Blood Cells Mol Dis* 2005; **34**: 226–8.

60. Castro O, Hasan O, Kaur K, Loyevsky M, Gordeuk V. Hemochromatosis in non-transfused African-American patient with sickle cell anemia. *Blood* 1998; **92** (suppl): 13b.

61. Collins TS, Arcasoy MO. Iron overload due to X-linked sideroblastic anemia in an African-American man. *Am J Med* 2004; **116**: 501–2.

62. Gordeuk VR. African iron overload. *Semin Hematol* 2002; **39**: 263–9.

63. Duane P, Raja KB, Simpson RJ, Peters TJ. Intestinal iron absorption in chronic alcoholics. *Alcohol Alcohol* 1992; **27**: 539–44.

64. Willner IR, Reuben A. Alcohol and the liver. *Curr Opin Gastroenterol* 2005; **21**: 323–30.

65. Fletcher LM, Powell LW. Hemochromatosis and alcoholic liver disease. *Alcohol* 2003; **30**: 131–6.

66. Barton JC, Acton RT, Richardson AK, Brissie RM. Stainable hepatic iron in 341 African-American adults at coroner/medical examiner autopsy. *BMC Clin Pathol* 2005; **5**: 2.

67. Alter MJ, Kruszon-Moran D, Nainan OV, *et al.* The prevalence of hepatitis C virus infection in the United States, 1988 through 1994. *N Engl J Med* 1999; **341**: 556–62.

68. Howell C, Jeffers L, Hoofnagle JH. Hepatitis C in African-Americans: summary of a workshop. *Gastroenterology* 2000; **119**: 1385–96.

69. Ioannou GN, Dominitz JA, Weiss NS, Heagerty PJ, Kowdley KV. Racial differences in the relationship between hepatitis C infection and iron stores. *Hepatology* 2003; **37**: 795–801.

70. Falck-Ytter Y, Younossi ZM, Marchesini G, McCullough AJ. Clinical features and natural history of non-alcoholic steatosis syndromes. *Semin Liver Dis* 2001; **21**: 17–26.

71. Caldwell SH, Harris DM, Patrie JT, Hespenheide EE. Is NASH underdiagnosed among African-Americans? *Am J Gastroenterol* 2002; **97**: 1496–500.

72. Mokdad AH, Ford ES, Bowman BA, *et al.* Prevalence of obesity, diabetes, and obesity-related health risk factors, 2001. *JAMA* 2003; **289**: 76–9.

73. Schafer AI, Cheron RG, Dluhy R, *et al.* Clinical consequences of acquired transfusional iron overload in adults. *N Engl J Med* 1981; **304**: 319–24.

74. Brown KE, Khan CM, Zimmerman MB, Brunt EM. Hepatic iron overload in blacks and whites: a comparative autopsy study. *Am J Gastroenterol* 2003; **98**: 1594–8.

75. Cotler SJ, Bronner MP, Press RD, *et al.* End-stage liver disease without hemochromatosis associated with elevated hepatic iron index. *J Hepatol* 1998; **29**: 257–62.

76. Ludwig J, Hashimoto E, Porayko MK, Moyer TP, Baldus WP. Hemosiderosis in cirrhosis: a study of 447 native livers. *Gastroenterology* 1997; **112**: 882–8.

77. Strasser SI, Kowdley KV, Sale GE, McDonald GB. Iron overload in bone marrow transplant recipients. *Bone Marrow Transplant* 1998; **22**: 167–73.

78. Pietrangelo A. Non-invasive assessment of hepatic iron overload: are we finally there? *J Hepatol* 2005; **42**: 153–4.

79. Dawkins FW, Gordeuk VR, Snively BM, *et al.* African-Americans at risk for increased iron stores or liver disease. *Am J Med* 2007; **120**: 734–9.

80. Barton JC, Alford TJ, Bertoli LF, Barton NH, Edwards CQ. Histochemically demonstrable hepatic iron excess in African-Americans [abstract]. *Blood* 1995; **86**: **128a**.

81. Phatak PD, Sham RL, Raubertas RF, *et al.* Prevalence of hereditary hemochromatosis in 16 031 primary care patients. *Ann Intern Med* 1998; **129**: 954–61.

82. Adams PC, Reboussin DM, Barton JC, *et al.* Hemochromatosis and iron-overload screening in a racially diverse population. *N Engl J Med* 2005; **352**: 1769–78.

83. Yang Q, McDonnell SM, Khoury MJ, Cono J, Parrish RG. Hemochromatosis-associated mortality in the United States from 1979 to 1992: an analysis of Multiple-Cause Mortality Data. *Ann Intern Med* 1998; **129**: 946–53.

84. Barton JC, Acton RT, Anderson LE, Alexander CB. A comparison between whites and blacks with severe multi-organ iron overload identified in 16 152 autopsies. *Clin Gastroenterol Hepatol* 2009; **7**: 781–5.e2.

85. Bassett ML. Iron and hepatitis C: beginning to make sense. *J Gastroenterol Hepatol* 2007; **22**: 1703–4.

86. Desai TK, Jamil LH, Balasubramaniam M, Koff R, Bonkovsky HL. Phlebotomy improves therapeutic response to interferon in patients with chronic hepatitis C: a meta-analysis of six prospective randomized controlled trials. *Dig Dis Sci* 2008; **53**: 815–22.

87. Barton JC, McDonnell SM, Adams PC, *et al.* Management of hemochromatosis. Hemochromatosis Management Working Group. *Ann Intern Med* 1998; **129**: 932–9.

88. Gordeuk VR, McLaren CE, Looker AC, Hasselblad V, Brittenham GM. Distribution of transferrin saturations in the African-American population. *Blood* 1998; **91**: 2175–9.

89. Schnitzler CM, MacPhail AP, Shires R, Schnaid E, Mesquita JM, Robson HJ. Osteoporosis in African hemosiderosis: role of alcohol and iron. *J Bone Miner Res* 1994; **9**: 1865–73.

Hereditary atransferrinemia

Hereditary atransferrinemia (OMIM #209300) is a rare disorder characterized by severe quantitative or functional deficiency of transferrin. As a consequence, there is reduced delivery of iron to erythroid cells in the marrow, reduced hemoglobin synthesis, increased iron absorption, and severe iron overload of parenchymal organs.

History

In 1961, Heilmeyer and colleagues described atransferrinemia in a girl who had severe hypochromic anemia at age 3 months and severe, progressive generalized iron overload.[1] Patients from other countries with similar abnormalities have been reported subsequently, and explanatory mutations in the gene that encodes transferrin (*TF*; chromosome 3q21) have been demonstrated in four cases. A similar disorder discovered in inbred mice is due to a splice-site mutation in *Tf*, the ortholog of *TF* in humans.[2,3] Cases of acquired or secondary atransferrinemia or hypotransferrinemia have also been described in patients with diverse underlying conditions.

Clinical description

Manifestations of anemia are the most common clinical abnormalities in patients with hereditary atransferrinemia (Table 19.1). Several probands have had pallor, fatigue, or severe hypochromic, microcytic anemia at birth or in infancy.[1,4] An Italian infant also had hypovolemia, metabolic acidosis, and persistent fetal circulation.[5] Pallor and anemia were discovered for the first time at age 7 years in a patient from Japan,[6] and at age 20 years in a patient from the US.[4] Most patients have had a systolic ejection murmur attributed to chronic anemia.[4] One patient had mild hepatomegaly.[7] One 20-year-old American woman presented with heavy menstrual bleeding and had a history of hypothyroidism ascribed to iron

overload; she later developed hypogonadotrophic hypogonadism and osteoporosis.[8] Several patients have had growth retardation,[4,9] although early diagnosis and treatment with plasma or purified transferrin was associated with normal growth.[10] One Slovak patient developed arthropathy and cirrhosis of synovial membranes in childhood,[11] and by age 27 years she had hemosiderosis of heart, liver, anterior pituitary gland, and thyroid gland attributed to inadequate treatment with plasma.[12] She was living at age 34 years.[13] One patient had hypospadias.[14] Two patients died in childhood of refractory congestive heart failure, two others died of infections, another died of congestive heart failure, and another drowned while swimming.[4]

Laboratory abnormalities

The most distinctive and consistent laboratory abnormalities of hereditary atransferrinemia in untreated patients are associated with either quantitative or functional deficiency of transferrin (Table 19.1). All untreated patients have hypoferremia. Immunologic assays of plasma or serum transferrin have detected low concentrations of immunoreactive transferrin in all cases (0–5 μmol/L; normal 25–40 μmol/L).[4] Accordingly, the total serum iron-binding capacity is also low, and has ranged from 4.1–14.0 μmol/L (normal 24–81 μmol/L). In untreated patients, plasma iron clearance, a function of transferrin, is normal or moderately accelerated,[4,7] and transferrin-mediated incorporation of iron into hemoglobin is diminished.[7] Characteristics of anemia have varied somewhat in probands at diagnosis. Anemia is usually moderate or severe, and thus the red blood cell count and hemoglobin level are decreased. There is microcytosis, hypochromia, anisocytosis, poikilocytosis, and reticulocytopenia.[4,7] Stainable iron is markedly reduced or absent in the bone marrows of patients untreated with plasma or purified transferrin.[4,10]

Most patients have evidence of iron overload (Table 19.1). Serum ferritin levels are markedly elevated,[4] an attribute that may occur in neonates.[10] Absorption of inorganic iron from the gastrointestinal tract is normal or increased.[7] This emphasizes that transferrin is not essential for absorption of iron from the intestine.[7] Much iron that enters plasma is deposited in non-hematopoietic tissues by non-transferrin-mediated iron uptake mechanisms.[4] Iron is deposited in excessive amounts in hepatocytes and Kupffer cells.[15] At autopsy, there was iron overload

and fibrosis of the liver, pancreas, thyroid, myocardium, and kidneys in two cases.[4] The patients who died of congestive heart failure had also received numerous transfusions of erythrocytes.[4]

The serum transferrin concentrations of parents and other relatives who have a single deleterious *TF* allele are approximately one-half normal values.[7,10–13] In these subjects, red blood cell counts, hemoglobin levels, plasma iron disappearance times, half-lives of plasma transferrin, red blood cell iron uptake percentages, and absorption of orally administered inorganic iron are typically normal.[7,10–13]

Table 19.1. Clinical and laboratory features of hereditary atransferrinemia

Presentation in infancy to young adulthood
Occurrence in kinships consistent with autosomal recessive inheritance
Hypochromic, microcytic anemia, either moderate or severe
Hypoferremia, low serum transferrin, and low serum total iron-binding capacity
Markedly increased serum ferritin levels
Lack of stainable bone marrow iron
Progressive iron overload of liver and other parenchymal organs
Reversal of anemia after infusion of normal plasma or purified transferrin

Genetics

Patients have been described from Germany,[1] Slovakia,[11–13] Japan,[6,7,9] Mexico,[16,17] France,[18] Samoa,[15] Italy,[5] US,[8] and Turkey.[10] Two siblings have been described in each of the kinships from Japan and Mexico. In all kinships, it is assumed that atransferrinemia was transmitted as an autosomal recessive disorder. This assumption has been substantiated in four kinships in which deleterious *TF* mutations have been demonstrated (Table 19.2). Consanguinity has been reported or inferred in some kinships.[1,10,13] This is consistent with demonstration of homozygosity for a deleterious *TF* allele in two respective probands.[10,13] There is no known relationship between the various kinships in which hereditary atransferrinemia has been reported, and this agrees with the different

Table 19.2. Transferrin (*TF*) genotypes in hereditary atransferrinemia[a]

TF genotype	Clinical presentation	Country	Reference
Compound heterozygosity for A477P (exon 12; 1429G→C) and 188fsX215 (exon 5; 562_571del 572_580dup)[b,c]	20-year-old woman with anemia, heavy menstrual bleeding	US	8
Compound heterozygosity for E394K (exon 9; 1180 G→A) and inferred maternal null allele[d]	7-year-old boy with new onset of pallor	Japan	6,7,9
Homozygosity for D77N (exon 3; 229G→A)[c]	2-month-old girl with severe anemia	Slovakia	11–13
Homozygosity for C137Y (exon 4; 410A→G)[c]	4-month-old girl with severe anemia	Turkey	10

Notes: [a]Mutations are indicated as cDNA nucleotide substitutions (or other alterations). We used the recommended nomenclature[34,35] in which the A of the upstream ATG is counted as nucleotide number 1 and the initiator methionine is amino acid number 1,[13] as suggested by Beutler and colleagues.[8,13]
[b]*TF* A477P involves a highly conserved site. *TF* 188fsX215 resulted in a stop codon 27 amino acids downstream.[8]
[c]Reported or previously unreported non-deleterious *TF* polymorphisms, especially single nucleotide polymorphisms, were also discovered in these patients.[8,10]
[d]No mutation was found in either the coding region or the exon-intron boundaries, suggesting an abnormality in the transcription or stability of mRNA of maternal allele origin.

deleterious *TF* mutations detected across the kinships (Table 19.2).

Deleterious *TF* alleles are typically not detected in population samples ("private" mutations).[8,10,13] In a Portuguese kinship, a transferrin null allele was discovered in a case of disputed paternity. The mother and putative father were heterozygous for transferrin null alleles and their transferrin levels were 40%–41% of normal.[19] Their child was homozygous for the respective null alleles and had a serum transferrin level of 35 mg/dL (12.5% of normal) at age 15–20 months, although it was not reported whether this child had iron overload.[19] Null transferrin alleles have also been described in German and Finnish kinships.[20–22]

Polymorphisms of *TF* are common,[23] and some patients with hereditary atransferrinemia have had known or previously unreported *TF* polymorphisms, in addition to deleterious *TF* alleles.[8,13] An investigation of five different transferrin variants was undertaken to determine their effect(s) on hemoglobin level, mean corpuscular volume, serum ferritin level, percent transferrin saturation, or unsaturated iron-binding capacity in subjects with defined *HFE* genotypes (919 persons undergoing health screening, 113 patients with hemochromatosis phenotypes). These five *TF* polymorphisms were not associated with any significant changes in iron metabolism, nor did they appear to influence the expression of hemochromatosis.[23]

Genotype–phenotype correlations

Phenotypic heterogeneity in patients with hereditary atransferrinemia is due in part to *TF* genotype (Table 19.2). In a Japanese case, an isoelectric focusing of serum proteins demonstrated that the patient and his father both had variant transferrin. This result suggested that the patient was a compound heterozygote who inherited a variant paternal *TF* allele that encoded the mutant transferrin and a null allele of maternal origin.[6,9] DNA analysis confirmed that the patient and his father shared a variant *TF* gene bearing a GAA to AAA transition at codon 394. This nucleotide substitution causes a non-conservative amino acid change from glutamate to lysine in amino acid residue 375 of transferrin protein (Table 19.2). This missense mutation is predicted to cause a conformational change in the coiled region of the carboxy-terminal iron-binding lobe of transferrin.[9] As for the maternal null allele, no mutation was found in either the coding region or the exon-intron boundaries, suggesting an abnormality in the transcription or stability of mRNA of maternal allele origin.[9]

Protein analysis suggested that an Italian patient had two different *TF* deleterious alleles that caused two distinct abnormalities. One allele caused low expression of apparently normal transferrin that probably allowed survival of the patient in the early years of life. The other allele produced transferrin with abnormal biochemical characteristics.[5] It was inferred that the proband was a compound heterozygote for each of the two deleterious *TF* alleles, although Southern blot analysis did not detect gross deletions or rearrangements of *TF*.[5] In the Slovak case, severe anemia and other manifestations occurred in early infancy.[11,12] Substitution of a polar asparagine residue for a negatively charged aspartate residue in the region of the transferrin molecule encoded by exon 3 of *TF* appears to have abrogated severely the synthesis or secretion of functional transferrin (Table 19.2).[13] The Turkish patient had compound heterozygosity for a *TF* mutation that altered a highly conserved amino acid residue of transferrin and a *TF* stop-codon mutation, explaining her severe phenotype at an early age (Table 19.2).[10]

Treatment

There are two treatment goals in patients with hereditary atransferrinemia: (1) restoration of iron-normal erythropoiesis; and (2) prevention or alleviation of iron overload. Iron-deficient erythropoiesis can be treated satisfactorily with periodic infusion of normal plasma or purified apotransferrin.[7,12] Infusion of either normal plasma or purified transferrin is followed in 10–14 days by reticulocytosis and a subsequent rise in hemoglobin concentration.[8] Individual infusions increase plasma transferrin concentration for less than 1 week. Erythroblasts maturing during this time acquire sufficient iron to synthesize normal levels of hemoglobin, enter the circulation, and circulate for approximately 4 months.[4] Therefore, this treatment is usually given once or twice each month. After several months, hemoglobin levels and erythrocyte indices become normal.[4,8] Anemia associated with otherwise untreated hereditary atransferrinemia does not respond to administration of supplemental iron.[1,7,10] Erythrocyte transfusion increases iron overload.

Early diagnosis and treatment with plasma or purified transferrin can prevent iron overload due to repeated erythrocyte transfusion and increased intestinal absorption of iron. In a 4-month-old girl from Turkey, a markedly elevated serum ferritin concentration declined to normal levels over 1 year with plasma infusions; she was not treated with phlebotomy or chelation therapy. This indicates that excessive iron stores at diagnosis were reduced solely by improved erythropoiesis. In other patients, serum ferritin concentration and tissue iron stores remained elevated despite infusions of plasma or purified transferrin, and they required treatment with chelating agents, phlebotomy, or both.[5,8,9,13] The American patient was treated with a monthly 500 mL phlebotomy followed immediately by intravenous infusion of one single-donor unit of normal human plasma obtained from a small group of volunteers to diminish risk of viral hepatitis; this treatment was continued for more than 10 years. After 120 phlebotomies, she had normal erythrocyte measures, was depleted of excess iron (serum ferritin <11 pmol/L), and had no apparent complications of treatment.[4,8] The two Japanese patients have been treated with 1–2 g of highly purified apotransferrin intravenously every 3–4 months for 4–7 years without development of anti-transferrin antibodies.[6,7,9,24] Purified transferrin reduces the risk of hepatitis associated with infusion of whole plasma, although this product is not presently available for therapy in the US. One of the Japanese patients no longer needs infusions of purified apotransferrin.[24] The patient from Italy was treated with deferoxamine.[5]

Acquired atransferrinemia

Nephrotic syndrome

Acquired or secondary cases of atransferrinemia or hypotransferrinemia have been described in patients with nephrotic syndrome.[25,26] This condition is characterized by marked urinary losses of albumin, transferrin, erythropoietin, immunoglobulins, and other intermediate-size plasma proteins.[27] Transferrinuria and increased transferrin loss cause hypotransferrinemia and, in some cases, iron-deficiency anemia. Dissociation of iron from filtered transferrin in renal tubular fluid of low pH could promote tubulointerstitial injury through the iron-catalyzed generation of oxygen free radicals.[27] Renal siderosis is also a feature

of hereditary atransferrinemia.[4] Renal injury by iron could account in part for the role of proteinuria as a risk factor for the progression of renal functional impairment in patients with nephrotic syndrome. Some children with nephrotic syndrome also have hypogammaglobulinemia, due to excessive urinary losses of immunoglobulins. At low concentrations of serum from patients with nephrotic syndrome, lymphocyte uptake of tritiated thymidine in vitro was directly proportional to the serum transferrin concentration. Addition of transferrin restored the ability of patients' sera to support normal in vitro lymphocyte proliferation.[28] These results suggest that hypotransferrinemia might adversely affect in vivo lymphocyte function and immunity in patients with nephrotic syndrome.

Iron supplementation and nutritional support are indicated in patients with nephrotic syndrome, severe transferrinuria, and iron-deficiency anemia. Transferrin synthesis is increased in patients with nephrotic syndrome, but is insufficient to compensate for urinary losses.[29] There is a significant relationship between transferrin synthesis and serum levels of either C-reactive protein or iron.[29] Accordingly, it is unlikely that inflammation suppresses or that iron deficiency stimulates increased transferrin synthesis in these patients. The correlation between transferrin synthesis and albumin synthesis suggests that transferrin synthesis is a component of a general response in hepatic protein synthesis in the nephrotic syndrome.[29] Correction or amelioration of proteinuria, when possible, is the ideal approach to maximize plasma transferrin concentrations and to reverse associated complications.[27,29] Acquired atransferrinemia has also been reported in a patient with erythroleukemia.[30]

Antitransferrin antibodies

Transferrin-IgG antitransferrin immune complexes caused an iron overload disorder in a 71-year-old woman.[31] She had extreme hyperferremia (serum iron 143 μmol/L; ~800 μg/dt), a feature that distinguishes this case from those of hereditary atransferrinemia. Hemosiderin was not detectable in her bone marrow macrophages, her proportions of erythrocytes and sideroblasts were lower, and radioiron utilization by her erythroid cells was decreased. She had cirrhosis associated with hepatic iron overload, bronzed skin that contained hemosiderin, and diabetes mellitus. She had an autoantibody with transferrin specificity that produced a circulating immune complex that bound serum iron. Immuno-suppressive therapy induced a partial remission of her disorder that included improvement in her general sense of well-being, an increase in transferrin levels unbound to autoantibody, a decrease in serum iron levels, an increase in erythrocyte production, and dis-appearance of hemosiderin in the liver.[31] Three other patients had monoclonal IgG with anti-transferrin specificity associated with hyperferremia, extremely high serum transferrin levels, and elevated transferrin saturation values.[32,33] One had low urinary hepcidin levels and developed iron-limited erythropoiesis, hyperferritinemia, and increased hepatic iron depos-ition.[33] The other two patients had normal serum ferritin levels and did not develop anemia.[32]

References

1. Heilmeyer L, Keller W, Vivell O, Betke K, Woehler F, Keiderling W. [Congenital atransferrinemia.] *Schweiz Med Wochenschr* 1961; **91**: 1203.

2. Bernstein SE. Hereditary hypotransferrinemia with hemosiderosis, a murine disorder resembling human atransferrinemia. *J Lab Clin Med* 1987; **110**: 690–705.

3. Trenor CC, III, Campagna DR, Sellers VM, Andrews NC, Fleming MD. The molecular defect in hypotransferrinemic mice. *Blood* 2000; **96**: 1113–18.

4. Fairbanks VF, Brandhagen DJ. Disorders of iron transport and storage. In: Beutler E, Lichtman MA, Coller BS, Kipps TJ, Seligsohn U, eds. *Williams Hematology*. New York, McGraw-Hill. 2001; 489–502.

5. Goldwurm S, Casati C, Venturi N, *et al.* Biochemical and genetic defects underlying human congenital hypotransferrinemia. *Hematol J* 2000; **1**: 390–8.

6. Sakata T. [A case of congenital atransferrinemia.] *Shonika Shinryo* 1969.

7. Goya N, Miyazaki S, Kodate S, Ushio B. A family of congenital atransferrinemia. *Blood* 1972; **40**: 239–45.

8. Beutler E, Gelbart T, Lee P, Trevino R, Fernandez MA, Fairbanks VF. Molecular characterization of a case of atransferrinemia. *Blood* 2000; **96**: 4071–4.

9. Asada-Senju M, Maeda T, Sakata T, Hayashi A, Suzuki T. Molecular analysis of the transferrin gene in a patient with hereditary hypotransferrinemia. *J Hum Genet* 2002; **47**: 355–9.

10. Aslan D, Crain K, Beutler E. A new case of human atransferrinemia with a previously undescribed mutation in the transferrin gene. *Acta Haematol* 2007; **118**: 244–7.

11. Cap J, Lehotska V, Mayerova A. [Congenital atransferrinemia in a 11-month-old child.] *Cesk Pediatr* 1968; **23**: 1020–5.

12. Hromec A, Payer J, Jr., Killinger Z, Rybar I, Rovensky J. [Congenital atransferrinemia.] *Dtsch Med Wochenschr* 1994; **119**: 663–6.

13. Knisely AS, Gelbart T, Beutler E. Molecular characterization of a third case of human atransferrinemia. *Blood* 2004; **104**: 2607.

14. Goldwurm S, Biondi A. Case of congenital hypotransferrinemia suggests that tissue hypoxia during fetal development may cause hypospadias. *Am J Med Genet* 2000; **95**: 287–90.

15. Hamill RL, Woods JC, Cook BA. Congenital atransferrinemia. A case report and review of the literature. *Am J Clin Pathol* 1991; **96**: 215–18.

16. Loperena L, Dorantes S, Medrano E, *et al.* [Hereditary atransferrinemia.] *Bol Med Hosp Infant Mex* 1974; **31**: 519–35.

17. Dorantes-Mesa S, Marquez JL, Valencia-Mayoral P. [Iron overload in hereditary atransferrinemia.] *Bol Med Hosp Infant Mex* 1986; **43**: 99–101.

18. Walbaum R. [Congenital transferrin deficiency.] *Lille Med* 1971; **16**: 1122–4.

19. Espinheira R, Geada H, Mendonca J, Reys L. Alpha-1-antitrypsin and transferrin null alleles in the Portuguese population. *Hum Hered* 1988; **38**: 372–4.

20. Weidinger S, Cleve H, Schwarzfischer F, Postel W, Weser J, Gorg A. Transferrin subtypes and variants in Germany; further evidence for a Tf null allele. *Hum Genet* 1984; **66**: 356–60.

21. Püshel K, Krüger A, Soder R. Further evidence of a silent Tf allele. *Int Congr Soc Forens Haemog (Vienna)* 1987.

22. Lukka M, Enholm C. A silent transferrin allele in a Finnish family. *Hum Hered* 1985; **35**: 157–60.

23. Lee PL, Ho NJ, Olson R, Beutler E. The effect of transferrin polymorphisms on iron metabolism. *Blood Cells Mol Dis* 1999; **25**: 374–9.

24. Hayashi A, Wada Y, Suzuki T, Shimizu A. Studies on familial hypotransferrinemia: unique clinical course and molecular pathology. *Am J Hum Genet* 1993; **53**: 201–13.

25. Oliva G, Dominici G, Latini P, Cozzolino G. [Atransferrinemic nephrotic syndrome. Clinical contribution and etiopathogenetic evaluation.] *Minerva Med* 1968; **59**: 1297–309.

26. Gaston Morata JL, Rodriguez CA, Urbano JF, Gonzalez MF, Ampuero AJ. [Atransferrinemia secondary to hepatic cirrhosis, hemochromatosis,

and nephrotic syndrome.] *Rev Esp Enferm Apar Dig* 1982; **62**: 491–5.

27. Vaziri ND. Erythropoietin and transferrin metabolism in nephrotic syndrome. *Am J Kidney Dis* 2001; **38**: 1–8.

28. Warshaw BL, Check IJ, Hymes LC, DiRusso SC. Decreased serum transferrin concentration in children with the nephrotic syndrome: effect on lymphocyte proliferation and correlation with serum immunoglobulin levels. *Clin Immunol Immunopathol* 1984; **33**: 210–19.

29. Prinsen BH, de Sain-van der Velden MG, Kaysen GA, *et al.* Transferrin synthesis is increased in nephrotic patients insufficiently to replace urinary losses. *J Am Soc Nephrol* 2001; **12**: 1017–25.

30. Hitzig WH, Schmid M, Betke K, Rothschild M. [Erythroleukemia with hemoglobin disorders and disorders of iron metabolism.] *Helv Paediatr Acta* 1960; **15**: 203–22.

31. Westerhausen M, Meuret G. Transferrin-immune complex disease. *Acta Haematol* 1977; **57**: 96–101.

32. Alyanakian MA, Taes Y, Bensaid M, *et al.* Monoclonal immunoglobulin with antitransferrin activity: a rare cause of hypersideremia with increased transferrin saturation. *Blood* 2007; **109**: 359–61.

33. Forni GL, Girelli D, Lamagna M, *et al.* Acquired iron overload associated with antitransferrin monoclonal immunoglobulin: a case report. *Am J Hematol* 2008; **83**: 932–4.

34. den Dunnen JT, Antonarakis SE. Mutation nomenclature extensions and suggestions to describe complex mutations: a discussion. *Hum Mutat* 2000; **15**: 7–12.

35. Antonarakis SE. Recommendations for a nomenclature system for human gene mutations. Nomenclature Working Group. *Hum Mutat* 1998; **11**: 1–3.

Chapter 20

Divalent metal transporter-1 (*SLC11A2*) iron overload

Divalent metal transporter-1 (DMT1) is a member of the "natural-resistance-associated macrophage protein" (*Nramp*) family. DMT1 is upregulated by dietary iron deficiency, is expressed strongly on the microvillus membranes of duodenal enterocytes at the villus tips, and is a key mediator of iron absorption.[1,2] DMT1 also mediates iron transfer from endosomes into the cytosol of developing erythroid cells. The *SLC11A2* gene that encodes DMT1 is located on chromosome 12q13 (OMIM *604653).[3]

In 1964, Shahidi and colleagues described a brother and sister of French-Canadian descent who had hypochromic, microcytic anemia. These siblings also had elevated serum iron concentrations, massive deposition of iron in hepatocytes, and absence of stainable iron in the bone marrow. These children apparently had no defect in transferrin or heme synthesis. Two of their siblings appeared to have normal iron phenotypes.[4] In 2004 and 2005, Priwitzerova and colleagues described a Czech female in a consanguineous kinship who came to medical attention at age 3 months because she had a syndrome of abnormal iron metabolism characterized by severe hypochromic, microcytic anemia, erythroid hyperplasia, abnormal erythroid maturation, elevated serum iron concentration, normal to slightly increased serum ferritin level, and markedly increased serum transferrin receptor levels.[5,6] In 2005, Mims and colleagues reported that this woman was homozygous for a mutation in *SLC11A2*.[7]

Clinical description

Clinical observations in patients with two *SLC11A2* mutations are limited. In one case, left ventricular hypertrophy was detected before birth, and birth weight was low.[8] Pallor is presumed to have been present in all reported cases.[9] Lack of physical vigor was mentioned in one case.[8] Enlargement of the liver and spleen were not detected in one patient,[8] but mild hepatomegaly and splenomegaly were reported in another case.[9]

Genetics and pathophysiology

The anemia–iron overload syndrome associated with inheritance of two abnormal *SLC11A2* alleles is transmitted as an autosomal recessive trait. Consanguinity was reported in one of the three families in which this syndrome appeared and was associated with homozygosity for a missense mutation of *SLC11A2*.[5] Each of the three kinships had European ancestry (Czech, Italian, and French, respectively), although this may reflect an increased awareness of hemochromatosis and other iron overload disorders due to the predominance of *HFE* mutations in European peoples. Five pathogenic mutations have been described in three probands with the clinical syndrome. The Czech patient was homozygous for *SLC11A2* E399D. The ultimate nucleotide of exon 12 of *SLC11A2* encodes a highly conserved glutamic acid residue that was changed to an aspartic acid residue due to the E399D missense mutation. The predominant effect of this mutation was preferential skipping of exon 12 during processing of pre-messenger RNA (mRNA).[6] The E399D substitution has no effect on protein expression and function in vitro,[6] and was stable and had normal targeting and trafficking to the membrane.[10] This suggests that the mutated protein has a modest amount of activity in vivo.[10] In the Italian patient, a 3-bp deletion in *SLC11A2* intron 4 (c.310–3_5del CTT) resulted in a splicing abnormality. The second abnormal allele in this patient was the missense mutation R416C.[9] In vitro studies indicate that R416C is a "loss-of-function" mutation.[11] The French proband was a compound heterozygote with a GTG deletion in exon 5, leading to the V114 in-frame deletion in transmembrane domain 2, and the missense mutation G212V in exon 8.[8] Variability of function of mutant DMT1 proteins largely accounts for the phenotypic heterogeneity that has been observed among the few reported patients with DMT1 anemia–iron overload syndrome.

The microcytic anemia (*mk*) mouse and the Belgrade rat (*b*) have the same *Slc11a2* missense mutation (G185R).[12,13] Animals that are homozygous for G185R demonstrate severe microcytic anemia at birth, diminished intestinal iron absorption, and defective erythroid iron utilization. In rodents with DMT1 mutations, iron absorption is decreased.[12,13] There is little expression of DMT1 at the apical membrane in *mk/mk* mice. The G185R mutation impairs the transport properties of DMT1, and may affect the membrane targeting of DMT1 protein in *mk/mk* enterocytes. In *mk/mk* mice, the loss of DMT1 function is paralleled by a great increase in expression of the defective protein. This is consistent with a feedback regulation of DMT1 expression by iron stores.

In patients with *SLC11A2* mutations, iron from dietary sources, supplemental iron, and erythrocyte transfusion probably contribute to the development of iron overload. This suggests that intestinal absorption of iron in humans with DMT1 anemia–iron overload syndrome differs from that in *mk* mice and *b* rats. In humans, iron absorption may be increased despite decreased function of DMT1, perhaps due to increased expression of greater numbers of mutant protein molecules in absorptive enterocytes.[8] Proton coupling to DMT1 increases its affinity for Fe^{2+}, although DMT1 can mediate facilitative Fe^{2+} transport in the absence of a proton gradient.[14] Human intestinal absorption probably compensates for deficient ferrous iron uptake by absorbing inorganic iron via alternate pathways, or by absorbing heme iron.[5,15] The positive effect of oral iron supplementation on the hemoglobin concentration in one patient with DMT1 anemia–iron overload syndrome indicates that ferrous iron supplements are absorbed effectively from the small intestine.[8] Erythrocyte transfusion contributes to iron overload, although the reported extent of transfusion varies across these patients.[5,6,8,9]

The most prominent consequence of impaired DMT1 function in humans is impaired erythropoiesis due to decreased *SLC11A2* expression and decreased iron uptake in erythroid cells. Accordingly, the severity of anemia and the age at which iron overload develops is probably attributable in part to the particular *SLC11A2* genotype. Hypochromic, microcytic anemia is present from birth. Examination of the bone marrow reveals erythroid hyperplasia with defective hemoglobinization of intermediate and late normoblasts and absence of sideroblasts in the bone marrow.[9] Stainable marrow iron was absent in the Shahidi case.[4] *SLC11A2* E399D was expressed in reduced quantities in hematopoietic cells in vitro, and *SLC11A2* R416C exhibited almost no function in vitro. This would explain the severe depression of iron uptake by erythroid cells of the corresponding patients. Serum iron levels and transferrin saturation are high.[5] Soluble transferrin receptor levels are elevated.[5] A striking reduction of DMT1 protein in peripheral blood mononuclear cells was demonstrated by Western blot analysis in one case.[9]

In patients with DMT1 anemia–iron overload syndrome, serum ferritin levels are mildly elevated and increase progressively with age, although the levels may be lower than expected for the degree of hepatic iron overload.[5,6,8,9] The age at which hepatic iron overload becomes apparent is variable, although hepatic iron deposition is probably progressive in all cases. In one patient, hepatic iron overload was observed at the age 5 years.[9] In another patient, hepatic iron overload was documented at age 19 years.[7] Mild elevation of serum activities of hepatic transaminases may be a relatively early indicator of accumulation of excessive hepatic iron.[5] Excessive iron deposition is observed in hepatocytes and Kupffer cells.[7,9] Cirrhosis has not been described. Hepatocyte iron uptake in persons with *SLC11A2* mutations may occur because there is much non-transferrin bound iron, although this is unproven. An alternative hypothesis is that a defective DMT1 in hepatocyte endosomal compartments impairs iron efflux toward the cytosol, leading to intracellular accumulation of iron in a compartment that does not trigger ferritin synthesis and/or secretion.[8]

In experimental studies, the reported effects of iron overload and iron depletion on the expression of *SLC11A2* in hepatocytes are disparate, and do not necessarily correspond to those observed in humans with DMT1 anemia-iron overload syndrome. In normal rats, DMT1 protein staining was observed on hepatocyte plasma membranes, with highest values in the iron-loaded animals, lower values in control animals, and none after iron depletion.[16] DMT1 in normal liver and hepatoma cells in vitro was preferentially located in cytoplasm, but weakly on cell surfaces. In addition, iron depletion of hepatoma cells increased their membrane expression of DMT1, suggesting that intracellular iron levels regulate DMT1 expression in hepatocytes via the iron regulatory protein/iron-responsive element system.[17]

SLC11A2 mutations have been investigated as possible "modifiers" of iron overload phenotypes in persons with hemochromatosis associated with *HFE* C282Y homozygosity. In one study, *SLC11A2* mutations were sought using sequencing in C282Y homozygotes with clinical disease, in C282Y homozygotes with normal or low serum ferritin levels and no iron overload disease, in persons without common *HFE* mutations who had high ferritin and transferrin saturation levels, and in normal control subjects without common *HFE* mutations.[18] No *SLC11A2* mutations were found that explained differences in iron phenotypes in these subjects.[18] In another study, the presence of four specific mutations/polymorphisms within the *SLC11A2* gene (1245T/C, 1303C/A, IVS4 + 44C/A, IVS15Ex16–16C/G) was evaluated in C282Y homozygotes and in control subjects without common *HFE* mutations using standard PCR techniques.[19] There were no significant differences in the allele frequencies of the IVS4 + 44C/A, 1303C/A, 1254T/C, and IVS15Ex16–16C/G polymorphisms in the patient cohort and in the control cohort. The commonest haplotypes identified were CCTC: IVS4C + 44C, 1303C, 1254T, IVS15ex16–16C; ACCC: IVS4C + 44A, 1303C, 1254C, IVS15ex16–16C, ACTG: IVS4C + 44A, 1303C, 1254T, IVS15ex16–16G. Similarly, there were no significant differences in the frequencies of these three haplotypes in the patient cohorts (regardless of the degree of hepatic iron deposition) and in the control cohort. Accordingly, it appears that common *SLC11A2* polymorphisms do not influence hemochromatosis phenotypes in persons with *HFE* C282Y homozygosity. In French-Canadian subjects with restless leg syndrome (RLS), a disorder characterized by abnormal brain iron metabolism, sequencing of *SLC11A2* from selected patients did not detect pathogenic mutation(s).[20] Further studies did not find any association between ten single nucleotide polymorphisms (SNPs), spanning the entire *SLC11A2* gene region, and the presence or absence of RLS. Two *SLC11A2* intronic SNPs were positively associated with RLS in patients with a history of anemia.[20]

Laboratory findings

Complete blood counts and measurement of serum iron, transferrin saturation, and serum ferritin should be performed in all suspected cases. Severe anemia with markedly subnormal mean corpuscular volume and mean corpuscular hemoglobin and normal or decreased red blood cell counts have been observed in all cases.[5,8,9] The occurrence of iron-deficient erythropoiesis (in the presence of elevated serum iron and transferrin saturation levels) is verified by the demonstration of markedly elevated levels of soluble transferrin receptor and free erythrocyte protoporphyrin. Reticulocyte counts were normal to slightly elevated in one case.[5] Bone marrow smears of imprint specimens should include staining for general cytologic detail (Wright/Giemsa staining) and to demonstrate ferric iron (Perls' technique). Erythroid hyperplasia, decreased hemoglobinization of erythroid cells, decreased or absent sideroblasts, and decreased or absent macrophage iron are typical. Specimens of liver obtained by percutaneous biopsy technique can be analyzed for histology, stainable iron (Perls' technique), and iron content using atomic absorption spectrometry. Hepatic iron overload was detected in one case with superconducting quantum interference susceptometry (SQUID) technique, and in another case with magnetic resonance imaging (MRI).[8,9]

Family screening

All patients with two abnormal *SLC11A2* alleles described to date have had hypochromic, microcytic anemia at birth. The presence of anemia, elevated serum iron and transferrin saturation levels, and elevated soluble transferrin receptor levels should suffice to make a tentative diagnosis at an early age in siblings of index patients. Serum ferritin levels are predicted to be normal in the youngest patients, and to rise over a period of years. The development of iron overload is a relatively late consequence. Therefore, using iron overload as a diagnostic criterion in siblings of probands is not timely. Pathogenic *SLC11A2* alleles described to date appear to be "private" mutations, and thus consanguinity may increase the risk that DMT1 anemia–iron overload syndrome will occur. Parents, offspring, and some siblings of probands are heterozygous or are presumed to be heterozygous for an abnormal *SLC11A2* allele, and typically have normal serum iron measures[4] and do not develop iron overload. If direct sequencing or other testing to detect a *SLC11A2* missense mutation or deletion is available, this should be used to evaluate family members.

Treatment

All reported patients have been treated with erythrocyte transfusion,[5,6,8,9] although most have not required regular transfusion like that required by patients with beta-thalassemia. In one case, the proband required blood transfusions until erythropoietin treatment allowed transfusion independence when hemoglobin levels between 75 and 95 g/L (7.5 and 9.5 g/dL) were achieved.[9] Continuous oral iron supplementation resulted in a rise of hemoglobin concentration of 10 to 20 g/L with a striking improvement of quality of life.[8] These observations suggest that therapeutic phlebotomy to alleviate iron overload may be feasible in some cases, but that iron-poor erythropoiesis may also be ameliorated to some extent by iron overload or administration of oral iron supplements. There are no reports of iron chelation therapy in this disorder. In mice, the L-type calcium channel blocker nifedipine increases DMT1-mediated cellular iron transport 10- to 100-fold at concentrations between 1 and 100 μM. Nifedipine causes this effect by prolonging the iron-transporting activity of DMT1, and thus mobilizes iron from the livers of mice with primary and secondary iron overload and enhances its urinary iron excretion.[21] It is speculative that modulation of DMT1 function by L-type calcium channel blockers could be used to treat iron-deficient erythropoiesis and progressive iron overload in persons with *SLC11A2* mutations.

References

1. Gunshin H, Mackenzie B, Berger UV, *et al.* Cloning and characterization of a mammalian proton-coupled metal-ion transporter. *Nature* 1997; **388**: 482–8.

2. Hubert N, Hentze MW. Previously uncharacterized isoforms of divalent metal transporter (DMT)-1: implications for regulation and cellular function. *Proc Natl Acad Sci USA* 2002; **99**: 12345–50.

3. Vidal S, Belouchi AM, Cellier M, Beatty B, Gros P. Cloning and characterization of a second human *NRAMP* gene on chromosome 12q13. *Mamm Genome* 1995; **6**: 224–30.

4. Shahidi NT, Nathan DG, Diamond LK. Iron deficiency anemia associated with an error of iron metabolism in two siblings. *J Clin Invest* 1964; **43**: 510–21.

5. Priwitzerova M, Pospisilova D, Prchal JT, *et al.* Severe hypochromic microcytic anemia caused by a congenital defect of the iron transport pathway in erythroid cells. *Blood* 2004; **103**: 3991–2.

6. Priwitzerova M, Nie G, Sheftel AD, Pospisilova D, Divoky V, Ponka P. Functional consequences of the human *DMT1* (*SLC11A2*) mutation on protein expression and iron uptake. *Blood* 2005; **106**: 3985–7.

7. Mims MP, Guan Y, Pospisilova D, *et al.* Identification of a human mutation of *DMT1* in a patient with microcytic anemia and iron overload. *Blood* 2005; **105**: 1337–42.

8. Beaumont C, Delaunay J, Hetet G, Grandchamp B, de Montalembert M, Tchernia G. Two new human *DMT1* gene mutations in a patient with microcytic anemia, low ferritinemia, and liver iron overload. *Blood* 2006; **107**: 4168–70.

9. Iolascon A, d'Apolito M, Servedio V, Cimmino F, Piga A, Camaschella C. Microcytic anemia and hepatic iron overload in a child with compound heterozygous mutations in DMT1 (*SCL11A2*). *Blood* 2006; **107**: 349–54.

10. Lam-Yuk-Tseung S, Mathieu M, Gros P. Functional characterization of the E399D *DMT1/NRAMP2/SLC11A2* protein produced by an exon 12 mutation in a patient with microcytic anemia and iron overload. *Blood Cells Mol Dis* 2005; **35**: 212–16.

11. Lam-Yuk-Tseung S, Camaschella C, Iolascon A, Gros P. A novel R416C mutation in human *DMT1* (*SLC11A2*) displays pleiotropic effects on function and causes microcytic anemia and hepatic iron overload. *Blood Cells Mol Dis* 2006; **36**: 347–54.

12. Fleming MD, Trenor CC, III, Su MA, *et al.* Microcytic anaemia mice have a mutation in *Nramp2*, a candidate iron transporter gene. *Nat Genet* 1997; **16**: 383–6.

13. Fleming MD, Romano MA, Su MA, Garrick LM, Garrick MD, Andrews NC. *Nramp2* is mutated in the anemic Belgrade (*b*) rat: evidence of a role for Nramp2 in endosomal iron transport. *Proc Natl Acad Sci USA* 1998; **95**: 1148–53.

14. Mackenzie B, Ujwal ML, Chang MH, Romero MF, Hediger MA. Divalent metal-ion transporter DMT1 mediates both H+ -coupled Fe2+ transport and uncoupled fluxes. *Pflugers Arch* 2006; **451**: 544–58.

15. Shayeghi M, Latunde-Dada GO, Oakhill JS, *et al.* Identification of an intestinal heme transporter. *Cell* 2005; **122**: 789–801.

16. Trinder D, Oates PS, Thomas C, Sadleir J, Morgan EH. Localization of divalent metal transporter-1 (DMT1) to the microvillus membrane of rat duodenal enterocytes in iron deficiency, but to hepatocytes in iron overload. *Gut* 2000; **46**: 270–6.

17. Shindo M, Torimoto Y, Saito H, *et al.* Functional role of DMT1 in transferrin-independent iron uptake by human hepatocyte and hepatocellular carcinoma cell, HLF. *Hepatol Res* 2006; **35**: 152–62.

18. Lee P, Gelbart T, West C, Halloran C, Beutler E. Seeking candidate mutations that affect iron homeostasis. *Blood Cells Mol Dis* 2002; **29**: 471–87.

19. Kelleher T, Ryan E, Barrett S, O'Keane C, Crowe J. *DMT1* genetic variability is not responsible for phenotype variability in hereditary hemochromatosis. *Blood Cells Mol Dis* 2004; **33**: 35–9.

20. Xiong L, Dion P, Montplaisir J, *et al.* Molecular genetic studies of *DMT1* on 12q in French-Canadian restless legs syndrome patients and families. *Am J Med Genet B Neuropsychiatr Genet* 2007; **144**: 911–17.

21. Ludwiczek S, Theurl I, Muckenthaler MU, *et al.* Ca^{2+} channel blockers reverse iron overload by a new mechanism via divalent metal transporter-1. *Nat Med* 2007; **13**: 448–54.

Iron overload associated with thalassemia syndromes

Introduction

Thalassemia comprises a diverse group of heritable disorders that decrease the synthesis of one or more globin chains. Specific thalassemia syndromes are named by the affected globin chain(s) or the causative mutation(s).[1] Thalassemia is prevalent in some areas of the world, especially those in which malaria is or was endemic such as the Mediterranean region or southeast Asia. Many thalassemia mutations cause anemia, the severity of which varies with thalassemia or co-inherited hemoglobinopathy genotype, and the consequent effect on globin and hemoglobin synthesis. The most prevalent subtypes of thalassemia that cause severe anemia are beta-thalassemia major or double heterozygosity for beta-thalassemia and hemoglobin (Hb) E. The details of thalassemia genetics, laboratory and clinical phenotypes, and general management are presented in other comprehensive resources.[1–3]

Iron overload in persons with severe thalassemia syndromes is a major cause of morbidity due to endocrinopathy (especially hypogonadism and diabetes mellitus), liver disease, and cardiomyopathy. Many patients have increased susceptibility to severe or recurrent infections due to bacteria and other microbes (Chapter 7). Cardiomyopathy due to cardiac siderosis is the leading cause of death in patients with severe beta-thalassemia. Iron overload in patients with thalassemia is usually caused by increased absorption of dietary iron and retention of additional iron from chronic erythrocyte transfusion administered to alleviate severe anemia.[3] This chapter is devoted principally to iron overload and related abnormalities in patients with severe thalassemia.

Development of iron overload
Mechanisms that enhance iron absorption

In severe beta-thalassemia, deficient globin-chain production results in anemia and ineffective erythropoiesis. The expression and secretion of growth/differentiation factor 15 (GDF15), a member of the transforming growth factor-beta superfamily, is increased during erythroblast maturation.[4,5] Healthy volunteers had mean GDF15 serum concentrations of 450 ± 50 pg/mL. In comparison, individuals with beta-thalassemia syndromes had elevated GDF15 serum levels (mean $66\,000 \pm 9600$ pg/mL; range $4800–248\,000$ pg/mL; $P < 0.05$) that were positively correlated with serum levels of soluble transferrin receptor, erythropoietin, and ferritin.[4] Serum from thalassemia patients suppressed hepcidin mRNA expression in primary human hepatocytes, and depletion of GDF15 reversed hepcidin suppression.[4] These results suggest that GDF15 over expression arising from an expanded erythroid compartment contributes to accumulation of iron in the absence of blood transfusions in persons with thalassemia syndromes by inhibiting hepcidin expression.[4,5]

Erythroblast expression of a second molecule named twisted gastrulation (TWSG1) is another potential erythroid regulator of hepcidin. Transcriptome analyses suggest TWSG1 is produced during the earlier stages of erythropoiesis. Hepcidin suppression assays demonstrated inhibition by TWSG1 as measured by quantitative polymerase chain reaction (PCR) in dosed assays (1–1000 ng/mL TWSG1).[6] In human cells, TWSG1 suppressed hepcidin indirectly by inhibiting the signaling effects and associated hepcidin up-regulation by bone morphogenic proteins 2 and 4 (BMP2/BMP4).[6] In murine hepatocytes, hepcidin expression was inhibited by murine Twsg1 in the absence of additional BMP.[6] In vivo studies of Twsg1 expression were performed in healthy and thalassemic mice. Twsg1 expression was significantly increased in the spleen, bone marrow, and liver of the thalassemic animals. These data demonstrate that twisted gastrulation protein interferes with BMP-mediated hepcidin expression and may act with GDF15 to dysregulate iron homeostasis in thalassemia syndromes.[6]

Effects of thalassemia phenotypes

Iron overload develops rapidly in patients with thalassemia major, most of whom require regular erythrocyte transfusion therapy at an early age. Some patients with beta-thalassemia intermedia also develop iron overload. Thalassemia intermedia includes a wide and heterogeneous spectrum of globin defects, including homozygosity for β-mild mutations, double heterozygosity for β-thalassemia/HbE, double heterozygosity for β-mild and β-severe mutations, and compound heterozygosity for β-thalassemia and beta-globin chain variants such as HbE or HbC.[2,7] In patients with thalassemia intermedia who have not been transfused or who are transfused infrequently, iron overload, if any, develops slowly and is related principally to increased iron absorption due to ineffective erythropoiesis.[8] Most persons with beta-thalassemia minor do not develop iron overload unless they have coincidental abnormalities such as hemochromatosis-associated genotypes that increase iron absorption.[9,10] One patient with beta-thalassemia minor died of iron overload caused by chronic ingestion of iron supplements.[10]

Zimmerman *et al.* quantified red blood cell indices, serum iron measures, non-transferrin-bound iron, and GDF15 levels in Thai women heterozygous for beta-thalassemia, alpha-thalassemia 1, or HbE, and in control subjects and double beta-thalassemia/HbE heterozygotes.[11] Fractional iron absorption was measured from meals fortified with [57]Fe-labeled ferrous sulfate, and iron utilization was measured by the infusion of [58]Fe-labeled ferric citrate. The investigators observed that iron utilization was approximately 15% lower in alpha-thalassemia 1 and beta-thalassemia heterozygotes than in controls. When corrected for differences in serum ferritin, absorption was significantly higher in the alpha- and beta-thalassemia groups, but not the HbE heterozygotes, than in controls. Beta-thalassemia/HbE double heterozygotes had lower iron utilization and higher iron absorption and body iron than did controls. Non-transferrin-bound iron and GDF15 were higher in the double heterozygotes, but not in the other groups, than in the controls. They concluded that dietary iron absorption is not adequately down-regulated in alpha-thalassemia 1 and beta-thalassemia heterozygotes with ineffective erythropoiesis, despite a modest increase in body iron stores.[11]

Alpha-thalassemia is common in the Mediterranean region and in southeast Asia, where the predominant lesion is a deletion of one or more of the four gene loci responsible for alpha-globin chain production. In persons with alpha-thalassemia who have two or three alpha-globin genes that are normally functional, anemia and iron overload are rare. In US blacks, the overall gene frequency for alpha-thalassemia was estimated to be 0.07.[12] The −3.7 kb alpha-thalassemia deletion typical of alpha-thalassemia in African-Americans accounts for about one-third of the difference in the hemoglobin levels of African-Americans and whites.[13] The mean hemoglobin, mean corpuscular volume, and transferrin saturation levels of African-Americans were lower than those of whites; mean serum ferritin levels were higher.[13] Nonetheless, iron overload in African-Americans is very uncommon and not causally related to alpha-thalassemia (Chapter 18). In HbH disease, only one alpha-globin gene is normally functional, and the three mutant alpha-globin genes have reduced function. Excess alpha chains, precipitated in tetramers, cause hemolysis of circulating erythrocytes, but there is little ineffective erythropoiesis. Unless regularly transfused, most patients with HbH disease do not develop severe iron overload. Unusual patients with HbH disease and iron overload may have non-*HFE* hemochromatosis.[14]

Chronic erythrocyte transfusion

Each unit of red blood cells delivers 200–250 mg of iron via transfusion (Chapter 36). In patients without compensatory blood loss or treatment of iron overload, 10–20 units or more of transfused erythrocytes increases the risk of organ injury and dysfunction due to iron overload.

Thalassemia and *HFE* mutations

Some persons inherit hemochromatosis-associated *HFE* mutations and thalassemia syndromes, although the genes for these respective disorders are located on different chromosomes. It is plausible that there is synergy of co-inherited hemochromatosis and thalassemia alleles that could increase iron absorption, leading to more severe iron overload and possibly to a modification of the natural history of the illnesses of affected patients.[15]

Hemochromatosis patients with thalassemia alleles

In northern Italian subjects, Piperno *et al.* demonstrated that the beta-thalassemia trait aggravates the clinical picture of *HFE* C282Y homozygotes, favoring higher rates of iron accumulation and the development of severe iron-related complications. This implies that the otherwise mild risk of iron overload in some patients with *HFE* hemochromatosis-associated genotypes could be increased by co-inheritance of beta-thalassemia trait.[16] In another study of hemochromatosis subjects with *HFE* C282Y from Italy, Arruda *et al.* reported that beta-thalassemia trait might increase the severity of iron overload.[17] A C282Y homozygote with beta-thalassemia trait developed severe iron overload with complications after he ingested 153 g of inorganic iron as supplements over several years. His estimated fractional absorption of iron from the supplements was 20.9%.[9]

Severe thalassemia patients with *HFE* alleles

In a study of patients with severe thalassemia from Italy, the allele frequencies of C282Y and H63D were respectively 1.4% and 12.7% in patients and 1.1% and 11.4% in controls.[18] No case of C282Y homozygosity was recorded among these patients. There were no significant differences of serum ferritin, liver iron concentration, or the age at initiation of chelation in patients with and without *HFE* mutations, although a single patient with H63D homozygosity was severely iron-loaded. Longo *et al.* concluded that the presence of a single HFE mutation does not influence the severity of iron loading in thalassemia patients who follow a regular transfusion and chelation program.[18] In a study of southwest Iranian patients who required transfusion for beta-thalassemia and in control subjects, Karimi *et al.* reported that the H63D mutation was present with an allele frequency of 0.10 in newborns, 0.082 in normal adults, and 0.080 in the beta-thalassemia major populations, respectively. They observed no differences between normal adults and thalassemia major patients, suggesting that H63D does not increase mortality in beta-thalassemia. *HFE* C282Y and S65C were not detected in this study population.[19]

Thalassemia intermedia patients and *HFE* alleles

In a report from New Delhi, Sharma *et al.* studied 63 patients with thalassemia intermedia, including 48 subjects with beta-homozygous/heterozygous thalassemia intermedia and 15 with beta-thalassemia/HbE; age and transfusions were similar in both groups. Six

(12.5%) of the former and two (13.3%) of the latter were heterozygous for H63D; one H63D heterozygote was a 51-year-old man who had clinical features of hemochromatosis. Serum ferritin levels greater than 500 ng/dL were observed in all patients (100%) with H63D, and in 12/42 (28.6%) of patients without H63D ($P = 0.002$). Sharma *et al.* concluded that thalassemia intermedia patients with co-existent *HFE* H63D have a higher likelihood of developing iron overload and may require early iron chelation.[20]

Thalassemia trait and *HFE* alleles

In populations of Caucasian origin where hemochromatosis and thalassemia are common, the co-existence of the two disorders is not rare. For example, in northern Italy where the prevalence of *HFE* C282Y is about 10% and of beta-thalassemia alleles is approximately 3%, the expected probability of double heterozygosity for these two traits is 0.003. Studies from persons with beta-thalassemia trait in several populations summarized below suggest that the effect of common *HFE* alleles on iron metabolism, if any, is not great.

Piperno *et al.* studied serum iron measures in Italian persons heterozygous for *HFE* C282Y with and without beta-thalassemia trait. Their findings do not support the hypothesis that the association of the beta-thalassemia trait with a single C282Y or H63D allele might lead to iron overload.[16] Melis *et al.* evaluated the effect of the H63D mutation on the ferritin levels of 152 healthy Italian men who were heterozygous for beta-thalassemia.[21] Forty-five men were H63D heterozygotes and four were H63D homozygotes. Ferritin levels (mean ± SD) were 250 ± 138 μg/L in men with *HFE* wild-type genotype; 295 ± 186 μg/L in H63D heterozygotes; and 389 ± 75 μg/L in H63D homozygotes. Mean serum ferritin was significantly higher in men with H63D homozygosity than in men with a *HFE* wild-type genotype. This suggests that the H63D mutation may have a modulating effect on iron absorption.[21]

Martins *et al.* evaluated the effect of *HFE* C282Y, H63D, and S65C on iron measures of 101 Portuguese adults heterozygous for beta-thalassemia and 101 normal control subjects.[22] The respective allele frequencies of C282Y (1.5% vs. 3.5%), H63D (15.3% vs. 18.3%), and S65C (1.0% vs. 1.5%) did not differ significantly between beta-thalassemia carriers and normal controls. Serum iron levels and transferrin saturation were

235

increased in beta-thalassemia carriers heterozygous for H63D mutation ($P = 0.029$ and $P = 0.009$, respectively). The number of subjects with C282Y or S65C mutations was too low to conclude their effect on the iron status.

Garewal et al. determined the allele frequency of HFE C282Y and H63D and iron measures in 215 persons with beta-thalassemia trait and 60 normal control subjects in a north Indian population. The overall allele frequency of H63D was 9.09%; three subjects were H63D homozygotes. The difference in mean serum ferritin levels of persons with and without H63D was not significant in either group of subjects. Haplotyping of the homozygous H63D alleles revealed a pattern identical to that of Europeans. C282Y was not detected. Garewal et al. concluded that the presence of H63D does not increase serum ferritin in persons who have beta-thalassemia trait.[23]

Two Italian subjects with beta-thalassemia trait, hepatitis C, and iron overload were heterozygous for the HAMP promoter mutation −72C→T.[24]

Clinical manifestations

Severe anemia, transfusion dependency, ineffective erythropoiesis, and increased iron absorption appear in early infancy. All patients develop iron overload due to the combined effects of ineffective erythropoiesis and chronic erythrocyte transfusion.[25] Extramedullary hematopoiesis contributes to hepatomegaly, splenomegaly, and bone deformities. The rate of iron accumulation due to transfusion is 20–40 mg/d (0.3–0.7 mg/kg per day).[26] Regardless, periodic erythrocyte transfusion is necessary to sustain life, and decreases cardiomegaly, hepatomegaly, splenomegaly, and bone and orthodontic abnormalities, promotes growth until adolescence, and improves well-being.

Complications of iron overload in patients with severe thalassemia syndromes are similar to those in other patients with iron overload (Chapter 5), except that iron overload develops very early in life in severe thalassemia and resembles that in early age-of-onset hemochromatosis due to HJV mutations (Chapter 13). Hypogonadism was diagnosed in 55% of 578 patients with severe thalassemia who had reached the age of puberty: 83.5% of females and 78.6% of males with hypogonadism were receiving hormone replacement therapy.[27] Consequences of hypogonadism include subnormal growth, osteoporosis, delayed puberty, and infertility.[27–37] Some patients develop hypothyroidism or hypoparathyroidism.[38,39] Cardiac

iron overload is a major cause of morbidity and mortality.[40–43] Hepatic cirrhosis and primary liver cancer are also common, especially in patients with hepatitis C.[44] In the absence of adequate chelation therapy for iron overload, life expectancy is significantly shortened.[45] Timely institution of chelation therapy can increase survival significantly.[46] Therefore, regular monitoring for iron overload is necessary in all patients.

Management of iron overload

The Italian Society of Hematology commissioned a project to produce recommendations for the use of new technologies and iron chelators in thalassemia major and related disorders.[47] Providing recommendation for management of iron overload in thalassemia syndromes involves decisions that are multifactorial, and the metrics of which are variable and difficult to define accurately. In an attempt to consider all the factors that may affect these decisions, analytical hierarchy process, a multiple-criteria decision-making technique,[47] was applied in this study. The study design was graded using the system elaborated by the Scottish Intercollegiate Guideline Network (SIGN), which grades at the top metanalyses and randomized clinical trials. Other details of the study of the Italian Society of Hematology, including grading of tests and their prognostic value, are reported in their guidelines paper.[47] Herein, guidelines synthesized from this work are reproduced because they represent comprehensive, objective, practical, and outcomes-based advisories for medical practitioners involved in the care of patients with thalassemia major and related disorders with estimations of their respective levels of evidence. Additional discussion of topics pertinent to iron overload in thalassemia syndromes are presented in other chapters of this handbook, including diagnosis (Chapter 4), complications (Chapter 5), and management (Chapter 36).

Measures of body iron load requiring initiation of iron chelation therapy (Italian Society of Hematology)

"Patients with thalassemia major or related disorders in the early transfusional period, and with a known transfusional history, need to have serum ferritin levels determined 1–2 months apart in order to have a baseline value of iron load to use for initiating iron chelation therapy. Patients over 5 years of age and with an unknown previous transfusion history and/or inappropriate chelation therapy should have both serum ferritin and liver iron concentrations determined in order to plan iron chelation therapy. Liver biopsy with iron measurement by atomic absorption spectroscopy remains the gold standard for the assessment of liver iron concentration. Evidence of the accuracy of non-invasive methods for assessment of liver iron concentration is sufficient to recommend MRI technology as a feasible alternative to liver biopsy. R2 sequences and individual local calibration are recommended. SQUID remains a method to be reserved for experimental use since there is no calibration homogeneity and liver iron concentration could be underestimated."

When to start iron chelation therapy (Italian Society of Hematology)

"The panel judged that in children who have been regularly transfused, iron chelation should be started after they have received more than 10 units of blood, or with serum ferritin levels of >1000 μg/mL. In patients with an unknown previous transfusional history or inappropriate chelation therapy, iron chelation should be started when liver iron content is over the normal range of the method used."

First-line therapy in regularly transfused patients (Italian Society of Hematology)

"Children who start iron chelation therapy before 6 years of age, when the body iron burden is always modest, and in whom the goal of chelation therapy is the prophylactic maintenance of iron balance, should receive iron chelation with deferoxamine (level D). The better compliance of oral compounds make these new drugs attractive. The option of oral chelators in first-line therapy should, for the moment, be considered investigational and should only be performed within clinical trials or registries."

Monitoring iron chelation (Italian Society of Hematology)

"Patients undergoing iron chelation should receive periodic monitoring of serum ferritin. With a trend of increasing serum ferritin or decreasing serum ferritin below 1000 ng/mL, liver iron content should be assessed in order to avoid under- or over-treatment. Patients who have received determination of liver iron content before starting chelation therapy should repeat liver iron content every year during chelation therapy. In patients with a poor chelation history or in which liver iron content documents non-optimal chelation therapy, T2* MRI heart iron content should be monitored every year."

Switching to an alternative iron chelation therapy in patients uncompliant, intolerant, or refractory to DFO therapy (Italian Society of Hematology)

"For patients with evidence of non-compliance to deferoxamine, or with severe adverse effects from deferoxamine which preclude its use, but without existing or pending severe iron overload, an oral iron chelator should be used as an alternative to deferoxamine therapy (level D). The lack of studies comparing deferiprone with deferasirox in thalassemia major or related disorders did not allow the panel to recommend one of them on the basis of scientific evidence on long-term efficacy. The panel felt justified in recommending deferasirox as the alternative therapy to deferoxamine on the basis of its better safety profile compared with deferiprone (level D). Deferiprone should be considered in the case of resistance or intolerance to deferasirox (level D). Patients who develop severe iron overload (serum ferritin >3000 μg/mL maintained for 3 months at least, liver iron content higher than 15 mg/g dry weight, or heart T2*<12 ms) or overt iron-related cardiomyopathy (left ventricular ejection fraction <55%, arrhythmias, cardiac failure) should receive "intensive" or "combined" iron chelation therapy. The panel judged that the first choice for combined therapy is deferoxamine associated with deferiprone (level B). Patients who develop life-threatening cardiomyopathy should receive continuous intensive or combined chelation therapy."

"Ex-thalassemic" patients

Bone marrow transplantation (BMT) cures severe beta-thalassemia in some patients.[48] During BMT, some patients continue to be treated with iron chelation.[49] Patients who have undergone successful BMT have been called "ex-thalassemic after BMT," a term that underscores the cure of the genetic abnormality but maintenance of residual signs of organ damage

237

due to iron overload and dysfunction acquired during the pretransplant years.[50] Iron overload that persists after BMT is a major cause of morbidity and mortality. Cardiac function improves significantly after post-transplant treatment to reduce iron stores.[51] Myocardial and hepatic T2* magnetic resonance evaluation reveals significant reductions in the iron content of heart and liver in "ex-thalassemic" patients who had undergone iron depletion therapy.[52] In some patients in whom BMT has cured thalassemia, cirrhosis may be reversible after iron removal treatment.[53]

Spontaneous improvement

In early studies, spontaneous reversibility of liver iron overload, once the need for transfusions ceased when a functioning marrow graft had been established, was observed in the youngest patients, aged 1–8 years, whereas iron excess remained at the end of follow-up in many patients aged 9–15 years.[54] Possible explanations for this phenomenon include increased utilization of iron for hemoglobin synthesis, iron requirements for growth and development (especially in younger patients), laboratory iron losses during post-BMT monitoring, and increased unavoidable loss of iron typical of persons with iron overload of diverse causes.

Lucarelli *et al.* analyzed the extent and fate of tissue iron overload in 151 "ex-thalassemic after BMT" patients, according to the risk factors of hepatomegaly, hepatic portal fibrosis, and inadequate chelation therapy.[50] Serum ferritin concentrations decreased and unbound iron-binding capacity (UIBC) increased slowly during the years after the transplant. When analyzed according to risk group (assigned at the time of the transplant), serum ferritin and UIBC levels returned within the normal ranges only in the low-risk group (without hepatomegaly or portal fibrosis, and with adequate chelation pre-BMT). Ferritin and UIBC were still abnormal 7 years after the transplant in the moderate-risk group (those with one or two risk factors), and highly abnormal in the high-risk group (all three risk factors), indicating persistence of, respectively, moderate and severe iron overload at the time of transplant. In "ex-thalassemic" patients who were studied before and yearly after the transplant, the extent of iron overload, as judged by staining of liver biopsy samples, decreased during the years after transplant.[48] The degree of iron deposition and rate of post-BMT linear growth seem to influence rate of post-BMT decrease in tissue iron overload in different risk groups at the time of BMT.[48] Most patients who undergo BMT are transplanted with bone marrow or hematopoietic stem cells from first-degree relatives, many of whom are heterozygotes for beta-thalassemia or *HFE* alleles. Accordingly, some "ex-thalassemic" patients may have slightly increased iron absorption post-BMT.

Therapeutic phlebotomy

After BMT, "ex-thalassemic" patients have normal erythropoiesis capable of producing a hyperplastic response to phlebotomy so that this procedure can be contemplated as a method of mobilizing iron from overloaded tissues.[55] Angelucci *et al.* reported that 41 "ex-thalassemic" patients (mean age 16 ± 2.9 years) with prolonged follow-up (range 2–7 years) after BMT were submitted to a moderate intensity phlebotomy program (6 mL/kg blood withdrawal at 14-day intervals) to reduce iron overload. Serum ferritin decreased from a median of 2587 μg/L (range 2129–4817 μg/L) to 280 μg/L (range 132–920 μg/L) ($P < 0.0001$). Mean total transferrin increased from 2.34 ± 0.37 (SD) g/L to 2.9 ± 0.66 g/L ($P = 0.0001$). Mean transferrin saturation decreased from 90% ± 14% (SD) to 39% ± 34% ($P < 0.0001$). Median liver iron concentration evaluated on liver biopsy specimens decreased from 20.8 mg/g dry weight (range 15.5–28.1 mg/g dry weight) to 3.0 mg/g dry weight (0.9–14.6 mg/g dry weight) ($P < 0.0001$). Alanine aminotransferase decreased from 5.2 ± 3.4 to 1.6 ± 1.2 times the upper reference limit ($P < 0.0001$). The histological grading for chronic hepatitis (histology activity index) decreased from 4.2 ± 2.4 to 2.3 ± 1.8 ($P < 0.0001$). The investigators concluded that phlebotomy is a safe, efficient, and widely applicable method to decrease iron overload in "ex-thalassemic" patients.[55]

Mariotti *et al.* evaluated the reversibility of subclinical cardiac dysfunction during phlebotomy therapy to achieve iron depletion treatment (phlebotomy) in 32 "ex-thalassemic" patients cured of thalassemia by BMT.[51] These patients had altered left ventricular diastolic function and contractility, but they did not have clinical manifestations of heart failure. Seventeen patients underwent sequential echocardiographic evaluations during the phlebotomy program. After completion of the program, indices of contractility and diastolic function became normal.[51]

Iron chelation therapy

In eight patients undergoing BMT to cure severe thalassemia, intravenous deferoxamine therapy during BMT did not affect the engraftment parameters or the incidence of infections or graft-vs.-host disease.[49] No adverse effects were observed during the therapy. Therefore, patients with thalassemia major and heavy iron overload may be candidates for intravenous chelation therapy during the transplant period.[49]

Giardini *et al.* studied 18 heavily iron-loaded patients who had become "ex-thalassemics" after BMT with subcutaneous desferrioxamine therapy for 5–20 months.[56] The investigators observed reductions in serum ferritin concentrations, transferrin saturation values, and stainable liver iron obtained in follow-up biopsies. Serum concentrations of hepatic enzymes demonstrated trends toward normal values in all cases. Local skin reactions to desferrioxamine were the only toxicities observed. The investigators concluded that iron chelation is safe and effective therapy to reduce iron deposits in "ex-thalassemics" and represents a valid alternative to phlebotomy in selected patients.

References

1. Weatherall DJ. *The Thalassaemia Syndromes*. Oxford, Blackwell Scientific Publications, 2001.

2. Pippard MJ, Callender ST, Warner GT, Weatherall DJ. Iron absorption and loading in beta-thalassaemia intermedia. *Lancet* 1979; **2**: 819–21.

3. Pippard MJ. Secondary iron overload. In: Brock JHH, Powell LW, Halliday JW, Pippard MJ, eds. *Iron Metabolism in Health and Disease*. London, WB Saunders Co. Ltd. 1994; 271–309.

4. Tanno T, Bhanu NV, Oneal PA, *et al.* High levels of GDF15 in thalassemia suppress expression of the iron regulatory protein hepcidin. *Nat Med* 2007; **13**: 1096–101.

5. Vaulont S, Labie D. [Erythroblasts-derived GDF15 supresses hepcidin in thalassemia.] *Med Sci (Paris)* 2008; **24**: 139–41.

6. Tanno T, Porayette P, Sripichai O, *et al.* Identification of TWSG1 as a second novel erythroid regulator of hepcidin expression in murine and human cells. *Blood* 2009; **114**: 181–6.

7. Camaschella C, Mazza U, Roetto A, *et al.* Genetic interactions in thalassemia intermedia: analysis of beta-mutations, alpha-genotype, gamma-promoters, and beta-LCR hypersensitive sites 2 and 4 in Italian patients. *Am J Hematol* 1995; **48**: 82–7.

8. Bowdler AJ, Huehns ER. Thalassaemia minor complicated by excessive iron storage. *Br J Haematol* 1963; **9**: 13–24.

9. Barton JC, Lee PL, West C, Bottomley SS. Iron overload and prolonged ingestion of iron supplements: clinical features and mutation analysis of hemochromatosis-associated genes in four cases. *Am J Hematol* 2006; **81**: 760–7.

10. Barton JC, Acton RT, Anderson LE, Alexander CB. A comparison between whites and blacks with severe multi-organ iron overload identified in 16 152 autopsies. *Clin Gastroenterol Hepatol* 2009; **7**: 781–5.

11. Zimmermann MB, Fucharoen S, Winichagoon P, *et al.* Iron metabolism in heterozygotes for hemoglobin E (HbE), alpha-thalassemia 1, or beta-thalassemia and in compound heterozygotes for HbE/beta-thalassemia. *Am J Clin Nutr* 2008; **88**: 1026–31.

12. Johnson CS, Tegos C, Beutler E. Alpha-Thalassemia: prevalence and hematologic findings in American Blacks. *Arch Intern Med* 1982; **142**: 1280–2.

13. Beutler E, West C. Hematologic differences between African-Americans and whites: the roles of iron deficiency and alpha-thalassemia on hemoglobin levels and mean corpuscular volume. *Blood* 2005; **106**: 740–5.

14. Chim CS, Chan V, Todd D. Hemosiderosis with diabetes mellitus in untransfused Hemoglobin H disease. *Am J Hematol* 1998; **57**: 160–3.

15. Edwards CQ, Skolnick MH, Kushner JP. Coincidental non-transfusional iron overload and thalassemia minor: association with HLA-linked hemochromatosis. *Blood* 1981; **58**: 844–8.

16. Piperno A, Mariani R, Arosio C, *et al.* Haemochromatosis in patients with beta-thalassaemia trait. *Br J Haematol* 2000; **111**: 908–14.

17. Arruda VR, Agostinho MF, Cancado R, Costa FF, Saad ST. Beta-thalassemia trait might increase the severity of hemochromatosis in subjects with the C282Y mutation in the HFE gene. *Am J Hematol* 2000; **63**: 230.

18. Longo F, Zecchina G, Sbaiz L, Fischer R, Piga A, Camaschella C. The influence of hemochromatosis mutations on iron overload of thalassemia major. *Haematologica* 1999; **84**: 799–803.

19. Karimi M, Yavarian M, Delbini P, *et al.* Spectrum and haplotypes of the *HFE* hemochromatosis gene in Iran: H63D in beta-thalassemia major and the first E277K homozygous. *Hematol J* 2004; **5**: 524–7.

20. Sharma V, Panigrahi I, Dutta P, Tyagi S, Choudhry VP, Saxena R. *HFE* mutation H63D predicts risk of iron overload in thalassemia intermedia irrespective of blood transfusions. *Indian J Pathol Microbiol* 2007; **50**: 82–5.

21. Melis MA, Cau M, Deidda F, Barella S, Cao A, Galanello R. H63D mutation in the *HFE* gene increases

iron overload in beta-thalassemia carriers. *Haematologica* 2002; **87**: 242–5.

22. Martins R, Picanç I, Fonseca A, *et al.* The role of *HFE* mutations on iron metabolism in beta-thalassemia carriers. *J Hum Genet* 2004; **49**: 651–5.

23. Garewal G, Das R, Ahluwalia J, Marwaha RK. Prevalence of the H63D mutation of the *HFE* in north India: its presence does not cause iron overload in beta-thalassemia trait. *Eur J Haematol* 2005; **74**: 333–6.

24. Valenti L, Pulixi EA, Arosio P, *et al.* Relative contribution of iron genes, dysmetabolism, and hepatitis C virus (HCV) in the pathogenesis of altered iron regulation in HCV chronic hepatitis. *Haematologica* 2007; **92**: 1037–42.

25. Kattamis A, Papassotiriou I, Palaiologou D, *et al.* The effects of erythropoetic activity and iron burden on hepcidin expression in patients with thalassemia major. *Haematologica* 2006; **91**: 809–12.

26. Porter JB. Practical management of iron overload. *Br J Haematol* 2001; **115**: 239–52.

27. Borgna-Pignatti C, Rugolotto S, De Stefano P, *et al.* Survival and disease complications in thalassemia major. *Ann NY Acad Sci* 1998; **850**: 227–31.

28. Origa R, Fiumana E, Gamberini MR, *et al.* Osteoporosis in beta-thalassemia: clinical and genetic aspects. *Ann NY Acad Sci* 2005; **1054**: 451–6.

29. Shalitin S, Carmi D, Weintrob N, *et al.* Serum ferritin level as a predictor of impaired growth and puberty in thalassemia major patients. *Eur J Haematol* 2005; **74**: 93–100.

30. Borgna-Pignatti C, Rugolotto S, De Stefano P, *et al.* Survival and complications in patients with thalassemia major treated with transfusion and deferoxamine. *Haematologica* 2004; **89**: 1187–93.

31. Vogiatzi MG, Macklin EA, Trachtenberg FL, *et al.* Differences in the prevalence of growth, endocrine and vitamin D abnormalities among the various thalassaemia syndromes in north America. *Br J Haematol* 2009; **146**: 546–56.

32. Gamberini MR, De Sanctis, V, Gilli G. Hypogonadism, diabetes mellitus, hypothyroidism, hypoparathyroidism: incidence and prevalence related to iron overload and chelation therapy in patients with thalassaemia major followed from 1980 to 2007 in the Ferrara Centre. *Pediatr Endocrinol Rev* 2008; **6** Suppl 1: 158–69.

33. Kyriakou A, Savva SC, Savvides I, *et al.* Gender differences in the prevalence and severity of bone disease in thalassaemia. *Pediatr Endocrinol Rev* 2008; **6** Suppl 1: 116–22.

34. Vogiatzi MG, Macklin EA, Fung EB, *et al.* Bone disease in thalassemia: a frequent and still unresolved problem. *J Bone Miner Res* 2009; **24**: 543–57.

35. Fung EB, Harmatz PR, Lee PD, *et al.* Increased prevalence of iron-overload associated endocrinopathy in thalassaemia versus sickle-cell disease. *Br J Haematol* 2006; **135**: 574–82.

36. Skordis N, Michaelidou M, Savva SC, *et al.* The impact of genotype on endocrine complications in thalassaemia major. *Eur J Haematol* 2006; **77**: 150–6.

37. De Sanctis, V, Eleftheriou A, Malaventura C. Prevalence of endocrine complications and short stature in patients with thalassaemia major: a multicenter study by the Thalassaemia International Federation (TIF). *Pediatr Endocrinol Rev* 2004; **2** Suppl 2: 249–55.

38. Chern JP, Lin KH. Hypoparathyroidism in transfusion-dependent patients with beta-thalassemia. *J Pediatr Hematol Oncol* 2002; **24**: 291–3.

39. Filosa A, Di Maio S, Aloj G, Acampora C. Longitudinal study on thyroid function in patients with thalassemia major. *J Pediatr Endocrinol Metab* 2006; **19**: 1397–404.

40. Borgna-Pignatti C, Cappellini MD, De Stefano P, *et al.* Cardiac morbidity and mortality in deferoxamine- or deferiprone-treated patients with thalassemia major. *Blood* 2006; **107**: 3733–7.

41. Efthimiadis GK, Hassapopoulou HP, Tsikaderis DD, *et al.* Survival in thalassaemia major patients. *Circ J* 2006; **70**: 1037–42.

42. Schafer AI, Cheron RG, Dluhy R, *et al.* Clinical consequences of acquired transfusional iron overload in adults. *N Engl J Med* 1981; **304**: 319–24.

43. Tanner MA, Galanello R, Dessi C, *et al.* Myocardial iron loading in patients with thalassemia major on deferoxamine chelation. *J Cardiovasc Magn Reson* 2006; **8**: 543–7.

44. Borgna-Pignatti C, Vergine G, Lombardo T, *et al.* Hepatocellular carcinoma in the thalassaemia syndromes. *Br J Haematol* 2004; **124**: 114–17.

45. Borgna-Pignatti C, Rugolotto S, De Stefano P, *et al.* Survival and complications in patients with thalassemia major treated with transfusion and deferoxamine. *Haematologica* 2004; **89**: 1187–93.

46. Gabutti V, Piga A. Results of long-term iron-chelating therapy. *Acta Haematol* 1996; **95**: 26–36.

47. Angelucci E, Barosi G, Camaschella C, *et al.* Italian Society of Hematology practice guidelines for the management of iron overload in thalassemia major and related disorders. *Haematologica* 2008; **93**: 741–52.

48. Lucarelli G, Clift RA, Galimberti M, *et al.* Marrow transplantation for patients with thalassemia: results in class 3 patients. *Blood* 1996; **87**: 2082–8.

49. Gaziev D, Giardini C, Angelucci E, *et al.* Intravenous chelation therapy during transplantation for thalassemia. *Haematologica* 1995; **80**: 300–4.

50. Lucarelli G, Angelucci E, Giardini C, *et al.* Fate of iron stores in thalassaemia after bone marrow transplantation. *Lancet* 1993; **342**: 1388–91.

51. Mariotti E, Angelucci E, Agostini A, Baronciani D, Sgarbi E, Lucarelli G. Evaluation of cardiac status in iron-loaded thalassaemia patients following bone marrow transplantation: improvement in cardiac function during reduction in body iron burden. *Br J Haematol* 1998; **103**: 916–21.

52. Mavrogeni S, Gotsis ED, Berdousi E, *et al.* Myocardial and hepatic T2* magnetic resonance evaluation in ex-thalassemic patients after bone marrow transplantation. *Int J Cardiovasc Imaging* 2007; **23**: 739–45.

53. Muretto P, Angelucci E, Lucarelli G. Reversibility of cirrhosis in patients cured of thalassemia by bone marrow transplantation. *Ann Intern Med* 2002; **136**: 667–72.

54. Muretto P, Del Fiasco S, Angelucci E, De Rosa F, Lucarelli G. Bone marrow transplantation in thalassemia: modifications of hepatic iron overload and associated lesions after long-term engrafting. *Liver* 1994; **14**: 14–24.

55. Angelucci E, Muretto P, Lucarelli G, *et al.* Treatment of iron overload in the "ex-thalassemic." Report from the phlebotomy program. *Ann NY Acad Sci* 1998; **850**: 288–93.

56. Giardini C, Galimberti M, Lucarelli G, *et al.* Desferrioxamine therapy accelerates clearance of iron deposits after bone marrow transplantation for thalassaemia. *Br J Haematol* 1995; **89**: 868–73.

Chapter 22

Iron overload associated with hemoglobinopathies

The major cause of iron overload in persons with severe hemoglobinopathies is repeated transfusion of erythrocytes. Because body mechanisms to excrete iron are extremely limited, the short-term benefits of chronic transfusion are followed by the eventual development of iron overload and associated disorders. In some patients, especially those who also have thalassemia alleles (Chapter 21), dietary iron absorption is increased due to suppression of hepcidin production as a consequence of increased erythropoiesis or to mutations in iron regulatory genes. Prevention and treatment of iron overload in this heterogeneous group of patients has emerged as another clinical challenge in their management.

History

The advent of safe transfusion practices and the availability of erythrocytes for transfusion in some areas of the world during the twentieth century was associated with the development of iron overload in patients with several types of chronic anemia, including hemoglobinopathies. For more than five decades, the episodic use of erythrocyte transfusion to prevent or alleviate complications of hemolysis and intravascular sickling in African-Americans with sickle cell disease has increased. For more than three decades, systematic chronic erythrocyte transfusion has been used to decrease the incidence of recurrent stroke and premature death in sickle cell disease, especially in children. Hemoglobinopathy E, sometimes co-inherited with beta-thalassemia alleles, is very common in some Asian countries. Many patients require periodic erythrocyte transfusions to alleviate chronic severe anemia. Worldwide, chronic erythrocyte transfusion and improvement in other treatment modalities increase quality and length of life in some patients with severe hemoglobinopathy syndromes. Nonetheless, transfusion iron overload

was not widely recognized as a problem until 1981 when Schafer and colleagues reported details of 15 patients with severe non-thalassemia anemia.[1]

Clinical description

Patients who have received less than 12–15 units of packed erythrocytes (approximately ≤3 g Fe; serum ferritin concentration ≤1000 µg/L) typically have no symptoms attributable to iron overload. With iron overload of greater severity, weakness, malaise, and fatigue become increasingly prevalent. Some patients develop non-specific abnormalities such as palpitations, tachycardia, dyspnea on exertion, or mild hepatomegaly that suggest iron overload of the heart or liver. With severe iron overload, symptoms and signs of congestive heart failure, cirrhosis, diabetes mellitus, or cutaneous hyperpigmentation may appear. Some patients develop unusual or frequent infections, often by bacteria that require large quantities of iron. In children who have received much transfusion, growth retardation and delayed sexual development are common.

In many patients, manifestations of iron overload mimic those of the underlying severe hemoglobinopathy. For example, sickle cell disease causes chronic anemia of variable severity, diverse complications caused mainly by intravascular erythrocyte sickling, and increased susceptibility to infection in patients without iron overload. The clinical manifestations vary widely according to genotype, and differ greatly among patients with the same genotype. Chronic anemia alone may cause palpitations, tachycardia, or dyspnea on exertion. Repeated infarction of the myocardium or liver due to intravascular sickling can stimulate or potentiate the effects of severe iron overload. Autosplenectomy, neutrophil and macrophage abnormalities, and other host conditions may lead to increased frequency or severity of infections in patients with or without iron overload. In combined hemoglobinopathy/thalassemia syndromes such as double heterozygosity for hemoglobin E and beta-thalassemia, severe chronic anemia is the major clinical problem in untransfused patients. Other abnormalities related to chronic anemia or extramedullary hematopoiesis include leg ulcers, bone deformities, variable degrees of splenomegaly and hypersplenism, and compression of the brain or spinal cord due to tumorous masses of extramedullary hematopoietic tissue. Transfused patients with sickle cell disease had a significantly lower prevalence of diabetes mellitus, hypogonadism, and growth failure than patients with severe thalassemia.[2] The prevalence of these complications in patients with sickle cell disease with and without regular transfusion therapy did not differ significantly, suggesting that the underlying disease may modulate iron-related endocrine injury.[2]

In a natural history study, transfused patients with sickle cell disease were hospitalized more frequently than non-transfused sickle cell disease patients or subjects with severe thalassemia.[3] Among the transfused patients with sickle cell disease, those who died began transfusion earlier (age 12 years vs. 25 years) and chelation therapy later (age 14 years vs. 27 years) than did those who survived. The death rate in this sample of transfused adults with either sickle cell disease or severe thalassemia was three times greater than that of the general US population.[3] Another study analyzed the clinical and autopsy findings in 141 adult African-Americans with sickle cell disease.[4] The mean age at death was 36 ± 11 years. Leading circumstances of death included pulmonary hypertension (26%), sudden death (23%), renal failure (23%), infection (18%), thromboembolism (15%), cardiac diagnoses (12%), cirrhosis (11%), pneumonia or acute chest syndrome (10%), bleeding (8%), and iron overload (7%). When circumstances of deaths that occurred after 1991 were compared to those that occurred in 1991 or earlier, pulmonary hypertension was significantly more common patients who died in 1992 or later. Significant associations were also found between pulmonary hypertension and thromboembolism, and between cirrhosis and iron overload.[4]

Genetics

Hemoglobin comprises two polypeptide subunits derived from genes in the alpha gene cluster on chromosome 16 and two polypeptide subunits derived from genes in the beta gene cluster on chromosome 11, along with a heme moiety. Severe hemoglobinopathies are caused by mutations in the genes that encode the alpha or beta-globin chains. Such mutations affect primarily qualitative aspects of normal adult hemoglobin (Hb A). This tetramer consists of two alpha chains and two beta chains ($\alpha_2\beta_2$). Hemoglobin S (Hb S) is the most common hemoglobinopathy worldwide and is the predominant hemoglobin in persons with sickle cell disease. This disease-producing polymorphism alters the beta-globin chain, giving the molecule the globin structure, $\alpha_2\beta^S_2$. Hb S heterozygotes have no anemia and few, if any, clinical manifestations. "Classical" sickle cell disease is due to homozygosity for the Hb S mutation (sickle cell anemia). The Hb S polymorphism is best known in natives of sub-Saharan Africa and their descendants. Analyses of linked polymorphisms and other haplotype characteristics demonstrate that this mutation arose at least twice in west and other areas of sub-Saharan Africa. The Hb S allele also arose independently in the Near and Middle East and in India. For reasons that are incompletely understood, sickle cell anemia and other sickling syndromes are sometimes more severe in persons of sub-Saharan African descent than in persons of other ancestry with the same hemoglobinopathy genotype.

Hemoglobin E (Hb E), the second most common hemoglobinopathy worldwide, is also caused by a beta-globin gene mutation. Hb E is especially common in southeast Asia. Heterozygosity is benign; homozygosity for Hb E results in mild hemolytic anemia and splenomegaly. Hemoglobin C (Hb C), is common in persons of sub-Saharan African descent. Heterozygosity for Hb C is benign; homozygous Hb C disease ($\alpha_2\beta^C_2$) is associated with mild hemolytic anemia and splenomegaly. Patients with Hb SC disease are compound heterozygotes for single Hb S and Hb C mutations that are inherited from their respective parents. They have a sickling disorder that is generally similar to that in patients with sickle cell anemia for which transfusion therapy may be required. Many other hemoglobinopathy syndromes are caused by compound heterozygosity for Hb S and an alpha or another beta-globin chain mutation.[5] These conditions are much less prevalent worldwide than Hb SS or Hb SC disease, although some are common in certain regions. Uncommon hemoglobinopathy syndromes associated with iron overload include Hb S/Hb D-Punjab, Hb D, and Hb Olympia.[6–8]

243

Thalassemia genes variably reduce alpha or beta-globin chain production, respectively. Therefore, the co-inheritance of hemoglobin mutations and thalassemia alleles results in disorders in which there are both quantitative and qualitative abnormalities of Hb A. Patients with Hb S/beta-thalassemia inherit an allele for Hb S from one parent and an allele for beta-thalassemia from the other, and thus are double heterozygotes. This condition also causes a clinical phenotype of sickle cell disease, the severity of which is determined largely by the quantity of Hb A produced by the beta-thalassemia allele. If the thalassemia allele produces no normal hemoglobin (β^0-thalassemia), the condition (Hb S/β^0-thalassemia) is clinically indistinguishable from "classical" sickle cell anemia ($\alpha_2\beta^S_2$). Other patients produce a small amount of Hb A and thus have Hb S/β^+-thalassemia that is less severe than sickle cell anemia. In addition, there are many genetic variants of β^0-thalassemia and β^+-thalassemia alleles, many with clinically appreciable or distinctive manifestations.[5,9] Double heterozygosity for Hb E and beta-thalassemia alleles causes one of the most important hemoglobinopathies in the world. This condition is sometimes classified as moderately severe thalassemia (thalassemia intermedia), although many patients have a clinical syndrome indistinguishable from that of severe beta-thalassemia. The severity of the clinical phenotype varies greatly according to genetic heterogeneity of thalassemia alleles and other factors, some of which are not understood.[5,9]

Laboratory findings

Evaluation of abnormal hemoglobin or thalassemia

Electrophoresis techniques are the routine means of identifying hemoglobin variants. These methods induce differential migration of normal and abnormal hemoglobin components due to dissimilarities in their molecular charge. Proportions of the hemoglobin components can also be quantified. Migration patterns are diagnostic characteristics of many common hemoglobinopathy syndromes in patients who require chronic transfusion therapy, especially those with Hb SS, Hb SC, Hb S/β-thalassemia, Hb C/β-thalassemia, or Hb E/β-thalassemia.

In patients with Hb S/β^0-thalassemia, electrophoresis shows no Hb A. Patients with Hb S/β^+-thalassemia have an amount of Hb A that depends on the level of function of their β^+-thalassemia allele. Altogether, electrophoresis in Hb S/β-thalassemia reveals 60%–90% Hb S, 0%–30% Hb A, increased levels of Hb $A_{2(\alpha_2\delta_2)}$, and 1%–15% Hb $F_{(\alpha_2\gamma_2)}$. In Hb C/β^+-thalassemia there is 65%–80% Hb C; the remainder is Hb A and 2%–5% Hb F. In Hb C/β^0-thalassemia, Hb A is absent. Many patients with Hb E/β-thalassemia have β^0-thalassemia alleles. Electrophoresis shows Hb E, a high percentage of Hb F ($\sim$50%), and usually no Hb A. In patients with Hb E/β-thalassemia who have β^+-thalassemia alleles, Hb A is present in variable amounts.

Tentative laboratory diagnoses must be corroborated by evaluation of erythrocyte morphology, erythrocyte counts and indices, presence or absence of splenomegaly, red blood survival estimates, and details of patient and family history. Comparison of unusual patient electrophoresis specimens with samples from first-degree family members or unrelated patients with defined hemoglobinopathy or thalassemia disorders is often helpful. In unusual cases, referral of patient specimens and those of first-degree family members to university reference laboratories for additional electrophoresis procedures or DNA-based analyses is necessary.

Evaluation of iron overload

Monitoring patients who receive regular erythrocyte transfusions is commonly performed by measuring their serum ferritin concentration every 3 months. In African-American children with sickle cell disease in a stroke prevention trial, Files and colleagues reported that serum ferritin levels increased linearly with cumulative transfusion volume during the first four ferritin measurements, but the rate of increase varied widely among patients.[10] Rates of increase varied similarly among patients who received exclusively simple transfusions with packed erythrocytes and in patients who received exchange transfusions. Ferritin levels continued to increase linearly after the first four measurements in 40%, but there was a plateau before serum ferritin reached 3000 µg/L in the remaining 60%. The ferritin level never reached 3000 ng/dL in 20% of those with a linear increase. Intra-patient correlation declined at transfusion volumes of more than 250 mL of transfused erythrocytes/kg.[10]

Direct assessments of iron stores are needed in many patients because the correlation of serum ferritin levels with organ iron content and iron overload severity is imperfect.[10] Hepatic iron stores in a specimen of liver obtained by percutaneous biopsy can be quantified using atomic absorption spectrometry and otherwise evaluated with histochemical staining techniques to highlight iron deposits, fibrosis, and other microanatomical features. Non-invasive evaluation of liver and cardiac iron content can also be performed using MRI techniques (Chapter 4). T2 relaxation time is a reliable method for the assessment of iron deposition in the liver in patients with sickle cell disease; results for the heart become reliable only after there is heavy iron deposition.[11] In a few locations, estimates of liver and cardiac iron content can be made using a superconducting quantum interference device (SQUID) (Chapter 4). Additional tests of target organ function are often indicated to assess management needs.[12] Routine clinical measurement of serum concentrations of hepatic enzymes, glucose, and pituitary trophic hormones or performance of electrocardiography and other heart-related functional studies are helpful, but are no substitute for measuring serum ferritin levels or organ iron content.

Evaluation of iron regulatory genes

DNA-based evaluation is indicated in patients with hemoglobinopathy who develop iron overload that is disproportionately great for the extent of previous erythrocyte transfusion, and in patients whose phenotype or family characteristics suggest hemochromatosis or other heritable iron overload disorder. There are limited observations in this area of interest.

African-Americans comprise a large, diverse subpopulation group in which sickle cell disease is common. Heterozygosity and homozygosity for HFE C282Y occurs in approximately 2.2% and 0.01%, respectively, of African-Americans; these genotypes are due to admixture with whites.[13,14] In African-American patients with sickle cell disease, the prevalence of the common HFE C282Y and H63D mutations is similar to that observed in African-American control subjects.[15] These mutations were not associated with the degree of iron overload in patients with sickle cell disease receiving chronic transfusion therapy.[15]

Hb E syndromes are very common in Thailand.[16] Viprakasit and colleagues evaluated 380 normal controls from Bangkok for the HFE C282Y, H63D, and IVS5+1 G→A alleles.[16] They also determined HFE genotypes in 70 patients with homozygous Hb E disease and correlated their genotypes with levels of serum ferritin. They observed a mean H63D allele frequency of 3% (range 1%–5%) and a single individual who was heterozygous for the HFE splice site mutation IVS5+1 G→A. HFE C282Y was not detected. Among Hb E homozygotes, there was no significant difference in mean serum ferritin level in those with, and in those without, HFE H63D. Hb E homozygotes have mild hemolytic anemia and do not require routine erythrocyte transfusion. The mean serum ferritin concentrations in these subjects (137 ± 78 μg/L vs. 116 ± 128 μg/L, respectively) confirms that they had little or no iron overload. The paucity of these HFE mutations in the Thai population indicate that they are unlikely to explain hyperferritinemia and iron loading in individuals with Hb E-related disorders.[16] Likewise, HFE C282Y or other pathogenic HFE mutations are rare in many other racial and ethnic groups worldwide.[13,17–19] This suggests that these mutations probably do not influence substantially the risk that other non-European whites with severe hemoglobinopathy or hemoglobinopathy/thalassemia syndromes will develop non-transfusion iron overload.

African-Americans with non-transfusion iron overload who were heterozygous for HFE C282Y, Hb S, Hb C, or alpha or beta-thalassemia alleles had more severe iron overload, on the average, than did those without these alleles.[20] A non-transfused African-American man with sickle cell disease and hemochromatosis-like iron overload had human leukocyte antigen haplotypes typical of northern Europeans,[21] suggesting that he had HFE hemochromatosis. Another non-transfused African-American man with sickle cell anemia developed iron overload.[22] A promoter mutation of the ALAS2 gene that encodes erythrocyte-specific aminolevulinic acid synthase was detected in one woman with sickle cell anemia who had iron overload that was inadequately explained by erythrocyte transfusion.[23]

Hepcidin, a low-molecular weight peptide produced in the liver, is the major, direct regulator of iron absorption from the intestine and iron release from macrophage and hepatocyte stores. The receptor of hepcidin is ferroportin, an iron exporter expressed on enterocytes (basolateral surfaces), macrophages, hepatocytes, and placental cells. In health, hepcidin binds to ferroportin and promotes its internalization and destruction within cells and their consequent retention of iron. Relative or absolute deficiency of hepcidin permits increased iron absorption from enterocytes and increased ferroportin export of iron from macrophages into plasma. Abnormal hepcidin metabolism in some patients with hemoglobinopathy or thalassemia increases iron absorption from the intestine, thereby exacerbating iron overload due to erythrocyte transfusion. These results are consistent with observations in a 1979 report of inorganic iron absorption in five subjects with thalassemia major and one with thalassemia intermedia.[24] Iron absorption increased as the hemoglobin concentration decreased, although iron absorption was much higher at any given hemoglobin level in the subject with thalassemia intermedia than in the subjects with thalassemia major. In the latter, ~10% of iron was absorbed at hemoglobin concentrations of 9–10 g/dL and ~2.7% at hemoglobin concentrations between 11–13 g/dL. The percentage of iron absorbed could be predicted from the nucleated red blood cell count.[24]

In children with sickle cell anemia, urine levels of hepcidin were suppressed and inversely associated with the rate of erythropoiesis.[25] In patients with thalassemia major, there was a significant positive correlation of liver hepcidin mRNA levels with hemoglobin concentration and an inverse correlation with erythropoiesis measures. Urine hepcidin levels were disproportionately suppressed for the severity of iron overload. This suggests that hepcidin expression is regulated mainly by increased erythropoietic activity, rather than by the severity of iron overload.[26] In thalassemia intermedia, increased erythropoiesis is associated with severe hepcidin deficiency. The relative lack of hepcidin causes increased absorption of dietary iron, relative iron depletion of macrophages, and somewhat lower serum ferritin concentrations. In thalassemia major, transfusions decreased the rate of erythropoiesis and increase iron overload, thereby promoting relatively higher hepcidin levels. In the presence of higher hepcidin levels, dietary iron absorption is moderated and macrophages retain iron, contributing to higher serum ferritin levels.[27] During erythroblast maturation, there is increased expression and secretion of growth/differentiation factor 15 (GDF15), a member of the transforming growth factor-beta superfamily. Serum from thalassemia patients suppressed hepcidin mRNA expression in primary human hepatocytes, and depletion of GDF15 reversed hepcidin suppression. These results suggest that GDF15 over expression arises from an expanded erythroid compartment and contributes to iron overload in thalassemia syndromes by inhibiting hepcidin expression.[28]

Geographic distribution and prevalence

The prevalence of iron overload in patients with severe hemoglobinopathy depends primarily on the availability and administration of transfusion, and the co-inheritance of thalassemia alleles. Approximately 1 in 625 African-American neonates are homozygous for Hb S. Sickle cell anemia is much less prevalent in older African-Americans than in neonates due to early mortality associated with the disease. In African-American adults, the prevalence of Hb SC is approximately the same as that of Hb SS.[5] Hb S/β-thalassemia occurs mainly in persons of sub-Saharan African native ancestry (including those in the US and the Caribbean), in Mediterranean peoples (especially in Greece, Italy, and Turkey), in the Middle East, and in parts of India.[5,9,29] Other less common types of sickle cell disease contribute to the overall prevalence of sickling disorders in African-Americans and in other population subgroups.[5]

Stroke, a major complication of sickle cell disease, affects approximately 11% of patients by age 20 years;[30] at-risk patients can be identified by transcranial Doppler examinations. Regular transfusions significantly reduce the incidence of stroke in at-risk children, but risk increases after transfusions are discontinued.[31–33] Some patients receive transfusions to alleviate other complications. Transfusion iron overload is an important cause of morbidity and mortality in such patient populations.[4,34] In contrast, only 27% of Senagalese patients with sickle cell anemia who made regular visits to a specialty clinic and staff received erythrocyte transfusions (typically for specific complications), but collectively the patients had infrequent medical problems, good levels of socioeconomic function, and increased longevity.[35]

Hb C/β-thalassemia occurs mainly in sub-Saharan African natives and their ancestors; the Hb C/β⁰-thalassemia variant is associated with severe anemia and splenomegaly. Hb E/β-thalassemia is very common in Thailand and in southeast Asia, including Malaysia, Indonesia, and Burma, and in parts of the Indian subcontinent.[5,9,36–39] Prevalence estimates are lacking for most regions, although large case series have been reported. In 1969, for example, Wasi and colleagues estimated that there were probably

~49 000 patients or potential patients with this disorder in Thailand alone.[36] In 1966, Chatterjea reported 526 cases in Indian Hindus in Calcutta, and another 48 cases in Bengalese Muslims.[40]

Prevention and treatment

Prevention

Iron absorption is increased in many patients with severe hemoglobinopathy or thalassemia due to a relative or absolute decrease in their hepcidin levels. This suggests that decreasing dietary iron absorption may significantly reduce the rate of iron loading in such patients. de Alarçon and colleagues measured iron absorption in five subjects with thalassemia major and one with thalassemia intermedia.[24] Tea reduced inorganic iron absorption by 41%–95%. Corresponding findings have been reported in patients with *HFE* hemochromatosis, in whom there is also a relative decrease in hepcidin levels.[41] These observations indicate that patients with severe hemoglobinopathy or thalassemia should not consume excessive dietary iron or take iron supplements.

Cazzola and colleagues demonstrated that moderate transfusion may allow more effective prevention of iron loading in patients with severe thalassemia than hypertransfusion, with higher likelihood of spontaneous pubertal development and without producing excessive expansion of erythropoiesis.[42] Patients with severe hemoglobinopathies, with or without thalassemia alleles, are likely to respond in a similar manner. In patients with sickle cell disease, rates of increase in serum ferritin levels varied similarly among 23 patients who received exclusively simple transfusion with packed erythrocytes and in five patients who received exchange transfusions.[10] Altogether, this suggests that a moderate rate of transfusion is more important in ameliorating severe anemia and in slowing the rate of iron accumulation than is the manner in which the erythrocytes are transfused. Nonetheless, leukodepleted, washed, or frozen red blood cells should be administered to patients receiving chronic transfusion therapy to avoid various transfusion reactions.

One approach to the prevention of transfusion iron overload is the selective transfusion of young erythrocytes (neocytes).[43] Young red blood cells are less dense and have a longer life-span than do erythrocytes in routine donor units because the latter contain a greater proportion of older, more dense erythrocytes (gerocytes). Radiochromium studies in splenectomized thalassemia major patients revealed an average half-life of 47 days for neocytes stored in the frozen state and an average half-life of 30 days for standard frozen red blood cells.[43] Thus, it was proposed that neocytes could decrease the frequency or quantity of red blood cell transfusion by approximately 50% in patients with sickle cell disease or severe thalassemia, and thus forestall the development of transfusion iron overload.[43,44] A two-period study compared transfusions of standard erythrocytes versus neocytes in the same group of 18 severe thalassemia patients.[45] There was a reduction in transfusion requirements in all patients during the neocyte period of the study. The total annually transfused red blood cells and concomitant iron delivery by transfusion were reduced by approximately 20%, respectively, but the outcomes varied across patients. Seven of the 18 patients had a relatively large reduction in blood consumption (25%–35%), nine others had reductions of 11%–22%, and two others had less than 10% reduction.[45] Altogether, it is possible to produce neocyte-enriched erythrocyte units for transfusion using a variety of techniques in special blood centers. The neocytes have a higher survival rate in vivo than do normal donor erythrocytes. Nonetheless, studies involving substantial numbers of patients have not shown sufficient positive results to justify the expense and technical expertise required to produce neocyte-enriched units on a broad scale.[46]

Treatment

Patients with severe hemoglobinopathy or thalassemia are intolerant of therapeutic phlebotomy because they have severe anemia. Therefore, treatment of iron overload in such cases has necessarily focused on strategies to mobilize and remove excessive iron, particularly that stored in vital target organs, especially the heart, liver, and anterior pituitary gland. The mainstay of such treatments is iron chelating drugs.

Deferoxamine (desferrioxamine, DFO), a parenterally administered iron chelator, has been used for many years to treat patients with sickle cell disease. Because the half-life of DFO is very short, standard treatment involves a stringent infusion routine that is necessary for optimal iron chelation and excretion. Treatment should begin by the time the serum ferritin level is 1000 µg/L. The initial dose is usually 20 mg/kg 5 nights each week given subcutaneously using a portable infusion pump. Oral vitamin C (100 mg daily in small children; 200 mg daily in older children or adults) increases iron excretion in patients receiving DFO therapy.[47] DFO mobilizes iron deposited in parenchymal cells and macrophages; iron mobilization from the heart occurs less rapidly than that from the liver and other sites.[48] Urinary iron excretion often wanes after several consecutive days of DFO infusion, but usually returns to higher rates after several days off therapy. Lack of patient compliance and physician dissatisfaction are major impediments to successful DFO therapy in patients with sickle cell disease.[49] Even in patients who are fully compliant with DFO treatment, chronic transfusion permits few "vacations" from DFO treatment. These realities have led to intensive efforts to develop satisfactory oral iron chelators.

Deferiprone (DFP) is an oral iron chelator approved in many countries for treatment of iron overload in severe beta-thalassemia; it is not presently available in the US. During short-term treatment, DFP can maintain negative iron balance in patients who require transfusion. In addition, DFP can remove pathologic iron deposits from sickle cells in vitro and in vivo. At "standard" doses, DFP significantly reduced serum ferritin levels and measures of hepatic iron content.[50] Regardless, there was no significant correlation of serum ferritin levels, liver and heart iron measures, and left ventricular ejection fraction. Compliance with DFP therapy was good, and there were no significant adverse effects.[50] It has been proposed that deferasirox could eventually replace DFO as the "standard" therapy for iron overload associated with sickle cell anemia.[51]

Deferasirox (DFX) is a once-daily, oral iron chelator developed for treating transfusion iron overload. The kidney was a potential target organ of DFX toxicity in preclinical and clinical studies,[52] and some some patients with sickle cell disease have impaired renal function.[53] The safety and tolerability of DFX in pediatric and adult patients with sickle cell disease was generally good. Some patients experienced transient nausea, vomiting, diarrhea, abdominal pain, or skin rash. DFX therapy was sometimes associated with mild non-progressive increases in serum creatinine and reversible elevations in serum concentrations of hepatic enzymes. Discontinuation rates from DFX (11.4%) and DFO (11.1%) were similar. Over 1 year, similar dose-dependent reductions in liver iron concentrations were observed with DFX and DFO.

Prospective trials are needed to assess if DFP at 100 mg/kg per day can be given long term with safety, and if it will result in more effective iron chelation in patients inadequately treated with 75 mg/kg per day. Results of DFX monotherapy and doublet therapy with DFO and either DFP or DFX are needed to determine if cardiac iron deposits are more susceptible to chelation with these oral drugs than with DFO, and if cardiac mortality rates can be reduced further, especially in patients with severe thalassemia syndromes. Randomized trials designed to compare DFP and DFX therapy will help to refine presently available knowledge regarding optimal use of these drugs. Long-term survival and safety data for DFP and DFX therapy of young persons are needed, including investigations to determine the molecular basis of adverse events of oral chelation therapy such as agranulocytosis, arthralgias, elevated hepatic transaminase levels, and elevated serum creatinine concentrations.[52,54]

Erythrocytapheresis can be used as an automated method of erythrocyte exchange, especially in patients with sickle cell disease at risk for stroke. Treatment reduces Hb S levels, prevents further iron accumulation, decreases body iron burdens, and eliminates the need for DFO therapy in some patients, including children.[4,34,55–59] Long-term erythrocytapheresis therapy was associated with significantly greater cardiac dysfunction than was detected in non-transfused patients, possibly due to greater pretreatment iron overload in patients managed with erythrocytapheresis.[60]

References

1. Schafer AI, Cheron RG, Dluhy R, et al. Clinical consequences of acquired transfusional iron overload in adults. *N Engl J Med* 1981; **304**: 319–24.

2. Fung EB, Harmatz PR, Lee PD, et al. Increased prevalence of iron-overload associated endocrinopathy in thalassaemia versus sickle cell disease. *Br J Haematol* 2006; **135**: 574–82.

3. Fung EB, Harmatz P, Milet M, et al. Morbidity and mortality in chronically transfused subjects with thalassemia and sickle cell disease: A report from the multicenter study of iron overload. *Am J Hematol* 2007; **82**: 255–65.

4. Darbari DS, Kple-Faget P, Kwagyan J, Rana S, Gordeuk VR, Castro O. Circumstances of death in adult sickle cell disease patients. *Am J Hematol* 2006; **81**: 858–63.

5. Bunn HF, Forget BG. *Hemoglobin: Molecular, Genetic and Clinical Aspects*. Philadelphia, WB Saunders Company, 1986.

6. Wearer GA, Rahbar S, Ellsworth CA, de Alarçon PA, Forbes GB, Beutler E. Iron overload in three generations of a family with hemoglobin Olympia, *Gastroenterology* 1984; **87**: 695–702.

7. Eriksson S, Lindmark B, Hanik L. A Swedish family with alpha 1-antitrypsin deficiency, haemochromatosis, haemoglobinopathy D and early death in liver cirrhosis. *J Hepatol* 1986; **2**: 65–72.

8. Jiskoot PM, Halsey C, Rivers R, Bain BJ, Wilkins BS. Unusual splenic sinusoidal iron overload in sickle cell/haemoglobin D-Punjab disease. *J Clin Pathol* 2004; **57**: 539–40.

9. Weatherall DJ, Clegg JB. The β and δβ thalassaemias in association with structural haemoglobin variants. *The Thalassaemia Syndromes*. Oxford, Blackwell Scientific Publications. 1981; 320–95.

10. Files B, Brambilla D, Kutlar A, *et al.* Longitudinal changes in ferritin during chronic transfusion: a report from the Stroke Prevention Trial in Sickle Cell Anemia (STOP). *J Pediatr Hematol Oncol* 2002; **24**: 284–90.

11. Voskaridou E, Douskou M, Terpos E, *et al.* Magnetic resonance imaging in the evaluation of iron overload in patients with beta-thalassaemia and sickle cell disease. *Br J Haematol* 2004; **126**: 736–42.

12. Barton JC, McDonnell SM, Adams PC, *et al.* Management of hemochromatosis. Hemochromatosis Management Working Group. *Ann Intern Med* 1998; **129**: 932–9.

13. Adams PC, Reboussin DM, Barton JC, *et al.* Hemochromatosis and iron-overload screening in a racially diverse population. *N Engl J Med* 2005; **352**: 1769–78.

14. Barton JC, Acton RT, Dawkins FW, *et al.* Initial screening transferrin saturation values, serum ferritin concentrations, and *HFE* genotypes in whites and blacks in the Hemochromatosis and Iron Overload Screening Study. *Genet Test* 2005; **9**: 231–41.

15. Jeng MR, Adams-Graves P, Howard TA, Whorton MR, Li CS, Ware RE. Identification of hemochromatosis gene polymorphisms in chronically transfused patients with sickle cell disease. *Am J Hematol* 2003; **74**: 243–8.

16. Viprakasit V, Vathesathokit P, Chinchang W, *et al.* Prevalence of *HFE* mutations among the Thai population and correlation with iron loading in haemoglobin E disorder. *Eur J Haematol* 2004; **73**: 43–9.

17. Merryweather-Clarke AT, Pointon JJ, Shearman JD, Robson KJ. Global prevalence of putative haemochromatosis mutations. *J Med Genet* 1997; **34**: 275–8.

18. Mortimore M, Merryweather-Clarke AT, Robson KJ, Powell LW. The haemochromatosis gene: a global perspective and implications for the Asia-Pacific region. *J Gastroenterol Hepatol* 1999; **14**: 838–43.

19. Pointon JJ, Viprakasit V, Miles KL, *et al.* Hemochromatosis gene (*HFE*) mutations in southeast Asia: a potential for iron overload. *Blood Cells Mol Dis* 2003; **30**: 302–6.

20. Barton JC, Acton RT, Rivers CA, *et al.* Genotypic and phenotypic heterogeneity of African-Americans with primary iron overload. *Blood Cells Mol Dis* 2003; **31**: 310–19.

21. Conrad ME. Sickle cell disease and hemochromatosis. *Am J Hematol* 1991; **38**: 150–2.

22. Castro O, Hasan O, Kaur K, Loyevsky M, Gordeuk V. Hemochromatosis in non-transfused African-American patient with sickle cell anemia. *Blood* 1998; **92** (suppl): 13b.

23. Barton JC, Lee PL, Bertoli LF, Beutler E. Iron overload in an African-American woman with SS hemoglobinopathy and a promoter mutation in the X-linked erythroid-specific 5-aminolevulinate synthase (*ALAS2*) gene. *Blood Cells Mol Dis* 2005; **34**: 226–8.

24. de Alarcon PA, Donovan ME, Forbes GB, Landaw SA, Stockman JA, III. Iron absorption in the thalassemia syndromes and its inhibition by tea. *N Engl J Med* 1979; **300**: 5–8.

25. Kearney SL, Nemeth E, Neufeld EJ, *et al.* Urinary hepcidin in congenital chronic anemias. *Pediatr Blood Cancer* 2007; **48**: 57–63.

26. Kattamis A, Papassotiriou I, Palaiologou D, *et al.* The effects of erythropoetic activity and iron burden on hepcidin expression in patients with thalassemia major. *Haematologica* 2006; **91**: 809–12.

27. Origa R, Galanello R, Ganz T, *et al.* Liver iron concentrations and urinary hepcidin in beta-thalassemia. *Haematologica* 2007; **92**: 583–8.

28. Tanno T, Bhanu NV, Oneal PA, *et al.* High levels of GDF15 in thalassemia suppress expression of the iron regulatory protein hepcidin. *Nat Med* 2007; **13**: 1096–101.

29. Serjeant GR, Ashcroft MT, Serjeant BE. The clinical features of haemoglobin SC disease in Jamaica. *Br J Haematol* 1973; **24**: 491–501.

30. Ohene-Frempong K, Weiner SJ, Sleeper LA, *et al.* Cerebrovascular accidents in sickle cell disease: rates and risk factors. *Blood* 1998; **91**: 288–94.

31. Adams RJ, McKie VC, Brambilla D, *et al.* Stroke prevention trial in sickle cell anemia. *Control Clin Trials* 1998; **19**: 110–29.

32. Adams RJ, Brambilla DJ, Granger S, *et al.* Stroke and conversion to high risk in children screened with

transcranial Doppler ultrasound during the STOP Study. *Blood* 2004; **103**: 3689–94.

33. Lee MT, Piomelli S, Granger S, *et al.* Stroke Prevention Trial in Sickle Cell Anemia (STOP): extended follow-up and final results. *Blood* 2006; **108**: 847–52.

34. Ballas SK. Iron overload is a determinant of morbidity and mortality in adult patients with sickle cell disease. *Semin Hematol* 2001; **38**: 30–6.

35. Diop S, Mokono SO, Ndiaye M, Toure Fall AO, Thiam D, Diakhate L. [Homozygous sickle cell disease in patients above 20 years of age: follow-up of 108 patients in Dakar.] *Rev Med Interne* 2003; **24**: 711–15.

36. Wasi P, Na-Nakorn S, Pootrakul S, *et al.* Alpha- and beta-thalassemia in Thailand. *Ann NY Acad Sci* 1969; **165**: 60–82.

37. Rees DC, Styles L, Vichinsky EP, Clegg JB, Weatherall DJ. The hemoglobin E syndromes. *Ann NY Acad Sci* 1998; **850**: 334–43.

38. Agarwal S, Gulati R, Singh K. Hemoglobin E-beta-thalassemia in Uttar Pradesh. *Indian Pediatr* 1997; **34**: 287–92.

39. Khanh NC, Thu LT, Truc DB, Hoa DP, Hoa TT, Ha TH. Beta-thalassemia/Haemoglobin E disease in Vietnam. *J Trop Pediatr* 1990; 43–5.

40. Chatterjea JB. Haemoglobinopathies, glucose-6-phosphate dehydrogenase deficiency and allied problems in the Indian subcontinent. *Bull World Health Organ* 1966; **35**: 837–56.

41. Kaltwasser JP, Werner E, Schalk K, Hansen C, Gottschalk R, Seidl C. Clinical trial on the effect of regular tea drinking on iron accumulation in genetic haemochromatosis. *Gut* 1998; **43**: 699–704.

42. Cazzola M, Borgna-Pignatti C, Locatelli F, Ponchio L, Beguin Y, De Stefano P. A moderate transfusion regimen may reduce iron loading in beta-thalassemia major without producing excessive expansion of erythropoiesis. *Transfusion* 1997; **37**: 135–40.

43. Klein HG. Transfusions with young erythrocytes (neocytes) in sickle cell anemia. *Am J Pediatr Hematol Oncol* 1982; **4**: 162–5.

44. Anderson J, Lay H. Neocyte transfusions for thalassemia major. *Transfusion* 1982; **22**: 539.

45. Spanos T, Ladis V, Palamidou F, *et al.* The impact of neocyte transfusion in the management of thalassaemia. *Vox Sang* 1996; **70**: 217–23.

46. Montoya AF. Neocyte transfusion: a current perspective. *Transfus Sci* 1993; **14**: 147–56.

47. Pippard MJ, Letsky EA, Callender ST, Weatherall DJ. Prevention of iron loading in transfusion-dependent thalassaemia. *Lancet* 1978; **1**: 1178–81.

48. Anderson LJ, Wonke B, Prescott E, Holden S, Walker JM, Pennell DJ. Comparison of effects of oral deferiprone and subcutaneous desferrioxamine on myocardial iron concentrations and ventricular function in beta-thalassaemia. *Lancet* 2002; **360**: 516–20.

49. Treadwell MJ, Law AW, Sung J, *et al.* Barriers to adherence of deferoxamine usage in sickle cell disease. *Pediatr Blood Cancer* 2005; **44**: 500–7.

50. Voskaridou E, Douskou M, Terpos E, *et al.* Deferiprone as an oral iron chelator in sickle cell disease. *Ann Hematol* 2005; **84**: 434–40.

51. Okpala I. Investigational agents for sickle cell disease. *Expert Opin Investig Drugs* 2006; **15**: 833–42.

52. Barton JC. Deferasirox Novartis. *Curr Opin Investig Drugs* 2005; **6**: 327–35.

53. Vichinsky E, Onyekwere O, Porter J, *et al.* A randomized comparison of deferasirox versus deferoxamine for the treatment of transfusional iron overload in sickle cell disease. *Br J Haematol* 2007; **136**: 501–8.

54. Barton JC. Chelation therapy for iron overload. *Curr Gastroenterol Rep* 2007; **9**: 74–82.

55. Adams DM, Schultz WH, Ware RE, Kinney TR. Erythrocytapheresis can reduce iron overload and prevent the need for chelation therapy in chronically transfused pediatric patients. *J Pediatr Hematol Oncol* 1996; **18**: 46–50.

56. Hartwig D, Schlager F, Bucsky P, Kirchner H, Schlenke P. Successful long-term erythrocytapheresis therapy in a patient with symptomatic sickle cell disease using an arterio-venous fistula. *Transfus Med* 2002; **12**: 75–7.

57. Hilliard LM, Williams BF, Lounsbury AE, Howard TH. Erythrocytapheresis limits iron accumulation in chronically transfused sickle cell patients. *Am J Hematol* 1998; **59**: 28–35.

58. Kim HC, Dugan NP, Silber JH, *et al.* Erythrocytapheresis therapy to reduce iron overload in chronically transfused patients with sickle cell disease. *Blood* 1994; **83**: 1136–42.

59. Singer ST, Quirolo K, Nishi K, Hackney-Stephens E, Evans C, Vichinsky EP. Erythrocytapheresis for chronically transfused children with sickle cell disease: an effective method for maintaining a low hemoglobin S level and reducing iron overload. *J Clin Apher* 1999; **14**: 122–5.

60. Raj AB, Condurache T, Bertolone S, Williams D, Lorenz D, Sobczyk W. Quantitative assessment of ventricular function in sickle cell disease: effect of long-term erythrocytapheresis. *Pediatr Blood Cancer* 2005; **45**: 976–81.

Chapter 23

Iron overload associated with pyruvate kinase deficiency

Pyruvate kinase (PK) deficiency (OMIM #266200) is caused by mutations in the *PKLR* gene that encodes PK (chromosome 1q21). This disorder is the most common erythrocyte enzyme defect that causes hereditary non-spherocytic hemolytic anemia.[1,2] It is transmitted as an autosomal recessive trait. On the basis of gene frequency, it was estimated that the prevalence of homozygous PK deficiency is 51 cases per million in the US white population.[3] Based on data in a health registry, it was estimated that the prevalence of PK deficiency in northern England is 3.3 per million.[4] PK deficiency has a worldwide distribution, but may be more common among individuals of northern European descent. Herein, the pathophysiology of PK deficiency is discussed. The clinical manifestations of this disorder are reviewed with emphasis on the complication of iron overload.

Etiology and pathogenesis

Mature erythrocytes depend on the glycolytic production of adenosine triphosphate (ATP) to meet metabolic requirements. Deficiencies in several glycolytic enzymes can result in hemolytic anemia. These types of hemolytic anemia are not associated with a distinctive morphologic abnormality of erythrocytes, and thus are known collectively as congenital non-spherocytic hemolytic anemias. Most of these disorders are rare and are transmitted as autosomal recessive disorders.

PK deficiency is the most common erythrocyte glycolytic enzymopathy.[1,2] The predominant PK isoenzyme present in erythrocytes is the R form, encoded by *PKLR*. Multiple mutations can lead to PK deficiency, and the type of mutation may determine in part the severity of the clinical phenotype.

The cause of hemolysis is presumed to be the lack of cellular ATP that, over time, leads to cell lysis. Spleens removed from persons with PK deficiency reveal large numbers of reticulocytes rather than senescent erythrocytes. The reason that some reticulocytes are entrapped by the spleen whereas others survive normally is unclear. This phenomenon may be a random event, or it may be due to variation in PK activity in individual reticulocytes.

Clinical and laboratory manifestations

Fatigue, decreased physical endurance, pallor, anemia, jaundice, and splenomegaly are typical manifestations of PK deficiency. Skin ulcers occur infrequently, but may affect multiple members of the same kindred.[5] The severity of anemia and hemolysis in persons with PK deficiency is variable, ranging from mild compensated anemia to severe life-threatening hemolysis requiring regular erythrocyte transfusions.[1,2] Macrocytosis and reticulocytosis are prominent in come cases. Shrunken, spiculated erythrocytes or acanthocytes are sometimes present. In other cases, the blood smear may not reveal significant abnormalities. The osmotic fragility test is normal and the autohemolysis test is usually abnormal; as many as 50% of erythrocytes may lyse after incubation in saline for 48 hours. Individuals in the same kindred usually have similar degrees of hemolysis, anemia, and PK laboratory phenotypes, although PK analyses vary widely across kinships. Prenatal or neonatal mortality may lower the frequency with which PK deficiency is found in the population at large. Under diagnosis or misdiagnosis is also likely, even when PK assays are performed.[3,4]

Many patients with PK deficiency develop iron overload,[6–8] and this complication may be severe in young patients who have not received transfusion.[9] In typical cases, both transferrin saturation and serum ferritin levels are elevated.[6–8] Excessive iron is deposited predominantly in hepatocytes. Magnetic resonance imaging can be used to estimate liver iron concentrations.[9] Some patients develop cirrhosis due to severe hepatic iron loading.[8]

Genetics

Patients with PK deficiency in consanguineous kinships are usually homozygotes for a single *PKLR* allele.[10] Founder effects for some *PKLR* mutations have been identified in genetically isolated populations.[11,12] In case series of PK deficiency, diverse mutations, many novel, have been reported.[13–15] Thus, many patients with PK deficiency are compound heterozygotes for two different pathogenic *PKLR* alleles.

Iron overload

Etiology

Iron overload may occur in persons with PK deficiency who have received few or no red blood cell transfusions.[6,7,16] Increased absorption of iron is mediated by ineffective erythropoiesis through growth development factor 15 (GDF15), a bone marrow-derived factor that abrogates hepcidin-mediated protection from iron overload under conditions of increased or ineffective erythropoiesis.[17] (Chapter 2). In PK deficiency, serum hepcidin concentrations are positively correlated with hemoglobin and negatively with serum GDF15 levels.[17] Some reports suggest that ingestion of large doses of ascorbic acid may enhance iron absorption and increase the risk of iron overload in some patients.[18,19]

Non-transfused PK deficiency subjects with *HFE* C282Y or H63D had serum ferritin and transferrin saturation values significantly higher than those with a wild-type *HFE* genotype.[20] Of 12 adult non-transfused patients with increased iron measures, one was a C282Y homozygote, one was a compound C282Y/H63D heterozygote, three were H63D heterozygotes, and seven had a normal *HFE* genotype. Serum ferritin and transferrin saturation were not related to hemoglobin, reticulocyte, and bilirubin measures.[20] Serum ferritin concentration was independently associated with age and gender, but not with splenectomy and *HFE* genotypes. The retrospective evaluation of the iron status profile of ten patients (three with abnormal and seven with wild-type *HFE* genotypes) with at least 10 years of follow-up showed that overt iron accumulation requiring iron chelation had occurred only in the three patients with *HFE* mutations (two of whom were splenectomized).[20] Chronic erythrocyte transfusion exacerbates iron overload caused by increased absorption in some patients.

Management

Serum iron measures should be monitored in all patients with PK deficiency and anemia; magnetic resonance imaging of the liver can be used to estimate liver iron concentrations.[9] Splenectomy controls or alleviates anemia, hemolysis, and complications such as cholelithiasis in some patients. A paradoxical increase in reticulocytosis sometimes occurs after splenectomy despite improvement in erythrocyte survival and decrease in markers of hemolysis (e.g. hyperbilirubinemia). Iron absorption and transfusion requirements may decrease in patients who experience benefits of splenectomy.

Therapeutic phlebotomy can be performed carefully in patients whose hemoglobin level is normal or in whom anemia is mild. Erythropoietin levels are presumed to be elevated in persons with PK deficiency who have hemolysis, as they are in animal models of PK deficiency.[21] There are some reports of cases in which erythropoietin was administered to patients with PK deficiency with the intent of increasing their hemoglobin levels and thus enable phlebotomy therapy.[22,23] The potential advantages of such an approach, if any, have not been carefully studied in large numbers of patients. In many patients, therapeutic phlebotomy is not feasible because anemia is too severe. In such cases, iron chelation therapy should be considered (Chapter 36).

References

1. Zanella A, Fermo E, Bianchi P, Valentini G. Red cell pyruvate kinase deficiency: molecular and clinical aspects. *Br J Haematol* 2005; **130**: 11–25.

2. Zanella A, Bianchi P, Fermo E. Pyruvate kinase deficiency. *Haematologica* 2007; **92**: 721–3.

3. Beutler E, Gelbart T. PK deficiency prevalence and the limitations of a population-based survey. *Blood* 2000; **96**: 4006.

4. Carey PJ, Chandler J, Hendrick A, *et al*. Prevalence of pyruvate kinase deficiency in northern European population in the north of England. Northern Region Haematologists Group. *Blood* 2000; **96**: 4005–6.

5. Muller-Soyano A, Tovar de Roura E, Duke PR, *et al*. Pyruvate kinase deficiency and leg ulcers. *Blood* 1976; **47**: 807–13.

6. Salem HH, van der Weyden MB, Firkin BG. Iron overload in congenital erythrocyte pyruvate kinase deficiency. *Med J Aust* 1980; **1**: 531–2.

7. Zanella A, Berzuini A, Colombo MB, *et al*. Iron status in red cell pyruvate kinase deficiency: study of Italian cases. *Br J Haematol* 1993; **83**: 485–90.

8. Hilgard P, Gerken G. Liver cirrhosis as a consequence of iron overload caused by hereditary non-spherocytic hemolytic anemia. *World J Gastroenterol* 2005; **11**: 1241–4.

9. Andersen FD, d'Amore F, Nielsen FC, van Solinge W, Jensen F, Jensen PD. Unexpectedly high but still asymptomatic iron overload in a patient with pyruvate kinase deficiency. *Hematol J* 2004; **5**: 543–5.

10. Kanno H, Fujii H, Hirono A, Miwa S. cDNA cloning of human R-type pyruvate kinase and identification of a single amino acid substitution (Thr384–Met) affecting enzymatic stability in a pyruvate kinase variant (PK Tokyo) associated with hereditary hemolytic anemia. *Proc Natl Acad Sci USA* 1991; **88**: 8218–21.

11. Muir WA, Beutler E, Wasson C. Erythrocyte pyruvate kinase deficiency in the Ohio Amish: origin and characterization of the mutant enzyme. *Am J Hum Genet* 1984; **36**: 634–9.

12. Larochelle A, De Braekeleer M, Marceau D, de Medicis E. *Miami Short Reports. Advances in Gene Technology: The Molecular Biology of Human Genetic Disease.* New York, IRL Press, 1991.

13. Baronciani L, Beutler E. Molecular study of pyruvate kinase deficient patients with hereditary non-spherocytic hemolytic anemia. *J Clin Invest* 1995; **95**: 1702–9.

14. Baronciani L, Bianchi P, Zanella A. Hematologically important mutations: red cell pyruvate kinase (2nd update). *Blood Cells Mol Dis* 1998; **24**: 273–9.

15. Pissard S, Max-Audit I, Skopinski L, *et al.* Pyruvate kinase deficiency in France: a 3-year study reveals 27 new mutations. *Br J Haematol* 2006; **133**: 683–9.

16. Boivin P, Galand C. [Iron overload in congenital hemolytic anemia caused by pyruvate kinase deficiency. A major late complication.] *Presse Med* 1990; **19**: 1087–90.

17. Finkenstedt A, Bianchi P, Theurl I, *et al.* Regulation of iron metabolism through GDF15 and hepcidin in pyruvate kinase deficiency. *Br J Haematol* 2009; **144**: 789–93.

18. Rowbotham B, Roeser HP. Iron overload associated with congenital pyruvate kinase deficiency and high dose ascorbic acid ingestion. *Aust NZ J Med* 1984; **14**: 667–9.

19. Bett JH, Wilkinson RK, Boyle CM. Iron overload associated with congenital pyruvate kinase deficiency and high dose ascorbic acid ingestion. *Aust NZ J Med* 1985; **15**: 270.

20. Zanella A, Bianchi P, Iurlo A, *et al.* Iron status and *HFE* genotype in erythrocyte pyruvate kinase deficiency: study of Italian cases. *Blood Cells Mol Dis* 2001; **27**: 653–61.

21. Richard RE, Weinreich M, Chang KH, Ieremia J, Stevenson MM, Blau CA. Modulating erythrocyte chimerism in a mouse model of pyruvate kinase deficiency. *Blood* 2004; **103**: 4432–9.

22. Zachee P, Staal GE, Rijksen G, De Bock R, Couttenye MM, De Broe ME. Pyruvate kinase deficiency and delayed clinical response to recombinant human erythropoietin treatment. *Lancet* 1989; **1**: 1327–8.

23. Vukelja SJ. Erythropoietin in the treatment of iron overload in a patient with hemolytic anemia and pyruvate kinase deficiency. *Acta Haematol* 1994; **91**: 199–200.

Iron overload associated with congenital dyserythropoietic anemias

The term congenital dyserythropoietic anemia (CDA) encompasses a group of rare heritable disorders characterized by anemia, ineffective erythropoiesis, structural and functional abnormalities of erythroblasts and mature erythrocytes, and increased iron absorption. CDA type I is the second most prevalent subtype (OMIM #224120). CDA type II is the most common subtype (OMIM #224100). CDA type II is often described by the acronym HEMPAS (hereditary erythroblastic multinuclearity with positive acidifed serum test). The clinical manifestations of these two subtypes of CDA are reviewed herein with an emphasis on the complication of iron overload.

General characteristics

Characteristics shared by patients with various subtypes of CDA include ease of fatigue, pallor, scleral icterus, jaundice, and splenomegaly. Some patients have abnormal fingernails or toenails, abnormal shapes or size of bones in the feet, or scoliosis. Circulating erythrocytes are often macrocytic and may have abnormal expression of membrane antigens. The bone marrow typically reveals erythroid hyperplasia, CDA erythroblasts are often enlarged, and have abnormal nuclear contours, nuclear fragmentation (karyorrhexis), or multinuclearity. In some patients with CDA, the rate of erythrocyte destruction is increased, resulting in anemia, reticulocytosis, and hyperbilirubinemia.

Congenital dyserythropoietic anemia type I (OMIM #224120)

Clinical manifestations

The median age at diagnosis is about 17 years (range birth to about age 45 years).[1] In a study of 70 Israeli Bedouin patients with CDA type I, 64% had identifiable abnormalities at birth.[2] The most common abnormalities among these 45 newborns were anemia (100%), hepatomegaly (65%), jaundice (53%), small size for gestational age (24%), pulmonary hypertension (15%), direct hyperbilirubinemia, elevated serum levels of hepatic transaminases (13%), and transient thrombocytopenia (6%). Eighty percent of newborns required red blood cell transfusion during the first month of life. After age 4 months, 11% still required transfusions.[2] Anemia was more severe in women than in men.[3]

Physical examination abnormalities may include any combination of the following: patches of brown skin discoloration, *pectus carinatum* (pigeon chest deformity), scoliosis with duplication of vertebrae, splenomegaly (~80% of patients), hypoplasia or absence of fingernails or toenails, syndactyly, or missing fingers or toes or extra metatarsal bones (acrodysostosis).[1,4–6]

Laboratory abnormalities

Blood smears reveal abnormal variation in the size of red blood cells (anisocytosis), abnormal variation in the shape of red blood cells (poikilocytosis), stippled red cells containing RNA precipitated during staining, and the presence of nucleated red blood cells.[1,4] Reticulocyte indices and serum levels of indirect-reacting (unconjugated) bilirubin are typically elevated, consistent with hemolysis. Microscopic examination of the bone marrow reveals erythroid hyperplasia; megaloblastic erythroblasts; abnormal shapes and increased numbers of nuclei in erythroblasts; and occasional erythroblasts with multiple nuclei that are connected by thin chromatin bridges. Erythroblasts demonstrate S-phase arrest.[5] Electron microscopy of erythroblasts shows a characteristic "Swiss cheese" appearance of the nuclear chromatin.[1,4,5] Granulocytopoiesis and megakaryocytopoiesis is normal. Some macrophages in the bone marrow appear filled with lipid material.

Iron abnormalities

Iron overload in excess of the amount transfused with red blood cells occurs in most patients with CDA type I. The severity of iron loading is highly variable. Serum ferritin values in many iron-loaded adults with CDA type I are 600–1500 µg/mL. Liver biopsy specimens reveal heavy iron deposition in both hepatocytes and Kupffer cells.[7]

It was presumed for a long time that ineffective erythropoiesis in CDA type I stimulates increased iron absorption that causes non-transfusion iron overload.[4,7] A subsequent study revealed that hepcidin production was suppressed in a patient with CDA type I.[8] In another report, mean levels of growth development factor 15 (GDF15) were approximately 40-fold higher in patients with CDA type I than in healthy volunteer control subjects.[9] GDF15 levels were correlated significantly with measures of hepcidin-25, serum ferritin, and hepcidin-25/ferritin ratios. These results demonstrate that patients with CDA type I express very high levels of serum GDF15, and that GDF15 contributes to the inappropriate suppression of hepcidin. This would explain increased iron absorption in CDA type I.[9] HFE genotypes that account for increased iron absorption are not usually detected in patients with CDA type I,[3,7] although an unusual patient was homozygous for HFE C282Y.[10]

Clinical course

The course of CDA type I is often indolent but some patients develop heart failure, liver failure, or infections. Chronic hyperbilirubinemia may contribute to the development of gallstones and cholecystitis. Delayed puberty is common in adolescents with CDA type I.[3] Adults with this disorder are fertile. Splenectomy does not result in improvement of hemoglobin parameters.[4] Five patients were treated with interferon alpha-2a, and all responded with a rise in hemoglobin concentration of 2.5 to 3.5 g/dL. Ages at death range from the neonatal period to age 57 years.[3] Reported causes of death in patients with CDA type I include heart or liver failure, severe iron overload, invasive squamous cell carcinoma, and septicemia.

Genetics

CDA type I is inherited as an autosomal recessive condition that is due to mutations in the CDAN1 gene (chromosome 15q15.1–q15.3) that encodes codanin-1. In the fruit fly Drosophila, the orthologous gene product is thought to be important in cell cycling and survival. In humans, codanin-1 is a cell cycle-regulated protein active in the S phase,[11] but its precise function remains unknown.

Patients with CDA type I have been described in European, Arab, and French Polynesian kinships. The clinical features of patients who have sporadic CDA type I are heterogeneous.[5] This could be explained by the CDAN1 genotype heterogeneity in sporadic cases.[12] In Israeli Bedouins, a single founder missense mutation (CDAN1 R1040W) was identified in a large number of cases and could explain the phenotype similarity observed in many affected persons.[2] The majority of other reported pathogenic CDAN1 mutations are missense alleles; others are either splice-site or nonsense mutations.[5] Null mutations that would result in the absence of any activity of the codanin-1 gene product have not been reported, suggesting that absence of the gene product may be lethal. Mutations in a gene not linked to chromosome 15q may produce a phenocopy of CDA type I.[12]

Treatment

Anemia

Red blood cell transfusions usually are required in neonates. The hematocrit often stabilizes at 24%–33% in older patients, so transfusions may not be required. Treatment with vitamins, erythropoietin, or prednisone does not improve the anemia of patients with CDA-type I. Splenectomy does not induce durable elevation of hemoglobin and hematocrit values, although it may decrease hemolysis in some patients.[4] Some patients who underwent splenectomy developed thrombocytosis and resultant splanchnic or other serious deep vein thromboses.[4]

Therapy with recombinant interferon-α2a therapy has been tested in patients who have CDA type I and II. In six patients who received either interferon-α2a (9 million units weekly), or pegylated interferon-α2a (50 µg weekly), all experienced a rise in their plasma hemoglobin concentration of 2.5 to 3.5 g/dL (increased hematocrit of 7%–10%).[2] The hemoglobin increased 4 weeks after the initiation of therapy. In two patients who discontinued interferon therapy, hemoglobin values declined to pre-treatment values.[2] The serum and erythrocyte ferritin levels of a 9-year-old patient treated with interferon decreased progressively, and remained inversely correlated with hemoglobin levels.

Repeated liver biopsies revealed that hepatic iron overload resolved.[13] Other investigators observed that patients with CDA type I obtained no benefit from interferon therapy.[14]

Iron overload

Iron loading is expected to occur independent of transfusions. Phlebotomy therapy is tolerated by some patients whose anemia is not severe. Phlebotomy therapy may involve the withdrawal of 200–400 mL of whole blood every 4–6 weeks, rather than the much more aggressive phlebotomy schedule that is preferred for *HFE* hemochromatosis patients who have normal hemoglobin levels and rates of erythropoiesis. Iron chelation with either deferoxamine or deferiprone has been employed to deplete the excessive iron stores of patients with CDA type I, usually starting when the serum ferritin concentration reaches 1000 µg/mL.[4,15]

Congenital dyserythropoietic anemia type II (OMIM #224100)

Clinical manifestations

The mean age at presentation was 5 years (1 month to 25 years) in 98 patients with CDA type II.[16] The age at diagnosis ranged from age 4 months to 65 years (average 16 years old). One patient in a different series was not diagnosed until age 78 years.[17] The wide range of ages between the time of the first presentation of symptoms and the age at which the diagnosis is established indicates that there is difficulty in recognizing this rare disorder. The most common presenting symptom or sign is jaundice (53%).

Laboratory abnormalities

At diagnosis, 66% of patients have anemia. Characteristics of anemia include mean hemoglobin concentration of approximately 8.3 g/dL; average mean corpuscular volume of 86 fL; and mean absolute reticulocyte count of 109×10^9/L. The average serum total bilirubin concentration was elevated (4.6 mg/dL). Individuals in whom the diagnosis was established after age 16 years had an average hemoglobin concentration of 10.1 g/dL. The result of hemoglobin electrophoresis in adults with CDA type II is expected to reveal a predominance of normal hemoglobin A.

Blood smears of patients who have CDA type II reveal prominent anisocytosis, poikilocytosis, and basophilic stippling of erythrocytes. The mean corpuscular volume is usually normal, not increased. Red blood cell survival in the circulation is about 20% to 50% shorter than in normal persons. Red blood cells from patients with CDA type II lyse readily in acidified serum, in contrast to those of normal subjects, and thus the acidified serum test can be used as a diagnostic aid. CDA type II red blood cells agglutinate in the presence of serum that contains an IgM antibody that reacts with the fetal *i* protein that persists on their surface membranes. Serum that contains anti-*I* also agglutinates red blood cells of patients who have CDA type II. The erythrocytes of some patients who have some other types of anemia (e.g. sickle cell anemia) that have persistence of the fetal *i* and *I* antigens are not expected to undergo agglutination when mixed with serum that contains anti-*i* or anti-*I* antibodies. Erythrocytes from patients with CDA type II do not undergo increased lysis in an isotonic solution of sucrose (the sucrose lysis test).[1] White blood cell counts and platelet counts typically are normal in CDA type II.

The bone marrow reveals severe erythroid hyperplasia characteristic of ineffective erythropoiesis. Erythroid precursors are not megaloblastic, but 20%–45% of erythroblasts contain two nuclei; some are multinucleate.[17] Granulocytopoiesis and megakaryocytopoiesis are normal. Lipid-laden macrophages are present in most patients. Electron microscopy shows a double membrane inside the cytoplasmic membrane of bone marrow erythroblasts; this represents persistent endoplasmic reticulum.[17]

Some patients with CDA type II were mistakenly diagnosed to have thalassemia, hereditary spherocytosis, hemolytic anemia, iron deficiency and hepatitis, hemoglobinopathy C, thiamine-responsive anemia with diabetes and deafness, pyruvate kinase deficiency, congenital myelodysplasia, folate or vitamin B_{12} deficiency, acute myelogenous leukemia, hairy cell leukemia, or infection with parvovirus B19.[1,4] Many of these disorders can be distinguished from CDA type II by age at presentation, history, physical examination findings, or the results of laboratory evaluation.

Clinical course

Among 64 neonates with CDA type II, 15 (23%) had a hemoglobin concentration less than 8 g/dL; two-thirds of these infants required red blood cell transfusions. Splenomegaly occurred in 68 of 88 infants (77%). Jaundice was present in 55% of infants. Sixteen percent had gallstones. Unlike CDA type I, congenital malformations are unusual in CDA type II. Growth is usually normal in children and adolescents who have CDA type II. Gallstones were identified in 22 of 39 (56%) of patients younger than age 40.[17] Aplastic crises due parvovirus B19 have been observed in some patients.[18] Rarely, paravertebral extramedullary hematopoietic tissue develops.[17] Among adults with CDA type II, 6% were transfusion-dependent; of these, 60% were heterozygous for β-thalassemia alleles.[16] Some patients with CDA type II die of multi-organ iron overload.[17]

Iron overload

Iron loading occurs independently of transfusions due to increased absorption of iron associated with ineffective erythropoiesis.[19–21] This is presumed to be mediated by increase GDF15 expression and hepcidin suppression as has been demonstrated in CDA type I. Serum transferrin saturation and ferritin levels are usually elevated.[17,19,20,22,23] In an exceptional case, serum ferritin levels were normal, but the iron content of liver and spleen biopsy specimens was approximately 6–12 times normal.[21] Liver biopsy specimens reveal severe iron deposition in hepatocytes and in Kupffer cells. Non-transfusion iron overload in CDA type II is not typically related to inheritance of common HFE alleles.[4,19,23] Red blood cell transfusions increase iron overload in some cases.

Genetics

CDA type II is inherited as an autosomal recessive trait that is due to mutations in the SEC23B gene located on chromosome 20q11.2. SEC23B encodes an essential component of coat protein complex II (COPII)-coated vesicles that transport secretory proteins from the endoplasmic reticulum (ER) to the Golgi complex.[24] Schwarz et al. demonstrated that SEC23B RNA expression was increased relative to SEC23A expression during in vitro erythroid differentiation of CD34+ blood cells exposed to erythropoietin. In seeded stable CD34+ cells, the relative expression levels were equal. Short hairpin RNA (shRNA)-mediated suppression of SEC23B expression recapitulated the cytokinesis defect typical of CDA type II, including an increase in binucleate

erythrocytes with twice the normal amount of DNA, suggesting a defect in cytokinesis.[24] Knockdown of zebrafish sec23b also leads to aberrant erythrocyte development. These results provide in vivo evidence for SEC23B selectivity in erythroid differentiation and show that SEC23A and SEC23B, although highly related paralogous secretory COPII components, are non-redundant in erythrocyte maturation.[24]

Two relatively common mutations have been detected in unrelated persons with CDA type II: In affected members of seven unrelated families, Schwarz et al. identified a homozygous 325G→A transition in exon 4 of the SEC23B gene, resulting in a glutamine 109 to lysine (E109K) substitution in the N-terminal zinc finger domain. Two other probands were compound heterozygotes for SEC23B E109K and another pathogenic mutation. SEC23B E109K was not identified in 237 healthy individuals. Haplotype analysis did not identify a founder effect. In vitro functional expression studies showed that the E109K protein was unstable, with less than 5% of protein detectable compared to wild-type SEC23B.[24] Affected members of ten unrelated families with CDAII were compound heterozygotes for two mutations in the SEC23B gene. All families had a heterozygous 40C→T transition in exon 2, resulting in an arginine14 to tryptophan (R14W) substitution at the interface of the zinc finger domain and SEC23B core fold. In vitro functional expression studies showed that the R14W protein was also unstable, and there was less than 5% of the amount of protein expressed by wild type SEC23B. Mutations found in compound heterozygosity with R14W included R530W (exon 14); R264X (exon 7); and R324X (exon 8).[24] Some patients with CDA type II phenotypes have a disorder that cannot be mapped to chromosome 20q11.2.[16]

Treatment

Anemia

Some children with CDA type II require transfusion, but repeated transfusions are not required by most adults. Splenectomy increases hemoglobin values, decreases serum bilirubin levels, and eliminates the need for transfusions, but does not prevent further iron loading.[16,17] Erythropoietin has not been found to be effective in people who have CDA type II. Interferon therapy did not alleviate anemia in three patients.[14]

Iron overload

Iron-loaded patients have been treated with iron chelation drugs, splenectomy, phlebotomy, and with interferon.[14,22,23,25] Iron depletion therapy was initiated in 16 patients aged 7 to 36 years.[17] Thirteen patients were treated with deferoxamine in doses recommended for treatment of secondary hemochromatosis in thalassemia major.[17] Treatment was usually begun when serum ferritin reached a concentration of 1000 μg/L. Age at initiation of deferoxamine therapy ranged from 7 to 35 years (mean, 20 years; median, 21 years).[17] Reduction of elevated serum ferritin concentrations was achieved in all patients, and normal ferritin concentrations (below 300 μg/L) were reached in all patients with satisfactory compliance.[17]

Three splenectomized patients underwent regular phlebotomies of 200 to 300 mL every 4–6 weeks, with normalization of ferritin and transferrin iron saturation.[17] Two Czech brothers with CDA type II with mild anemia and severe hepatic iron overload were treated by splenectomy at age 15 years and age 23 years, respectively, and later by monthly removal of 400 mL whole blood for 3 years. Their initial serum ferritin values of 1131 μg/L and 1450 μg/L decreased to 447 μg/L and 457 μg/L. Their hemoglobin values remained unchanged.[23]

References

1. Wickramasinghe SN, Wood WG. Advances in the understanding of the congenital dyserythropoietic anaemias. *Br J Haematol* 2005; **131**: 431–46.

2. Shalev H, Kapelushnik J, Moser A, Dgany O, Krasnov T, Tamary II. A comprehensive study of the neonatal manifestations of congenital dyserythropoietic anemia type I. *J Pediatr Hematol Oncol* 2004; **26**: 746–8.

3. Shalev H, Kapleushnik Y, Haeskelzon L, *et al.* Clinical and laboratory manifestations of congenital dyserythropoietic anemia type I in young adults. *Eur J Haematol* 2002; **68**: 170–4.

4. Heimpel H, Schwarz K, Ebnother M, *et al.* Congenital dyserythropoietic anemia type I (CDA I): molecular genetics, clinical appearance, and prognosis based on long-term observation. *Blood* 2006; **107**: 334–40.

5. Tamary H, Dgany O, Proust A, *et al.* Clinical and molecular variability in congenital dyserythropoietic anaemia type I. *Br J Haematol* 2005; **130**: 628–34.

6. Goede JS, Benz R, Fehr J, Schwarz K, Heimpel H. Congenital dyserythropoietic anemia type I with bone abnormalities, mutations of the *CDAN I* gene, and

7. significant responsiveness to alpha-interferon therapy. *Ann Hematol* 2006; **85**: 591–5.

8. Chrobak L, Hulek P, Nozicka J. [Congenital dyserythropoietic anemia-type II (CDA-II) in three siblings with long-term follow-up and iron overload.] *Acta Medica (Hradec Kralove) Suppl* 2004; **47**: 29–33.

9. Papanikolaou G, Tzilianos M, Christakis JI, *et al.* Hepcidin in iron overload disorders. *Blood* 2005; **105**: 4103–5.

10. Tamary H, Shalev H, Perez-Avraham G, *et al.* Elevated growth differentiation factor 15 expression in patients with congenital dyserythropoietic anemia type I. *Blood* 2008; **112**: 5241–4.

11. Fargion S, Valenti L, Fracanzani AL, *et al.* Hereditary hemochromatosis in a patient with congenital dyserythropoietic anemia. *Blood* 2000; **96**: 3653–5.

12. Noy-Lotan S, Dgany O, Lahmi R, *et al.* Codanin-1, the protein encoded by the gene mutated in congenital dyserythropoietic anemia type I (*CDAN1*), is cell cycle-regulated. *Haematologica* 2009; **94**: 629–37.

13. Ahmed MR, Chehal A, Zahed L, *et al.* Linkage and mutational analysis of the *CDAN1* gene reveals genetic heterogeneity in congenital dyserythropoietic anemia type I. *Blood* 2006; **107**: 4968–9.

14. Lavabre-Bertrand T, Ramos J, Delfour C, *et al.* Long-term alpha interferon treatment is effective on anaemia and significantly reduces iron overload in congenital dyserythropoiesis type I. *Eur J Haematol* 2004; **73**: 380–3.

15. Marwaha RK, Bansal D, Trehan A, Garewal G. Interferon therapy in congenital dyserythropoietic anemia type I/II. *Pediatr Hematol Oncol* 2005; **22**: 133–8.

16. Smithson WA, Perrault J. Use of subcutaneous deferoxamine in a child with hemochromatosis associated with congenital dyserythropoietic anemia, type I. *Mayo Clin Proc* 1982; **57**: 322–5.

17. Iolascon A, Delaunay J, Wickramasinghe SN, Perrotta S, Gigante M, Camaschella C. Natural history of congenital dyserythropoietic anemia type II. *Blood* 2001; **98**: 1258–60.

18. Heimpel H, Anselstetter V, Chrobak L, *et al.* Congenital dyserythropoietic anemia type II: epidemiology, clinical appearance, and prognosis based on long-term observation. *Blood* 2003; **102**: 4576–81.

19. Heimpel H, Wilts H, Hirschmann WD, *et al.* Aplastic crisis as a complication of congenital dyserythropoietic anemia type II. *Acta Haematol* 2007; **117**: 115–18.

20. Van Steenbergen W, Matthijs G, Roskams T, Fevery J. Non-iatrogenic haemochromatosis in congenital dyserythropoietic anaemia type II is not related to

C282Y and H63D mutations in the *HFE* gene: report on two brothers. *Acta Clin Belg* 2002; **57**: 79–84.

20. Halpern Z, Rahmani R, Levo Y. Severe hemochromatosis: the predominant clinical manifestation of congenital dyserythropoietic anemia type II. *Acta Haematol* 1985; **74**: 178–80.

21. Faruqui S, Abraham A, Berenfeld MR, Gabuzda TG. Normal serum ferritin levels in a patient with HEMPAS syndrome and iron overload. *Am J Clin Pathol* 1982; **78**: 97–101.

22. Hovinga JA, Solenthaler M, Dufour JF. Congenital dyserythropoietic anaemia type II (HEMPAS) and haemochromatosis: a report of two cases. *Eur J Gastroenterol Hepatol* 2003; **15**: 1141–7.

23. Chrobak L. Successful treatment of iron overload with phlebotomies in two siblings with congenital dyserythropoietic anemia type II (CDA-II). *Acta Medica (Hradec Kralove)* 2006; **49**: 193–5.

24. Schwarz K, Iolascon A, Verissimo F, *et al.* Mutations affecting the secretory COPII coat component SEC23B cause congenital dyserythropoietic anemia type II. *Nat Genet* 2009; **41**: 936–40.

25. Vassiliadis T, Garipidou V, Perifanis V, *et al.* A case of successful management with splenectomy of intractable ascites due to congenital dyserythropoietic anemia type II-induced cirrhosis. *World J Gastroenterol* 2006; **12**: 818–21.

Chapter 25

Hereditary sideroblastic anemias

X-linked sideroblastic anemias (XLSA) are characterized by impaired mitochondrial iron metabolism, "ringed" sideroblasts and increased erythropoiesis. In some cases, these disorders cause parenchymal iron overload similar to that of hemochromatosis.[1] Increased iron absorption is upregulated by relative or absolute suppression of hepcidin expression presumably mediated by ineffective erythropoiesis through growth/differentiation factor 15 (GDF15). Iron overload in some patients is exacerbated by erythrocyte transfusion. Mutations in the *ALAS2* gene that encodes erythroid-specific 5-aminolevulinate synthase (ALA synthase) account for most cases (OMIM #300751), although rare mutations in other genes on the X chromosome or elsewhere also cause sideroblastic anemia phenotypes and variable degrees of iron loading. Anemia in two-thirds of patients with *ALAS2* mutations can be alleviated with simple, nontransfusion therapy. Early recognition and treatment of iron accumulation prevents irreversible organ damage. Informal experience suggests that XLSA may be more common than is generally recognized.

ALAS2 sideroblastic anemia
History

In 1945, Thomas Cooley described the first cases of XLSA in two brothers from a large family in which the inheritance of the condition was documented through six generations.[2,3] Additional observations in this family and description of a new kinship were published by Rundles and Falls in 1946.[4] In 1956, Harris and co-workers reported the first case of "pyridoxine-responsive anemia."[5] Ringed sideroblasts were described by Bjorkman in 1956 (Fig. 25.1).[5] Byrd and Cooper coined the term "hereditary iron-loading anemia" in 1961.[6] The term "sideroblastic anemia" was adopted in 1965.[7] By this time, the association of anemia sometimes responsive to pyridoxine and iron overload were widely recognized.[7,8] In a sequence of discoveries, *ALAS2* was localized to chromosome X, subregion Xp11.21.[9-11] In 1994, Cotter and colleagues demonstrated a *ALAS2* missense mutation in members of the family first reported by Cooley.[3]

Clinical description

Most patients have symptoms or signs of anemia, although these finding are heterogeneous across patients. Some have severe anemia in infancy or early childhood, whereas others have mild anemia that is discovered late in adulthood. In members of the same kinship, the severity of anemia may vary greatly according to sex and other factors. Iron overload unrelated to transfusion develops in most patients, and is often manifest at the time of diagnosis of anemia. Mild enlargement of the liver or spleen may be present. Impaired growth or development occur in severely affected children.[12] In a few cases, abnormal heart rhythms or evidence of cardiomyopathy occur as late consequences of severe iron overload. Neurologic symptoms or abnormalities are not caused by known *ALAS2* mutations.

Laboratory findings
Characteristics of anemia

Hypochromic anemia due to impaired hemoglobin synthesis and ineffective erythropoiesis occurs in almost all patients (Fig. 25.1). Its severity varies widely across patients and within kinships,[8,13] and sometimes increases with age.[8] In men, macrocytosis is typically present. In women with severe skewed X-inactivation that strongly favors expression of the abnormal *ALAS2* allele, macrocytosis is also typical. In heterozygous women in whom there is balanced expression of both normal and abnormal *ALAS2* alleles, dimorphism of erythrocyte size is common, although the microcytic

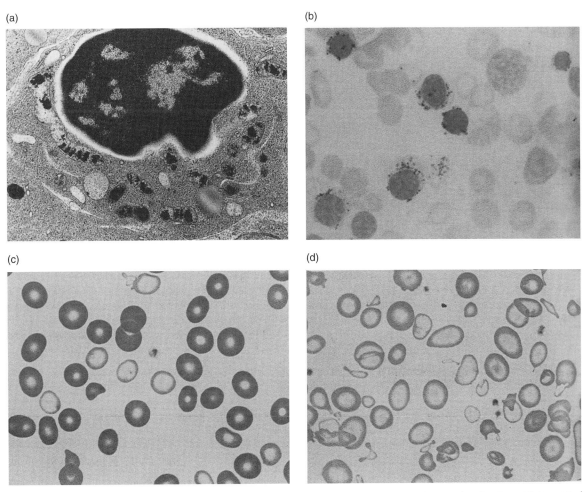

Fig. 25.1. Features of sideroblastic anemia. (a) Electron micrograph of an erythroblast with iron-laden mitochondria. From S.S. Bottomley.[1] Taken from James C. Barton and Corwin Q. Edwards (eds), **Hemochromatosis: Genetics, Pathophysiology, Diagnosis and Treatment**, Cambridge University Press 2000. (b) Bone marrow smear with ringed sideroblasts (Prussian blue stain). From S.S. Bottomley.[1] Taken from James C. Barton and Corwin Q. Edwards (eds), **Hemochromatosis: Genetics, Pathophysiology, Diagnosis and Treatment**, Cambridge University Press 2000. (c) and (d) Blood smears of mild and severe sideroblastic anemia, respectively (Wright stain). From S.S. Bottomley.[1] Taken from James C. Barton and Corwin Q. Edwards (eds), **Hemochromatosis: Genetics, Pathophysiology, Diagnosis and Treatment**, Cambridge University Press 2000. Reproduced with permission. See plate section for color version.

component may be small.[14] In severe anemia, aniso-cytosis, poikilocytosis, leptocytes, or Pappenheimer bodies are present on Wright/Giemsa-stained blood films (Fig. 25.1); Perls' staining of bone marrow may reveal siderocytes. Leukocyte and platelet values are usually normal, but may be decreased in the presence of splenomegaly (hypersplenism).[8]

Increased production of erythropoietin promotes erythroid hyperplasia, defective erythroblasts are destroyed within the marrow, and reticulocytosis is not observed.[1] These features are reflected in the ferrokinetic abnormalities of increased plasma iron turnover rate and reduced incorporation of iron into circulating erythrocytes, and in an increased erythropoietic component of the "early-label" bilirubin peak, leading to hyperbilirubinemia and excessive urobilinogen excretion.[1] Erythrocyte survival is normal or slightly reduced, and hemolysis occurs predominantly in the medullary space.[1] The free erythrocyte porphyrin level is typically normal or low.[5,15] Patients with sideroblastic anemia and elevated free erythrocyte porphyrin levels probably have a disorder other than XLSA.

Bone marrow examination is necessary for certain diagnosis. Late-stage erythroblasts typically show

261

delayed cytoplasmic maturation due to decreased hemoglobinization. Iron deposits (as ferric phosphate and ferric hydroxide) readily detected by light microscopy occur in erythroblast mitochondria in all patients. Iron-laden mitochondria tend to assume a perinuclear distribution in late erythroblasts. Prussian blue-positive granules form a distinctive full or partial ring around the nucleus of the erythroid precursor cells ("ringed" sideroblasts). Mitochondrial iron accumulation in XLSA is caused by decreased ALA synthase activity that leads to insufficient generation of protoporphyrin to utilize the iron delivered to erythroblasts.[1,8] Iron deposition in marrow macrophages is also increased in most untreated patients. Nuclear abnormalities typical of congenital dyserythropoietic anemias or myelodysplasia are lacking in erythroblasts and in other myeloid precursor cells.

Iron overload

This feature is characterized by increased iron saturation of serum transferrin and by elevated serum ferritin concentration.[6,8,16–18] The severity of overload is closely related to the degree of marrow erythroid hyperplasia and the patient's age,[17,19] but not to the severity of anemia. Best estimates of the degree of iron overload are obtained by measuring the iron concentration in liver specimens obtained by biopsy. In non-transfused patients, specimens stained with Perls' (Prussian blue) technique are indistinguishable from those in hemochromatosis. There is preferential deposition of iron in hepatocytes, and fibrosis or micronodular cirrhosis are present in advanced cases. Cirrhosis is often discovered in the third or fourth decade in untreated patients,[8] and can occur in asymptomatic patients with mild anemia.[19–21] Serum concentrations of hepatic transaminases are often mildly elevated, but often understate the severity of iron overload or the presence of cirrhosis. Primary liver cancer has been reported in one patient.[13] Diabetes mellitus or abnormal glucose tolerance may or may not be related to iron overload; skin hyperpigmentation is uncommon.[8]

Iron overload that cannot be ascribed to transfusion in most patients with *ALAS2* XLSA can only be explained by increased iron absorption. This has been documented in a small number of cases.[19,22,23] Increased iron absorption is presumably upregulated by relative or absolute suppression of hepcidin expression presumably mediated by ineffective erythropoiesis through increased expression and secretion of growth/differentiation factor GDF15, as is the case for acquired forms of sideroblastic anemia due to myelodysplasia.[24] Altogether, this indicates that the accumulation of iron in the absence of blood transfusions may result from inappropriate suppression of the iron-regulating peptide hepcidin by an erythropoietic mechanism.[25]

Genetics

Mutations in *ALAS2* account for most cases (Table 25.1). Most are missense mutations that result in single amino acid changes in ALA synthase, the first enzyme of the heme biosynthesis pathway that catalyzes the pyridoxal 5′-phosphate-dependent condensation of glycine and succinyl-CoA to yield 5′-aminolevulinic acid. The same *ALAS2* promoter region mutation was detected in two unrelated kinships, and premature stop-codon and *de novo* frameshift mutations, respectively, were identified in two other families (Table 25.1). Approximately two-thirds of probands are hemizygous men.[8] In apparently rare cases, hemizygous males do not have an XLSA phenotype.[26] The remaining third of patients comprise heterozygous women who have variable degrees of unbalanced inactivation of chromosome X.[8,27] In some kinships, men and women are affected, and pedigree analysis may suggest autosomal dominant transmission of disease (Fig. 25.2).[8] In other kinships, only heterozygous women are affected, hinting that the mutation is fatal *in utero* or in early life to male hemizygotes (Fig. 25.3).[15,19,28,29] In kinships in which there is hereditary anemia, early detection of anemia and iron overload in asymptomatic relatives is important. This is facilitated by constructing a pedigree to determine possible modes of genetic transmission, and by DNA analysis of persons in kindreds with identified *ALAS2* mutations. In kindreds with X-linked anemia without identifiable *ALAS2* mutations, another chromosome X locus is implicated.[30,31]

ALAS2 mutations associated with XLSA are uncommon, and most XLSA kinships are not consanguineous. Most mutations are "private" (not found in the general population). A possible exception is *ALAS2* P520L, an allele detected in several iron overload kinships, some with anemia and others without.[32] P520L alone has no anemia- or iron-associated phenotype, but it acts by an unknown mechanism to modify the severity of other heritable iron overload disorders.[32]

Table 25.1. *ALAS2* mutations associated with X-linked sideroblastic anemia[a]

Amino acid change	Anemia	Pyridoxine responsiveness	Reference
M154I	?	?	83
D159Y	severe	partial	84
D159N	?	partial	85
T161A	?	?	86
F165L	severe	partial	3
R170S	severe	partial	8
R170C	?	partial	87
R170H	mild	none	43
R170L	severe	partial	88
A172T	severe	complete	89
D190V	moderate	none	33
Y199H	moderate	partial	39
R204Term	severe	none	90,91
R204Q	severe	partial	35
R227C	moderate	none	91
S251P	severe	?	92
D263N	severe	probable	8
C276W	severe	none	91
I289T	severe	responsive	93
C291S	severe	complete	94
K299Q	severe	complete	89
G351R	moderate	complete	8
T388S	severe	complete	94
C395Y	severe	complete	27
G398D	severe	none	91
R411C	severe	partial	34,39,95
R411H	moderate	partial	91
G416D	moderate	partial	96
M426V	severe	complete	33
R436W	severe	none	91,97
R448Q	mild to moderate	none/partial	39,87,96
R452S	moderate	partial	96
R452C	mild	partial	39,87,96
R452H	mild to severe	none/partial	8,40,87,98
I476N	severe	complete	36

Table 25.1. (*cont.*)

Amino acid change	Anemia	Pyridoxine responsiveness	Reference
CD506–507(-C)	severe	none	99
T508S	moderate	?	8
R517C	severe	none	91
P520L[b]	anemia absent	anemia absent	32
H524D	severe	partial	100
R560H	severe	partial	32
S568G	moderate to severe	partial	35
C→G at nt(-)206[c]	mild	none/partial	38,61

Notes: [a]Adapted in part from Bottomley.[8]
[b]P520L alone has no phenotype, but modifies the severity of other heritable iron overload disorders. In one family, P520L occurred on the same haplotype as *ALAS2* R560H (Fig. 25.3).[32]
[c]This promoter mutation was associated with sideroblastic anemia and iron overload in Welsh and African-American kinships. In the former, ALAS2 mRNA levels in the proband's erythroid precursors were reduced 87%. The mutation occurred in or near three different putative transcription factor binding sites of unknown importance; the region affected by the mutation may be a receptor for an erythroid regulatory element.

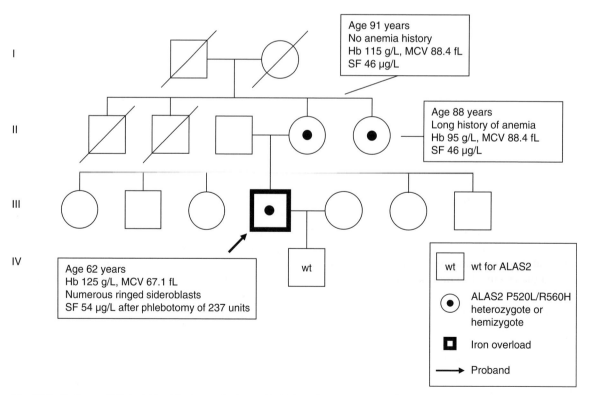

Fig. 25.2. Pedigree of X-linked sideroblastic anemia due to *ALAS2* P520L/R560H in a *cis* configuration. The proband was treated with ~170 units of erythrocyte transfusion until age 34 years when sideroblastic anemia was diagnosed. His anemia responded to pyridoxine, and he was treated with pyridoxine and phlebotomy thereafter. Hb = hemoglobin; MCV = mean corpuscular volume; SF = serum ferritin. Adapted from Lee *et al.*[32]

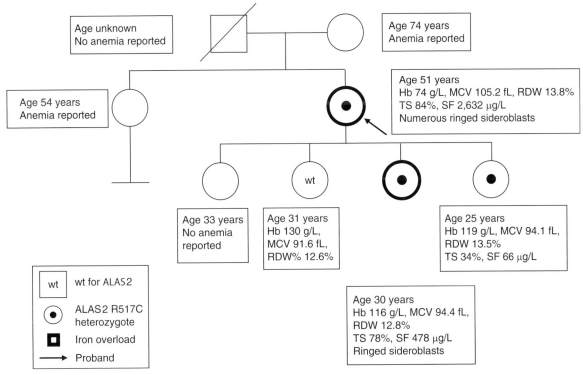

Fig. 25.3. Pedigree of X-linked sideroblastic anemia due to *ALAS2* R517C in which all affected family members are women. The proband did not have *HFE* C282Y or H63D. Her anemia did not respond to pyridoxine; iron overload was treated with deferoxamine. Hb = hemoglobin; MCV = mean corpuscular volume; RDW = red blood cell distribution width; TS = transferrin saturation; SF = serum ferritin.

In one family, *ALAS2* P520L occurred on the same haplotype as *ALAS2* R560H.[32] Mutations in the triplet codon for the arginine-452 residue of ALA synthase and a promoter mutation appear to have arisen independently in unrelated kindreds (Table 25.1). Many reported kinships have been Caucasian, although this disorder has also been described in Japanese,[33–35] Chinese,[36] and African-Americans.[12,37,38] *ALAS2* mutation analysis or gene sequencing is not available commercially, although some research laboratories will perform this testing. Routine clinical laboratory methods and pedigree analysis are sufficient for diagnosis and management in most kinships.

Common *HFE* coding region mutations occur in some patients with XLSA. In a summary of 50 patients, the prevalence of the *HFE* alleles C282Y and H63D was similar to that in general white populations.[1] Nonetheless, co-inheritance of common *HFE* mutations may affect the iron overload phenotype primarily due to XLSA. In one Caucasian kinship, iron overload was more severe in C282Y homozygotes who had *ALAS2* P520L than in C282Y homozygous family members without P520L.[32] There was a significantly higher frequency of co-inheritance of *HFE* C282Y in 18 unrelated XLSA hemizygotes than in a normal population.[39] A man with *ALAS2* Y199H and severe, early-onset iron overload also had C282Y homozygosity.[39] This suggests that co-inheritance of C282Y may increase the severity of abnormalities that lead to the diagnosis of XLSA. *HFE* C282Y or H63D have been reported in other Caucasians with XLSA.[40] In contrast, C282Y and H63D were not detected in Japanese patients with XLSA.[1,41] These *HFE* alleles, especially C282Y, are rare in the general Japanese population. HFE protein does not seem to be involved directly in the pathogenesis of anemia or iron overload in persons with XLSA.[8]

Prevention and treatment

Anemia. Many patients with XLSA have been reported as patients with pyridoxine-responsive anemia. It is presumed that an increased supply of 5′-pyridoxal phosphate, the essential co-factor for ALA synthase, enhances its impaired binding to some mutants of the enzyme.[1] Most pathogenic *ALAS2* mutations alter catalytic or substrate-binding domains of the enzyme.

Regardless, pyridoxine responsiveness or other phenotype attributes cannot be correlated reliably with specific mutations.[8,42] Except for the response to pyridoxine therapy, there are no distinct clinical, hematologic, or biochemical differences between pyridoxine-responsive and refractory forms of XLSA.[8,43]

Approximately one-third of patients with XLSA respond to pyridoxine supplements; "effective" doses vary widely. Typical oral doses are 50 mg three or four times daily, although higher doses are tolerated well. In some patients, anemia is corrected, others respond partially, and still others have no response (Table 25.1).[8] Varying degrees of pyridoxine responsiveness have been observed in members of the same kindred.[8] Patients who achieve a response to pyridoxine should continue treatment indefinitely. Interruption of therapy for a few months permits the severity of anemia to increase; responses to subsequent courses of pyridoxine are sometimes less than those originally observed. In patients with megaloblastic features on bone marrow examination or in those with low serum or erythrocyte folate levels, daily supplementation with this nutrient is indicated. In some patients, anemia became less severe after iron overload was alleviated.[1,35,39,44–46] All patients should avoid taking iron supplements. Patients whose anemia does not respond satisfactorily to other measures require erythrocyte transfusion.

Iron overload. Measurement of the serum ferritin level is the most practical means of monitoring the severity of iron overload after analysis of liver biopsy specimens has demonstrated this complication. When the serum ferritin reaches 500–1000 µg/L or in any patient with evidence of liver or cardiac injury, therapy to prevent progression of iron overload or to diminish its severity must be initiated.[1,8] In patients with pyridoxine-responsive anemia that is mild or moderate, phlebotomy is feasible. Phlebotomy volumes must be lower and intervals between phlebotomy sessions must greater than are typical for management of *HFE* hemochromatosis. Special precautions may be needed in patients with relative contraindications to therapeutic phlebotomy such as heart disease.[44,45] Phlebotomy therapy should be continued on a regular basis indefinitely to prevent iron reaccumulation.

In patients with severe anemia, in those who require regular erythrocyte transfusions, or in patients otherwise intolerant of phlebotomy, the parenteral iron chelator deferoxamine (DFO) should be prescribed (Chapter 36). Continuous infusion of DFO is necessary, and effective rates of iron excretion occur with daily 12- to 24-hour infusions administered subcutaneously or intravenously.[1,8] The goal of DFO therapy is to maintain serum ferritin <500 µg/L, but the progress of long-term treatment is best assessed with follow-up analysis of hepatic iron content.[47] Iron removal with DFO is enhanced by ascorbate; intake of the vitamin should be limited to 200 mg daily.[1] A few patients with *ALAS2* XLSA have been treated with the oral chelation agent deferiprone in clinical trials, but control of hepatic iron levels was not sustained in a substantial proportion of study participants.[48] Informal experience in one patient *ALAS2* XLSA suggests that the oral chelation drug deferasirox was effective, and thus deferasirox should be considered for management of iron overload in patients who cannot tolerate or are non-compliant with DFO therapy.

Regular consumption of tea significantly decreases the absorption of dietary inorganic iron in patients with severe beta-thalassemia or *HFE* hemochromatosis.[49,50] The central underlying mechanism for increased iron absorption in these conditions and in XLSA is the same (relative or absolute deficiency of hepcidin expression). Hence, it is rational to recommend regular consumption of tea to patients with XLSA and iron overload to decrease iron absorption. This strategy does not affect the excretion of iron that has already been absorbed. Treatment of severe hereditary or congenital sideroblastic anemia with bone marrow or stem cell transplantation in a few young patients was successful.[51–53]

ABCB7 sideroblastic anemia and iron overload

Hereditary sideroblastic anemia with ataxia (XLSA/A) is characterized by hypochromic, microcytic anemia, non-progressive cerebellar ataxia manifest in infancy or early childhood, and lack of systemic iron overload. This rare disorder is due to mutations in the gene *ABCB7* on chromosome X that encodes ATP-binding cassette, subfamily B, member 7. The family of ABC transporters consists of a large group of adenosine triphosphate-dependent transmembrane proteins that specifically transport a wide variety of substrates across cell and organelle membranes.[54–56]

Many genetic disorders result from alterations in the ability of these proteins to transport diverse substrates.[57] *ABCB7* is an ortholog of the yeast *ATM1* gene, the product of which localizes to the mitochondrial inner membrane and is involved in iron homeostasis. ABCB7 functions as a mitochondrial iron-sulfur (Fe/S) cluster transporter.

History

In 1985, Pagon and colleagues described four males in two generations of one family and a fifth male from an unrelated family who had sideroblastic anemia and a non-progressive spinocerebellar syndrome that differed from previously reported forms of X-linked sideroblastic anemia (XLSA).[58] Raskind and colleagues mapped the putative gene for this disorder by linkage analysis to the long arm of chromosome X (Xq13).[59] Cox and colleagues demonstrated that locus heterogeneity of X-linked forms of sideroblastic anemia excluded the *ALAS2* locus from the minimal region containing the putative XLSA/A gene.[30] In subsequent reports, different *ABCB7* missense mutations have been described in each of three XLSA/A kinships.[31,57,60]

Clinical description

Characteristic neurologic abnormalities include non-progressive cerebellar ataxia, diminished deep tendon reflexes, and lack of co-ordination. The proband in one kinship had a low birthweight, mild post-natal growth retardation, substantially impaired gross motor and cognitive development, inability to sit unsupported until age 4, and difficulty walking. He used simple language from age 5, and exhibited severe, static intellectual development. After four decades, there has been no evidence of progression of ataxia or intellectual impairment, and his general physical and mental health was good.[57] A brother had a similar phenotype. Their heights as adults were subnormal. The brothers had cerebellar signs including nystagmus, dysarthria, past pointing, and dysdiadochokinesis. Tendon reflexes could not be elicited at the elbows or ankles and were diminished at the knees. Plantar responses were flexor. Cutaneous photosensitivity was not observed or reported.[57] Heterozygous females do not exhibit neurologic abnormalities. Most affected males and heterozygous females have mild pallor. Abnormalities typical of iron overload or its complications are absent.

Laboratory findings

Neurologic studies. In one proband, CT scans of the brain at age 18 showed striking, selective cerebellar hypoplasia.[57]

Anemia and iron studies

In all reported kinships, affected males have mild-moderate, hypochromic, microcytic anemia. Mean corpuscular hemoglobin (MCH) levels are ~20 pg and mean corpuscular volumes (MCV) are ~60 fL. The red blood cell distribution width (RDW) is moderately increased. Heterozygous females in one family did not have anemia or erythrocyte dimorphism,[58] whereas heterozygous females in another kinship had dimorphic anemia, markedly increased RDW, MCH ~27 pg, and MCV ~81 fL.[57] Soluble transferrin receptor levels are normal or increased.[61] Total erythrocyte protoporphyrin is increased.[57,58] Bone marrow examination reveals ringed sideroblasts without other significant abnormalities. Saturation of serum transferrin with iron is normal; serum ferritin levels are normal or slightly increased.[57] In the few reported cases, there has been no evidence of increased parenchymal iron stores.

Genetics

The three families with documented pathogenic *ABCB7* mutations have been Caucasian; there was no consanguinity in these kindreds. The kinships show typical disease manifestations in males hemizygous for *ABCB7* mutations, no abnormalities in their siblings without *ABCB7* mutations, and mild erythrocyte abnormalities in their heterozygous mothers. This suggests that routine hematologic studies can be used to identify heterozygous women. No heterozygous women with neurologic manifestations due to skewed X-inactivation have been reported, but differences in lyonization could account for anemia phenotype disparities in hemizygous women in two kinships.[58,61] Each novel *ABCB7* missense mutation occurred in exon 10 and each changed a highly conserved amino acid (Table 25.2). Each mutation affected a relatively short span of 34 consecutive amino acids in a region of the protein involved in binding and transport of substrate. These respective *ABCB7* mutations were not detected in population control subjects.[31,57,60]

ABCB7 positively regulates the expression of extra-mitochondrial thioredoxin and the intramitochondrial iron–sulfur-containing protein, ferrochelatase,

Table 25.2. *ABCB7* mutations associated with X-linked sideroblastic anemia and ataxia[a]

Amino acid change	Reference
I400M	31
V411L	60
E433K	57

Note: [a]Each *ABCB7* missense mutation occurred in exon 10 and each changed a highly conserved amino acid. Each mutation affected a span of 34 consecutive amino acids in a region of the protein involved in binding and transport of substrate. These mutations were not detected in population control subjects.[31,57,60]

in erythroid precursors, and thus influences normal heme synthesis.[62,63] The precise mechanism by which *ABCB7* mutations impair neurologic development or lead to neurologic injury is unknown, although abnormal mitochondrial iron metabolism in neural cells is involved in the pathogenesis of Friedreich ataxia (Chapter 29).

Prevention and treatment

No means of early detection or prevention of XLSA/A are known. Hypochromic, microcytic anemia is present from birth, and may be a harbinger of this disorder. Hemizygous males with neurologic abnormalities may require special accommodations in upbringing and education. Anemia is not responsive to pyridoxine therapy.[57] Non-transfusion iron overload has not developed in reported cases, and anemia is not severe enough to require repeated erythrocyte transfusion.

GLRX sideroblastic anemia and iron overload

Normal erythropoiesis depends on iron-reactive protein (IRP) function and production of iron–sulfur (Fe/S) clusters. Zebrafish *shiraz* mutants have defective production of Fe/S clusters with consequent deficient hemoglobin synthesis, defective hematopoiesis, severe hypochromic anemia, and lethality.[64] These fish have a large deletion encompassing the *GLRX5* gene[64] that encodes a 156 amino acid mitochondrial enzyme belonging to an antioxidant protein family that is highly conserved in eukaryotes. The *shiraz* phenotype suggested sideroblastic anemia and iron overload in some humans could be explained by corresponding mutations.[65]

History

In 2007, Camaschella and colleagues described a man in his 60s who had sideroblastic anemia, severe iron overload, cirrhosis, diabetes mellitus, and hyperpigmentation.[65] He had an explanatory, pathogenic mutation in the *GLRX5* gene. Located on chromosome 5q14,[66] *GLRX5* encodes glutaredoxin, a glutathione (GSH)-dependent hydrogen donor for ribonucleotide reductase that also catalyzes glutathione-disulfide oxidoreduction reactions in the presence of NADPH and glutathione reductase.[67]

Clinical description

All observations in this disorder were reported from a single case.[65] He reported that he had been well until age 44 when he developed diabetes mellitus. At presentation at age 60, he had jaundice, dark skin, and marked liver and spleen enlargement, and appeared severely ill. His hepatomegaly was much more severe than that in patients with pathogenic *ALAS2* mutations. He did not have neurologic abnormalities.[65]

Laboratory findings

Before transfusion, he had anemia (hemoglobin 57.0–88.6 g/L), hypochromia (mean corpuscular hemoglobin 16–23 pg), microcytosis (mean corpuscular volume 51–59 fL), reticulocytopenia, and elevated levels of transferrin saturation, serum ferritin (1100–1324 µg/L), indirect bilirubin, and liver transaminases. Liver iron content estimated by SQUID was 3576 µg/g wet weight (reference <400 µg/g wet weight). Urinary iron excretion after deferoxamine administration (DFO) was increased. Levels of haptoglobin and hemoglobin A_2 were subnormal. Moderate thrombocytopenia was attributed to hypersplenism. Bone marrow examination performed before his referral revealed erythroid hyperplasia, abundant iron, and a normal karyotype. He had evidence of cirrhosis, insulin-dependent diabetes mellitus, and hypogonadism. Re-evaluation of the bone marrow after DFO treatment revealed 12% ringed sideroblasts and 20% mitochondrial ferritin-positive erythroblasts. Mutations of alpha- and beta-thalassemia genes or *DMT1* were not detected.[65]

Genetics

This patient's kinship was consanguineous (his parents were first cousins). This suggested that he had an autosomal recessive disorder. Sequencing of his *GLRX5* gene using genomic DNA revealed that he was homozygous for an A→G transition at position 294 in the third nucleotide of the last codon of *GLRX5* exon 1. The CAA→CAG substitution does not change the encoded glutamine at position 98. However, the change affects the penultimate nucleotide of exon 1, and therefore it was predicted that the mutation would interfere with correct RNA splicing.[65] Amplification products of *GLRX5* cDNA from the patient's blood mononuclear cells were much lower than in controls. Analysis of *GLRX* expression by quantitative RT-PCR showed significantly decreased levels in the proband than in healthy subjects. Compatible with a splicing defect, unspliced fragments encompassing the exon-intron junctions were amplified from the patient's cDNA.[65]

Aconitase and H-ferritin levels were low and transferrin receptor level was high in the patient's lymphoblastoid cell line, compatible with increased IRP1-binding. Based on the biochemical and clinical phenotype, it was hypothesized that IRP2, less degraded by low levels of heme, contributed to the repression of erythroblast ferritin and ALA synthase and thereby increased mitochondrial iron deposition. It was also hypothesized that iron chelation could redistribute iron to erythroblast cytosol, decrease IRP2 excess, and improve heme synthesis and anemia.[65]

Treatment

Folic acid and pyridoxine supplementation were ineffective. Iron chelation was started with subcutaneous DFO at 30 mg/kg with a portable pump for 10 hours daily. Clinical improvement was noticed within 6 months. Serum ferritin level and liver iron concentration decreased, whereas hemoglobin levels consensually increased until transfusions and iron chelation were stopped.

Other types of hereditary sideroblastic anemia

Thiamine-responsive megaloblastic anemia syndrome (TRMA), also known as Rogers syndrome,[68] is an early-onset, autosomal recessive disorder defined by megaloblastic anemia, diabetes mellitus, and sensorineural deafness. TRMA is due to mutations in the gene *SLC19A2* (chromosome 1q23.3) that encodes thiamine transporter protein 1. A variety of *SLC19A2* mutations have been identified in patients

with TRMA.[69,70] Patients represent diverse race/ethnicity groups. Clinical phenotypes are also heterogeneous. Anemia, mild or moderate, is typically macrocytic, although some patients have normocytic anemia.

Pancytopenia has been reported in some cases. Bone marrow examination reveals megaloblastic erythroid precursors, some of which are ringed sideroblasts. Non-transfusion systemic iron overload seems unreported. The anemia in many patients responds to daily pharmacologic doses of thiamine. Relapses of anemia occur after thiamine treatment is discontinued. In one patient, insulin requirements also decreased with thiamine replacement.[71]

Mild hypochromic, microcytic anemia is common in persons with erythropoietic protoporphyria, a heterogeneous disorder due to mutations in the *FECH* gene (chromosome 18q21.3) that encodes ferrochelatase. Bone marrow examination in a few patients revealed ringed sideroblasts.[72,73] Because the bone marrow is not routinely evaluated in persons with erythropoietic protoporphyria, the prevalence of ringed sideroblasts in this disorder may be greater than presently recognized.

Mitochondrial myopathy and sideroblastic anemia (MLASA) is a rare autosomal recessive oxidative phosphorylation disorder specific to skeletal muscle and bone marrow that is due to mutations in the gene *PSU1* (chromosome 12q24.33) that encodes pseudouridine synthase-1.[74–81] Mitochondrial DNA is normal.[79] Several MLASA kinships have been consanguineous; the disorder has been reported in several race/ethnicity groups. MLASA is characterized by myopathy, lactic acidosis, and sideroblastic anemia. Many patients present in childhood with progressive exercise intolerance and later develop high-output cardiomyopathy. Some patients have neurologic or somatic abnormalities. Deposition of iron within the mitochondria of bone marrow erythroblasts has been observed by electron microscopy. Irregular and enlarged mitochondria with paracrystalline inclusions were also seen on electron microscopy of muscle.[79] Sideroblastic anemia is typically mild and does not require treatment, although some patients have severe anemia and require transfusion.[78]

Pearson marrow–pancreas syndrome comprises refractory sideroblastic anemia, vacuolization of marrow precursors, and exocrine pancreatic dysfunction, and is due to mutations or deletions of mitochondrial DNA (Chapter 26).

Patients or families with unexplained sideroblastic anemia, some with other abnormalities, have been reported.[8] Modes of inheritance of these disorders vary across kinships, but explanatory genes and mutations have not been identified. Primary defects in mitochondrial oxidative phosphorylation, thiamine metabolism, and iron–sulfur cluster biosynthesis have been implicated in some of these cases of apparently constitutional sideroblastic anemias that may secondarily affect heme metabolism.[82]

References

1. Bottomley SS. Iron overload in sideroblastic and other non-thalassemic anemias. In: Barton JC, Edwards CQ, eds. *Hemochromatosis: Genetics, Pathophysiology, Diagnosis and Treatment.* Cambridge, Cambridge University Press. 2000; 442–52.

2. Cooley TB. A severe type of hereditary anemia with elliptocytosis. Interesting sequence of splenectomy. *Am J Med Sci* 1945; **209**: 568.

3. Cotter PD, Rucknagel DL, Bishop DF. X-linked sideroblastic anemia: identification of the mutation in the erythroid-specific delta-aminolevulinate synthase gene (*ALAS2*) in the original family described by Cooley. *Blood* 1994; **84**: 3915–24.

4. Rundles RW, Falls HF. Hereditary (sex-linked) anemia. *Am J Med Sci* 1946; **211**: 641–58.

5. Harris JW, Whittington RM, Weisman R, Jr., Horrigan DL. Pyridoxine responsive anemia in the human adult. *Proc Soc Exp Biol Med* 1956; **91**: 427–32.

6. Byrd RB, Cooper T. Hereditary iron-loading anemia with secondary hemochromatosis. *Ann Intern Med* 1961; **55**: 103–23.

7. Mollin DL. Sideroblasts and sideroblastic anaemia. *Br J Haematol* 1965; **11**: 41–8.

8. Bottomley SS. Sideroblastic anemias. In: Greer JP, Foerster J, Lukens JN, Rogers GM, Paraskevas F, Glader BE, eds. *Wintrobe's Clinical Hematology.* Philadelphia, Lippincott Williams & Wilkins. 2004; 1011–33.

9. Aoki Y, Urata G, Takaku F. Aminolevulinic acid synthetase activity in erythroblasts of patients with primary sideroblastic anemia. *Nippon Ketsueki Gakkai Zasshi* 1973; **36**: 74–7.

10. Astrin KH, Bishop DF. Assignment of human erythroid delta-aminolevulinate synthase (*ALAS2*) to the X chromosome [abstract]. *Cytogenet Cell Genet* 1989; **51**: 953–4.

11. Cotter PD, Willard HF, Gorski JL, Bishop DF. Assignment of human erythroid delta-aminolevulinate synthase (*ALAS2*) to a distal subregion of band Xp11.21 by PCR analysis of somatic cell hybrids containing X; autosome translocations. *Genomics* 1992; **13**: 211–12.

12. Prasad AS, Tranchida L, Konno ET, *et al.* Hereditary sideroblastic anemia and glucose-6-phosphate dehydrogenase deficiency in a Negro family. *J Clin Invest* 1968; **47**: 1415–24.

13. Barton JC, Lee PL. Disparate phenotypic expression of *ALAS2* R452H (nt 1407G→A) in two brothers, one with severe sideroblastic anemia and iron overload, hepatic cirrhosis, and hepatocellular carcinoma. *Blood Cells Mol Dis* 2006; **36**: 342–6.

14. Pinkerton PH. X-linked hypochromic anemia. *Lancet* 1967; **1**: 1106–7.

15. Pasanen AV, Salmi M, Vuopio P, Tenhunen R. Heme biosynthesis in sideroblastic anemia. *Int J Biochem* 1980; **12**: 969–74.

16. Hathway D, Harris JW, Stenger RJ. Histopathology of the liver in pyridoxine-responsive anemia. *Arch Pathol* 1967; **83**: 175–9.

17. Cazzola M, Barosi G, Bergamaschi G, *et al.* Iron loading in congenital dyserythropoietic anaemias and congenital sideroblastic anaemias. *Br J Haematol* 1983; **54**: 649–54.

18. Bottomley SS, Wasson EG, Wise PD. Role of the hemochromatosis *HFE* gene mutation(s) in the iron overload of herditary sideroblastic anemia [abstract]. *Blood* 1997; **90** (Suppl 1): 11b.

19. Peto TE, Pippard MJ, Weatherall DJ. Iron overload in mild sideroblastic anaemias. *Lancet* 1983; **1**: 375–8.

20. Marcus RE. Iron overload in mild sideroblastic anaemia. *Lancet* 1983; **1**: 1276–7.

21. Bottomley SS. Sideroblastic anemia: death from iron overload. *Hosp Pract (Off Ed)* 1991; **26** Suppl 3: 55–6.

22. Pippard MJ, Weatherall DJ. Iron absorption in non-transfused iron loading anaemias: prediction of risk for iron loading, and response to iron chelation treatment, in beta-thalassaemia intermedia and congenital sideroblastic anaemias. *Haematologia (Budap)* 1984; **17**: 17–24.

23. Pippard MJ, Callender ST, Warner GT, Weatherall DJ. Iron absorption in iron-loading anaemias: Effect of subcutaneous desferrioxamine infusions. *Lancet* 1977; **2**: 737–9.

24. Ramirez JM, Schaad O, Durual S, *et al.* Growth differentiation factor 15 production is necessary for normal erythroid differentiation and is increased in refractory anaemia with ringed sideroblasts. *Br J Haematol* 2009; **144**: 251–62.

25. Tanno T, Bhanu NV, Oneal PA, *et al.* High levels of GDF15 in thalassemia suppress expression of the iron regulatory protein hepcidin. *Nat Med* 2007; **13**: 1096–101.

26. Cazzola M, May A, Bergamaschi G, Cerani P, Ferrillo S, Bishop DF. Absent phenotypic expression of X-linked sideroblastic anemia in one of two brothers with a novel *ALAS2* mutation. *Blood* 2002; **100**: 4236–8.

27. Cazzola M, May A, Bergamaschi G, Cerani P, Rosti V, Bishop DF. Familial-skewed X-chromosome inactivation as a predisposing factor for late-onset X-linked sideroblastic anemia in carrier females. *Blood* 2000; **96**: 4363–5.

28. Lee GR, MacDiarmid WD, Cartwright GE, Wintrobe MM. Hereditary, X-linked, sideroachrestic anemia. The isolation of two erythrocyte populations differing in Xga blood type and porphyrin content. *Blood* 1968; **32**: 59–70.

29. Weatherall DJ, Pembrey ME, Hall EG, Sanger R, Tippett P, Gavin J. Familial sideroblastic anaemia: problem of Xg and X chromosome inactivation. *Lancet* 1970; **2**: 744–8.

30. Cox TC, Kozman HM, Raskind WH, May BK, Mulley JC. Identification of a highly polymorphic marker within intron 7 of the *ALAS2* gene and suggestion of at least two loci for X-linked sideroblastic anemia. *Hum Mol Genet* 1992; **1**: 639–41.

31. Allikmets R, Raskind WH, Hutchinson A, Schueck ND, Dean M, Koeller DM. Mutation of a putative mitochondrial iron transporter gene (*ABC7*) in X-linked sideroblastic anemia and ataxia (XLSA/A). *Hum Mol Genet* 1999; **8**: 743–9.

32. Lee PL, Barton JC, Rao SV, Acton RT, Adler BK, Beutler E. Three kinships with *ALAS2* P520L (c. 1559 C → T) mutation, two in association with severe iron overload, and one with sideroblastic anemia and severe iron overload. *Blood Cells Mol Dis* 2006; **36**: 292–7.

33. Furuyama K, Fujita H, Nagai T, *et al.* Pyridoxine refractory X-linked sideroblastic anemia caused by a point mutation in the erythroid 5-aminolevulinate synthase gene. *Blood* 1997; **90**: 822–30.

34. Furuyama K, Uno R, Urabe A, *et al.* R411C mutation of the *ALAS2* gene encodes a pyridoxine-responsive enzyme with low activity. *Br J Haematol* 1998; **103**: 839–41.

35. Harigae H, Furuyama K, Kimura A, *et al.* A novel mutation of the erythroid-specific delta-aminolaevulinate synthase gene in a patient with X-linked sideroblastic anaemia. *Br J Haematol* 1999; **106**: 175–7.

36. Cotter PD, Baumann M, Bishop DF. Enzymatic defect in "X-linked" sideroblastic anemia: molecular evidence for erythroid delta-aminolevulinate synthase deficiency. *Proc Natl Acad Sci USA* 1992; **89**: 4028–32.

37. Collins TS, Arcasoy MO. Iron overload due to X-linked sideroblastic anemia in an African-American man. *Am J Med* 2004; **116**: 501–2.

38. Barton JC, Lee PL, Bertoli LF, Beutler E. Iron overload in an African-American woman with SS hemoglobinopathy and a promoter mutation in the X-linked erythroid-specific 5-aminolevulinate synthase (*ALAS2*) gene. *Blood Cells Mol Dis* 2005; **34**: 226–8.

39. Cotter PD, May A, Li L, *et al.* Four new mutations in the erythroid-specific 5-aminolevulinate synthase (*ALAS2*) gene causing X-linked sideroblastic anemia: increased pyridoxine responsiveness after removal of iron overload by phlebotomy and coinheritance of hereditary hemochromatosis. *Blood* 1999; **93**: 1757–69.

40. Koc S, Bishop DF, LiL. Iron overload in pyridoxine-responsive X-linked sideroblastic anemia: greater severity in a heterozygote than in her hemizygoous brother [abstract]. *Blood* 1997; **90** (suppl): 16b.

41. Furuyama K, Kondo M, Fujita H, Hayashi N, Anderson KE, Sassa S. Absence of C282Y and H63D mutations of the hemochromatosis gene in Japanese patients with sideroblastic anemia. *Am J Hematol* 1999; **61**: 276.

42. Shoolingin-Jordan PM, Al Daihan S, Alexeev D, *et al.* 5-Aminolevulinic acid synthase: mechanism, mutations and medicine. *Biochim Biophys Acta* 2003; **1647**: 361–6.

43. May A, Bishop DF. The molecular biology and pyridoxine responsiveness of X-linked sideroblastic anaemia. *Haematologica* 1998; **83**: 56–70.

44. Bottomley SS, Muller-Eberhard U. Pathophysiology of heme synthesis. *Semin Hematol* 1988; **25**: 282–302.

45. Hines JD. Effect of pyridoxine plus chronic phlebotomy on the function and morphology of bone marrow and liver in pyridoxine-responsive sideroblastic anemia. *Semin Hematol* 1976; **13**: 133–40.

46. Weintraub LR, Conrad ME, Crosby WH. Iron-loading anemia. Treatment with repeated phlebotomies and pyridoxine. *N Engl J Med* 1966; **275**: 169–76.

47. Olivieri NF, Brittenham GM. Iron-chelating therapy and the treatment of thalassemia. *Blood* 1997; **89**: 739–61.

48. Hoffbrand AV, AL Refaie F, Davis B, *et al.* Long-term trial of deferiprone in 51 transfusion-dependent iron-overloaded patients. *Blood* 1998; **91**: 295–300.

49. de Alarcon PA, Donovan ME, Forbes GB, Landaw SA, Stockman JA, III. Iron absorption in the thalassemia syndromes and its inhibition by tea. *N Engl J Med* 1979; **300**: 5–8.

50. Kaltwasser JP, Werner E, Schalk K, Hansen C, Gottschalk R, Seidl C. Clinical trial on the effect of regular tea drinking on iron accumulation in genetic haemochromatosis. *Gut* 1998; **43**: 699–704.

51. Ayas M, Al Jefri A, Mustafa MM, Al Mahr M, Shalaby L, Solh H. Congenital sideroblastic anaemia successfully treated using allogeneic stem cell transplantation. *Br J Haematol* 2001; **113**: 938–9.

52. Gonzalez MI, Caballero D, Vazquez L, *et al*. Allogeneic peripheral stem cell transplantation in a case of hereditary sideroblastic anaemia. *Br J Haematol* 2000; **109**: 658–60.

53. Urban C, Binder B, Hauer C, Lanzer G. Congenital sideroblastic anemia successfully treated by allogeneic bone marrow transplantation. *Bone Marrow Transplant* 1992; **10**: 373–5.

54. Higgins CF. ABC transporters: from micro-organisms to man. *Annu Rev Cell Biol* 1992; **8**: 67–113.

55. Higgins CF. The ABC of channel regulation. *Cell* 1995; **82**: 693–6.

56. Dean M, Allikmets R. Evolution of ATP-binding cassette transporter genes. *Curr Opin Genet Dev* 1995; **5**: 779–85.

57. Bekri S, Kispal G, Lange H, *et al*. Human *ABC7* transporter: gene structure and mutation causing X-linked sideroblastic anemia with ataxia with disruption of cytosolic iron-sulfur protein maturation. *Blood* 2000; **96**: 3256–64.

58. Pagon RA, Bird TD, Detter JC, Pierce I. Hereditary sideroblastic anaemia and ataxia: an X linked recessive disorder. *J Med Genet* 1985; **22**: 267–73.

59. Raskind WH, Wijsman E, Pagon RA, *et al*. X-linked sideroblastic anemia and ataxia: linkage to phosphoglycerate kinase at Xq13. *Am J Hum Genet* 1991; **48**: 335–41.

60. Maguire A, Hellier K, Hammans S, May A. X-linked cerebellar ataxia and sideroblastic anaemia associated with a missense mutation in the *ABC7* gene predicting V411L. *Br J Haematol* 2001; **115**: 910–17.

61. Bekri S, May A, Cotter PD, *et al*. A promoter mutation in the erythroid-specific 5-aminolevulinate synthase (*ALAS2*) gene causes X-linked sideroblastic anemia. *Blood* 2003; **102**: 698–704.

62. Kispal G, Csere P, Prohl C, Lill R. The mitochondrial proteins Atm1p and Nfs1p are essential for biogenesis of cytosolic Fe/S proteins. *EMBO J* 1999; **18**: 3981–9.

63. Taketani S, Kakimoto K, Ueta H, Masaki R, Furukawa T. Involvement of ABC7 in the biosynthesis of heme in erythroid cells: interaction of ABC7 with ferrochelatase. *Blood* 2003; **101**: 3274–80.

64. Wingert RA, Galloway JL, Barut B, *et al*. Deficiency of glutaredoxin 5 reveals Fe-S clusters are required for vertebrate haem synthesis. *Nature* 2005; **436**: 1035–9.

65. Camaschella C, Campanella A, De Falco L, *et al*. The human counterpart of zebrafish *shiraz* shows sideroblastic-like microcytic anemia and iron overload. *Blood* 2007; **110**: 1353–8.

66. Padilla CA, Bajalica S, Lagercrantz J, Holmgren A. The gene for human glutaredoxin (*GLRX*) is localized to human chromosome 5q14. *Genomics* 1996; **32**: 455–7.

67. Padilla CA, Martinez-Galisteo E, Barcena JA, Spyrou G, Holmgren A. Purification from placenta, amino acid sequence, structure comparisons and cDNA cloning of human glutaredoxin. *Eur J Biochem* 1995; **227**: 27–34.

68. Porter FS, Rogers LE, Sidbury JB, Jr. Thiamine-responsive megaloblastic anemia. *J Pediatr* 1969; **74**: 494–504.

69. Raz T, Labay V, Baron D, *et al*. The spectrum of mutations, including four novel ones, in the thiamine-responsive megaloblastic anemia gene SLC19A2 of eight families. *Hum Mutat* 2000; **16**: 37–42.

70. Labay V, Raz T, Baron D, *et al*. Mutations in *SLC19A2* cause thiamine-responsive megaloblastic anaemia associated with diabetes mellitus and deafness. *Nat Genet* 1999; **22**: 300–4.

71. Lagarde WH, Underwood LE, Moats-Staats BM, Calikoglu AS. Novel mutation in the *SLC19A2* gene in an African-American female with thiamine-responsive megaloblastic anemia syndrome. *Am J Med Genet A* 2004; **125**: 299–305.

72. Scott AJ, Ansford AJ, Webster BH, Stringer HC. Erythropoietic protoporphyria with features of a sideroblastic anaemia terminating in liver failure. *Am J Med* 1973; **54**: 251–9.

73. Rademakers LH, Koningsberger JC, Sorber CW, Baart de la Faille H, Van Hattum J, Marx JJ. Accumulation of iron in erythroblasts of patients with erythropoietic protoporphyria. *Eur J Clin Invest* 1993; **23**: 130 8.

74. Zeharia A, Fischel-Ghodsian N, Casas K, *et al*. Mitochondrial myopathy, sideroblastic anemia, and lactic acidosis: an autosomal recessive syndrome in Persian Jews caused by a mutation in the *PUS1* gene. *J Child Neurol* 2005; **20**: 449–52.

75. Bykhovskaya Y, Casas K, Mengesha E, Inbal A, Fischel-Ghodsian N. Missense mutation in pseudouridine synthase 1 (*PUS1*) causes mitochondrial myopathy and sideroblastic anemia (MLASA). *Am J Hum Genet* 2004; **74**: 1303–8.

76. Casas K, Bykhovskaya Y, Mengesha E, *et al*. Gene responsible for mitochondrial myopathy and sideroblastic anemia (MSA) maps to chromosome 12q24.33. *Am J Med Genet A* 2004; **127**: 44–9.

77. Casas KA, Fischel-Ghodsian N. Mitochondrial myopathy and sideroblastic anemia. *Am J Med Genet A* 2004; **125**: 201–4.

78. Fernandez-Vizarra E, Berardinelli A, Valente L, Tiranti V, Zeviani M. Nonsense mutation in pseudouridylate synthase 1 (*PUS1*) in two brothers affected by myopathy, lactic acidosis and sideroblastic anaemia (MLASA). *J Med Genet* 2007; **44**: 173–80.

79. Inbal A, Avissar N, Shaklai M, *et al*. Myopathy, lactic acidosis, and sideroblastic anemia: a new syndrome. *Am J Med Genet* 1995; **55**: 372–8.

80. Patton JR, Bykhovskaya Y, Mengesha E, Bertolotto C, Fischel-Ghodsian N. Mitochondrial myopathy and sideroblastic anemia (MLASA): missense mutation in the pseudouridine synthase 1 (*PUS1*) gene is associated with the loss of tRNA pseudouridylation. *J Biol Chem* 2005; **280**: 19 823–8.

81. Rawles JM, Weller RO. Familial association of metabolic myopathy, lactic acidosis and sideroblastic anemia. *Am J Med* 1974; **56**: 891–7.

82. Fleming MD. The genetics of inherited sideroblastic anemias. *Semin Hematol* 2002; **39**: 270–81.

83. Zhu P, Wang M, Shi Y, *et al*. [Pathogenic gene linkage analysis and hemopoietic characteristics in a kindred with sideroblastic anemia.] *Zhonghua Yi Xue Yi Chuan Xue Za Zhi* 1999; **16**: 22–5.

84. Hurford MT, Marshall-Taylor C, Vicki SL, *et al*. A novel mutation in exon 5 of the *ALAS2* gene results in X-linked sideroblastic anemia. *Clin Chim Acta* 2002; **321**: 49–53.

85. Furuyama K, Harigae H, Kinoshita C, *et al*. Late-onset X-linked sideroblastic anemia following hemodialysis. *Blood* 2003; **101**: 4623–4.

86. Zhu P, Bu D. [A novel mutation of the *ALAS2* gene in a family with X-linked sideroblastic anemia.] *Zhonghua Xue Ye Xue Za Zhi* 2000; **21**: 478–81.

87. Furuyama K, Sassa S. Multiple mechanisms for hereditary sideroblastic anemia. *Cell Mol Biol (Noisy-le-grand)* 2002; **48**: 5–10.

88. Edgar AJ, Vidyatilake HM, Wickramasinghe SN. X-linked sideroblastic anaemia due to a mutation in the erythroid 5-aminolaevulinate synthase gene leading to an arginine170 to leucine substitution. *Eur J Haematol* 1998; **61**: 55–8.

89. Cotter PD, May A, Fitzsimons EJ, *et al*. Late-onset X-linked sideroblastic anemia. Missense mutations in the erythroid delta-aminolevulinate synthase (*ALAS2*) gene in two pyridoxine-responsive patients initially diagnosed with acquired refractory anemia and ringed sideroblasts. *J Clin Invest* 1995; **96**: 2090–6.

90. Anderson KE, Sassa S, Bishop DF, Desnick RJ. Disorders of heme biosynthesis: X-linked sideroblastic anemia and the porphyrias. In: Scriver CR, Beaudet AL, Sly WS, Valle D, Childs B, Kinzler KW, Vogelstein B, eds. *The Metabolic and Molecular Bases of Inherited Disease*. New York, McGraw-Hill 2001; 2991–3062.

91. Bottomley SS, Wise PD, Wasson EG, Carpenter NJ. X-linked sideroblastic anemia in ten female probands due to *ALAS2* mutations and skewed X chromosome inactivation [abstract]. *Am J Hum Genet* 1998; **63** (suppl): A352.

92. Rivera CE, Heath AP. Identification of a new mutation in erythroid-specific 5-aminolevulinate synthase in a patient with congential sideroblastic anemia [abstract]. *Blood* 1999; **94** (suppl): 19b.

93. Percy MJ, Cuthbert RJ, May A, McMullin MF. A novel mutation, Ile289Thr, in the *ALAS2* gene in a family with pyridoxine responsive sideroblastic anaemia. *J Clin Pathol* 2006; **59**: 1002.

94. Prades E, Chambon C, Dailey TA, Dailey HA, Briere J, Grandchamp B. A new mutation of the *ALAS2* gene in a large family with X-linked sideroblastic anemia. *Hum Genet* 1995; **95**: 424–8.

95. Bishop DF, Cotter PD, May A. A novel mutation in exon 9 of the erythroid 5-aminolevulinate synthase gene shows phenotypic variablility lead to X-linked sideroblastic anemia in two unrelated male children but to the late-onset form of this disorder in an unrelated female [abstract]. *Am J Hum Genet* 1996; **59** (suppl): A248.

96. Bottomley SS, May BK, Cox TC, Cotter PD, Bishop DF. Molecular defects of erythroid 5-aminolevulinate synthase in X-linked sideroblastic anemia. *J Bioenerg Biomembr* 1995; **27**: 161–8.

97. Aivado M, Gattermann N, Rong A, *et al*. X-linked sideroblastic anemia associated with a novel *ALAS2* mutation and unfortunate skewed X-chromosome inactivation patterns. *Blood Cells Mol Dis* 2006; **37**: 40–5.

98. Edgar AJ, Losowsky MS, Noble JS, Wickramasinghe SN. Identification of an arginine[452] to histidine substitution in the erythroid 5-aminolaevulinate synthetase gene in a large pedigree with X-linked hereditary sideroblastic anaemia. *Eur J Haematol* 1997; **58**: 1–4.

99. Cortesao E, Vidan J, Pereira J, Goncalves P, Ribeiro ML, Tamagnini G. Onset of X-linked sideroblastic anemia in the fourth decade. *Haematologica* 2004; **89**: 1261–3.

100. Edgar AJ, Wickramasinghe SN. Hereditary sideroblastic anaemia due to a mutation in exon 10 of the erythroid 5-aminolaevulinate synthase gene. *Br J Haematol* 1998; **100**: 389–92.

Pearson marrow–pancreas syndrome

Pearson marrow–pancreas syndrome (OMIM #557000) is an uncommon, heterogeneous disorder caused by deletions or duplications of mitochondrial DNA (mtDNA).[1] First reported in 1979,[2] this disorder presents in neonates or infants and is characterized by refractory sideroblastic anemia with vacuolization of marrow precursors, exocrine pancreatic dysfunction, and metabolic acidosis. Consequent multisystem mitochondrial cytopathy results in inadequate ATP generation for cellular energy requirements and secondary accumulation of iron in mitochondria.[3]

Clinical and laboratory manifestations

Pearson syndrome causes multiple abnormalities that are evident in neonates or infants. Anemia, usually macrocytic, was present in 82% of 55 patients.[3] Typical values of hematocrit are 15%–18%. Some patients have neutropenia or thrombocytopenia. The bone marrow is either normocellular or hypocellular. Ringed sideroblasts are present, and there is vacuolization of marrow erythroblasts and delayed erythroid maturation. Some patients develop splenic atrophy.

Pancreatic exocrine insufficiency was observed in 31% of 55 patients before age 4 years.[3] This results in malabsorption, and thus fat is present in stools. The presence of persistent metabolic (lactic) acidosis suggests that affected patients have a mitochondrial disorder. 3-Methylglutaconic aciduria may be a useful marker for Pearson syndrome.[4] Muscle biopsy may reveal ragged-red fibers that lack cytochrome C, an indicator of abnormal function of the respiratory chain that is typically due to deletions or duplications of mtDNA. Neuroimaging in some patients with Pearson syndrome reveals increased signal intensity over the basal ganglia, brainstem, cerebral hemispheres, or vermis.[3] This is attributed to increased mitochondrial iron retention in these areas of the brain.

Neurologic abnormalities were reported in 18 of 55 cases (33%). Available information in 11 of the 18 patients was sufficient to allow further analysis.[3] The most common abnormalities were developmental delay (6/11, 55%), ataxia (5/11, 45%), tremor (3/11, 27%), and hypotonia (2/11, 18%). Some children (3/11, 27%) developed Kearns–Sayre syndrome, others (3/11, 27%) developed Leigh syndrome, and one (11%) had features of both Kearns–Sayre syndrome (OMIM #530000) and Leigh syndrome (OMIM #256000).[3] The abnormalities in Kearns–Sayre syndrome include ptosis, external ophthalmoplegia, retinitis pigmentosa, and one or more of the following: cardiomyopathy, heart block, ataxia, weakness of the muscles of the pharynx and extremities and trunk, small stature, deafness, electroencephalographic abnormalities, and increased protein concentration in cerebrospinal fluid. The children who developed features of Leigh syndrome subsequently developed subacute necrotizing encephalomyelitis.

Some children with Pearson syndrome experience progression to a multisystem disorder that involves one or more of these complications: insulin-dependent diabetes mellitus, liver disease, splenic atrophy, retinitis pigmentosa, short stature, hypoparathyroidism, Fanconi renal syndrome or other renal tubular defects, cardiomyopathy, heart failure, ptosis, ophthalmoplegia, or other neurologic abnormalities. Bilateral zonular cataract and cardiomyopathy are unusual manifestations.[5,6]

Children with Pearson syndrome can be separated into two groups based on survival data: death occurs in one group before age 4; and other patients live to age 7 years or greater. In a study of 55 patients, 47% died by age 3 years, 58% by age 4 years.[3]

The most common causes of death are severe infections, liver failure, intracerebral hemorrhage, and encephalitis. At autopsy, pancreatic fibrosis was observed in some children who had pancreatic insufficiency; other patients had thyroid atrophy.

Genetics

Rotig *et al.* found partial deletion of the mitochondrial genome in a patient with Pearson syndrome. The deletions spanned 4977 base pairs, and included genes coding for four subunits of NADH dehydrogenase, one subunit of cytochrome oxidase, and one subunit of ATPase.[1] mtDNA heteroplasmy caused by deletions of various sizes has been demonstrated in other patients with clinical features consistent with Pearson syndrome.[7–10] Short repeats at the boundaries of the deleted mtDNA sequences may promote intramolecular recombination, deletions, or duplications.[11,12] In a study of nine unrelated children, including the patient originally reported by Pearson, Rotig *et al.* detected five different types of direct repeats at the boundaries of mtDNA deletions and provided evidence for conservation of the 3-prime-repeated sequence in the deletions.[11]

Most deletions of mtDNA occur as sporadic events in single family members; both sexes are affected. mtDNA heteroplasmy that causes relatively mild clinical manifestations may be transmitted as an autosomal dominant trait.[13,14]

Like Pearson syndrome, both Kearns–Sayre syndrome and Leigh syndrome are also caused by deletions of mtDNA. In a patient with features of Pearson syndrome who later developed features of Kearns–Sayre syndrome, there was mtDNA heteroplasmy for a deletion of 4.9 kb.[15] There was heteroplasmy for a deletion in mtDNA in a patient who recovered spontaneously from infantile sideroblastic anemia of the type associated with Pearson syndrome, but who subsequently developed features of Kearns–Sayre syndrome.[16] External ophthalmoplegia has been reported to occur in patients first diagnosed to have either Pearson syndrome or Kearns–Sayre syndrome. Progressive external ophthalmoplegia (OMIM #157640) is another autosomal dominant disorder due to mtDNA deletions in some cases.

Pearson syndrome is a heterogeneous condition that is not confined to bone marrow and pancreas, but rather it is a multi-organ disorder. The correlation of the genotypes and phenotypes of affected children with different mtDNA deletions or duplications is not especially strong, but accounts for the heterogeneity of Pearson syndrome and its overlap with other mtDNA deletion or duplication syndromes. mtDNA duplications, in contrast to dimerizations, may result in milder clinical phenotypes with Kearns–Sayre-like symptoms and permit greater life expectancy.[12] The tissue distribution and relative proportions of abnormal mtDNA molecules are probably important determinants of phenotype and clinical course.

Differential diagnosis

Persistent metabolic acidosis is a sign of several mitochondrial abnormalities. The major differential diagnoses of patients who may have Pearson syndrome include Kearns–Sayre syndrome, Leigh syndrome, and other disorders characterized by progressive external ophthalmoplegia.[17] Many types of progressive external ophthalmoplegia are due to mutations of DNA polymerase gamma involved in the replication of mtDNA, whereas others are due to alterations in nuclear DNA. The MERRF (myoclonus, epilepsy, ragged-red muscle fibers) syndrome is readily distinguished from the hematologic abnormalities, metabolic acidosis, and ragged-red fiber mitochondrial myopathy of Pearson syndrome. The sideroblastic anemia, bone marrow abnormalities, metabolic acidosis, and deletions of mtDNA in Pearson syndrome can be readily distinguished from the X-chromosome-linked sideroblastic anemia with ataxia that is caused by mutation of the *ABCB7* (ATP-binding cassette transporter protein, subfamily B, member 7) gene (Chapter 25).

Treatment

Management is supportive; randomized controlled treatment trials have not been reported. Many patients need erythrocyte transfusions soon after birth, although spontaneous recovery from infantile sideroblastic anemia in Pearson syndrome has been described.[16] Oral replacement of pancreatic enzymes is indicated in patients with pancreatic exocrine insufficiency. Oral antacids may control persistent metabolic acidosis. Oral supplements of multiple vitamins and cytochrome C by mouth have been used for treatment of some patients. Efforts to decrease mitochondrial iron deposition have not been reported.

Insulin therapy is required for children with severe diabetes mellitus. In patients with inadequate intake of food or fluids, gastrostomy or jejunostomy tubes can provide a route to deliver fluids and nutrition. Antibiotics may be required for bacterial infections. Children who have complete heart block can be treated with a permanent cardiac pacemaker. Some children with episodes of apnea need treatment with a mechanical ventilator. Many commonly prescribed medications may cause undesirable adverse effects in patients who have Pearson syndrome; these have been carefully reviewed.[17]

References

1. Rotig A, Colonna M, Bonnefont JP, *et al*. Mitochondrial DNA deletion in Pearson's marrow–pancreas syndrome. *Lancet* 1989; **1**: 902–3.

2. Pearson HA, Lobel JS, Kocoshis SA, *et al*. A new syndrome of refractory sideroblastic anemia with vacuolization of marrow precursors and exocrine pancreatic dysfunction. *J Pediatr* 1979; **95**: 976–84.

3. Lee HF, Lee HJ, Chi CS, Tsai CR, Chang TK, Wang CJ. The neurological evolution of Pearson syndrome: case report and literature review. *Eur J Paediatr Neurol* 2007; **11**: 208–14.

4. Gibson KM, Bennett MJ, Mize CE, *et al*. 3-Methylglutaconic aciduria associated with Pearson syndrome and respiratory chain defects. *J Pediatr* 1992; **121**: 940–2.

5. Cursiefen C, Kuchle M, Scheurlen W, Naumann GO. Bilateral zonular cataract associated with the mitochondrial cytopathy of Pearson syndrome. *Am J Ophthalmol* 1998; **125**: 260–1.

6. Krauch G, Wilichowski E, Schmidt KG, Mayatepek E. Pearson marrow–pancreas syndrome with worsening cardiac function caused by pleiotropic rearrangement of mitochondrial DNA. *Am J Med Genet* 2002; **110**: 57–61.

7. Rotig A, Cormier V, Blanche S, *et al*. Pearson's marrow–pancreas syndrome. A multisystem mitochondrial disorder in infancy. *J Clin Invest* 1990; **86**: 1601–8.

8. Majander A, Suomalainen A, Vettenranta K, *et al*. Congenital hypoplastic anemia, diabetes, and severe renal tubular dysfunction associated with a mitochondrial DNA deletion. *Pediatr Res* 1991; **30**: 327–30.

9. Baerlocher KE, Feldges A, Weissert M, Simonsz HJ, Rotig A. Mitochondrial DNA deletion in an 8-year-old boy with Pearson syndrome. *J Inherit Metab Dis* 1992; **15**: 327–30.

10. Superti-Furga A, Schoenle E, Tuchschmid P, *et al*. Pearson bone marrow–pancreas syndrome with insulin-dependent diabetes, progressive renal tubulopathy, organic aciduria and elevated fetal haemoglobin caused by deletion and duplication of mitochondrial DNA. *Eur J Pediatr* 1993; **152**: 44–50.

11. Rotig A, Cormier V, Koll F, *et al*. Site-specific deletions of the mitochondrial genome in the Pearson marrow–pancreas syndrome. *Genomics* 1991; **10**: 502–4.

12. Jacobs LJ, Jongbloed RJ, Wijburg FA, *et al*. Pearson syndrome and the role of deletion dimers and duplications in the mtDNA. *J Inherit Metab Dis* 2004; **27**: 47–55.

13. Shanske S, Tang Y, Hirano M, *et al*. Identical mitochondrial DNA deletion in a woman with ocular myopathy and in her son with Pearson syndrome. *Am J Hum Genet* 2002; **71**: 679–83.

14. Casademont J, Barrientos A, Cardellach F, *et al*. Multiple deletions of mtDNA in two brothers with sideroblastic anemia and mitochondrial myopathy and in their asymptomatic mother. *Hum Mol Genet* 1994; **3**: 1945–9.

15. McShane MA, Hammans SR, Sweeney M, *et al*. Pearson syndrome and mitochondrial encephalomyopathy in a patient with a deletion of mtDNA. *Am J Hum Genet* 1991; **48**: 39–42.

16. Larsson NG, Holme E, Kristiansson B, Oldfors A, Tulinius M. Progressive increase of the mutated mitochondrial DNA fraction in Kearns–Sayre syndrome. *Pediatr Res* 1990; **28**: 131–6.

17. Finsterer J. Overview on visceral manifestations of mitochondrial disorders. *Neth J Med* 2006; **64**: 61–71.

Acquired sideroblastic anemias

Acquired sideroblastic anemia is a heterogeneous group of disorders characterized by excessive accumulation of amorphous iron deposits in the mitochondria of erythrocyte precursors.[1] Ring sideroblasts, the *sine qua non* of sideroblastic anemia, are erythroblasts in Prussian blue-stained marrow aspirates that have numerous iron-positive mitochondria that occur in a perinuclear distribution. In sideroblastic anemia, typical ring sideroblasts have a full or partial ring and usually comprise more than 5% of all erythroblasts (Chapter 25, Fig. 25.1 a, b). Other erythroblasts in the same specimens may have markedly increased numbers of iron-positive mitochondria that do not form a perinuclear halo. Acquired sideroblastic anemias encompass two main categories: clonal hematopoietic stem cell disorders classified as myelodysplastic syndromes (MDS); and reversible types of sideroblastic anemia due to drugs, chemicals, or other factors. Heritable types of sideroblastic anemia are described in Chapter 25.

Acquired sideroblastic anemia due to myelodysplastic syndromes
Classification

Refractory anemia with ring sideroblasts (RARS) is characterized by erythroid dysplasia, mitochondrial accumulation of mitochondrial iron-containing ferritin (mitoferrin), defective erythroid maturation, and anemia; some patients also have elevated platelet counts. Other patients with MDS and ring sideroblasts are classified as having refractory cytopenias with multilineage dysplasia and ring sideroblasts (RCMD-RS). MDS in patients with either RARS or RCMD-RS may progress to excess marrow blasts (refractory anemia with excess blasts, RAEB) or acute leukemia.

Pathophysiology

Non-germline mutations in marrow stem cells underlie the pathogenesis of MDS, including MDS subcategories typically associated with ring sideroblasts. Cytogenetic analyses of marrow cells in some patients with RARS reveal trisomy 8 (+8) or deletion of the long arm of chromosome 20 (20q-),[2] although many patients have no cytogenetic abnormality demonstrable by conventional banding techniques.[3] An acquired mutation in the Janus Kinase 2 gene (*JAK2* V617F) occurs in some RARS patients, especially those with thrombocytosis.[4–6]

Erythroid intramedullary apoptosis is increased in RARS, and is initiated at the level of CD34+ stem cells; enhanced caspase activation at the stem cell level contributes to erythroid apoptosis.[7] Local iron-mediated toxicity probably adds to early erythroid cell death and ineffective erythropoiesis.[8] The rate of iron incorporation into hemoglobin is often decreased. In some cases, the basis of mitochondrial iron accumulation is decreased protoporphyrin synthesis. In other cases, defects in the heme biosynthetic pathway that affect the erythroid 5-aminolevulinate synthase isoform, or a mitochondrial iron transporter (ABCB7), or ferrochelatase, or flavin monooxygenase (a ferrireductase) have been reported.[9,10] Two patients with sideroblastic anemia had heteroplasmic point mutations in subunit I of mitochondrial cytochrome oxidase.[11] Regardless, no specific underlying molecular defect has been found in most cases.[9]

Growth/differentiation factor 15 (GDF15), a cytokine of the transforming growth factor-beta (TGF-β) family, is markedly upregulated in RARS patients; serum levels of GDF15 are also markedly increased.[12] In vitro studies demonstrate that production of GDF15 is erythroid-specific and depends on erythropoietin.[12] High GDF15 levels contribute to inappropriate suppression of hepcidin with consequent increase in iron absorption.[13–15]

Clinical features

Some patients present with symptoms of anemia or neutropenia; others are discovered to have anemia

277

incidental to medical evaluation for other conditions. In a series of 37 patients with RARS, the median age at diagnosis was 69 years (range 28–80 years).[3] Physical examination reveals no characteristic abnormality except pallor. There is no family history of anemia, hemochromatosis, or iron overload in most cases.

Laboratory features

In 37 patients with RARS, the mean hemoglobin concentration was 7.5 g/dL (range 4.0–11.9 g/dL); anemia was macrocytic in 84% and hypochromic in 46% of patients.[3] The reticulocyte index is decreased in most patients, indicating that production of erythrocytes is inappropriately low for the degree of anemia. Examination of the peripheral blood smear usually reveals dimorphism of erythrocytes with a predominance of macrocytes and smaller numbers of hypochromic, microcytic erythrocytes (Chapter 25, Fig. 25.1 c, d). The average mean corpuscular volume in 37 patients with RARS was 103 fL (range 86–125 fL).[3] Pappenheimer bodies and siderotic granules may occur in erythrocytes.

Leukocyte or platelet counts were abnormal in 10 of 37 patients (27%); some patients had subnormal histochemical scores for leukocyte alkaline phosphatase.[3] In RCMD and RAEB, dysplastic neutrophils and platelets are common and circulating immature forms are sometimes present.

Plasma iron and transferrin saturation were simultaneously increased in 21 of 37 subjects (57%) with RARS at initial evaluation. In all 19 patients in whom serum ferritin was measured at diagnosis of RARS, the value was elevated (geometric mean 684 μg/L; range 390–1550 μg/L). Fourteen of 15 patients who underwent liver biopsy had increased stainable iron.[3] By definition, all patients had increased stainable intramedullary iron and ring sideroblasts. Excessive numbers of iron-positive cytoplasmic granules (mitochondria) are present in the majority of marrow erythroid precursors. In contrast to hereditary sideroblastic anemia in which ring sideroblasts are usually late-stage erythroblasts, the ring sideroblasts in MDS often encompass all stages of erythroid cell development. Dyserythropoiesis and erythroid hyperplasia are present in most patients at diagnosis of RARS.[3] Erythropoietin levels are normal in patients with normal renal function, although erythropoietin levels may be inappropriately low for the degree of anemia. The prevalence of common heritable mutations of HFE (C282Y, H63D) in persons with RARS is similar to that in control subjects.[16]

Management

Patients without symptoms of sideroblastic anemia due to RARS or other MDS subtypes require no treatment. Such patients should be evaluated several times yearly to review symptoms and to perform complete blood counts and serum iron measures. Patients with symptoms due to anemia should undergo a therapeutic trial of oral pyridoxine (50 mg three or four times daily) and parenteral vitamin B_{12} (1 mg monthly). It may take several months for responses to become evident, although the proportion of patients who have salutary effects is very small. Anemia in some patients, especially those with RARS, responds to erythropoiesis-stimulating agents.[17–19] Recombinant erythropoietin and darbepoietin seem to be equally effective. Most patients require relatively high doses of these agents at regular intervals; missed treatments or infections are often associated with a rapid decline in hemoglobin levels. Regular erythrocyte transfusion is necessary in other patients, especially those with intolerable symptoms of anemia. Chemotherapy of carefully selected patients with azacytidine or decitabine sometimes improves production of erythrocytes, neutrophils, or platelets, especially in patients with bi- or tri-lineage hemocytopenias. MDS and deletion of chromosome 5q ("5q minus syndrome") often responds to lenalidomide therapy, although most of these patients do not have ring sideroblasts. Allogeneic marrow transplantation is appropriate for other patients.

Iron overload of variable severity is present at diagnosis in most patients with RARS.[3] Iron overload at diagnosis is usually presumed to be due to excessive iron absorption that occurs due to ineffective erythropoiesis and hepcidin suppression by excessive GDF15,[12–15] although some patients have been treated with supplemental iron in an attempt to correct anemia. Methods available for assessment of body iron stores (Chapter 4) are appropriate for patients with MDS. Patterns of parenchymal iron deposition are similar to those of HFE hemochromatosis.[20] Nonetheless, HFE mutation analysis is not routinely indicated in the absence of distinctive patient features of hemochromatosis or a family history of hemochromatosis or iron overload.

Many patients with MDS and iron overload report symptoms often attributed to iron overload.[21,22]

Iron overload progresses slowly in patients whose anemia responds to erythropoietin administration. In patients who require regular erythrocyte transfusion, iron overload is inevitable; its rate of progression is largely a function of the frequency of erythrocyte transfusion. Patients with MDS and iron overload may have a less favorable prognosis than MDS patients without iron overload.[23] A small proportion of patients with RARS die of iron overload complications (liver failure, cardiomyopathy), but most die of either neutropenia and infection or acute leukemia.[3]

The role of iron overload in the pathogenesis, abnormal hematopoiesis, symptoms, organ dysfunction, and longevity remains poorly defined in patients with MDS, with or without sideroblastic anemia. Phlebotomy therapy to alleviate iron overload is sometimes feasible in patients whose sideroblastic anemia responds well to pyridoxine or vitamin B_{12} supplementation or to therapy with erythropoietin or darbepoietin (Chapter 36). Supplemental iron should not be administered to patients with MDS in the absence of convincing evidence that they have iron deficiency. Chelation treatment of iron overload with parenteral deferoxamine, or oral deferiprone, or deferasirox should be considered in patients with favorable MDS subtypes, especially in patients with serum ferritin >1000 µg/L who have a life expectancy greater than 1 year.[24–26] General guidelines for chelation therapy are given in Chapter 36. Major uncertainties about the clinical importance of iron overload and the necessity for iron chelation therapy in patients with MDS who require chronic erythrocyte transfusion are unresolved.[27–29]

Acquired reversible sideroblastic anemia

Acquired sideroblastic anemia is sometimes due to chemical or physical agents, many of which cause sideroblastic anemia by interfering with protoporphyrin or heme synthesis. These types of anemia are characterized by ineffective erythropoiesis, populations of small, poorly hemoglobinized erythrocytes, and decreased erythrocyte survival. Awareness of these types of sideroblastic anemia is important because some patients can be treated or cured with relatively simple means. A thorough medical history is the most important means to identify the etiology of these conditions (Table 27.1).

Table 27.1. Reversible causes of acquired sideroblastic anemia

Anti-tuberculosis drugs: isoniazid, pyrazinamide, cycloserine
Lead
Chloramphenicol, thiamphenicol
Ethanol
Copper deficiency
malabsorption, parenteral nutrition
copper chelation therapy
zinc excess due to supplements, swallowed coins
Progesterone

Sideroblastic anemia due to anti-tuberculosis drugs

The first step of heme biosynthesis is the condensation of glycine and succinyl coenzyme A to form aminolevulinic acid (ALA). The reaction is catalyzed by ALA synthase and requires the presence of pyridoxal 5′-phosphate. ALA synthase is transcribed in a precursor form in the cytoplasm and transported to the inner membranes of mitochondria where it becomes active. Pyridoxal 5′-phosphate, derived from pyridoxine, is also necessary for the conversion of serine to glycine. Certain drugs used to treat tuberculosis can cause sideroblastic anemia because they are pyridoxine antagonists. These drugs include isoniazid,[30,31] pyrazinimide,[30,32,33] and cycloserine.[30,32,33] Anemia in most patients responds to discontinuation of the corresponding anti-tuberculosis drug, and to pyridoxine supplements. Transfusion is necessary in some cases.

Sideroblastic anemia due to lead intoxication

Lead intoxication of diverse sources causes anemia in children and adults because lead directly inhibits several enzymes essential for heme biosynthesis. The severity of anemia is generally proportional to the duration of lead exposure and to the severity of lead intoxication.[34,35] Sideroblastic anemia is common; basophilic stippling of blood erythrocytes is distinctive, especially in severe lead poisoning. Renal insufficiency may contribute to anemia in some cases. Blood lead levels are elevated. Increased urinary excretion of ALA and coproporphyrin III may occur;

porphobilinogen excretion is not usually increased.[34] Activities of ALA dehydratase, coproporphyrin oxidase, and ferrochelatase activities are reduced; ALA synthetase activity is increased. Erythrocyte protoporphyrin (free erythrocyte porphyrin (FEP) and zinc protoporphyrin (ZPP)) is increased.[34] The predominant treatment strategy is to avoid further lead exposure. Some patients, especially those with neurologic manifestations, lead "colic," or renal insufficiency require chelation therapy to remove lead.

Alcohol-induced sideroblastic anemia

Bone marrow toxicity due to ethanol causes megaloblastic changes in erythroblasts, ring sideroblasts, subnormal megakaryopoiesis, macrocytosis, and thrombocytopenia. Ring sideroblasts may be prominent, making distinction from MDS and heritable forms of sideroblastic anemia difficult in some cases. Vacuolated erythroid precursors occur in some cases.[36] Some patients with sideroblastic anemia have severe chronic alcoholism; others are binge drinkers. Consequently, some of them also have folate or pyridoxine deficiency, other nutritional deficits, and liver disease that contribute to anemia and related abnormalities. Ring sideroblasts and other abnormalities usually resolve within a few weeks of discontinuation of ethanol intake and reconstitution of nutritional deficits, although macrocytic anemia may persist in patients with chronic liver disease. Plasma levels of pyridoxal 5′-phosphate are low in some patients with chronic alcoholism, but these levels do not correspond with the appearance of ring sideroblasts in the marrow.[37,38] This may reflect, in part, the multitude of factors that eclipse to cause anemia in some patients with alcoholism. Most patients do not have or develop systemic iron overload. Patients found to have excessive hepatocyte iron and other evidence of iron overload should be evaluated for hemochromatosis.

Sideroblastic anemia due to chloramphenicol

Chloramphenicol and thiamphenicol sometimes cause reversible sideroblastic anemia.[39–41] In rabbits treated with chloramphenicol, there was decreased erythropoiesis and selective depletion of cytochromes a + a(3) and b attributed to decreased intra-mitochondrial synthesis. These proliferative and enzymatic abnormalities resolved simultaneously when chloramphenicol administration was discontinued.[40]

Sideroblastic anemia due to copper deficiency and zinc excess

Copper deficiency is rare because the recommended daily requirements for this nutrient are very low, and adequate amounts of copper are present in most diets. Copper is absorbed in the small intestine. Cytochrome c oxidase, ceruloplasmin, and hephaestin contain copper. Copper deficiency may occur after prolonged parenteral alimentation, in adults with short bowel and malabsorption syndromes, and in infants with marasmus.[42–45] Patients with Wilson disease or rheumatoid arthritis have developed sideroblastic anemia after they were treated with chelation drugs intended to remove copper (D-penicillamine, triethylene tetramine dihydrochloride).[46–48]

Zinc competitively inhibits copper absorption. Therefore, regular ingestion of large quantities of zinc, especially as supplements, can cause copper deficiency.[49–51] Children or adults who ingest coins or other objects that contain zinc may also develop sideroblastic anemia due to secondary copper deficiency.[49,52]

The severity of anemia is variable.[51] Many patients also have leukopenia or neutropenia. Serum copper and ceruloplasmin levels are usually subnormal; copper may be more sensitive for diagnosis. Serum zinc levels may be elevated in individuals whose anemia is due to absorption of excessive quantities of zinc. Examination of the bone marrow reveals ring sideroblasts and characteristic (but not pathognomonic) vacuoles in the erythroid and myeloid precursors. Chelation therapy to remove copper and supplemental zinc ingestion should be discontinued. Copper deficiency should be corrected. Ingested coins or other zinc-containing objects should be removed by endoscopy or surgery. Anemia and ring sideroblasts resolve after appropriate management, although some patients who ingest coins and other objects continue to do so. Patients with sideroblastic anemia due to copper deficiency or zinc excess do not typically have or develop systemic iron overload.

Sideroblastic anemia associated with progesterone

One woman developed sideroblastic anemia with iron overload shortly after the administration of progesterone on two separate occasions more than 15 years apart.[53] Treatment with folic acid, pyridoxine, or androgens corrected the anemia. In both instances, discontinuation of progesterone led to prompt disappearance of ring sideroblasts. In vitro, the patient's erythroid progenitors had enhanced sensitivity to progesterone.[53] Pyridoxal-5'-phosphate is an inhibitor of DNA-binding of glucocorticoid-, progesterone-, and estrogen-receptor complexes.[54]

Sideroblastic anemia associated with cancer chemotherapy and immunosuppressive drugs

Ring sideroblasts and dysplastic changes in marrow cells may develop in individuals who have received chemotherapeutic agents for management of malignancy, or immunosuppressive drugs such as cyclophosphamide, methotrexate, or azathioprine for treatment of autoimmune disorders. These hematologic abnormalities are usually due to MDS. Evaluation and management of these cases is described in the previous section on acquired sideroblastic anemia due to MDS.

Sideroblastic anemia associated with other conditions

Three patients with hypothermia had anemia with reduced normoblastic erythropoiesis, marked ringed sideroblasts, and thrombocytopenia; estimates of megakaryocyte numbers were normal. In two patients, erythropoiesis became normal and thrombocytopenia resolved after body temperature returned to normal.[55] Sideroblastic anemia has been described in some patients with chronic infection or inflammation; some of these have MDS.

References

1. Bottomley SS. Sideroblastic anaemia. *Clin Haematol* 1982; **11**: 389–409.

2. Bitran J, Golomb HM, Rowley JD. Idiopathic acquired refractory sideroblastic anemia: banded chromosome analysis in six patients. *Acta Haematol* 1977; **57**: 15–23.

3. Cazzola M, Barosi G, Gobbi PG, Invernizzi R, Riccardi A, Ascari E. Natural history of idiopathic refractory sideroblastic anemia. *Blood* 1988; **71**: 305–12.

4. Hellström-Lindberg E, Cazzola M. The role of *JAK2* Mutations in RARS and other MDS. *Hematology Am Soc Hematol Educ Program* **2008**; 2008: 52–9.

5. Steensma DP, Tefferi A. *JAK2* V617F and ringed sideroblasts: not necessarily RARS-T. *Blood* 2008; **111**: 1748.

6. Schmitt-Graeff AH, Teo SS, Olschewski M, *et al.* *JAK2* V617F mutation status identifies subtypes of refractory anemia with ringed sideroblasts associated with marked thrombocytosis. *Haematologica* 2008; **93**: 34–40.

7. Hellstrom-Lindberg E, Schmidt-Mende J, Forsblom AM, Christensson B, Fadeel B, Zhivotovsky B. Apoptosis in refractory anaemia with ringed sideroblasts is initiated at the stem cell level and associated with increased activation of caspases. *Br J Haematol* 2001; **112**: 714–26.

8. Martin FM, Prchal J, Nieva J, *et al.* Purification and characterization of sideroblasts from patients with acquired and hereditary sideroblastic anaemia. *Br J Haematol* 2008; **143**: 446–50.

9. Bottomley SS. Iron overload in sideroblastic and other non-thalassemic anemias. In: Barton JC, Edwards CQ, eds. *Hemochromatosis: Genetics, Pathophysiology, Diagnosis and Treatment*. Cambridge, Cambridge University Press. 2000; 442–52.

10. Barber M, Conrad ME, Umbreit JN, Barton JC, Moore EG. Abnormalities of flavin monooxygenase as an etiology for sideroblastic anemia. *Am J Hematol* 2000; **65**: 149–53.

11. Gattermann N, Retzlaff S, Wang YL, *et al.* Heteroplasmic point mutations of mitochondrial DNA affecting subunit I of cytochrome c oxidase in two patients with acquired idiopathic sideroblastic anemia. *Blood* 1997; **90**: 4961–72.

12. Ramirez JM, Schaad O, Durual S, *et al.* Growth differentiation factor 15 production is necessary for normal erythroid differentiation and is increased in refractory anaemia with ring sideroblasts. *Br J Haematol* 2009; **144**: 251–62.

13. Lakhal S, Talbot NP, Crosby A, *et al.* Regulation of growth differentiation factor 15 expression by intracellular iron. *Blood* 2009; **113**: 1555–63.

14. Tanno T, Bhanu NV, O'Neal PA, *et al.* High levels of GDF15 in thalassemia suppress expression of the iron regulatory protein hepcidin. *Nat Med* 2007; **13**: 1096–101.

15. Murphy PT, Mitra S, Gleeson M, Desmond R, Swinkels DW. Urinary hepcidin excretion in patients with low grade myelodysplastic syndrome. *Br J Haematol* 2009; **144**: 451–2.

16. Beris P, Samii K, Darbellay R, *et al.* Iron overload in patients with sideroblastic anaemia is not related to the presence of the haemochromatosis Cys282Tyr and His63Asp mutations. *Br J Haematol* 1999; **104**: 97–9.

17. Lindberg EH. Strategies for biology- and molecular-based treatment of myelodysplastic syndromes. *Curr Drug Targets* 2005; **6**: 713–25.

18. Tehranchi R, Fadeel B, Schmidt-Mende J, *et al.* Antiapoptotic role of growth factors in the myelodysplastic syndromes: concordance between in vitro and in vivo observations. *Clin Cancer Res* 2005; **11**: 6291–9.

19. Ljung T, Back R, Hellstrom-Lindberg E. Hypochromic red blood cells in low-risk myelodysplastic syndromes: effects of treatment with hemopoietic growth factors. *Haematologica* 2004; **89**: 1446–53.

20. Bottomley SS. Sideroblastic anemia: death from iron overload. *Hosp Pract (Off Ed)* 1991; **26** Suppl 3: 55–6.

21. Bennett JM. Consensus statement on iron overload in myelodysplastic syndromes. *Am J Hematol* 2008; **83**: 858–61.

22. Dreyfus F. The deleterious effects of iron overload in patients with myelodysplastic syndromes. *Blood Rev* 2008; **22** Suppl 2: S29–34.

23. Platzbecker U, Bornhauser M, Germing U, *et al.* Red blood cell transfusion dependence and outcome after allogeneic peripheral blood stem cell transplantation in patients with de novo myelodysplastic syndrome (MDS). *Biol Blood Marrow Transpl* 2008; **14**: 1217–25.

24. Wimazal F, Nosslinger T, Baumgartner C, Sperr WR, Pfeilstocker M, Valent P. Deferasirox induces regression of iron overload in patients with myelodysplastic syndromes. *Eur J Clin Invest* 2009; **39**: 406–11.

25. Messa E, Cilloni D, Messa F, Arruga F, Roetto A, Saglio G. Deferasirox treatment improved the hemoglobin level and decreased transfusion requirements in four patients with the myelodysplastic syndrome and primary myelofibrosis. *Acta Haematol* 2008; **120**: 70–4.

26. Metzgeroth G, Dinter D, Schultheis B, *et al.* Deferasirox in MDS patients with transfusion-caused iron overload—a phase-II study. *Ann Hematol* 2009; **88**: 301–10.

27. Maggio A. Light and shadows in the iron chelation treatment of haematological diseases. *Br J Haematol* 2007; **138**: 407–21.

28. Steensma DP. Myelodysplasia paranoia: Iron as the new radon. *Leuk Res* 2009; **33**: 1158–63.

29. DeLoughery TG. Iron: The fifth horseman of the apocalypse? *Am J Hematol* 2009; **84**: 263–4.

30. Verwilghen R, Reybrouck G, Callens L, Cosemans J. Antituberculous drugs and sideroblastic anaemia. *Br J Haematol* 1965; **II**: 92.

31. Sharp RA, Lowe JG, Johnston RN. Anti-tuberculous drugs and sideroblastic anaemia. *Br J Clin Pract* 1990; **44**: 706–7.

32. Hines JD, Grasso JA. The sideroblastic anemias. *Semin Hematol* 1970; **7**: 86–106.

33. Harris EB, MacGibbon BH, Mollin DL. Experimental sideroblastic anemia. *Br J Haematol* 1965; **11**: 99.

34. Lubran MM. Lead toxicity and heme biosynthesis. *Ann Clin Lab Sci* 1980; **10**: 402–13.

35. Schwartz J, Landrigan PJ, Baker EL, Jr., Orenstein WA, von Lindern IH. Lead-induced anemia: dose-response relationships and evidence for a threshold. *Am J Public Health* 1990; **80**: 165–8.

36. Conrad ME, Barton JC. Anemia and iron kinetics in alcoholism. *Semin Hematol* 1980; **17**: 149–63.

37. Hines JD, Cowan DH. Studies on the pathogenesis of alcohol-induced sideroblastic bone marrow abnormalities. *N Engl J Med* 1970; **283**: 441–6.

38. Pierce HI, McGuffin RG, Hillman RS. Clinical studies in alcoholic sideroblastosis. *Arch Intern Med* 1976; **136**: 283–9.

39. Beck EA, Ziegler G, Schmid R, Ludin H. Reversible sideroblastic anemia caused by chloramphenicol. *Acta Haematol* 1967; **38**: 1–10.

40. Firkin FC. Mitochondrial lesions in reversible erythropoietic depression due to chloramphenicol. *J Clin Invest* 1972; **51**: 2085–92.

41. Beck EA. [Blood damage due to chloramphenicol and thiamphenicol.] *Schweiz Med Wochenschr* 1975; **105**: 1078–80.

42. Graham GG, Cordano A. Copper depletion and deficiency in the malnourished infant. *Johns Hopkins Med J* 1969; **124**: 139–50.

43. Joffe G, Etzioni A, Levy J, Benderly A. A patient with copper deficiency anemia while on prolonged intravenous feeding. *Clin Pediatr (Phila)* 1981; **20**: 226–8.

44. Spiegel JE, Willenbucher RF. Rapid development of severe copper deficiency in a patient with Crohn's disease receiving parenteral nutrition. *J Parenter Enteral Nutr* 1999; **23**: 169–72.

45. Hirase N, Abe Y, Sadamura S, *et al.* Anemia and neutropenia in a case of copper deficiency: role of copper in normal hematopoiesis. *Acta Haematol* 1992; **87**: 195–7.

46. Condamine L, Hermine O, Alvin P, Levine M, Rey C, Courtecuisse V. Acquired sideroblastic anaemia during treatment of Wilson's disease with triethylene tetramine dihydrochloride. *Br J Haematol* 1993; **83**: 166–8.

47. Perry AR, Pagliuca A, Fitzsimons EJ, Mufti GJ, Williams R. Acquired sideroblastic anaemia induced by a copper-chelating agent. *Int J Hematol* 1996; **64**: 69–72.

48. Ramselaar AC, Dekker AW, Huber-Bruning O, Bijlsma JW. Acquired sideroblastic anaemia after aplastic anaemia caused by D-penicillamine therapy for rheumatoid arthritis. *Ann Rheum Dis* 1987; **46**: 156–8.

49. Broun ER, Greist A, Tricot G, Hoffman R. Excessive zinc ingestion. A reversible cause of sideroblastic anemia and bone marrow depression. *JAMA* 1990; **264**: 1441–3.

50. Ramadurai J, Shapiro C, Kozloff M, Telfer M. Zinc abuse and sideroblastic anemia. *Am J Hematol* 1993; **42**: 227–8.

51. Fiske DN, McCoy HE, III, Kitchens CS. Zinc-induced sideroblastic anemia: report of a case, review of the literature, and description of the hematologic syndrome. *Am J Hematol* 1994; **46**: 147–50.

52. Kumar A, Jazieh AR. Case report of sideroblastic anemia caused by ingestion of coins. *Am J Hematol* 2001; **66**: 126–9.

53. Brodsky RA, Hasegawa S, Fibach E, Dunbar CE, Young NS, Rodgers GP. Acquired sideroblastic anaemia following progesterone therapy. *Br J Haematol* 1994; **87**: 859–62.

54. Henrikson KP, Gross SC, Dickerman HW. Effect of pyridoxal 5′-phosphate on oligodeoxynucleotide binding of mouse uterine cytosol estradiol-receptor complexes. *Endocrinology* 1981; **109**: 1196–202.

55. O'Brien H, Amess JA, Mollin DL. Recurrent thrombocytopenia, erythroid hypoplasia and sideroblastic anaemia associated with hypothermia. *Br J Haematol* 1982; **51**: 451–6.

Hereditary aceruloplasminemia

Hereditary aceruloplasminemia (OMIM #604290) is a rare autosomal recessive disorder due to mutations of *Cp*, the gene that encodes the copper-binding protein ceruloplasmin (Cp). The first report of hereditary aceruloplasminemia was published in 1987 in Japan.[1] The patient was a 52-year-old woman who had a movement disorder that resembled Parkinson's disease, blepharospasm, retinal degeneration, and diabetes mellitus. Her serum immunofixation test revealed that her serum Cp concentration was very low. Computed tomography scanning revealed increased amounts of iron in her basal ganglia and liver. Subsequent histologic evaluation confirmed that there was increased iron in her basal ganglia and substantia nigra and in her liver, without increased copper.[1]

The frequency of homozygosity for deleterious *Cp* mutations in non-consanguineous marriages in Japan was estimated to be 1 per 2 000 000 population.[2] Aceruloplasminemia has been reported in several countries including Japan, China, Ireland, Belgium, France, Italy, and the US.[3] More Japanese patients have been reported than any other nationality. Altogether, about 60 patients with hereditary aceruloplasminemia have been described.[3]

Ceruloplasmin (Cp) biochemistry

Cp is a plasma metalloprotein, an alpha-2 glycoprotein polypeptide of 1046 amino acids. A member of the multi-copper oxidase enzyme family, Cp is the principal copper transport protein in plasma. Cp is synthesized in hepatocytes where it binds copper, and is thereafter secreted into plasma. About 95% of circulating plasma copper is bound to Cp; the remainder is bound to albumin, precuprein, and complexes of copper and amino acids. Each Cp molecule can bind and transport six atoms of copper. The Cp concentration of plasma responds as an acute-phase reactant to inflammation and pregnancy, and during treatment with estrogen.[4] The serum Cp level increases during treatment with some anticonvulsants (phenobarbital, phenytoin, carbamazepine, valproic acid).[5]

Cp functions as a ferroxidase, catalyzing the oxidation of ferrous to ferric iron in cells that store iron, including hepatocytes and macrophages. Ferric iron then passes into plasma and becomes bound to apotransferrin that transports iron to sites of normal physiologic function, principally to the bone marrow for hemoglobin synthesis, and to myoglobin and cytochromes (Chapter 2). In Cp deficiency, ferrous iron is not oxidized, so iron is not transported from storage cells into plasma. This results in accumulation of iron within storage cells. Cp must not be involved in the transport of iron from intestinal epithelia into plasma, because individuals with aceruloplasminemia become iron loaded.

Clinical manifestations

Aceruloplasminemia is associated with the accumulation of excessive storage iron in most tissues, including the occurrence of heavy iron deposits in the retina, liver, pancreas, and basal ganglia. A classic triad of retinal degeneration, diabetes mellitus, and neuropsychiatric disease is characteristic of aceruloplasminemia, but there is heterogeneity among affected individuals. Some patients have been observed to have microcytic anemia before the diagnosis of aceruloplasminemia was made. A psychological disorder, e.g. depression, may precede the onset of decreased cognitive ability and dementia.

Age of onset

The average age at the onset of symptoms or signs of illness is age 51 years (range 16–71 years).[3] Some affected individuals have lived until age 79 years. The most common published cause of death among homozygotes has been pneumonia; this is typical of patients who have advanced neurologic disorders.

Table 28.1. Prevalence of clinical manifestations of aceruloplasminemia[a,b]

Manifestation	Percent affected
Aceruloplasminemia	100
Subnormal serum copper level	100
Subnormal serum iron level	100
Elevated serum ferritin level	100
Retinal degeneration	93
Diabetes mellitus	89
Microcytic anemia	80
Ataxia	63
Involuntary movements	58
Parkinson features	30
Cognitive impairment	18

Note: [a,b]Compiled from observations of 45 patients[6] and 28 patients.[3]

Other published causes of death were heart failure, myocardial infarction, and pancreatic cancer.[3]

Physical examination

Neurologic abnormalities are common, and include decreased cognitive ability, retinal degeneration, tremors, facial dystonia, dysarthria, blepharospasm, chorea, and cerebellar ataxia. The frequency of manifestations reported in two studies of 45 and 28 patients with aceruloplasminemia, respectively, are displayed in Table 28.1.[3,6] Asymptomatic retinal degeneration, usually detected by funduscopic examination as patches of yellow atrophy in the retinal pigment epithelium, was present in 93% of patients. Ataxia and movement disorders occurred in 63% and 43% of patients, respectively.[3,6] Parkinsonism with rigidity and stiffness (30% of patients) and dementia (18% of patients) were also identified.

Laboratory findings

The most common laboratory abnormalities in 45 Japanese patients were absence of serum Cp, presence of diabetes mellitus (89%), microcytic anemia (80%), decreased serum iron concentration, and elevated serum ferritin concentration (Table 28.1).[3] Affected individuals also have increased amounts of iron the liver, brain, and cerebrospinal fluid. They also have increased concentrations of lipid peroxidation products in plasma, cerebrospinal fluid, and brain.[7-11] Excessive copper does not accumulate in the liver or brain.[1]

Histopathology

Liver biopsy specimens reveal heavy iron loading of hepatocytes and Kupffer cells, without copper overload. Most patients do not develop hepatic cirrhosis. Iron also accumulates in the beta-cells of the pancreatic islets. In the brain, iron accumulation is usually greatest in the globus pallidus; lesser quantities of iron occur in the putamen, cerebral cortex, and cerebellar cortex. Massive amounts of iron may accumulate in the astrocytes and neurons of the basal ganglia, where neuronal degeneration and dropout are most severe. In the cerebellum, Purkinje cells and astrocytes may become heavily iron loaded and damaged. The neurologic abnormalities that occur in patients with aceruloplasminemia correspond to the areas of the brain where excessive iron accumulates and causes injury and cell death. In contrast, iron deposition does not typically occur in the frontal cortex.

Magnetic resonance imaging (MRI)

Iron accumulation in the liver and affected areas of the brain result in decreased magnetic resonance signal intensity in T1- and T2-weighted images (Chapter 4). This decreased signal intensity (hypointensity) usually is most prominent in the corpus striatum, thalamus, and dentate nucleus. The iron-loaded liver and brain of individuals with aceruloplasminemia appear blacker or darker than normal due to the paramagnetic effect of the iron that accumulates in these sites. Magnetic resonance images of normal liver and brain are expected to appear whiter or less dark than iron-loaded areas. Functional metabolic neurologic imaging (photon emission tomography) of the brain of patients with aceruloplasminemia shows decreased metabolic activity in the basal ganglia, caudate nucleus, thalamus, cerebral cortex, and cerebellar cortex, all related to the increased amounts of iron and associated cellular injury.[3]

Genetics

The *Cp* gene that encodes Cp is located on the long arm of chromosome 3 (3q23–q24) and comprises 20 exons. About 40 *Cp* mutations have been reported in 60 patients in 46 families with aceruloplasminemia worldwide.[3,12] Many of the reported *Cp* mutations are "private," occurring in only one family.[2] In Japan, 4990 healthy adults were screened using serum Cp measurements. Subsequent *Cp* sequencing in subjects with subnormal serum Cp detected three mutations (5-bp insertion in exon 7, one heterozygote; one-bp deletion in exon 14, two heterozygotes; nonsense mutation in exon 15, one homozygote and two heterozygotes). The estimated frequency of these mutations was 70 per 100 000.[13] The mutations in aceruloplasminemia kindreds include nonsense, missense, base-pair insertions, base-pair deletions, and splice site, frame shift, and truncation stop-codon mutations involving different *Cp* exons and introns.[3] In a tabulation of 21 *Cp* mutations, abnormal variants were detected in 11 exons and 1 intron.[3]

Cp mutations in patients with aceruloplasminemia are diverse. Consequently, the only feasible way to substantiate a genetic diagnosis in newly diagnosed individuals is to sequence the *Cp* gene. This is neither commercially available nor practical for routine patient care. In contrast, most persons with *HFE* hemochromatosis with iron overload in many countries have the C282Y missense mutation, and thus a single, inexpensive mutation analysis will identify a high proportion of patients (Chapter 4).

Genotype–phenotype correlations

Neurologic complications and different *Cp* mutations have been reported in 28 homozygotes and 5 heterozygotes, but the authors were able to identify few informative genotype–phenotype correlations.[3] Many different *Cp* mutations cause a similar neurologic phenotype, and siblings with the same genotype may have a different neurologic phenotype.[3]

Some persons who are heterozygous for pathogenic *Cp* mutations develop tremors and cerebellar ataxia.[3] Heterozygotes usually have normal serum iron and ferritin concentrations; their serum Cp levels are intermediate between those of normal people and homozygotes.

Pathophysiology

All six copper-binding sites of Cp must be properly oriented in order for Cp to bind any copper atoms. Any mutation that distorts the normal Cp conformation prevents copper-binding and increases instability of Cp. Thus, abnormal Cp apoprotein lacks

ferroxidase activity, is not resistant to trypsin, and is rapidly degraded.[14] Some nonsense *Cp* mutations prevent the synthesis of Cp altogether. Other *Cp* mutations result in Cp molecules that cannot undergo normal proper folding. Such abnormal molecules remain within the endoplasmic reticulum, causing damage and cell death.[14,15]

Microcytic anemia is an important clinical problem in patients who have aceruloplasminemia. The absence of Cp (and its corresponding lack of ferroxidase activity) prevents oxidation of intracellular ferrous iron, so iron is not transported across cell membranes into plasma. As a consequence, the serum iron concentration is low, the percent saturation of transferrin with iron is low, and transferrin does not bind or transport an adequate amount of iron to the bone marrow for hemoglobin synthesis, even though there is abundant iron in macrophages and other cell types.

Neurologic abnormalities in some patients with aceruloplasminemia, such as extrapyramidal signs and cerebellar ataxia, can resemble those in patients with Parkinson's disease. Patients who have aceruloplasminemia often develop loss of intellectual function. Iron accumulates in the brain, including some cells of the basal ganglia, thalamus, putamen, caudate and dentate nuclei, substantia nigra, and cerebellum. Much iron can also accumulate in the cerebral cortex of patients with aceruloplasminemia. T1- and T2-weighted MRI reveals hypo-intensity in the iron-loaded areas of the brain. Iron also accumulates in the retina, pancreas, liver, heart, reticuloendothelial system, and other organs in patients with aceruloplasminemia.

A normal physiologic function of Cp is the prevention of lipid peroxidation. Iron-induced lipid peroxidation injury occurs in the absence of adequate Cp ferroxidase activity. Consequently, absence of Cp in neurons and retina results in lipid peroxidation, which in turn causes cell damage and death, followed by organ dysfunction. Neuronal injury in the retina causes a type of macular degeneration.

Differential diagnosis

Aceruloplasminemia is one of several heritable disorders characterized by neurodegeneration with brain iron accumulation, including Friedreich ataxia (Chapter 29), neuroferritinopathies (Chapter 31), and pantothenate kinase-associated neurodegeneration

(Chapter 30). Aceruloplasminemia and Wilson's disease (Chapters 4, 28) could be confused because neurologic abnormalities occur in patients with these respective disorders, and both disorders are inherited as autosomal recessive traits. Further, hypointensity in T2-weighted images of the brain and liver occur in each of these disorders due to the accumulation of iron and copper, respectively.

Wilson disease

Aceruloplasminemia is distinct from Wilson disease (Chapter 4). Aceruloplasminemia is not associated with increased copper storage, although serum Cp concentrations are low or undetectable. Patients with Wilson disease have increased copper storage and typically have subnormal serum Cp concentrations. In aceruloplasminemia, there is no excess excretion of urinary copper after administration of d-penicillamine, whereas d-penicillamine induces the urinary excretion of increased amounts of copper in persons with Wilson disease. In aceruloplasminemia, there is hepatic iron overload without copper accumulation or cirrhosis. In Wilson disease, there is heavy copper loading of the liver and cirrhosis. In aceruloplasminemia, the onset of neurologic abnormalities appear in adulthood, and hepatic failure does not occur as a consequence of iron overload. In Wilson disease, teenagers often develop neurologic disability and hepatic failure. Identification of mutations of the *Cp* gene confirm the diagnosis of aceruloplasminemia.

HFE hemochromatosis

Serum iron and ferritin concentrations are increased in hemochromatosis homozygotes, whereas patients with aceruloplasminemia have low serum iron and elevated serum ferritin levels. Serum Cp concentration is decreased in iron-loaded *HFE* hemochromatosis homozygotes; the Cp level returns to normal values after iron depletion.[16] Measuring serum Cp is not a useful phenotypic test for the evaluation of individuals who are suspected to have hemochromatosis. Similarly, measurement of serum Cp in *HFE* hemochromatosis homozygotes does not provide useful information for diagnosis, prognosis, or management. The presence of *CP* gene mutations and the absence of mutations of the *HFE* gene distinguish aceruloplasminemia from *HFE* hemochromatosis. Typical hemochromatosis patients do not accumulate excessive iron in the basal ganglia and do not develop retinal degeneration, movement disorders, cognitive disability, or dementia.

Other neurodegenerative disorders with brain iron accumulation

Aceruloplasminemia is associated with very low or undetectable serum Cp. This permits rapid distinction of aceruloplasminemia from neurologic degenerative disorders with brain iron accumulation due to mutations of genes other than *Cp* (Friedreich ataxia, neuroferritinopathies, or pantothenate kinase-associated neurodegeneration). Low or undetectable levels of serum Cp are not found in disorders due to mutations of mitochondrial DNA, Parkinson's disease, or Huntington's disease.

Menke disease

This disorder is an X-linked disorder characterized by inability of the intestine to absorb adequate copper and by low serum concentrations of Cp and copper in affected infants. Infants with Menke disease have so-called pili torti, scalp hairs that are twisted along their long axis. These hairs are easily broken, and are grey or silver. Affected infants fail to gain weight or thrive. Many experience seizures within the first days or months of life. Some have hypotonia and hypothermia. These children often die before age 3 years.[17] These features of Menke disease are very different from the decades-later onset of symptoms and signs in individuals who have hereditary aceruloplasminemia.

Utility of MRI

Both gradient echo T2* MRI and fast spin echo MRI can identify iron accumulation within the brain and are capable of distinguishing the four types of neurodegeneration associated with brain iron accumulation. These MRI methods can be used to select specific molecular tests to confirm the anticipated diagnosis.[18]

Treatment
Therapeutic phlebotomy

Phlebotomy therapy can be used to reduce body iron in aceruloplasminemia (Chapter 36). Patients with aceruloplasminemia usually have mild-moderate anemia (mean hemoglobin ~11 g/dL) with microcytosis.[3] This permits phlebotomy therapy to be performed, although the volume of blood removed at each session and the timing of repeat treatments must be carefully adjusted to hemoglobin concentration, body size, and tolerance of phlebotomy. In patients with very low hemoglobin levels or in those intolerant of blood removal, phlebotomy therapy is not feasible.

Deferoxamine chelation

Deferoxamine infusions are expected to deplete excessive hepatic storage iron.[13] Deferoxamine may be administered by subcutaneous infusion or by intravenous infusion[13,19] (Chapter 36). Some investigators treated aceruloplasminemia patients with intravenous infusions of deferoxamine, 500 mg during 1 hour, once or twice weekly for 6–10 months.[13] A marked decrease in serum ferritin concentration during deferoxamine therapy suggests that excessive hepatic iron stores have been mobilized and excreted. Some investigators reported MRI evidence that deferoxamine treatment mobilized iron from the liver or brain.[13] Other investigators found that deferoxamine therapy mobilized hepatic iron stores, but they did not observe MRI evidence of brain iron depletion.[20] There are no known reports of combination chelation therapy using either deferoxamine and deferiprone or deferoxamine and deferasirox to deplete excessive iron from the brain and the liver in patients with aceruloplasminemia. In patients with hemoglobin less than 9–10 g/dL, deferoxamine infusions exacerbate anemia.

Fresh-frozen plasma

In a report from Japan, a 54-year-old woman with aceruloplasminemia was treated with the combination of deferoxamine infusions and subsequently with fresh-frozen plasma that contained Cp and with deferoxamine.[21] The authors concluded that treatment with both deferoxamine and fresh-frozen plasma removed more iron than deferoxamine alone. The combination therapy resulted in decreased hepatic storage iron and improved neurologic function; the patient's previously abnormal electroencephalogram improved. Although neurologic function improved after this combination treatment, MRI T2-weighted images of the patient's brain did not appear to change.[21] There are no reports of controlled comparisons of deferoxamine therapy versus deferoxamine plus fresh-frozen plasma in patients who have aceruloplasminemia.

Zinc therapy

A 16-year-old girl with aceruloplasminemia developed a rapidly worsening neurodegenerative disorder that included dysarthria, spilling while drinking, deterioration of handwriting, abnormal ocular movements, intention tremor, involuntary arm movements, and unco-ordinated gait. One year after presentation, she became bedfast. Her liver biopsy revealed increased storage iron without excessive copper. She was heterozygous for a *Cp* mutation, but did not have a mutation of the *ATP7B* Wilson disease gene.[22] The authors treated her with oral zinc in an attempt to protect her brain from iron-generated free radical injury.[22] In addition, zinc induces the synthesis of metallothionein that can bind iron in intestinal epithelia that would then be sloughed subsequently, presumably preventing continued absorption of iron. She was treated with oral zinc sulfate, starting at 50 mg daily; during 1 month, the dose was increased to 50 mg four times daily.

This patient's neurologic function improved somewhat during the ensuing 18 months of follow-up.[22] She became able to sit up in a wheelchair and regained the ability to walk a few steps and to assist with some activities of daily living, such as eating, washing, and dressing herself. The authors did not report the appearance of a liver biopsy specimen after oral zinc therapy.[22] There are no reports of controlled trials of zinc therapy vs. other treatment for patients who have aceruloplasminemia.

References

1. Miyajima H, Nishimura Y, Mizoguchi K, Sakamoto M, Shimizu T, Honda N. Familial apoceruloplasmin deficiency associated with blepharospasm and retinal degeneration. *Neurology* 1987; **37**: 761–7.

2. Miyajima H, Kohno S, Takahashi Y, Yonekawa O, Kanno T. Estimation of the gene frequency of aceruloplasminemia in Japan. *Neurology* 1999; **53**: 617–19.

3. McNeill A, Pandolfo M, Kuhn J, Shang H, Miyajima H. The neurological presentation of ceruloplasmin gene mutations. *Eur Neurol* 2008; **60**: 200–5.

4. Cox DW. Factors influencing serum ceruloplasmin levels in normal individuals. *J Lab Clin Med* 1966; **68**: 893–904.

5. Tutor-Crespo MJ, Hermida J, Tutor JC. Assessment of copper status in epileptic patients treated with anticonvulsant drugs by measuring the specific oxidase activity of ceruloplasmin. *Epilepsy Res* 2003; **56**: 147–53.

6. Miyajima H. Genetic disorders affecting proteins of iron and copper metabolism: clinical implications. *Intern Med* 2002; **41**: 762–9.

7. Miyajima H, Takahashi Y, Serizawa M, Kaneko E, Gitlin JD. Increased plasma lipid peroxidation in patients with aceruloplasminemia. *Free Radic Biol Med* 1996; **20**: 757–60.

8. Miyajima H, Fujimoto M, Kohno S, Kaneko E, Gitlin JD. CSF abnormalities in patients with aceruloplasminemia. *Neurology* 1998; **51**: 1188–90.

9. Tajima K, Kawanami T, Nagai R, Horiuchi S, Kato T. Hereditary ceruloplasmin deficiency increases advanced glycation end products in the brain. *Neurology* 1999; **53**: 619–22.

10. Kohno S, Miyajima H, Takahashi Y, Suzuki H, Hishida A. Defective electron transfer in complexes I and IV in patients with aceruloplasminemia. *J Neurol Sci* 2000; **182**: 57–60.

11. Kono S, Miyajima H. Molecular and pathological basis of aceruloplasminemia. *Biol Res* 2006; **39**: 15–23.

12. Hofmann WP, Welsch C, Takahashi Y, *et al.* Identification and in silico characterization of a novel compound heterozygosity associated with hereditary aceruloplasminemia. *Scand J Gastroenterol* 2007; **42**: 1088–94.

13. Miyajima H, Takahashi Y, Kamata T, Shimizu H, Sakai N, Gitlin JD. Use of desferrioxamine in the treatment of aceruloplasminemia. *Ann Neurol* 1997; **41**: 404–7.

14. Hellman NE, Kono S, Mancini GM, Hoogeboom AJ, De Jong GJ, Gitlin JD. Mechanisms of copper incorporation into human ceruloplasmin. *J Biol Chem* 2002; **277**: 46 632–8.

15. Kono S, Suzuki H, Oda T, *et al.* Cys-881 is essential for the trafficking and secretion of truncated mutant ceruloplasmin in aceruloplasminemia. *J Hepatol* 2007; **47**: 844–50.

16. Laine F, Ropert M, Lan CL, *et al.* Serum ceruloplasmin and ferroxidase activity are decreased in *HFE* C282Y homozygote male iron-overloaded patients. *J Hepatol* 2002; **36**: 60–5.

17. Agertt F, Crippa AC, Lorenzoni PJ, *et al.* Menke's disease: case report. *Arq Neuropsiquiatr* 2007; **65**: 157–60.

18. McNeill A, Birchall D, Hayflick SJ, *et al.* T2* and FSE MRI distinguishes four subtypes of neurodegeneration with brain iron accumulation. *Neurology* 2008; **70**: 1614–19.

19. Loreal O, Turlin B, Pigeon C, *et al.* Aceruloplasminemia: new clinical, pathophysiological and therapeutic insights. *J Hepatol* 2002; **36**: 851–6.

20. Mariani R, Arosio C, Pelucchi S, *et al.* Iron chelation therapy in aceruloplasminaemia: study of a patient with a novel missense mutation. *Gut* 2004; **53**: 756–8.

21. Yonekawa M, Okabe T, Asamoto Y, Ohta M. A case of hereditary ceruloplasmin deficiency with iron deposition in the brain associated with chorea, dementia, diabetes mellitus, and retinal pigmentation: administration of fresh-frozen human plasma. *Eur Neurol* 1999; **42**: 157–62.

22. Kuhn J, Bewermeyer H, Miyajima H, Takahashi Y, Kuhn KF, Hoogenraad TU. Treatment of symptomatic heterozygous aceruloplasminemia with oral zinc sulphate. *Brain Dev* 2007; **29**: 450–3.

Friedreich ataxia and cardiomyopathy

Friedreich ataxia (OMIM #229300) is characterized by ataxia, cardiomyopathy, and accumulation of iron in mitochondria of the dentate nucleus of the cerebellum and of cardiac myocytes. Systemic iron overload does not occur. This is the most common type of heritable ataxia, and affects approximately 1 person per 30 000.

Clinical manifestations

Initial clinical evidence of Friedreich ataxia usually occurs in adolescents and adults less than 25 years of age. In 115 affected individuals in 90 families, the onset of symptoms occurred at mean age 10.5 years.[1] The symptoms and signs that appear during the first 5 years are ataxia of limbs and trunk, and absence of deep tendon reflexes. As the condtion worsens, additional characteristic findings develop, including dysarthria, hypotonia, scoliosis, a Babinski plantar extensor response, loss of position sense in toes, and loss of vibratory sensation in feet. Peripheral neuropathy adds a sensory component to gait ataxia. Affected individuals experience progressive loss of ability to walk, causing 95% to become chair bound by age 44 years.[1] Pes cavus is common, and is caused by nerve injury and consequent atrophy of intrinsic muscles of the feet.

Hypertrophic cardiomyopathy is present in two-thirds of the patients. This typically affects the interventricular septum or the wall of the left ventricle. In some patients, echocardiography demonstrates cardiac hypertrophy or decreased left ventricular ejection fraction before overt heart failure occurs. Heart failure is the most common cause of death in patients with Friedreich ataxia. Oculomotor abnormalities (nystagmus) develop in some patients. Decreased visual acuity may indicate the presence of optic nerve atrophy. Viewed by fundoscopy the optic disk is pale in such patients. Hearing loss occurs in 8%–13% of patients. Diabetes mellitus occurs in 10% of patients.

The neurologic abnormalities are due to degeneration of dorsal root ganglia, the posterior columns, the dorsal spinocerebellar tracts, Clarke column, and the lateral corticospinal tracts. Large myelinated axons of peripheral nerves and sensory neurons in dorsal root ganglia are affected. In some patients, atrophy of the cerebellum or medulla also occurs. Nerve conduction studies show axonal type of sensory neuropathy.[2] Magnetic resonance imaging (MRI) reveals atrophy of the cervical spinal cord. The prevalence of 14 neurologic abnormalities in Friedreich ataxia patients is displayed in Table 29.1.

Other degenerative neurologic disorders share some features with Friedreich ataxia. These include spinocerebellar ataxia, cerebellar degeneration, severe vitamin E deficiency, and some heritable sensory and motor neuropathies. Ataxia-telangiectasia, a different autosomal recessive disorder, shares the feature of cerebellar ataxia with Friedreich ataxia, but the former condition usually is associated with prominent telangiectases of the skin. Syphilitic tabes dorsalis is due to injury of the posterior columns and dorsal roots of the spinal cord, but not the dorsal spinocerebellar tracts and lateral corticospinal tracts. Vitamin B_{12} deficiency usually causes injury of posterior columns, dorsal roots, and dorsal spinocerebellar tracts, but not the lateral corticospinal tracts. Autosomal dominant spinocerebellar ataxias and some other acquired ataxias may be considered in the differential diagnosis. Acquired ataxias include post-viral cerebellar ataxia (recovery is usual), and alcoholic, paraneoplastic, and other autoimmune types of cerebellar degeneration. Historical features, physical examination findings, and laboratory evaluation often help to include or exclude further consideration of these different types of acquired ataxia.

Genetics

Friedreich ataxia is caused by mutations of the *FXN* gene (chromosome 9q13–21.1) that encodes

Table 29.1. Abnormalities in Friedreich ataxia patients (percent)[a]

Abnormality	Harding 1981 (115 patients)[1]	Durr 1996 (140 patients)[2]	Delatycki 2000 (83 patients)[4]
Gait ataxia	—	100	100
Limb ataxia	99	99	100
Dysarthria	97	91	95
Extensor plantar responses	89	79	74
Leg muscle weakness	88	67	—
Diminished vibratory sensation	73	78	88
Scoliosis	79	60	78
Cardiomyopathy	66[b]	63	65
Pes cavus	55	55	74
Sphincter disturbance	—	23	41
Diabetes	10	32	8
Decreased visual acuity	18	13	—
Hearing loss	8	13	—
Reflexes in legs present	1	12	2

Notes: [a]Adapted from Delatycki et al.[4]
[b]Significant electrocardiographic abnormalities.

the protein frataxin. This disorder is inherited as an autosomal recessive condition. There is an increased coefficient of consanguinity in at least one study of affected families.[1] Mutations of the first intron of the frataxin gene result in an expansion of the numbers of repeats of three nucleic acids: guanine; adenine; adenine (GAA). Most patients with Friedreich ataxia have 70–1500 GAA repeats in *FXN* intron 1, whereas normal individuals have only as many as 30 GAA intronic repeats.[3] In some patients with Friedreich ataxia, intronic GAA trinucleotide repeat sequences accumulate with age.

More than 90% of Friedreich ataxia patients are homozygous for *FXN* genes that contain excessive intronic triplet repeats. About 4% of patients are compound heterozygotes who have one *FXN* allele with excessive intronic GAA repeats, and one point mutation in the *FXN* gene.[3,4] Patients who have longer GAA expansions may experience earlier onset of symptoms and more rapid worsening of the disease than patients with shorter expansions.[2] In a study of 101 first-degree relatives of affected individuals, no neurologic abnormalities and no cardiomyopathy were identified.[1]

Pathophysiology

Frataxin is a mitochondrial protein that is involved in RNA processing and intramitochondrial iron metabolism. In its absence, iron–sulfur protein clusters are not produced, and normal heme synthesis does not occur.[5] Deficient frataxin activity thus causes the accumulation of iron within mitochondria. The generation of murine cell lines carrying a frataxin conditional allele were used to create murine cellular models depleted for endogenous frataxin and expressing missense-mutated human frataxin. These new cellular models reproduce all the biochemical phenotypes associated with Friedreich ataxia. Thus these models are important tools to gain new insights into the in vivo consequences of pathological missense mutations, and to screen compounds aimed at compensating frataxin deficiency.[6]

The cause of the neurologic and cardiac abnormalities is age-related accumulation of intronic GAA trinucleotide repeat sequences of the *FXN* gene in dorsal root ganglia. The activity of *FXN* in dorsal root ganglia of affected people is only 5%–30% of that observed in normal persons.[3] Dorsal root ganglia are sensitive to inadequate amounts of frataxin protein. Age-related expansion of the triplet repeat sequences causes the progressive degeneration of dorsal root ganglia and demyelination of axons in the posterior column of the spinal cord, and progressive loss of granule cells in the cerebellum. Iron consequently accumulates in mitochondria, causing inadequate mitochondrial respiratory chain activity, decreased cytosolic aconitase activity, production of free radicals, and oxidative damage. The trinucleotide repeat sequences are also thought to cause hypertrophic cardiomyopathy.

At the subcellular level, deficient frataxin activity results in inadequate expression of a mitochondrial protein chaperone involved in the formation of iron-sulfur clusters in mitochondria, and in the movement of the iron–sulfur clusters from mito-chondria into cytosol. Heme synthesis, also decreased due to subnormal activity of frataxin is related to decreased ferrochelatase activity. In the absence of normal frataxin activity, iron accumulates in mito-chondria. Therein, fibers proliferate, cristae degener-ate, and vacuoles accumulate. Oxidative injury then occurs in sensory neurons and in cardiac myocytes.[7,8] Cardiac myocytes undergo hypertrophy, and accumu-late myofibrils and excessive amounts of iron. Hepatic xanthine oxidase is dependent on some activity of iron–sulfur clusters. In the absence of adequate iron–sulfur clusters, xanthine oxidase activity is decreased, and thus uric acid synthesis is decreased.

Treatment

Beta blockade

A 12.5-year-old girl who had symptomatic hyper-trophic cardiomyopathy was treated with high-dose beta blockade (propranolol 120 mg daily). This induced a remission of her cardiac symptoms and electrocardiographic abnormalities. There was also a decrease in the thickness of her interventricular septum and the posterior wall of her left ventricle. These improvements persisted during 4.5 years of follow-up.[9]

Reduction of intramitochondrial oxyradicals

Oxidative injury due to free radicals is thought to cause the mitochondrial and neuronal abnormalities. Accordingly, there is a rationale for using free radical scavengers for treatment, including idebenone, iron chelation, and erythropoietin. The reasoning that led to consideration of each of these treatments was the goal of mobilizing excessive iron from mitochondria into plasma, thereby decreasing the production of reactive oxygen radicals within mitochondria.

Idebenone

This is a short-chain quinine analogue of coenzyme Q10 that acts as a scavenger of free radicals. This compound has been tested in several groups of Friedreich ataxia patients. Idebenone decreased the urinary excretion of 8-hydroxy-2-deoxyguanosine, a marker that correlates with oxidative stress.[10] In 2003, the results of a one-year, double-blind,

randomized, placebo-controlled trial of the effect of idebenone on the heart and on neurologic abnormal-ities in Friedreich ataxia patients was published.[11] None of the 29 patients had echocardiographic abnor-malities before participating in the study. Fifteen patients were randomized to the placebo group and 14 to the idebenone group. There was a 10% decrease in thickness of the interventricular septum and left ventricular mass in 5 of 14 patients treated with idebenone, whereas no significant cardiac change was observed in any of 15 patients who received placebo. The left ventricular ejection fraction did not increase in any patient.[11]

Iron chelation

Investigators in Jerusalem and France treated nine young patients with the bidentate iron chelator defer-iprone for 6 months. The patients were already taking idebenone.[5] The authors employed deferiprone because it readily permeates cell membranes. MRI scans of dentate nuclei was performed before and after 6 months of treatment with deferiprone. The results were compared to those of a group of nine Friedreich ataxia patients treated with idebenone but not deferiprone. The deferiprone was associated with MRI evidence of iron removal from the dentate nuclei. The chelation therapy was also associated with objective improvement in tests of manual dexterity and gait ataxia, and in subjective improvement of sensory peripheral neuropathy. The youngest patients experienced the greatest improvement in neurologic function.[5]

Additional investigation will be required to deter-mine if very early chelation therapy may prevent neurologic deterioration in patients who have Friedreich ataxia. Similarly, additional investigation is needed to determine if the combination of defer-iprone and deferoxamine will cause mobilization and excretion of excess myocardial iron, and prevent myocardial fibrosis and hypertrophy. Iron chelators in the 2-pyridylcarboxaldehyde isonicotinoyl hydra-zone class decrease mitochondrial iron in mice, and suggest additional types of chelators to test in Friedreich ataxia patients.[12]

Erythropoietin

Recombinant human erythropoietin may increase the expression of frataxin. Because frataxin expression is decreased in Friedreich ataxia, some investigators reasoned that erythropoietin administration might benefit patients with Friedreich ataxia. Erythropoietin increased the expression of frataxin in the cell types in vitro that are most affected in Friedreich ataxia, including neurons, cardiac myocytes, and fibroblasts.[13] It is anticipated that studies will be conducted to determine if erythropoietin therapy will decrease the neurologic and cardiac complications in patients who have Friedreich ataxia.

Until recently, only supportive care was available for the management of patients with Friedreich ataxia. It remains appropriate for physicians to arrange for patients to have physical therapy, occupational therapy, speech therapy, a four-pronged cane, a four-legged walker, or a wheelchair, as needed. Some patients with ataxia have been treated with types of centrally acting medications, such as buspirone, amantadine, and 5-hydroxytryptophan,[3,7,14] but these medications are no longer used routinely.

References

1. Harding AE. Friedreich's ataxia: a clinical and genetic study of 90 families with an analysis of early diagnostic criteria and intrafamilial clustering of clinical features. *Brain* 1981; **104**: 589–620.

2. Durr A, Cossee M, Agid Y, *et al*. Clinical and genetic abnormalities in patients with Friedreich's ataxia. *N Engl J Med* 1996; **335**: 1169–75.

3. Campuzano V, Montermini L, Lutz Y, *et al*. Frataxin is reduced in Friedreich ataxia patients and is associated with mitochondrial membranes. *Hum Mol Genet* 1997; **6**: 1771–80.

4. Delatycki MB, Williamson R, Forrest SM. Friedreich ataxia: an overview. *J Med Genet* 2000; **37**: 1–8.

5. Boddaert N, Quan Sang KH, Rotig A, *et al*. Selective iron chelation in Friedreich ataxia: biologic and clinical implications. *Blood* 2007; **110**: 401–8.

6. Calmels N, Schmucker S, Wattenhofer-Donze M, *et al*. The first cellular models based on frataxin missense mutations that reproduce spontaneously the defects associated with Friedreich ataxia. *PLoS One* 2009; 4: e6379.

7. Botez MI, Botez-Marquard T, Elie R, Pedraza OL, Goyette K, Lalonde R. Amantadine hydrochloride treatment in heredodegenerative ataxias: a double-blind study. *J Neurol Neurosurg Psychiatry* 1996; **61**: 259–64.

8. Simon D, Seznec H, Gansmuller A, *et al*. Friedreich ataxia mouse models with progressive cerebellar and sensory ataxia reveal autophagic neurodegeneration in dorsal root ganglia. *J Neurosci* 2004; **24**: 1987–95.

9. Kosutic J, Zamurovic D. High-dose beta-blocker hypertrophic cardiomyopathy therapy in a patient with Friedreich ataxia. *Pediatr Cardiol* 2005; **26**: 727–30.

10. Schulz JB, Dehmer T, Schols L, *et al*. Oxidative stress in patients with Friedreich ataxia. *Neurology* 2000; **55**: 1719–21.

11. Mariotti C, Solari A, Torta D, Marano L, Fiorentini C, Di Donato S. Idebenone treatment in Friedreich patients: 1-year-long randomized placebo-controlled trial. *Neurology* 2003; **60**: 1676–9.

12. Lovejoy DB, Kalinowski D, Bernhardt PV, Richardson DR. PCTH: a novel orally active chelator for the treatment of iron overload disease. *Hemoglobin* 2006; **30**: 93–104.

13. Sturm B, Stupphann D, Kaun C, *et al*. Recombinant human erythropoietin: effects on frataxin expression in vitro. *Eur J Clin Invest* 2005; **35**: 711–17.

14. Trouillas P, Serratrice G, Laplane D, *et al*. Levorotatory form of 5-hydroxytryptophan in Friedreich's ataxia. Results of a double-blind drug-placebo co-operative study. *Arch Neurol* 1995; **52**: 456–60.

Pantothenate kinase (*PANK2*)-associated neurodegeneration

In 1922, German investigators Hallervorden and Spatz reported a syndrome of neurologic and pathologic findings in a sibship of 12 individuals, among whom 5 siblings had progressive dysarthria and dementia. At autopsy, the investigators observed brown discoloration of the substantia nigra and the globus pallidus of the affected siblings.[1] Since the initial report, hundreds of individuals with this disorder have been reported, and most have mutations of the *PANK2* gene that encodes pantothenate kinase 2.[2] In 2001, this disorder was named pantothenate kinase-associated neurodegeneration, also known as neurodegeneration with brain iron accumulation (OMIM #234200). The brown discoloration of the brains of persons with pantothenate kinase-associated neurodegeneration is caused by the deposition of excessive quantities of iron. This condition occurs in approximately 3 per 1 000 000 people. In a university hospital autopsy series that was evaluated to identify iron overload disorders specifically, only one case of neurodegeneration with brain iron accumulation was found in 10 345 adults (age ≥21 years) and 1337 children (>1 year of age).[3]

Clinical manifestations

There is phenotypic heterogeneity in the clinical presentation of patients who have mutations of the *PANK2* gene. The report of an international study published in 2003 describes findings in 186 patients from 145 families, including clinical histories, physical examination findings, laboratory characteristics, extrapyramidal neurologic abnormalities, and magnetic resonance imaging evidence of iron deposition in the basal ganglia. The investigators identified and separated 123 patients from 98 families into three groups: (1) patients who presented with "classical" clinical findings, and had mutations of the *PANK2* gene; (2) those with an "atypical" disease presentation, but who had *PANK2* mutations; and (3) patients

whose presentation was atypical, and who had no mutations of the *PANK2* gene.[4] Three groups of patients with extrapyramidal neurologic abnormalities and increased iron in the brain are discussed here.[4]

Group 1 "Classical" disease presentation and *PANK2* mutations

In a report of 123 patients with sufficient clinical data to permit classification, 66 patients (54%) were considered to have "classical" disease.[4] The "classical" presentation included early age of onset (before age 10 years), rapid worsening of dystonia, severe disability by age 20 years, and magnetic resonance imaging (MRI) scans compatible with excessive deposition of iron in the basal ganglia. Among the 66 patients with the "classical" presentation, all had a mutation of the *PANK2* gene.

The mean age of onset of symptoms was 3.4 years (range 0.5–12 years). In 78% of the patients, symptoms at presentation involved gait and posture. Neurologic findings at some time in 98% of these 66 patients included extrapyramidal abnormalities with dystonia, rigidity, dysarthria, and choreoathetosis. Dystonia was present in 87% of the patients; this usually involved the muscles of the head and limbs. Later, dystonias of the spinal musculature occurred. Corticospinal tract abnormalities, present in 25%, included spasticity, hyperreflexia, and a Babinski (extensor) toe response. Decline in cognitive ability was present in 29% of patients; evidence of dementia was uncommon. Dysarthria occurred in 16% of patients. Patients did not have seizures.

Further investigation revealed that 66% of patients with the "classical" disease had electroretinographic or physical examination evidence of retinopathy. Atrophy of the optic nerve was detected in only 3% of patients. Acanthocytosis of red blood cells was present in 8% of the patients whose blood smears were evaluated.

Clinical deterioration did not occur at a predictable pace among the patients with "classical" disease. Some patients experienced steady decline in function; others experienced episodes of deterioration followed by 1 or 2 months of stability, after which further neurologic deterioration occurred. A characteristic finding was that 85% of the patients with "classical" disease became unable to walk within 15 years after the onset of symptoms.[4]

Group 2 "Atypical" disease presentation and *PANK2* gene mutations

Of the 123 patients studied, 57 had an "atypical" disease presentation. Among these 57 patients, 23 (40%) had mutations of the *PANK2* gene. The presentation of disease, the physical and laboratory findings, and the clinical course in these patients were more heterogeneous than in the patients who had the "classical" presentation. The mean age of onset of disease in the patients in this "atypical" disease presentation group was 13.7 years (range 1–28 years).

Dysarthria or repetition of words or phrases was a prominent early finding in these patients (39%). Although 73% of these patients had extrapyramidal abnormalities, dystonia and rigidity were not as severe, and did not worsen as rapidly, as in patients who presented with "classical" disease. Sixty-four percent of the patients with "atypical" presentations were able to walk as adults. Decline in cognitive function was very common, and was similar to that of frontotemporal dementia. One-third had psychiatric symptoms, personality changes, depression, violent outbursts, impulsivity, or emotional lability. Corticospinal tract involvement with spasticity, hyperreflexia, and extensor toe responses was present in 18% of the patients with "atypical" presentations.

Group 3 "Atypical" presentation without *PANK2* gene mutations

Of the 57 patients with "atypical" disease presentation, 34 did not have *PANK2* mutations. Among patients in this subgroup, the mean age of onset of disease was age 9.9 years (range 0.5–38 years). These patients had extrapyramidal and corticospinal neurologic findings that were similar to those of patients who had "classical" disease with *PANK2* mutations,

and to those of patients who had "atypical" disease presentation with *PANK2* mutations. None of the patients in the subgroup with "atypical" disease presentation without *PANK2* mutations had dysarthria, and none developed psychiatric symptoms.

Other clinical descriptions

Other publications report valuable information about the clinical presentation of other patients who have *PANK2* mutations. These articles provide additional insight into the similarities and differences in the symptoms and signs that occur in affected individuals.[5–7]

Pathophysiology

PANK2 encodes pantothenate kinase, a dimeric kinase that promotes phosphorylation of pantothenate and some other substrates. Pantothenate kinase catalyzes the initial and rate-limiting step in the synthesis of coenzyme A that is required for homeostasis within the matrix of normal mitochondria.[2,5,8]

In the absence of adequate activity of pantothenate kinase, mitochondrial synthesis of coenzyme A from its nutritional precursor pantothenate is reduced. It has been hypothesized that deficiency of pantothenate kinase results in the accumulation of cysteine that becomes oxidized in the presence of iron. This causes free radical production and injury of mitochondria and other organelles and membranes, leading to degeneration of neurons in the basal ganglia, retina, and optic nerve. This accounts for the symptoms and physical examination abnormalities of patients who have pantothenate kinase-associated neurodegeneration. Iron accumulation accompanies the neurodegeneration in the basal ganglia and the pars reticulata of the substantia nigra and globus pallidus.

Iron causes brown discoloration of the bilateral pars reticulata of the substantia nigra, the bilateral globus pallidus, and of the red and dentate nuclei. Iron deposits are visible in the same areas of the brain. Excessive iron in the globus pallidus can be demonstrated in vivo by MRI or ex vivo using iron staining. Staining routines that increase the sensitivity of the Perls' Prussian blue technique are used to evaluate non-heme ferric brain iron deposits.[9,10] The Turnbull blue reaction is used to identify ferrous iron in brain sections.[10] Neuronal axonal spheroids are also present.

Brain imaging

The diagnosis of pantothenate kinase-associated neurodegeneration has usually been made post-mortem. The description of MRI alterations in the basal ganglia[11-13] suggested the possibility of an in vivo diagnosis. Angelini and colleagues presented the clinical and MRI findings of 11 patients diagnosed as having pantothenate kinase-associated neurode-generation. This is consistent with the utility of MRI in detecting excess iron deposition in other organs (Chapter 4).

MRI of the brain of individuals who have pantothenate kinase-associated neurodegeneration often reveals the so-called "eye of the tiger" sign. This pattern in T2-weighted images is composed of an area of hyperintensity in the anteromedial portion of the overall hypointense globus pallidus. This sign is caused by the accumulation of iron bilaterally in the globus pallidus. The hypointensity (T2 shortening) of the globus pallidus is caused by iron accumulation. The hyperintensity, referred to as T2 prolongation, in the anteromedial area is thought to be caused by neuronal loss, gliosis, and edema in the globus palli-dus. MRI machines that have low magnet strength may not identify the increased amounts of iron in the globus pallidus. Magnets with 1.5 Tesla strength usu-ally identify increased pallidal iron. In the past, the "eye of the tiger" sign was considered to be pathogno-monic of iron accumulation in individuals who had pantothenate kinase-associated neurodegeneration. Recently, this sign was identified in subjects who did not have mutations of the pantothenate kinase 2 gene.[12] Interested readers can refer to recent discussions of this topic.[4,5,14-16]

Genotype–phenotype correlations

The syndrome of dystonia, progressive neurodegenera-tion, accumulation of iron in the globus pallidus, and mutations of the *PANK2* gene is typically transmitted as an autosomal recessive disorder.[2,17] The disorder has been reported almost exclusively from Europeans of various ethnic or national groups. *PANK2* is located on the short arm of chromosome 20 (chromo-some 20p13–p12.3).[2,17] The most common mutations of the *PANK2* gene in patients with pantothenate kinase-associated neurodegeneration are the missense mutations G411R, T418M, T528M, and G521R. These amino acid changes cause loss of function of the pantothenate kinase enzyme.[4,6,18] There is genotypic

heterogeneity in patients with this disorder. For example, some patients have only one identifiable *PANK2* mutation, whereas other patients have two *PANK2* mutations. This could be construed as semi-dominant heritability.

Some conditions that may mimic pantothenate kinase-associated neurodegeneration include Wilson disease; aceruloplasminemia; several enzymatic abnormalities of neuronal ceroid lipofuscinosis types 1–9 (referred to as Batten disease); deficiency of β-galactosidase; deficiency of ganglioside monosialic acid-1-hexosaminidase, also referred to as GM1-gangliosidase; neuroaxonal dystrophy; neuroferritino-pathy; Huntington disease; and HARP syndrome.

HARP syndrome

Neurodegeneration of the globus pallidus is charac-teristic of the so-called HARP syndrome—hypoprebe-talipoproteinemia, acanthocytosis, retinitis pigmentosa, and degeneration of the globus pallidus. This dis-order is also caused by *PANK2* mutations and is thus allelic to pantothenate kinase-associated neuro-degeneration. The most distinguishing feature of HARP syndrome is the decrease or absence of pre-beta-lipoproteins that can be detected on lipoprotein electrophoresis. Persons with HARP syndrome have normal levels of triglycerides, total cholesterol, and the low-density and the high-density lipoprotein subtypes of cholesterol. Retinal pigmentation in HARP syndrome is typically much greater than occurs in some patients who have pantothenate kinase-associated neurodegeneration. A common *PANK2* mutation that causes HARP syndrome is R371X; another is *PANK2* M327T. These mutations prevent synthesis of the normal pantothenate kinase 2 protein.

Treatment

There is no specific treatment for patients who have pantothenate kinase-associated neurodegeneration, and no management is known to cure the dystonias. Pantothenic acid (vitamin B5) is the substrate on which pantothenate kinase acts. The generally accepted minimum daily requirement of pantothenic acid is 10 mg. Some experts recommend that patients with pantothenate kinase-associated neurodegenera-tion take much higher doses of pantothenate in the form of pantothenic acid or as calcium pantothenate. There are no known controlled trials that have evalu-ated the putative value of this replacement therapy.

Some patients who take very high doses of oral pantothenate supplements (several grams daily for a few weeks) develop diarrhea, but there are no known serious complications of high-dose pantothenate intake.

Some oral medications, including baclofen and trihexyphenidyl, provide some patients with some relief. Baclofen, used as a muscle relaxant and antispasmodic, can also cause central nervous system depression. Baclofen is thought to act on monosynaptic and polysynaptic reflexes at the level of the spinal cord, perhaps by hyperpolarization of afferent terminals. Some patients have been treated with continuous intrathecal administration of baclofen using an infusion pump.[19] Abrupt withdrawal of intrathecal baclofen infusion can cause life-threatening complications[20] such as fever, altered mental status, rebound spasticity, muscle rigidity, and rhabdomyolysis.

Trihexyphenidyl is thought to act as an antispasmodic agent by directly relaxing smooth muscle, and by indirectly inhibiting the parasympathetic nervous system. The adverse effects of trihexyphenidyl are similar to those of atropine (dry mouth, nervousness, blurred vision, nausea, and dizziness), but usually are less pronounced. Levodopa, carbidopa, bromocryptine, and iron chelation therapy do not improve symptoms.[19]

Deep brain stimulation is an invasive procedure that relieves some of the dystonias in patients who have pantothenate kinase-associated neurodegeneration.[21,22] In this treatment, electrodes are placed in each globus pallidus to allow electrical stimulation of these structures. Deep brain stimulation has been tested in fewer patients with pantothenate kinase-associated neurodegeneration than in patients with other types of movement disorders such as Parkinson disease and different childhood dystonias. Ablation of the globus pallidus[23] or incision of the thalamus[24] have provided improvement in a few patients with intractable dystonia. The dystonias may recur within 1 year after pallidotomy or thalamotomy.

Patients with severe dystonia and osteopenia may experience bone fractures without trauma. It is important to provide adequate analgesia for these patients. Individuals who become unable to eat and drink adequately may benefit from a gastrostomy or jejunostomy tube to allow care providers to administer nutrition and fluids reliably.

References

1. Hallervorden J, Spatz H. *Eigenartige Erkrankung im extrapyramidalen System mit besonderer Beteiligung des Globus pallidus und der Substantia nigra: ein Beitrag zu den Beziehungen zwischen diesen beiden Zentren. Z Ges Neurol Psychiat* 1922; **79**: 254–302.

2. Zhou B, Westaway SK, Levinson B, Johnson MA, Gitschier J, Hayflick SJ. A novel pantothenate kinase gene (*PANK2*) is defective in Hallervorden–Spatz syndrome. *Nat Genet* 2001; **28**: 345–9.

3. Barton JC, Acton RT, Anderson LE, Alexander CB. A comparison between whites and blacks with severe multi-organ iron overload identified in 16 152 autopsies. *Clin Gastroenterol Hepatol* 2009; **7**: 781–5.

4. Hayflick SJ, Westaway SK, Levinson B, *et al.* Genetic, clinical, and radiographic delineation of Hallervorden–Spatz syndrome. *N Engl J Med* 2003; **348**: 33–40.

5. Hartig MB, Hortnagel K, Garavaglia B, *et al.* Genotypic and phenotypic spectrum of *PANK2* mutations in patients with neurodegeneration with brain iron accumulation. *Ann Neurol* 2006; **59**: 248–56.

6. Pellecchia MT, Valente EM, Cif L, *et al.* The diverse phenotype and genotype of pantothenate kinase-associated neurodegeneration. *Neurology* 2005; **64**: 1810–12.

7. Thomas M, Hayflick SJ, Jankovic J. Clinical heterogeneity of neurodegeneration with brain iron accumulation (Hallervorden–Spatz syndrome) and pantothenate kinase-associated neurodegeneration. *Mov Disord* 2004; **19**: 36–42.

8. Zhang YM, Rock CO, Jackowski S. Biochemical properties of human pantothenate kinase 2 isoforms and mutations linked to pantothenate kinase-associated neurodegeneration. *J Biol Chem* 2006; **281**: 107–14.

9. Nguyen-Legros J, Bizot J, Bolesse M, Pulicani JP. ["Diaminobenzidine black" as a new histochemical demonstration of exogenous iron (author's transl).] *Histochemistry* 1980; **66**: 239–44.

10. Morris CM, Candy JM, Oakley AE, Bloxham CA, Edwardson JA. Histochemical distribution of non-haem iron in the human brain. *Acta Anat (Basel)* 1992; **144**: 235–57.

11. Littrup PJ, Gebarski SS. MR imaging of Hallervorden–Spatz disease. *J Comput Assist Tomogr* 1985; **9**: 491–3.

12. Tanfani G, Mascalchi M, Dal Pozzo GC, Taverni N, Saia A, Trevisan C. MR imaging in a case of Hallervorden–Spatz disease. *J Comput Assist Tomogr* 1987; **11**: 1057–8.

13. Sethi KD, Adams RJ, Loring DW, el Gammal T. Hallervorden–Spatz syndrome: clinical and magnetic resonance imaging correlations. *Ann Neurol* 1988; **24**: 692–4.

14. Valentino P, Annesi G, Ciro Candiano CI, *et al.* Genetic heterogeneity in patients with pantothenate kinase-associated neurodegeneration and classic magnetic resonance imaging eye-of-the-tiger pattern. *Mov Disord* 2006; **21**: 252–4.

15. Zolkipli Z, Dahmoush H, Saunders DE, Chong WK, Surtees R. Pantothenate kinase 2 mutation with classic pantothenate-kinase-associated neurodegeneration without eye-of-the-tiger sign on MRI in a pair of siblings. *Pediatr Radiol* 2006; **36**: 884–6.

16. Hayflick SJ, Hartman M, Coryell J, Gitschier J, Rowley H. Brain MRI in neurodegeneration with brain iron accumulation with and without *PANK2* mutations. *AJNR Am J Neuroradiol* 2006; **27**: 1230–3.

17. Taylor TD, Litt M, Kramer P, *et al.* Homozygosity mapping of Hallervorden-Spatz syndrome to chromosome 20p12.3–p13. *Nat Genet* 1996; **14**: 479–81.

18. Matarin MM, Singleton AB, Houlden H. *PANK2* gene analysis confirms genetic heterogeneity in neurodegeneration with brain iron accumulation (NBIA) but mutations are rare in other types of adult neurodegenerative disease. *Neurosci Lett* 2006; **407**: 162–5.

19. Albright AL, Barry MJ, Fasick P, Barron W, Shultz B. Continuous intrathecal baclofen infusion for symptomatic generalized dystonia. *Neurosurgery* 1996; **38**: 934–8.

20. Zuckerbraun NS, Ferson SS, Albright AL, Vogeley E. Intrathecal baclofen withdrawal: emergent recognition and management. *Pediatr Emerg Care* 2004; **20**: 759–64.

21. Krause M, Fogel W, Tronnier V, *et al.* Long-term benefit to pallidal deep brain stimulation in a case of dystonia secondary to pantothenate kinase-associated neurodegeneration. *Mov Disord* 2006; **21**: 2255–7.

22. Castelnau P, Cif L, Valente EM, *et al.* Pallidal stimulation improves pantothenate kinase-associated neurodegeneration. *Ann Neurol* 2005; **57**: 738–41.

23. Justesen CR, Penn RD, Kroin JS, Egel RT. Stereotactic pallidotomy in a child with Hallervorden–Spatz disease. Case report. *J Neurosurg* 1999; **90**: 551–4.

24. Tsukamoto H, Inui K, Taniike M, *et al.* A case of Hallervorden–Spatz disease: progressive and intractable dystonia controlled by bilateral thalamotomy. *Brain Dev* 1992; **14**: 269–72.

Neuroferritinopathies

Neuroferritinopathy (OMIM #606159), also known as adult-onset basal ganglia disease, is a progressive movement disorder caused by mutations in the coding region of the ferritin light chain gene (*FTL*, chromosome 19q13.3–q13.4). Persons with neuroferritinopathy have abnormal ferritin light chain polypeptide, decreased serum ferritin concentrations, and accumulation of iron in the basal ganglia. Curtis and colleagues first described this syndrome in an English kinship in 2001. They also coined the commonly used term "neuroferritinopathy."[1] Subsequent identification and study of other subjects have revealed additional observations on the genotypes, phenotypes, and epidemiology associated with neuroferritinopathy.

Other mutations of the *FTL* coding region segregate with a syndrome that comprises hyperferritinemia, absence of iron overload, and absence of ocular cataracts. Mutations of the iron-responsive element of *FTL* cause a different clinical syndrome characterized by elevated levels of otherwise normal ferritin, cataracts due to ferritin light-chain deposition in the ocular lens, and absence of neurological abnormalities (Chapter 17).

History

In 2001, Curtis and colleagues described late-onset autosomal dominant dystonia that segregated with *FTL* 460insA in an English kinship.[1] In 2003, Chinnery, Curtis, and colleagues reported a French family in which some members had a similar clinical disorder and the same *FTL* mutation.[2] In 2007, Chinnery and colleagues compiled observations in 41 patients with neuroferritinopathy and *FTL* 460insA.[3] They presented between the ages of 38 and 58 years; some had chorea, others had focal dystonia, and others had an akinetic rigid Parkinsonian syndrome. Brain imaging showed basal ganglia cavitation that was confirmed at necropsy. Neuronal loss was accompanied by the formation of neuroaxonal spheroids with

intraneural and extraneural iron deposition. Serum ferritin levels were low in the presence of normal serum iron, transferrin, and hemoglobin levels. These results provided a direct link between a primary heritable disorder of iron storage metabolism and a late-onset neurodegenerative movement disorder (Table 31.1).[1–3]

Clinical description

At presentation in 41 subjects with *FTL* 460insA, the mean age of onset was 39 years.[3] One-half of subjects presented with focal-onset chorea, 43% with focal dystonia (more prevalent in legs than arms), and 8% with Parkinsonism. Blepharospasm and writer's cramp were early features in 10% of patients. Two individuals described marked diurnal variation of their lower limb dystonia with sleep benefit early in the disease course, and two had palatal tremor (palatal myoclonus). There was no significant relationship of mode of presentation to age or gender.[3]

Follow-up observations were available in 38 of the 41 subjects.[3] The presenting movement disorder, typically asymmetrical and involving the legs, remained the major phenotype in almost two-thirds of subjects. Oromandibular dyskinesia was observed in 65% of subjects, and caused tongue injury in three. Nearly two-thirds of subjects developed characteristic speech with dysarthrophonia, and action-specific dystonia involving symmetric frontalis and platysma contraction giving a startled appearance. The facial and orolingual dyskinesia appears to be a consistent finding, and is characteristic of neuroferritinopathy.[3] One-third of subjects developed facial hypomimia and bradykinesia not directly related to their dystonia. The majority of patients were ambulatory two decades after onset. Subjects with predominantly dystonic phenotype had the most severe physical disability. Forty percent of subjects had dysphagia that was effectively controlled with dietary advice in most

Table 31.1. Major characteristics of neuroferritinopathy

Mean age at presentation 39 years

Progressive, focal-onset chorea, focal dystonia (more prevalent in legs than arms), or Parkinsonism-like symptoms

Facial, orolingual dyskinesia is consistent, characteristic finding

Positive family history of similar neurologic disorder; autosomal dominant pattern

Serum ferritin level usually low; hemoglobin and serum iron levels usually normal

Brain iron deposition, predominantly in basal ganglia, detectable with gradient-echo MRI

Iron-positive intranuclear inclusions in brain, peripheral nerve, and skeletal muscle

Mutation, usually insertion, in *FTL* exon 4

No benefit from iron depletion

cases. Severe dystonic hypophonia and aphonia required speech amplification in some individuals. No patient had documented seizures.

Physical examination revealed normal fundoscopy and slit-lamp examination.[3] Brisk tendon reflexes were uncommon (13% in upper limbs, 18% in lower limbs), and no subjects developed overt spasticity. Cognitive features were subtle early in the disease course. The majority (56%) of patients whose symptoms began less than 10 years previously had normal psychometric profiles; one subject had a normal psychometric profile 36 years after onset. Others had mild defects of verbal fluency. Two subjects had features consistent with frontal/subcortical dementia (present 12 and 29 years after onset, respectively). Disinhibition and emotional lability were frequently noted even in the early stages. One individual presented with paranoid psychosis. Mini-Mental State Examination was not sensitive for the frontal/subcortical cognitive deficits.

Laboratory abnormalities

Complete blood counts, morphology of blood cells, routine biochemical testing, hemoglobin A1c levels, and serum creatine kinase levels were normal. Cerebrospinal analysis was typically normal. Fasting plasma and cerebrospinal fluid lactate levels were also normal.

Serum ferritin levels were below the range for iron deficiency in 82% of males, all postmenopausal females, and 23% of pre-menopausal females. Serial ferritin measurements remained below the lower reference limit. There was no relationship between age or disease duration and the serum ferritin level. Hemoglobin and serum iron levels were typically normal. Thus, subnormal serum ferritin measures are very prevalent in persons with neuroferritinopathy and provide a useful screening test in routine practice.

Electroretinography, electromyography, and peripheral nerve conduction studies were normal in selected subjects. Electroencephalography was typically normal. None of the subjects reported were shown to have symptomatic disease in organs other than the brain. The fine structural hallmarks of neuroferritinopathy are granular nuclear inclusions in neurons, oligodendroglial, and microglial cells with similar extracellular derivatives in the central nervous system, muscle, peripheral nerve, and skin.[4] There is morphologic evidence of both lipid peroxidation and abnormal nitration of proteins in putaminal neurons and glia, confirming the expected oxidative stress due to deposition of excessive iron. Mitochondria also have biochemical and immunohistochemical abnormalities, probably due to an imbalance in iron homeostasis that had a deleterious effect on the respiratory chain.[5]

Chinnery and colleagues reported that histochemical analyses on muscle biopsy specimens were typically normal or non-diagnostic.[3] In contrast, Schroder previously reported that granular nuclear inclusions had been described in perivascular cells of muscle and nerve biopsy specimens in a case with an apparently identical disease, formerly designated as "granular nuclear inclusion body disease."[6] The nuclear inclusions, at the light microscopic level, are iron-positive by histochemical reactions, and react in a specific manner with ferritin antibodies. By electron microscopy, these granules are 5–15 nm in diameter. A moderate peak of iron detectable by energy dispersive microanalysis of the granular nuclear inclusions in neuroferritinopathy may also be significant. These observations suggest that ferritinopathy or "granular nuclear inclusion body disease" can be diagnosed by a simple muscle or nerve biopsy without brain biopsy, autopsy, or molecular genetic testing of the considerable number of neurodegenerative diseases with similar symptoms.[6]

Gradient-echo brain magnetic resonance imaging (MRI) identifies all symptomatic cases of neuroferritinopathy, and can distinguish neuroferritinopathy from other heritable conditions characterized by brain iron accumulation.[7] With brain MRI, a characteristic pattern of signal change was observed in all subjects, consistent with iron deposition predominantly in the basal ganglia.[3] Even in an asymptomatic carrier, a characteristic pattern of iron deposition was seen on gradient echo sequences, consisting of loss of T2* signal within the dentate nuclei, red nuclei, substantia nigra, putamina, globi pallidi, thalami, caudate nuclei, and the Rolandic prefrontal cortex. In early cases, the only discernible abnormality on conventional spin echo MR sequences was mild reduction in T2 signal within the red nuclei and substantia nigra. In increasingly severe disease, T2* signal loss became more pronounced within the dentate nuclei, thalami, and globi pallidi, with abnormal T2 signal in the lentiform and caudate nuclei, mirroring areas of high signal on T1 signals in these locations, and indicating iron deposition. In subjects with more advanced disease, there was more pronounced focal signal abnormality within the globus pallidus, with central high T2 and FLAIR signal and peripheral high T1 signal, consistent with focal pre-cystic degeneration. In advanced cases, these foci showed internal cystic degeneration associated with generalized involutional changes and an excess of small vessel ischemic lesions. The MR findings were the same in two patients with palatal tremor as in other subjects.[3]

Genetics

All reported pathogenic *FTL* mutations associated with neuroferritinopathy are rare (Table 31.2).[1–3,5,8–13] *FTL* 460InsA was the first mutation reported and has been described in the greatest number of cases. Most of these cases occurred in a geographic cluster in Cumbria that was traced to a common ancestor.[1–3] *FTL* 460InsA has also been identified in other English[14] and French[2] patients. All reported pathogenic *FTL* mutations associated with neuroferritinopathy involve exon 4 of *FTL*. Most mutations are insertions in exon 4 that result in frameshifts. These mutations alter the reading frame, lengthen the C-terminus of ferritin

Table 31.2. Pathogenic *FTL* mutations in neuroferritinopathy

cDNA substitution[a]	Race/ethnicity	Reference
458dupA	French	17
460insA	English/Cumbrian; French	1,2,18
469_484dup16nt	Japanese	12
474G→A	Portuguese/Gypsy	11
498insTC	French	14
641_642dup4nt	Japanese	15
646insC	French Canadian/ Dutch	5

Note: [a]Each mutation occurs in exon 4 of *FTL*.

light chain polypeptide, and disrupt protein folding and stability. As a consequence, ferritin dodecahedron structure is altered, causing accumulation of ferritin and iron,[14] primarily in central neurons.

The expression of one of the two variant L-ferritins increases intracellular iron availability and sensitivity to oxidative damage.[4] Cremonesi and colleagues described a 52-year-old woman who had no history of iron deficiency anemia, neurologic dysfunction, nor cataract. Hematologic examination was normal except that serum and erythrocyte ferritin levels were decreased. She was heterozygous for the *FTL* ATG start codon mutation c.1A→G, predicted to disable protein translation and expression.[9] Taken together, these findings suggest that L-ferritin has no effect on systemic iron metabolism and also indicate that neuroferritinopathy is not a consequence of haploinsufficiency of L-ferritin, but likely results from gain-of-function mutations in the *FTL* gene.[9,14] A disorder similar to neuroferritinopathy in humans occurs in transgenic mice.[14]

Genotype–phenotype correlations

There are relatively few mutations and corresponding patient observations from which meaningful correlations can be established. Penetrance of *FTL* 460insA is nearly 100%.[3] Onset of chorea in middle age is common in patients with insertions in the 5′ portion of exon 4, whereas patients with insertions in the 3′ portion of exon 4 develop early-onset tremor.[15]

The clinical presentation of the patients with the *FTL* 498InsTC and 646InsC mutations fall within the spectrum described in patients with *FTL* 460InsA.[3] The patient with *FTL* 474G→A (the only single-nucleotide *FTL* substitution reported in neuroferritinopathy) had a relatively early age of presentation with Parkinsonism, ataxia, corticospinal signs, mild non-progressive cognitive deficit, and episodic psychosis, although his mother and younger brother also had *FTL* 474G→A, but had less severe neurological abnormalities.[11]

Persons heterozygous for the coding region mutation *FTL* T301I have elevated serum levels of glycosylated ferritin, report no specific symptoms, and lack iron overload, ocular cataracts, and neurologic abnormality.[16] It has been postulated that *FTL* T301I increases the efficacy of L-ferritin secretion by increasing the hydrophobicity of the N terminal "A" alpha helix.[16]

Treatment

Three patients with neuroferritinopathy and *FTL* 460insA have been treated with the intent of reducing brain iron stores.[3] Each was treated with monthly phlebotomy for 6 months. Thereafter, two had subcutaneous deferoxamine (4000 mg weekly for as long as 14 months); the third patient had oral deferiprone (2 g three times daily for 2 months). All three treatments caused profound and refractory iron depletion. The condition of one patient with generalized dystonia deteriorated greatly during treatment, and that of the other patients did not improve. Long-term benefits, perhaps with different treatment regimens, remain a possibility, especially in patients with no or minimal neurologic abnormalities. A variety of drugs were administered to patients with neuroferritinopathy and *FTL* 460insA for management of hyperkinesis or dystonia. Results were inconsistent; many patients had adverse effects.[3]

References

1. Curtis AR, Fey C, Morris CM, *et al.* Mutation in the gene encoding ferritin light polypeptide causes dominant adult-onset basal ganglia disease. *Nat Genet* 2001; **28**: 350–4.

2. Chinnery PF, Curtis AR, Fey C, *et al.* Neuroferritinopathy in a French family with late-onset dominant dystonia. *J Med Genet* 2003; **40**: e69.

3. Chinnery PF, Crompton DE, Birchall D, *et al.* Clinical features and natural history of neuroferritinopathy caused by the *FTL1* 460InsA mutation. *Brain* 2007; **130**: 110–19.

4. Levi S, Cozzi A, Arosio P. Neuroferritinopathy: a neurodegenerative disorder associated with L-ferritin mutation. *Best Pract Res Clin Haematol* 2005; **18**: 265–76.

5. Mancuso M, Davidzon G, Kurlan RM, *et al.* Hereditary ferritinopathy: a novel mutation, its cellular pathology, and pathogenetic insights. *J Neuropathol Exp Neurol* 2005; **64**: 280–94.

6. Schroder JM. Ferritinopathy: diagnosis by muscle or nerve biopsy, with a note on other nuclear inclusion body diseases. *Acta Neuropathol* 2005; **109**: 109–14.

7. McNeill A, Birchall D, Hayflick SJ, *et al.* T2* and FSE MRI distinguishes four subtypes of neurodegeneration with brain iron accumulation. *Neurology* 2008; **70**: 1614–19.

8. Costa MC, Teixeira-Castro A, Constante M, *et al.* Exclusion of mutations in the *PRNP, JPH3, TBP, ATN1, CREBBP, POU3F2* and *FTL* genes as a cause of disease in Portuguese patients with a Huntington-like phenotype. *J Hum Genet* 2006; **51**: 645–51.

9. Cremonesi L, Cozzi A, Girelli D, *et al.* Case report: a subject with a mutation in the ATG start codon of L-ferritin has no haematological or neurological symptoms. *J Med Genet* 2004; **41**: e81.

10. Foglieni B, Ferrari F, Goldwurm S, *et al.* Analysis of ferritin genes in Parkinson disease. *Clin Chem Lab Med* 2007; **45**: 1450–6.

11. Maciel P, Cruz VT, Constante M, *et al.* Neuroferritinopathy: missense mutation in *FTL* causing early-onset bilateral pallidal involvement. *Neurology* 2005; **65**: 603–5.

12. Ohta E, Nagasaka T, Shindo K, *et al.* Neuroferritinopathy in a Japanese family with a duplication in the ferritin light chain gene. *Neurology* 2008; **70**: 1493–4.

13. Wild EJ, Mudanohwo EE, Sweeney MG, *et al.* Huntington's disease phenocopies are clinically and genetically heterogeneous. *Mov Disord* 2008; **23**: 716–20.

14. Vidal R, Miravalle L, Gao X, *et al.* Expression of a mutant form of the ferritin light chain gene induces neurodegeneration and iron overload in transgenic mice. *J Neurosci* 2008; **28**: 60–7.

15. Kubota A, Hida A, Ichikawa Y, *et al.* A novel ferritin light chain gene mutation in a Japanese family with neuroferritinopathy: Description of

clinical features and implications for genotype–phenotype correlations. *Mov Disord* 2008; **24**: 441–5.

16. Kannengiesser C, Jouanolle AM, Hetet G, *et al.* A new missense mutation in the L-ferritin coding sequence associated with elevated levels of glycosylated ferritin in serum and absence of iron overload. *Haematologica* 2009; **94**: 335–9.

17. Devos D, Tchofo PJ, Vuillaume I, *et al.* Clinical features and natural history of neuroferritinopathy caused by the 458dupA *FTL* mutation. *Brain* 2009; **132** (**6**): e109.

18. Mir P, Edwards MJ, Curtis AR, Bhatia KP, Quinn NP. Adult-onset generalized dystonia due to a mutation in the neuroferritinopathy gene. *Mov Disord* 2005; **20**: 243–5.

GRACILE syndrome

GRACILE syndrome (OMIM #603358) is a rare lethal disorder of infants. The acronym GRACILE represents growth retardation, aminoaciduria, cholestasis, iron loading, and early death. This autosomal recessive disorder is caused by mutations of the *BCS1* gene on chromosome 2q33. The human *BCS1* gene encodes a homolog of *S. cerevisiae* bcs1 protein involved in the assembly of complex III (CIII) of the mitochondrial respiratory chain. GRACILE syndrome was first reported from Finland[1–3] where its estimated population frequency is 1 per 47 000 to 70 000 infants.[3–5] GRACILE syndrome has been identified in other geographic regions, but population prevalence estimates are not available for most other countries. Other mutations of *BCS1* result in clinical and laboratory phenotypes that differ from those of GRACILE syndrome.

Clinical manifestations

GRACILE syndrome has been identified by antenatal testing,[2] but the disorder is readily apparent in neonates and worsens soon after birth (Table 32.1). Growth retardation is a characteristic finding among affected infants. In a study from Finland, the median weight of 17 infants with GRACILE syndrome was 4 SD lower than the median weight in a group of normal infants.[3] All 17 infants had aminoaciduria and cholestasis. Plasma or serum concentrations of lactic acid were typically normal at birth; pH of umbilical cord blood was 7.3 or higher (reference <7.2). Fulminant lactic acidosis developed within 24 hours in all patients. Median lactate levels rose to 12 mmol/L (reference <1.8 mmol/L), and median blood pH values decreased to 7.00 (reference 7.35–7.45). None of the infants had hypotonia or seizures.[3]

Iron accumulates mainly in the liver. This occurs *in utero*, based on the finding of liver iron loading in a 14th week fetus, and the finding of hepatic iron overload in neonates.[2] The median values for transferrin saturation and serum ferritin concentration in six infants were 81% (normal infants, <60%) and 1314 μg/L (normal infants, <150 μg/L), respectively.[3] The median stainable liver iron was grade 3 (normal, grade 0 or 1) in the 13 infants so studied.[3] In the five infants whose hepatic iron concentration was measured, the median value was 5470 μg/g dry weight of liver (normal <2280 μg/g dry weight of liver).[3] Histologic examination demonstrated that iron does not accumulate in the brains of infants with GRACILE syndrome.[1]

Genetics

GRACILE syndrome is caused by homozygosity for missense mutations of the *BCS1* gene on chromosome 2q33; the gene has 7 exons.[4] The most common known pathogenic *BCS1* mutation is S78G (exon 2; nt232A→G). In one study, homozygosity for *BCS1* S78G was detected by direct sequencing in all Finnish patients with GRACILE syndrome.[3] Other *BCS1* mutations have been identified in patients with syndromic abnormalities that are dissimilar to those of GRACILE syndrome.[3,6–12]

The pathophysiology of iron accumulation is not clear, nor is it known if iron accumulation is directly attributable to mutations of the *BCS1* gene. BCS1 protein (419 amino acids) is a chaperone in the inner membrane of mitochondria that functions in the assembly of CIII of respirasomes, basic units of the electron transport chain (respiratory chain). BCS1 protein is ATP-dependent and maintains the pre-complex of CIII in a state that allows the assembly of Rieske iron–sulfur protein into complex III ubiquinol-cytochrome c oxidoreductase Qcr10p proteins that are required for normal function of the electron transport chain in mitochondria.[3,5,12] It seems likely, however, that the S78G alteration of *BCS1* disrupts the assembly of CIII and decreases the activity of the mitochondrial respirasomes, basic

Table 32.1. Abnormalities in 17 infants with GRACILE syndrome[a]

Abnormality	Percent
Growth retardation	100
Aminoaciduria	100
Cholestasis	100
Iron overload[b]	100
Lactic acidosis 24 hours after delivery	100
Early death	100

Notes: [a]Adapted from Visapää *et al.*[3] Similar findings were reported in eight other patients from Finland.[4]
[b]Thirteen subjects were tested.

units of the electron transport chain (respiration) in mitochondria; and that the decrease in CIII activity is associated with increased production of reactive oxygen species; and that the decreased activity of CIII results in the development of lactic acidosis.[3,5,12]

Differential diagnosis

Various genotypes and phenotypes occur in infants who have *BCS1* mutations that differ from the *BCS1* mutations detected in Finnish infants affected with GRACILE syndrome.[6–12] Some of the associated syndromes are described below.

Björnstad syndrome

This rare syndrome of sensorineural hearing loss and pili torti describes the condition of infants who are homozygous for *BCS1* mutations such as R306H, G35R, or R184C. These mutations have been mapped to chromosome 2q34–36, close to the site of mutations that cause the GRACILE syndrome.[7,8,12] The sensorineural hearing loss and pili torti in infants who have the Björnstad syndrome distinguish them from the clinical features of infants who have the GRACILE syndrome.

Progressive neurologic disease and tubulopathy

Two children with neurologic disease, lactic acidosis, and brittle, kinky hair were evaluated for *BCS1* mutations.[11] Neither child had liver disease.[11] One infant was born to unrelated parents from Italy. The child

had drug-resistant seizures, muscle hypotonia, severe psychomotor delay since infancy, and lactic acidosis. Neurologic disease progressed to quadriparesis by age 12 months. Brain MRI revealed marked cerebral atrophy and other abnormalities. The child died at age 4 years. She was a compound heterozygote for *BCS1* missense mutations R73C (exon 1) and F368I (exon 7).[11]

Another child had unrelated parents from Morocco. This child presented at age 9 months with psychomotor regression, hypotonia, and failure to thrive.[11] She developed spastic quadriparesis and lactic acidosis. An initial brain MRI was normal; at age 32 months; by MRI revealed symmetric atrophy of the brain and other abnormalities. At age 4 years, she had developed sensorineural hearing loss. She was a compound heterozygote for *BCS1* R183C (exon 3) and R184C (exon 3).[11]

Renal tubulopathy and liver disease

Two children in a Spanish family were evaluated because they had lactic acidosis, renal tubulopathy, liver disease, and severe failure to thrive.[10] Further investigation revealed that the children had a deficiency of CIII in the liver due to compound heterozygosity for *BCS1* mutations in exon 1 (the missense mutation R45C and a premature stop-codon mutation R56X).[10]

Renal tubulopathy, encephalopathy, and liver failure

Six children in four Turkish families developed lactic acidosis, encephalopathy, and liver dysfunction soon after birth.[9] Some of the children had microcephaly, deafness, blindness, hypotonia, hyperreflexia, or encephalopathy. One child was alive at age 9 years. Two children, one in each of two families, were born to consanguineous parents. de Lonlay *et al.* determined that the children had a several *BCS1* mutations involving four different exons, resulting in amino acid substitutions P99L, R155P, S227N, and V353M.[9] Brain MRI in some of the children was compatible with necrotizing encephalopathy that occurs in yet another mitochondrial disorder called Leigh syndrome (Chapter 26). The presence of neurologic disease and longer survival distinguishes these patients from infants with GRACILE syndrome.

Severe psychomotor retardation, extrapyramidal signs, athetosis, ataxia, and dementia

A non-lethal autosomal recessive neuromuscular syndrome was reported in an Israeli Bedouin family; parents of all 25 affected individuals were consanguineous.[13] During infancy, the affected boys and girls had delayed development, followed by extrapyramidal abnormalities, dystonia, athetosis, and ataxia at age 2–3 years. The children also had dementia with absent receptive and expressive communication, axial hypotonia, hyperreflexia in all limbs, and inability to walk independently. Cranial nerve function and ophthalmologic findings were normal. They had mild or moderate elevation of plasma lactate concentrations. Electroencephalography revealed non-specific generalized slowing. Brain MRI was performed in five patients, and showed symmetric abnormalities in basal ganglia, including increased density in the putamen and decreased density and size of the caudate nucleus and globus pallidus. The investigators found that the affected individuals did not have mutations of *BCS1*. Instead, they had homozygosity for the S45F mutation of the *UQCRQ* gene (chromosome 5q31), one of ten nuclear genes that encode proteins of mitochondrial CIII. *UQCRQ* S45F affected the encoding of ubiquinol-cytochrome c reductase in CIII, subunit VII.[13]

Other disorders

GRACILE syndrome is distinct from neonatal hemochromatosis (Chapter 33), neonatal viral hepatitis, neuroferritinopathies (Chapter 31), and other disorders that are sometimes associated with iron loading in infancy, and from other disorders caused by CIII abnormalities of the respiratory transport chain in mitochondria.

Treatment of GRACILE syndrome

Finnish infants were treated with alkalinization and other supportive measures. Despite intensive management, the median survival of the infants was 7 days; some infants died within hours after birth. All of the infants died by age 4 months.[3]

Infusions of apotransferrin followed by exchange transfusion were performed for 3 days in one affected infant and for 6 days in another.[14] Their pre-treatment transferrin saturation values were 100%. These treatments were started at age 3 weeks in one infant and at age 4 days in the other. One infant received three treatments between ages 3 and 6 weeks. The other infant received six treatments between ages 4 and 20 days. Infusions of apotransferrin elevated the serum transferrin concentration to high-normal adult values and decreased transferrin saturation. The apotransferrin infusions also cleared the plasma of non-transferrin-bound iron (bleomycin-detectable iron). There were no serious adverse effects. Nonetheless, these treatments did not prevent early death (ages 2 months and 2.5 months, respectively).[14]

References

1. Fellman V, Rapola J, Pihko H, Varilo T, Raivio KO. Iron-overload disease in infants involving fetal growth retardation, lactic acidosis, liver haemosiderosis, and aminoaciduria. *Lancet* 1998; **351**: 490–3.

2. Fellman V, Visapaa I, Vujic M, Wennerholm UB, Peltonen L. Antenatal diagnosis of hereditary fetal growth retardation with aminoaciduria, cholestasis, iron overload, and lactic acidosis in the newborn infant. *Acta Obstet Gynecol Scand* 2002; **81**: 398–402.

3. Visapaa I, Fellman V, Vesa J, *et al*. GRACILE syndrome, a lethal metabolic disorder with iron overload, is caused by a point mutation in *BCS1L*. *Am J Hum Genet* 2002; **71**: 863–76.

4. Fellman V. The GRACILE syndrome, a neonatal lethal metabolic disorder with iron overload. *Blood Cells Mol Dis* 2002; **29**: 444–50.

5. Fellman V, Lemmela S, Sajantila A, Pihko H, Jarvela I. Screening of *BCS1L* mutations in severe neonatal disorders suspicious for mitochondrial cause. *J Hum Genet* 2008; **53**: 554–8.

6. Morris AA, Taylor RW, Birch-Machin MA, *et al*. Neonatal Fanconi syndrome due to deficiency of complex III of the respiratory chain. *Pediatr Nephrol* 1995; **9**: 407–11.

7. Lubianca Neto JF, Lu L, Eavey RD, *et al*. The Björnstad syndrome (sensorineural hearing loss and pili torti) disease gene maps to chromosome 2q34–36. *Am J Hum Genet* 1998; **62**: 1107–12.

8. Selvaag E. Pili torti and sensorineural hearing loss. A follow-up of Björnstad's original patients and a review of the literature. *Eur J Dermatol* 2000; **10**: 91–7.

9. de Lonlay P, Valnot I, Barrientos A, *et al*. A mutant mitochondrial respiratory chain assembly protein causes complex III deficiency in patients with tubulopathy, encephalopathy, and liver failure. *Nat Genet* 2001; **29**: 57–60.

10. De Meirleir L, Seneca S, Damis E, *et al.* Clinical and diagnostic characteristics of complex III deficiency due to mutations in the *BCS1L* gene. *Am J Med Genet A* 2003; **121**A: 126–31.

11. Fernandez-Vizarra E, Bugiani M, Goffrini P, *et al.* Impaired complex III assembly associated with *BCS1L* gene mutations in isolated mitochondrial encephalopathy. *Hum Mol Genet* 2007; **16**: 1241–52.

12. Hinson JT, Fantin VR, Schonberger J, *et al.* Missense mutations in the *BCS1L* gene as a cause of the Björnstad syndrome. *N Engl J Med* 2007; **356**: 809–19.

13. Barel O, Shorer Z, Flusser H, *et al.* Mitochondrial complex III deficiency associated with a homozygous mutation in UQCRQ. *Am J Hum Genet* 2008; **82**: 1211–16.

14. Fellman V, von Bonsdorff L, Parkkinen J. Exogenous apotransferrin and exchange transfusions in hereditary iron-overload disease. *Pediatrics* 2000; **105**: 398–401.

Chapter 33

Neonatal hemochromatosis

Neonatal hemochromatosis (NH) is a heterogeneous group of disorders characterized by severe fetal or neonatal liver injury including cirrhosis, and hepatic and extrahepatic iron overload that occurs in a distribution similar to that of *HFE* hemochromatosis.[1] Extensive liver injury and dysfunction are the dominant clinical features. Fetal loss or early neonatal death is usual, although some children survive. Despite its rarity, NH is one of the most commonly recognized causes of liver failure in neonates, has a high recurrence rate in sibships, and is a frequent indication for liver transplantation in the first 3 months of life.[1–3] There is mounting evidence that many cases are caused by maternal alloimmunity against a fetal liver determinant. Treating at-risk mothers during pregnancy with intravenous IgG markedly decreases the risk and severity of NH in their subsequent offspring.[4] Other NH cases are due to other acquired conditions of the mother, to intrauterine infection, or to rare heritable disorders of the fetus.

History

In 1956, Kiaer and Olesen described a Danish kinship in which six of nine sibs died *in utero* or as neonates of a disorder consistent with NH.[5] In 1960, Fienberg reported two pairs of male siblings with "perinatal idiopathic hemochromatosis" and "giant cell hepatitis," and suggested that this condition was caused by an "inborn error of metabolism." In 1961, Laurendeau and colleagues described "idiopathic neonatal hemochromatosis" in two sisters. For several decades, most reports comprised single families in which there were one or several infants with NH. Reviews of large case series defined clinical features of NH further.[6–8] In 2005, Whitington hypothesized that many cases of NH are caused by maternal alloimmunity that injures fetal liver (Table 33.1).[9,10]

Clinical description

The gestational histories of women who have had an infant diagnosed with NH indicate that one of the most common presentations is late second and third trimester fetal loss.[4] Premature birth is common. Liver disease is usually apparent within hours after birth, but infrequently does not become apparent until days to weeks later.[10] In 16 patients, median age at diagnosis was 2 days (range 0–21 days). Median weight at the time of diagnosis was 2900 g (range 1520–4200 g).[8] Jaundice develops during the first few days after birth.[10] Most affected liveborn infants show non-specific evidence of fetal insult (i.e. intrauterine growth restriction and oligohydramnios), acute liver failure, and multiorgan failure. Edema, ascites, and oliguria are common. Twins may have disparate clinical findings.[11] Although iron is deposited in myocardial fibers, arrhythmia, or cardiomyopathy due to cardiac siderosis does not occur. Affected infants are frequently diagnosed mistakenly to have overwhelming sepsis of the newborn.

Laboratory findings

Typical histological abnormalities, including iron overload, may be present in early fetal life.[12] Iron deposition in the liver occurs before that in extrahepatic sites.[13,14] Iron measures at birth reveal non-specific abnormalities: elevated transferrin saturation, hypotransferrinemia, and hyperferritinemia (serum ferritin $>800\,\mu g/L$). In 16 NH patients, the median serum ferritin was $4179\,\mu g/L$, and median transferrin saturation was 99%.[8] In neonates, lip biopsy specimens prepared with Perls' stain can facilitate presumptive diagnosis. Hemosiderin is often present in the acini of minor salivary glands, although stain positivity or negativity seems unrelated to serum ferritin levels.[13] In mild cases, excessive iron may be confined to the liver.

Table 33.1. Causes of neonatal hemochromatosis[a]

Maternal alloimmunity, unknown antigen(s) (OMIM 231100)[4,9,31]

Neonatal lupus erythematosus syndrome (maternal anti-Ro/SS-A (OMIM #109092) and anti-Ro/SS-B autoantibodies (OMIM #109090))[39]

GRACILE syndrome (OMIM #660358)[4,12,25,26,40]

Δ-4–3-oxosteroid 5-beta-reductase deficiency (OMIM #235555)[27,28]

Cytomegalovirus infection[41]

Note: [a]Hepatic iron deposition has also been reported in some cases of Zellweger syndrome (OMIM #214100), hereditary tyrosinemia (OMIM +276700), leprechaunism (OMIM #246200),[42] and hemophagocytic lymphohistiocytosis (OMIM %267700; #603553; #603552; and #608898) of unspecified genetic type.[43]

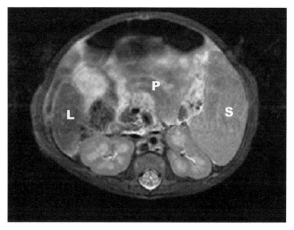

Fig. 33.1. MRI scan T2* gradient echo image of an infant with neonatal hemochromatosis. This 2900 g male infant was born in severe distress at 38-weeks gestation to a G1P0 healthy woman. Decreased fetal movement and oligohydramnios were noted at 36 weeks. The infant had liver failure at birth; refractory hypoglycemia and severe coagulopathy were the most prominent findings. Magnetic resonance imaging (MRI) performed at 8 days of age showed that the contracted liver (L) and pancreas (P) had reduced T2 signal intensity (dark) relative to spleen (S), diagnostic of excess iron in these tissues. Demonstrating extrahepatic siderosis in a newborn with severe liver disease fulfills the criteria for diagnosing neonatal hemochromatosis. Courtesy of Dr. Peter F. Whitington.

Hypoglycemia, marked coagulopathy, hypoalbuminemia, and anemia are prominent features. Most cases exhibit elevated serum levels of conjugated and non-conjugated bilirubin and plasma levels of ammonia. Serum aminotransferase concentrations are elevated, but are disproportionately low for the degree of hepatic injury. Circulating concentrations of alpha-fetoprotein (AFP) are very high, usually 100 000–600 000 µg/L. Both inappropriately low aminotransferase and high AFP levels could reflect the failure of the diseased liver to switch from fetal to neonatal metabolic patterns. Altogether, these abnormalities are typical of NH, but may occur in other severe fetal or neonatal liver injury syndromes.

Intrauterine (or postnatal) diagnosis of NH, regardless of etiology, is possible with magnetic resonance imaging (MRI) scanning using T2* gradient echo image (Chapter 4).[8,15,16] If the density of the fetal liver is less intense than that of maternal or fetal fat signal, hepatic iron overload should be suspected (Fig. 33.1). A prenatal diagnosis of the fetus for a mother of two previously deceased infants who died from GRACILE syndrome was made using haplotype analysis.[12] Duplex Doppler sonography does not provide information on iron overload, but shows abnormalities in the liver or blood-flow patterns associated with liver disease.[15]

At autopsy, most NH livers are small due to advanced cirrhosis. Abnormal histology includes hepatocellular necrosis, lobular disarray, intralobular fibrosis, hepatocyte multinuclearity, giant cell transformation, and cholestasis. Severe iron deposition is visualized in hepatocytes by Perls' technique; Kupffer cells contain little or no iron. Excess stainable iron is also present in thyroid follicular and renal distal tubular epithelia, pancreatic and salivary gland acini, adrenal glands, and myocardial fibers. Renal tubular dysgenesis has been reported in several cases.[17] Nonspecific morphologic abnormalities are sometimes observed in placentas.[7,18]

The apical microvilli of normal placental syncytiotrophoblasts (facing the mother) express transferrin and transferrin receptor. Syncytiotrophoblast cytoplasm contains ferritin, quantities of which increase in late gestation. The basolateral surfaces of placental cells (facing the fetus) contain an iron binder presumed to be ferroportin, the major iron exporter of syncytiotrophoblasts.[19–22] NH does not alter iron metabolism by dysregulating synthesis of transferrin receptor or ferritin.[23] There are no reports of ferroportin activity or mutation analyses in NH.

Elevated serum tyrosine levels in some infants with NH reflect markedly impaired hepatic metabolic function, not tyrosinemia.[10] Urine succinylacetone, typical of hereditary tyrosinemia, is absent in NH.[10] Blood or other cultures and evidence of chemical intoxication are almost always negative.

Genetics

Most reported fetuses or neonates with NH have been Caucasian, although this disorder also occurs in Asians and other race/ethnicity groups. There is clustering of NH in many kindreds, and the proportions of male and female fetuses or neonates with NH is approximately equal. This suggests that NH occurs as an autosomal recessive disorder in some families, especially consanguineous kinships.[7] In many kindreds, however, NH occurs with greater frequency among the offspring of mothers who have had a child with NH than would be expected if NH were a disorder transmitted by a simple autosomal recessive trait. Mothers have had fetuses or neonates with NH by two different fathers, but there are no reports of the same man having children with NH by different women.[7,24] Altogether, these observations indicate that some cases are due to a maternal factor expressed in gestation, or to a mitochondrial defect or other inherited factor expressed preferentially in women.[7] It seems unlikely that NH is an autosomal dominant disorder (with or without incomplete penetrance); there are no reports of NH survivors who later became the parents of children with NH.

Mendelian traits account for some NH phenotypes. GRACILE syndrome (OMIM #603358) (intrauterine growth retardation, aminoaciduria, cholestasis, iron overload, severe lactic acidosis, and early death), a rare autosomal recessive disorder due to mutations in the BCS1L gene on chromosome 2q33, is associated with a NH phenotype.[12,25,26] A few NH cases with an especially poor prognosis have been ascribed to delta 4-3-oxosteroid 5-beta-reductase deficiency (OMIM #235555), a primary genetic defect in bile acid synthesis.[27,28] On the other hand, there is no concordance of NH and human leukocyte antigen (HLA) types. Family members of affected neonates do not have major rearrangements or deletions of H- or L-apoferritin genes (FTH1, FTL), of transferrin receptor genes (TFR1, TFR2), or within HLA loci.[29] Sequence analysis of HFE, beta$_2$-microglobulin (B2M), and heme oxygenase genes (HMOX1, HMOX2) did not detect pathogenic mutations in NH families.[30] The clinical phenotype of NH differs greatly from that of juvenile or early age-of-onset hemochromatosis due to mutations in genes that encode ferroportin, hemojuvelin, hepcidin, or transferrin receptor-2 (SLC40A1, HJV, HAMP, and TFR2, respectively) (Chapters 12–15). In a 30-year follow-up of the 1956 Danish kindred of Kiaer and Olesen, Dalhøj and colleagues reported in 1990 that there was no evidence of hereditary hemochromatosis or other iron storage disease in the parents or surviving siblings.

Prevention and treatment

There is substantial clinical evidence that many NH cases are caused by an alloimmune mechanism(s); this hypothesis is supported by a mouse model of NH that simulates the human disorder.[9,31] The only presently identifiable mothers at risk to have infants with NH are those whose previous babies had NH. In a pivotal clinical trial, Whitington and colleagues assessed the effectiveness of high-dose intravenous immunoglobulin (IV IgG) administered during pregnancy in preventing or changing the severity of recurrent NH.[4] Women whose most recent pregnancy ended in documented NH were treated with IV IgG, 1 g/kg body weight weekly, from the 18th week until the end of their subsequent pregnancy. The outcomes of treated pregnancies were compared with outcomes of randomly selected previous affected pregnancies for each woman used as historical controls. Fifteen women were treated through 16 pregnancies. All pregnancies progressed uneventfully and resulted in live babies with normal physical examinations and birthweights appropriate for gestational age. Twelve babies had evidence of liver involvement with NH. Eleven had elevated serum levels of AFP and ferritin or AFP alone, including four who had coagulopathy (prothrombin time international normalized ratio >1.5); one had coagulopathy alone. All infants survived with medical management or no treatment, and were healthy at follow-up. Gestational IV IgG therapy was associated with significantly greater infant survival than in control pregnancies in the same mothers. Thus, this treatment of the mother appears to modify recurrent NH so that it is not lethal to the fetus or neonate. Favorable results with IV IgG therapy have been reported in additional patients, substantiating the hypothesis that many NH cases are due to fetal liver injury caused by a corresponding maternal alloantibody.[10]

Some mildly affected infants recover with supportive care. Exchange transfusions were used to treat one neonate with rapidly worsening coagulopathy. There was rapid clinical and laboratory improvement, after which a definitive diagnosis of NH was made. The patient was healthy 1 year later.[32] Three infants with GRACILE syndrome were treated with apotrans-ferrin and exchange transfusion. Their serum iron measures improved, but they had no apparent clinical benefit.[25] Adjunctive treatment of NH with an antioxidant-chelation "cocktail," consisting of deferox-amine, vitamin E, *N*-acetylcysteine, selenium, and prostaglandin-E1, did not change outcomes in a large series of patients with NH,[33] but may provide some benefit when applied early in mildly affected patients.[16] Nonetheless, this cocktail is widely used for NH in liver transplantation programs. Phlebotomy or chelation therapy are not feasible, given the severity of iron overload and other complications typical of NH.[34] Identifying the concurrence of renal tubular dysgenesis and NH is important if dialysis or liver transplantation is considered in infants with hepatic and renal failure.[17]

Orthotopic liver transplantation is the treatment of choice for patients with NH who are not responding to medical therapy.[2,8,35,36] Early referral to a tertiary care center is essential to increase survival of these children with a rare and otherwise fatal disease.[35] Many are treated with chelation "cocktail" as a conditioning and post-transplant regimen. The long-term survival is 50%–69%.[2,8,35–37] Deposition of iron in a liver allograft in a patient with NH has been reported.[38]

References

1. Knisely AS, Mieli-Vergani G, Whitington PF. Neonatal hemochromatosis. *Gastroenterol Clin North Am* 2003; **32**: 877–89, vi–vii.

2. Durand P, Debray D, Mandel R, *et al.* Acute liver failure in infancy: a 14-year experience of a pediatric liver transplantation center. *J Pediatr* 2001; **139**: 871–6.

3. Sundaram SS, Alonso EM, Whitington PF. Liver transplantation in neonates. *Liver Transpl* 2003; **9**: 783–8.

4. Whitington PF, Hibbard JU. High-dose immunoglobulin during pregnancy for recurrent neonatal haemochromatosis. *Lancet* 2004; **364**: 1690–8.

5. Kiaer W, Olesen M. [Hepatitis fetalis with perinatal death in 4 siblings.] *Ugeskr Laeger* 1956; **118**: 868–72.

6. Knisely AS, Magid MS, Dische MR, Cutz E. Neonatal hemochromatosis. *Birth Defects Orig Artic Ser* 1987; **23**: 75–102.

7. Kelly AL, Lunt PW, Rodrigues F, *et al.* Classification and genetic features of neonatal haemochromatosis: a study of 27 affected pedigrees and molecular analysis of genes implicated in iron metabolism. *J Med Genet* 2001; **38**: 599–610.

8. Grabhorn E, Richter A, Burdelski M, Rogiers X, Ganschow R. Neonatal hemochromatosis: long-term experience with favorable outcome. *Pediatrics* 2006; **118**: 2060–5.

9. Whitington PF, Malladi P. Neonatal hemochromatosis: is it an alloimmune disease? *J Pediatr Gastroenterol Nutr* 2005; **40**: 544–9.

10. Whitington PF. Fetal and infantile hemochromatosis. *Hepatology* 2006; **43**: 654–60.

11. Ekong UD, Kelly S, Whitington PF. Disparate clinical presentation of neonatal hemochromatosis in twins. *Pediatrics* 2005; **116**: e880–4.

12. Fellman V, Visapaa I, Vujic M, Wennerholm UB, Peltonen L. Antenatal diagnosis of hereditary fetal growth retardation with aminoaciduria, cholestasis, iron overload, and lactic acidosis in the newborn infant. *Acta Obstet Gynecol Scand* 2002; **81**: 398–402.

13. Hoogstraten J, de Sa DJ, Knisely AS. Fetal liver disease may precede extrahepatic siderosis in neonatal hemochromatosis. *Gastroenterology* 1990; **98**: 1699–701.

14. Smith SR, Shneider BL, Magid M, Martin G, Rothschild M. Minor salivary gland biopsy in neonatal hemochromatosis. *Arch Otolaryngol Head Neck Surg* 2004; **130**: 760–3.

15. Oddone M, Bellini C, Bonacci W, Bartocci M, Toma P, Serra G. Diagnosis of neonatal hemochromatosis with MR imaging and duplex Doppler sonography. *Eur Radiol* 1999; **9**: 1882–5.

16. Udell IW, Barshes NR, Voloyiannis T, *et al.* Neonatal hemochromatosis: radiographical and histological signs. *Liver Transpl* 2005; **11**: 998–1000.

17. Morris S, Akima S, Dahlstrom JE, Ellwood D, Kent A, Falk MC. Renal tubular dysgenesis and neonatal hemochromatosis without pulmonary hypoplasia. *Pediatr Nephrol* 2004; **19**: 341–4.

18. Elleder M, Chlumska A, Hadravska S, Pilat D. Neonatal (perinatal) hemochromatosis. *Cesk Patol* 2001; **37**: 146–53.

19. Parmley RT, Barton JC, Conrad ME. Ultrastructural, cytochemical, and radioautographic localization of placental iron. *Am J Pathol* 1981; **105**: 10–20.

20. Donovan A, Brownlie A, Zhou Y, *et al.* Positional cloning of zebrafish *ferroportin1* identifies a conserved vertebrate iron exporter. *Nature* 2000; **403**: 776–81.

21. Bradley J, Leibold EA, Harris ZL, *et al.* Influence of gestational age and fetal iron status on IRP activity and iron transporter protein expression in third-trimester human placenta. *Am J Physiol Regul Integr Comp Physiol* 2004; **287**: R894–901.

22. Bastin J, Drakesmith H, Rees M, Sargent I, Townsend A. Localization of proteins of iron metabolism in the

human placenta and liver. *Br J Haematol* 2006; **134**: 532–43.

23. Knisely AS, Harford JB, Klausner RD, Taylor SR. Neonatal hemochromatosis. The regulation of transferrin-receptor and ferritin synthesis by iron in cultured fibroblastic-line cells. *Am J Pathol* 1989; **134**: 439–45.

24. Verloes A, Temple IK, Hubert AF, *et al*. Recurrence of neonatal haemochromatosis in half sibs born of unaffected mothers. *J Med Genet* 1996; **33**: 444–9.

25. Fellman V. The GRACILE syndrome, a neonatal lethal metabolic disorder with iron overload. *Blood Cells Mol Dis* 2002; **29**: 444–50.

26. Visapaa I, Fellman V, Lanyi L, Peltonen L. *ABCB6* (*MTABC3*) excluded as the causative gene for the growth retardation syndrome with aminoaciduria, cholestasis, iron overload, and lactacidosis. *Am J Med Genet* 2002; **109**: 202–5.

27. Shneider BL, Setchell KD, Whitington PF, Neilson KA, Suchy FJ. Delta 4-3-oxosteroid 5-beta-reductase deficiency causing neonatal liver failure and hemochromatosis. *J Pediatr* 1994; **124**: 234–8.

28. Siafakas CG, Jonas MM, Perez-Atayde AR. Abnormal bile acid metabolism and neonatal hemochromatosis: a subset with poor prognosis. *J Pediatr Gastroenterol Nutr* 1997; **25**: 321–6.

29. Hardy L, Hansen JL, Kushner JP, Knisely AS. Neonatal hemochromatosis. Genetic analysis of transferrin-receptor, H-apoferritin, and L-apoferritin loci and of the human leukocyte antigen class I region. *Am J Pathol* 1990; **137**: 149–53.

30. Cox TM, Halsall DJ. Hemochromatosis—neonatal and young subjects. *Blood Cells Mol Dis* 2002; **29**: 411–17.

31. Whitington PF. Neonatal hemochromatosis: a congenital alloimmune hepatitis. *Semin Liver Dis* 2007; **27**: 243–50.

32. Timpani G, Foti F, Nicolo A, Nicotina PA, Nicastro E, Iorio R. Is exchange transfusion a possible treatment for neonatal hemochromatosis? *J Hepatol* 2007; **47**: 732–5.

33. Sigurdsson L, Reyes J, Kocoshis SA, Hansen TW, Rosh J, Knisely AS. Neonatal hemochromatosis: outcomes of pharmacologic and surgical therapies. *J Pediatr Gastroenterol Nutr* 1998; **26**: 85–9.

34. Jonas MM, Kaweblum YA, Fojaco R. Neonatal hemochromatosis: failure of deferoxamine therapy. *J Pediatr Gastroenterol Nutr* 1987; **6**: 984–8.

35. Rodrigues F, Kallas M, Nash R, *et al*. Neonatal hemochromatosis—medical treatment vs. transplantation: the King's experience. *Liver Transpl* 2005; **11**: 1417–24.

36. Heffron T, Pillen T, Welch D, *et al*. Medical and surgical treatment of neonatal hemochromatosis: single center experience. *Pediatr Transplant* 2007; **11**: 374–8.

37. Lund DP, Lillehei CW, Kevy S, *et al*. Liver transplantation in newborn liver failure: treatment for neonatal hemochromatosis. *Transplant Proc* 1993; **25**: 1068–71.

38. Egawa H, Berquist W, Garcia-Kennedy R, Cox K, Knisely AS, Esquivel CO. Rapid development of hepatocellular siderosis after liver transplantation for neonatal hemochromatosis. *Transplantation* 1996; **62**: 1511–13.

39. Schoenlebe J, Buyon JP, Zitelli BJ, Friedman D, Greco MA, Knisely AS. Neonatal hemochromatosis associated with maternal autoantibodies against Ro/SS-A and La/SS-B ribonucleoproteins. *Am J Dis Child* 1993; **147**: 1072–5.

40. Visapaa I, Fellman V, Vesa J, *et al*. GRACILE syndrome, a lethal metabolic disorder with iron overload, is caused by a point mutation in *BCS1L*. *Am J Hum Genet* 2002; **71**: 863–76.

41. Kershisnik MM, Knisely AS, Sun CC, Andrews JM, Wittwer CT. Cytomegalovirus infection, fetal liver disease, and neonatal hemochromatosis. *Hum Pathol* 1992; **23**: 1075–80.

42. Driscoll SG, Hayes AM, Levy HL. Neonatal hemochromatosis: evidence for autosomal recessive transmission [abstract]. *Am J Hum Genet* 1988; **43**: A232.

43. Parizhskaya M, Reyes J, Jaffe R. Hemophagocytic syndrome presenting as acute hepatic failure in two infants: clinical overlap with neonatal hemochromatosis. *Pediatr Dev Pathol* 1999; **2**: 360–6.

Chapter 34

Iron overload due to excessive supplementation

Iron overload occurs in some adults who have ingested iron supplements for prolonged intervals, and in some persons who have received excessive parenteral iron supplementation with iron–carbohydrate complexes.

Iron overload due to excessive oral iron supplements

One report included patients who reported that their only or predominant source of non-dietary iron was daily iron supplements that they had ingested for more than 5 years.[1] Patients who received either much parenteral iron or repeated erythrocyte transfusions were excluded. Most previously reported patients with iron overload due to iron supplements have been whites,[1] although an African-American case has been described.[2] Some patients were advised or elected to take iron because they had anemia. Other patients had types of anemia that may have enhanced iron absorption.[1] Iron measures, liver histology, and other features suggested that "hereditary hemochromatosis" caused or contributed to iron overload in some cases reported before the discovery of the gene *HFE*. In some cases, neither "hemochromatosis" nor a heritable type of anemia was apparent.[1]

Patient characteristics

Four patients ingested approximately 153, 547, 1341, and 4898 g of inorganic iron as supplements, respectively, over many years each.[1] Many patients developed endocrinopathy, arthropathy, hyperpigmentation, increased serum levels of hepatic transaminases, or cirrhosis without explanation other than iron overload, although some patients appeared to have no illness.[1] Among four patients,[1] one had *HFE* C282Y homozygosity and beta-thalassemia minor. Another had spherocytosis and no *HFE* coding region mutation. A third had no anemia, a normal *HFE* genotype, and no coding region mutation in *HAMP, SLC40A1,*

HJV, or *ALAS2*; she was heterozygous for the *TFR2* coding region mutation V583I (nt.1747G→A, exon 15). The fourth patient had no anemia and no coding region mutations in *HFE, TFR2, HAMP, SLC40A1, HJV,* or *ALAS2*.[1]

Iron absorption from supplements

Iron removed by phlebotomy in four patients was 32.4, 10.4, 15.2, and 4.0 g, respectively. Estimated absorption of iron from all ingested supplements in these patients was 20.9, 1.9, 1.1, and 0.08 percent, although it is unlikely that all iron absorbed over the intervals that these patients consumed iron supplements was derived from the supplements.[1]

Five normal subjects in an experiment took 65 mg of iron (as ferrous sulfate).[3] Within 24 hours after the first dose of iron, urinary hepcidin excretion increased 5.4-fold on average, but returned to the baseline levels by the next day, although the subjects continued taking iron supplements for 2 more days.[3] These observations imply that chronic ingestion of iron supplements leads to a net increase in iron absorption, even in persons without anemia or pathogenic mutations in hemochromatosis-associated genes,[1,4] although the fractional absorption of subsequent supplemental or food iron may be decreased due to hepcidin-mediated inhibition.

Prevalence of prolonged ingestion of supplemental iron

Seventeen of 120 patients (16 women and 1 man) in Norway with iron overload phenotypes had histories of oral iron intake lasting from 5 to 50 years; none had the *HFE* C282Y mutation.[4] In a survey of 2851 patients who reported that they had "hemochromatosis," 27% of respondents reported that they had used iron supplements for a median duration of 36 months before they were diagnosed to have "hemochromatosis."[5] Regardless, the extent to which prolonged ingestion of oral iron supplements contributes to the severity of iron overload in *HFE* C282Y homozygotes is unknown. It is also possible that some persons who ingest iron supplements for long periods without therapeutic indications do not develop iron overload.

Management

Only patients with documented iron deficiency, iron depletion, or chronic blood loss should ingest iron supplements. Physicians should supervise the effects and duration of supplemental iron therapy. Persons with hemochromatosis-associated mutations or some types of anemia may have increased risks to develop iron overload by ingesting iron supplements. Excess body iron in any form may be harmful and can lead to organ damage. Therefore, patients with iron overload from iron supplements who do not have severe anemia should also be treated with phlebotomy to remove the excess iron. Therapeutic phlebotomy is feasible and effective, and would prevent complications of iron overload. There is a positive correlation of $\log_{10}$ serum ferritin and the quantity of iron removed by phlebotomy in supplemental iron overload cases.[1]

Iron overload due to excessive parenteral iron–carbohydrate complexes

Iron complexed to a carbohydrate moiety such as dextran, sucrose, or gluconate is administered parenterally to treat iron deficiency in persons who have had suboptimal responses to oral iron therapy, who cannot tolerate oral iron supplements, or who have iron or blood loss that cannot be reconstituted adequately by using oral iron supplements alone. Most patients who require parenteral iron receive it by intravenous infusion, because relatively large quantities of iron can be administered in single treatments. Intramuscular iron therapy has been largely abandoned because relatively little iron can be administered with each injection. Unwarranted therapy with parenteral iron, regardless of the route of administration, can cause iron overload with the consequent possibility of organ injury and dysfunction.

Metabolism of iron from parenteral iron–carbohydrate complexes

After intravenous injection, iron–carbohydrate complexes are removed from the circulation by macrophages

that subsequently cleave iron from its carbohydrate ligand. Much injected iron is immediately incorporated into the bone marrow. Liver uptake occurs over a relatively long interval.[6] The iron is incorporated into ferritin/hemosiderin, or released into the circulation where it is bound to transferrin. The iron therefore becomes available to developing erythrocytes for hemoglobin synthesis or to other iron-depleted cells. The carbohydrate ligands are either metabolized or excreted. Negligible amounts of iron are lost via the urinary or alimentary pathways after administration of iron–carbohydrate complexes. The major portion of parenterally injected iron–carbohydrate complexes is assimilated within 72 hours; most of the remaining iron is incorporated into hemoglobin over the ensuing 2–4 weeks.[6,7] After intramuscular injection, iron dextran is removed from the injection site into the capillaries and lymphatic channels, and is metabolized in a manner similar to that of intravenously injected iron–carbohydrate complexes.

Patient characteristics

There are two general categories of patients who develop systemic iron overload due to the intravenous injection of iron–carbohydrate complexes: (1) patients who require chronic hemodialysis; and (2) persons who require protracted treatment with total parenteral nutrition (TPN). One unusual patient developed iron overload after prolonged intramuscular injection of iron dextran.[8] Administration of excessive quantities of parenteral iron is unlikely to be associated with any acute manifestations. Physical examination often reveals little or no specific sign of iron overload. Typical clinical laboratory findings include normal or elevated serum iron and transferrin saturation levels, hyperferritinemia, and increased hepatic iron levels estimated in percutaneous biopsy specimens by Perls' staining or atomic absorption spectrometry. Magnetic resonance imaging can detect elevated hepatic iron levels.

Patients who require chronic hemodialysis

Many patients treated with chronic hemodialysis receive regular infusions of intravenous iron–carbohydrate complexes because they have anemia due to chronic erythrocyte loss via hemodialysis apparatus and laboratory specimens. Nonetheless, early studies revealed that iron overload was common among such patients. In 1978, Pitts and colleagues reported an analysis of autopsy data on 24 chronic hemodialysis patients who had received varying doses of parenteral iron dextran. Hemosiderosis was common in those who received high total doses of iron, but absent in patients who received little or no iron. Organ dysfunction secondary to tissue iron deposition was not observed in any case.[9] In 1984, Murray and colleagues reported that 24 of 40 spleens surgically removed from maintenance hemodialysis patients (60%) showed massive iron loading; there was a significant direct, correlation between iron loading and the amount of intravenous iron dextran administered.[10]

Intravenous iron treatment of adults on chronic hemodialysis therapy improves their response to erythropoietin therapy and facilitates achievement of target values of hemoglobin and hematocrit. Excessive treatment, exposes patients to risks related to iron overload and oxidative stress.[11] International treatment guidelines generally recommend that intravenous iron be discontinued when serum ferritin is greater than 500–1000 μg/L. Serum ferritin values in the range of 200–2000 μg/L occur in chronic hemodialysis patients due to non-iron-related factors such as malnutrition and chronic inflammation.[12]

Many children with end-stage renal disease on chronic hemodialysis have iron deficiency. In one study, children with iron deficiency were initially treated with 3.0 mg Fe/kg body weight/dialysis of iron sucrose, but later this dose was reduced to 1 mg Fe/kg body weight/dialysis due to the rapid development of severe hyperferritinemia. Normally iron replete children were treated with 0.3 mg Fe/kg body weight/dialysis iron sucrose, and those with possible iron overload were not given iron sucrose. This indicates that a dosage of 1 mg Fe/kg body weight/dialysis and 0.3 mg Fe/kg body weight/dialysis seem appropriate for correction and maintenance therapy for children with iron deficiency and normal iron repletion, respectively.[13]

Some investigators have attempted to ascertain possible effects of inheritance of common hemochromatosis alleles on the development or progression iron overload in chronic hemodialysis patients treated with transfusion, infusion of iron-carbohydrate complexes, or both. Early studies of the human leukocyte antigen (HLA) alleles A*03, A*07, and B*14 as surrogate markers for hemochromatosis mutations revealed conflicting results.[14,15] Interpretation of these studies is confounded further by the present understanding that the prevalence of these HLA polymorphisms is significantly greater in HFE C282Y homozygotes than in general white populations,[16] but that most persons with these alleles do not have hemochromatosis or have hemochromatosis mutations.[17] In one multivariate analysis of chronic hemodialysis patients in a prospective study, however, the presence of common HFE mutations was associated with a reduced risk of death and a lower amount of erythropoietin and iron necessary to support erythropoiesis than was observed in persons without common HFE mutations.[18] This could be explained in part by the greater transport of iron into erythrocytes in persons with HFE C282Y homozygosity and heterozygosity than in those without C282Y,[19] and the increased rate of red blood cell turnover associated with C282Y homozygosity that may be due to iron-induced erythrocyte injury.[20]

Patients who receive chronic TPN

Most patients with iron overload due to parenteral administration of iron–carbohydrate complexes have been children who received TPN for long periods. Cohen and colleagues reported that correlation of clinical data with hepatic histopathology from 31 infants defined the chronologic progression of liver disease with long-term TPN that includes iron–carbohydrate complexes.[21] Steatosis and a prominent eosinophil component in portal-tract extramedullary hematopoiesis appeared during the first 5 days of TPN. The former persisted for 90 days, and the latter for 3 weeks. Canalicular cholestasis was detected after 10 days in 84% of the livers studied, and bile duct proliferation was observed in 64% of the livers after 3 weeks of TPN. Moderate to severe portal fibrosis occurred after only 90 days. Lipofuscin-like pigment and hemosiderin were each demonstrated in 90% of the livers studied. One patient developed micronodular cirrhosis after only 5 months of TPN.[21] In another study, Ben Hariz and colleagues evaluated the iron status of 30 children aged 1 to 18 years who received TPN for an average of 43 months with iron intakes of 100 μg/kg per day. Twelve children had serum ferritin levels greater than 300 μg/L, and eight had levels greater than 800 μg/L. Levels of serum ferritin and transferrin saturation were positively correlated ($r = 0.81$; $P < 0.01$). The serum ferritin level was positively correlated with TPN duration and with the total iron intake ($r = 0.68$; $P < 0.01$). Of 13 liver biopsy specimens, six revealed excessive iron deposition.[22]

Miscellaneous complications

Modest iron storage levels may increase the risk of bacteremia among hemodialysis patients who receive intravenous iron therapy.[23] This is consistent with broad clinical experience in patients with end-stage kidney disease undergoing chronic hemodialysis or peritoneal dialysis.[24–28] The risk for infection with *Vibrio vulnificus* and other marine vibrios may be especially great.[25–30] Some studies have suggested that intravenous therapy with iron–carbohydrate complexes and hyperferritinemia may increase the incidence of atherosclerosis, especially in patients with common *HFE* mutations.[31,32]

Sarcomas sometimes develop at the sites of intramuscular injection of iron dextran or other iron carbohydrate complexes.[33–37] Most patients were injected in the buttocks, and did not have or develop systemic iron overload as a consequence of the injections. Sarcomas have been induced by similar injections in experimental animals.[38] Extant reports of nine such sarcomas in humans were reviewed by Fielding and colleagues in 1977.[38] It was estimated that the latent period for development of sarcoma after intramuscular iron injection in man is 15–20 years. Fielding concluded that soft tissue sarcomas of the buttocks are not rare, that in only one case associated with iron dextran injection were the data sufficiently strong to support the probability of iron–dextran-induced sarcoma, and that on the basis of this single case a causal relationship of sarcoma and iron–carbohydrate complex injection in humans could not be made.[38] A high proportion of patients who receive intramuscular iron injections experience local discomfort or discoloration, or develop atrophy of subcutaneous tissue.

Management

Prevention is a crucial management strategy for iron overload due to parenteral iron–carbohydrate complexes. Only patients with documented iron deficiency, iron depletion, or chronic blood loss should receive parenteral iron supplements. It is important to ensure that persons with hemoglobinopathies, beta-thalassemia, or other forms of chronic, refractory anemia are not mistakenly diagnosed to have iron deficiency and thus are incorrectly treated with parenteral (or oral) iron.

In a report of parenteral iron therapy of chronic hemodialysis patients, it was concluded that the current published literature is inadequate for developing evidence-based guidelines for surveillance of possible iron overload, and that clinical judgment is critical to weigh the risks and benefits of intravenous iron treatment in the context of individual patients.[11] In children who require chronic hemodialysis, a dose rate of 1 mg Fe/kg body weight/dialysis and 0.3 mg Fe/kg body weight/dialysis seemed to be appropriate for replacement and maintenance therapy for those with iron deficiency and normal iron repletion, respectively.[13] Serum ferritin concentrations should be monitored regularly in all patients receiving chronic iron replacement therapy. Serum ferritin levels greater than 1000 ng/mL strongly suggest that iron overload is present, regardless of the underlying or associated disorders. Liver biopsy or MRI imaging should be performed to evaluate this possibility before more parenteral iron is administered. Physicians and pharmacists should supervise the dose, duration, and effects of parenteral iron therapy given alone or as part of hemodialysis or TPN regimens. In children receiving chronic TPN, parenteral iron should be less than 100 µg Fe/kg body weight per day.[22]

The detection of iron overload is an absolute indication to cease the administration of parenteral iron. In patients treated with end-stage renal insufficiency, hemodialysis removes iron predominantly from hemoglobin.[39] In contrast, removal of iron dextran by dialysis is negligible.[40,41] Iron overload in patients who require chronic hemodialysis has been treated with erythropoietin and therapeutic phlebotomy, resulting in major reductions in serum ferritin and hepatic iron levels.[42] Excess iron stores can also be removed by combination therapy with the parenteral iron chelator deferoxamine (2 g/dialysis given intravenously) and by hemodialysis itself until serum ferritin and hepatic iron levels return to safe levels.[39] Either of these treatments may take many months to reduce iron levels significantly, and thus managing physicians should be persistent in applying them. The oral iron chelator deferiprone causes iron excretion predominantly via the urine, and thus is not a rational choice for therapy of patients with iron overload who require chronic hemodialysis. Although approximately 85% of iron is excreted in the feces in persons who take the iron chelator deferasirox, this medication is relatively contraindicated in persons with renal disorders. Published trials of either of these drugs have included only patients with chronic anemia and transfusion iron overload unassociated with chronic hemodialysis. Physiologic excretory mechanisms for iron are very limited, but result in the daily loss of greater amounts of iron in persons with iron overload than in those who are normally iron replete. This could explain the decrease of iron overload due to intramuscular injections in one patient over many years who received no specific treatment.[8]

References

1. Barton JC, Lee PL, West C, Bottomley SS. Iron overload and prolonged ingestion of iron supplements: clinical features and mutation analysis of hemochromatosis-associated genes in four cases. *Am J Hematol* 2006; **81**: 760–7.

2. Barton JC, Acton RT, Rivers CA, *et al.* Genotypic and phenotypic heterogeneity of African–Americans with primary iron overload. *Blood Cells Mol Dis* 2003; **31**: 310–19.

3. Nemeth E, Rivera S, Gabayan V, *et al.* IL-6 mediates hypoferremia of inflammation by inducing the synthesis of the iron regulatory hormone hepcidin. *J Clin Invest* 2004; **113**: 1271–6.

4. Bell H, Berg JP, Undlien DE, *et al.* The clinical expression of hemochromatosis in Oslo, Norway. Excessive oral iron intake may lead to secondary hemochromatosis even in *HFE* C282Y mutation negative subjects. *Scand J Gastroenterol* 2000; **35**: 1301–7.

5. McDonnell SM, Preston BL, Jewell SA, *et al.* A survey of 2851 patients with hemochromatosis: symptoms and response to treatment. *Am J Med* 1999; **106**: 619–24.

6. Beshara S, Lundqvist H, Sundin J, *et al.* Kinetic analysis of ^{52}Fe-labelled iron(III) hydroxide-sucrose complex following bolus administration using positron emission tomography. *Br J Haematol* 1999; **104**: 288–95.

7. Watson Pharma Inc. *Package insert for InFeD*® (*Iron dextran injection USP*). 2008.

8. Saven A, Beutler E. Iron overload after prolonged intramuscular iron therapy. *N Engl J Med* 1989; **321**: 331–2.

9. Pitts TO, Barbour GL. Hemosiderosis secondary to chronic parenteral iron therapy in maintenance hemodialysis patients. *Nephron* 1978; **22**: 316–21.

10. Murray JA, Slater DN, Parsons MA, Fox M, Smith S, Platts MM. Splenic siderosis and parenteral iron dextran in maintenance haemodialysis patients. *J Clin Pathol* 1984; **37**: 59–64.

11. Fishbane S, Kalantar-Zadeh K, Nissenson AR. Serum ferritin in chronic kidney disease: reconsidering the upper limit for iron treatment. *Semin Dial* 2004; **17**: 336–41.

12. Kalantar-Zadeh K, Rodriguez RA, Humphreys MH. Association between serum ferritin and measures of inflammation, nutrition and iron in haemodialysis patients. *Nephrol Dial Transpl* 2004; **19**: 141–9.

13. Leijn E, Monnens LA, Cornelissen EA. Intravenous iron supplementation in children on hemodialysis. *J Nephrol* 2004; **17**: 423–6.

14. Quereda C, Teruel JL, Lamas S, Marcen R, Matesanz R, Ortuno J. HLA antigens and serum ferritin in hemodialysis patients. *Nephron* 1987; **45**: 104–10.

15. Carrera F, Andrade JC, Silva FJ, Simoes J. Serum ferritin and hemochromatosis alleles in chronic hemodialysis patients. *Nephron* 1988; **50**: 196–8.

16. Barton JC, Acton RT. HLA-A and -B alleles and haplotypes in hemochromatosis probands with *HFE* C282Y homozygosity in central Alabama. *BMC Med Genet* 2002; **3**: 9.

17. Witte DL, Crosby WH, Edwards CQ, Fairbanks VF, Mitros FA. Practice guideline development task force of the College of American Pathologists. Hereditary hemochromatosis. *Clin Chim Acta* 1996; **245**: 139–200.

18. Valenti L, Valenti G, Como G, et al. *HFE* genotype influences erythropoiesis support requirement in hemodialysis patients: a prospective study. *Am J Nephrol* 2008; **28**: 311–16.

19. Barton JC, Bertoli LF, Rothenberg BE. Peripheral blood erythrocyte parameters in hemochromatosis: evidence for increased erythrocyte hemoglobin content. *J Lab Clin Med* 2000; **135**: 96–104.

20. Feeney GP, Carter K, Masters GS, Jackson HA, Cavil I, Worwood M. Changes in erythropoiesis in hereditary hemochromatosis are not mediated by HFE expression in nucleated red cells. *Haematologica* 2005; **90**: 180–7.

21. Cohen C, Olsen MM. Pediatric total parenteral nutrition. Liver histopathology. *Arch Pathol Lab Med* 1981; **105**: 152–6.

22. Ben Hariz M, Goulet O, De Potter S, *et al.* Iron overload in children receiving prolonged parenteral nutrition. *J Pediatr* 1993; **123**: 238–41.

23. Teehan GS, Bahdouch D, Ruthazer R, Balakrishnan VS, Snydman DR, Jaber BL. Iron storage indices: novel predictors of bacteremia in hemodialysis patients initiating intravenous iron therapy. *Clin Infect Dis* 2004; **38**: 1090–4.

24. Boelaert JR, van Landuyt HW, Valcke YJ, *et al.* The role of iron overload in *Yersinia enterocolitica* and *Yersinia pseudotuberculosis* bacteremia in hemodialysis patients. *J Infect Dis* 1987; **156**: 384–7.

25. Klontz KC, Lieb S, Schreiber M, Janowski HT, Baldy LM, Gunn RA. Syndromes of *Vibrio vulnificus* infections. Clinical and epidemiologic features in Florida cases, 1981–1987. *Ann Intern Med* 1988; **109**: 318–23.

26. Taylor R, McDonald M, Russ G, Carson M, Lukaczynski E. *Vibrio alginolyticus* peritonitis associated with ambulatory peritoneal dialysis. *Br Med J (Clin Res Ed)* 1981; **283**: 275.

27. Stabellini N, Camerani A, Lambertini D, *et al.* Fatal sepsis from *Vibrio vulnificus* in a hemodialyzed patient. *Nephron* 1998; **78**: 221–4.

28. Bullen JJ. Bacterial infections in hemochromatosis. In: Barton JC, Edwards CQ, eds. *Hemochromatosis: Genetics, Pathophysiology, Diagnosis, and Treatment.* Cambridge, Cambridge University Press. 2000; 381–6.

29. Gholami P, Lew SQ, Klontz KC. Raw shellfish consumption among renal disease patients. A risk factor for severe *Vibrio vulnificus* infection. *Am J Prev Med* 1998; **15**: 243–5.

30. Barton JC, Coghlan ME, Reymann MT, Ozbirn TW, Acton RT. *Vibrio vulnificus* infection in a hemodialysis patient receiving intravenous iron therapy. *Clin Infect Dis* 2003; **37**: e63-7.

31. Reis KA, Guz G, Ozdemir H, *et al.* Intravenous iron therapy as a possible risk factor for atherosclerosis in end-stage renal disease. *Int Heart J* 2005; **46**: 255–64.

32. Valenti L, Valenti G, Como G, *et al. HFE* gene mutations and oxidative stress influence serum ferritin, associated with vascular damage, in hemodialysis patients. *Am J Nephrol* 2007; **27**: 101–7.

33. Grasso P. Sarcoma after intramuscular iron injection. *Br Med J* 1973; **2**: 667.

34. MacKinnon AE, Bancewicz J. Sarcoma after injection of intramuscular iron. *Br Med J* 1973; **2**: 277–9.

35. [no authors listed] Sarcoma after intramuscular iron injection. *Br Med J* 1976; **2**: 233–4.

36. Greenberg G. Sarcoma after intramuscular iron injection. *Br Med J* 1976; **1**: 1508–9.

37. Robertson AG, Dick WC. Intramuscular iron and local oncogenesis. *Br Med J* 1977; **1**: 946.

38. Fielding J. Does sarcoma occur in man after intramuscular iron? *Scand J Haematol Suppl* 1977; **32**: 100–4.

39. Baker LR, Barnett MD, Brozovic B, *et al.* Hemosiderosis in a patient on regular hemodialysis: treatment by desferrioxamine. *Clin Nephrol* 1976; **6**: 326–8.

40. Manuel MA, Stewart WK, Clair Neill GD, Hutchinson F. Loss of iron-dextran through cuprophane membrane of a disposable coil dialyser. *Nephron* 1972; **9**: 94–8.

41. Hatton RC, Portales IT, Finlay A, Ross EA. Removal of iron dextran by hemodialysis: an in vitro study. *Am J Kidney Dis* 1995; **26**: 327–30.

42. Onoyama K, Nakamura S, Yamamoto M, *et al.* Correction of serious iron overload in a chronic hemodialysis patient by recombinant human erythropoietin and removal of red blood cells: confirmation by follow-up liver biopsy. *Nephron* 1990; **56**: 325–8.

Chapter 35

Localized iron overload

Localized iron overload can sometimes occur in the lungs (pulmonary hemosiderosis) and the kidneys (renal hemosiderosis).

Pulmonary hemosiderosis

Idiopathic pulmonary hemosiderosis (IPH) (also known as Ceelen–Gellerstedt syndrome) is a rare disorder of unknown etiology characterized by recurrent episodes of diffuse alveolar hemorrhage and accumulation of storage iron in the lung parenchyma.[1–5] It is most common in children (age 1 to 7 years) but can also occur in adults.[2–5] Clinical manifestations of IPH include pulmonary symptoms (hemoptysis, dyspnea, cough), parenchymal lesions on chest X-ray, and iron deficiency anemia of unknown cause.[1–5] Diagnosis depends on exclusion of other disorders, such as inflammatory pulmonary capillaritis, in which diffuse alveolar hemorrhage is a cardinal sign.[2] The clinical course of IPH is variable; in chronic cases, the localized iron overload can result in pulmonary fibrosis, and death can sometimes occur due to pulmonary hemorrhage.[3–5] Treatment includes supportive therapy and administration of corticosteroids that can be combined with other immunosuppressive agents, such as azathioprine.[2–5] Successful resolution of some cases of IPH with immunosuppressive drugs suggests that an immunologic mechanism could be involved in the pulmonary capillary damage underlying alveolar bleeding which, in turn, leads to pulmonary iron accumulation.[3–5]

Hematite miners and other workers chronically exposed to iron ore dust may develop iron overload of the lungs and adjacent lymph nodes, but serum iron measures are usually normal.[6]

Renal hemosiderosis

Marked iron accumulation in the kidneys is rare in hemochromatosis, but when present, storage iron is usually located in cells of the tubules, particularly the convoluted tubules.[7] The most common causes of severe renal hemosiderosis are multiple blood transfusions and recurrent intravascular hemolysis.[8–11] In these situations, most excess iron is found in the proximal convoluted tubules. Mild to moderate renal iron accumulation does not produce significant pathology, whereas severe iron overload can result in tubular atrophy and interstitial fibrosis.[8–11] The precise mechanism of iron-induced renal damage is not clear, but it is likely to involve iron-mediated oxidative injury (Chapter 3). Renal siderosis may be minimized by ongoing chelation therapy in patients receiving multiple transfusions, and by treating the underlying conditions in individuals with recurrent intravascular hemolysis.[8–11]

Iron overload may be responsible for renal dysfunction in patients with thalassemia who have received multiple transfusions.[12] In diseases that cause intravascular hemolysis (such as paroxysmal nocturnal hemoglobinuria or mechanical hemolysis due to prosthetic cardiac valves), excess storage iron may accumulate in the renal cortex.[9–11] Intravascular hemolysis results in the direct release of hemoglobin into the plasma. When the amount of released hemoglobin exceeds the binding capacity of plasma haptoglobin, hemoglobin is filtered through the glomerulus. It is reabsorbed in the proximal convoluted tubules, where it is degraded and its liberated iron is stored as ferritin and hemosiderin.[9,10] Intravascular hemolysis does not result in iron accumulation in other organs.[9] In patients with intravascular hemolysis, acute renal failure is usually associated with more pronounced iron accumulation.[9]

References

1. Mundt E, Kriegel EM. Idiopathic pulmonary hemosiderosis; Ceelen–Gellerstedt syndrome. *Dtsch Arch Klin Med* 1952; **199**: 275–83.

2. Susarla SC, Fan LL. Diffuse alveolar hemorrhage syndromes in children. *Curr Opin Pediatr* 2007; **19**: 314–20.

3. Deniz O, Ongürü O, Ors F, *et al.* Idiopathic pulmonary hemosiderosis in an adult patient responded well to corticosteroid therapy. *Tuberk Toraks* 2007; **55**: 77–82.

4. Airaghi L, Ciceri L, Giannini S, Ferrero S, Meroni PL, Tedeschi A. Idiopathic pulmonary hemosiderosis in an adult. Favorable response to azathioprine. *Monaldi Arch Chest Dis* 2001; **56**: 211–13.

5. Willms H, Gutjahr K, Juergens UR, *et al.* Diagnostics and therapy of idiopathic pulmonary hemosiderosis. *Med Klin (Munich)* 2007; **102**: 445–50.

6. Laflamme L, Blank VL. Age-related accident risks: longitudinal study of Swedish iron ore miners. *Am J Ind Med* 1996; **30**: 479–87.

7. Barton JC, Bertoli LF. Histochemistry of iron and iron-associated proteins in hemochromatosis. In: Barton JC, Edwards CQ, eds. *Hemochromatosis. Genetics, Pathophysiology, Diagnosis and Treatment.* Cambridge, Cambridge University Press. 2000; 200–18.

8. Salim S, Asad H, Kumar MS, *et al.* Renal siderosis in donor allograft: Pathologic and clinical sequelae. *Am J Transplant* 2004; **4**: 1717–19.

9. Pardo-Mindán FJ, Diez J, Esparza N, Robledo C. Renal siderosis in patients with heart-valve prostheses: Clinical implications. *Nephrol Dial Transplant* 1990; **5**: 847–50.

10. Lee JW, Kim SH, Yoon CJ. Hemosiderin deposition on the renal cortex by mechanical hemolysis due to malfunctioning prosthetic cardiac valve: report of MR findings in two cases. *J Comput Assist Tomogr* 1999; **23**: 445–7.

11. Roubidoux MA. MR of the kidneys, liver, and spleen in paroxysmal nocturnal hemoglobinuria. *Abdom Imag* 1994; **19**: 168–73.

12. Koliakos G, Papachristou F, Koussi A, Perifanis V, Tsatra I, Souliou E. Urine biochemical markers of early renal dysfunction are associated with iron overload in beta-thalassaemia. *Clin Lab Haematol* 2003; **25**: 105–9.

Chapter 36

Management of iron overload

Iron overload is characterized by excessive iron deposition in and consequent injury and dysfunction of target organs, especially the heart, liver, anterior pituitary, pancreas, and joints (Chapter 5). Because physiologic mechanisms to excrete iron are very limited, patients with iron overload and its complications need safe, effective therapy that is compatible with their co-existing medical conditions. Worldwide, prevention of death due to cardiac siderosis is the most important potential benefit of therapy. The incidence of cardiac complications is greatest in patients with beta-thalassemia major and other heritable anemias treated with multiple transfusions. The liver is the primary target organ of iron overload in hemochromatosis and African iron overload, although maintaining normal hepatic function is important in all patients with iron overload. Preventing injury to endocrine organs is critical in children with iron overload. Successful treatment or prevention of iron overload increases quality of life and survival in many patients.[1]

Therapeutic phlebotomy removes iron as hemoglobin, and is thus suitable for treatment of patients with iron overload without severe anemia in whom erythropoiesis is fundamentally normal (Table 36.1). Many reports substantiate the effectiveness, outcomes, and safety of phlebotomy therapy in *HFE* hemochromatosis and allied disorders. Chelation therapy employs drugs that preferentially bind excess iron and increase its excretion (Table 36.1). Some dietary maneuvers may decrease the absorption of dietary iron, and may be useful as adjunctive therapy for some patients with iron overload, although such treatments do not diminish body iron burdens. In this chapter, techniques for the management of iron overload are discussed.

Therapeutic phlebotomy

Therapeutic phlebotomy removes excess iron and maintains low normal body iron stores. This was the first successful treatment for iron overload due to

hemochromatosis, and is still the preferred treatment because it is safe, effective, and economical.[2] Approximately 1% of *HFE* C282Y homozygotes develop severe iron overload;[3] some other C282Y homozygotes and some persons with *HFE* C282Y/H63D, *HFE* H63D/H63D, or novel *HFE* genotypes develop iron overload of lesser degrees. *HFE* mutations contribute to the abnormal iron phenotypes of some patients with porphyria cutanea tarda, non-alcoholic steatohepatitis, or chronic hepatitis C (Table 36.2). Phlebotomy prevents serious complications of iron overload in these disorders when used before iron overload becomes severe, and is useful for the management of other iron overload disorders in patients without severe anemia. One unit of blood (450–500 mL) from persons with normal levels of hemoglobin contains 200–250 mg of iron.[2] Phlebotomy treatment prevents all known complications of iron overload in hemochromatosis when applied appropriately in patients diagnosed before target organ injury has occurred.

Patient selection

Early studies demonstrated that the survival of adults with hemochromatosis who were treated with therapeutic phlebotomy was longer than that of those who were not treated. Since then, it has been regarded as unacceptable to conduct clinical trials in which persons with hemochromatosis or other iron overload conditions might receive placebo "treatment." Consequently, no randomized study has been performed to prove survival benefits of therapeutic phlebotomy in persons with other iron overload conditions. In addition, the experience with phlebotomy in the management of some primary iron overload disorders is limited. Nonetheless, it is recommended that all persons with iron overload who do not have severe anemia receive therapeutic phlebotomy and management similar to that recommended for *HFE* C282Y homozygotes (Table 36.2).[2]

Table 36.1. Treatments for iron overload[a]

Treatment	Iron overload disorders	Usual route of treatment	Advantages	Principal route/form of iron elimination	Compliance with treatment	Disadvantages	Adverse effects
Phlebotomy	*HFE* hemochromatosis, porphyria cutanea tarda, post-transplant, post-chemotherapy, overload due to supplements, other disorders with normal erythropoiesis	Venipuncture	Much clinical experience; effective, widely available, safe, inexpensive	Blood as hemoglobin	Excellent for iron depletion; good for maintenance	Requires repeated visits to health care facility	Transient hypovolemia; fatigue; increases iron absorption; iron deficiency if monitoring inadequate
Erythrocytapheresis	Hemochromatosis, sickle cell disease	Venipuncture	Rapid, safe	Blood as hemoglobin	Excellent	Limited clinical experience; requires special apparatus, careful patient selection; limited availability; expensive	Transient hypovolemia; fatigue; increases iron absorption
Deferoxamine (DFO) chelation	Beta-thalassemia major, intermedia; sickle cell disease; MDS; rare anemias	Subcutaneous infusion	Much clinical experience; widely available	Urine as chelate	Fair	Inadequate chelation of cardiac iron in some cases; expensive	Reactions at infusion sites; hearing, vision, growth, skeletal abnormalities; zinc deficiency; *Yersinia* infection

Agent	Indications	Route	Advantages	Excretion	Compliance	Disadvantages	Adverse effects
Deferiprone (DFP) chelation	Beta-thalassemia major, intermedia; sickle cell disease; MDS; rare anemias	Oral	Much clinical experience; good chelation of cardiac and hepatic iron; widely available	Urine as chelate	Excellent	Moderate expense; inadequate chelation of cardiac iron in some cases	Agranulocytosis; transient neutropenia; arthralgias; erosive arthritis; zinc deficiency; mild gastrointestinal symptoms
Deferasirox (DFX) chelation	Beta-thalassemia major, intermedia; sickle cell disease; MDS; rare anemias	Oral	Good chelation of hepatic iron; no growth abnormalities in children	Stool as chelate	Excellent	Expensive; limited availability; no clear benefit for patients with iron-induced cardiomyopathy	Skin rash; non-progressive elevation of serum creatinine; mild gastrointestinal symptoms; mild transaminase elevations; rare hearing, vision abnormalities; severe (sometimes fatal) liver, kidney, or marrow toxicity

Note: [a] Adapted from Barton.[1] MDS = myelodysplastic syndromes.

Table 36.2. Iron overload disorders managed with therapeutic phlebotomy

Disorder	Reference(s)
HFE hemochromatosis	2
HFE hemochromatosis and Wilson disease	114,115
HJV, TFR2, HAMP, or *SLC40A1* hemochromatosis[a]	116
African iron overload	117
African-American iron overload	118–120
Porphyria cutanea tarda	121
Hereditary anemias[b]	15,122–125
Transfusion iron overload after bone marrow transplantation for thalassemia	4
Iron overload after bone marrow transplantation for hereditary sideroblastic anemia	83
Transfusion iron overload after succesful treatment of hematologic malignancies	5
Iron overload due to prolonged ingestion of iron supplements	29
Non-alcoholic fatty liver disease	126
Hepatitis C	127,128
Diabetes mellitus, insulin-resistance associated with hyperferritinemia	129–131

Notes: [a]Patients with juvenile hemochromatosis phenotypes, especially those with cardiomyopathy, may benefit from simultaneous treatment with iron chelation drugs.
[b]Most untransfused patients with hereditary spherocytosis and iron overload also have hemochromatosis. Some patients with hereditary anemia undergoing therapeutic phlebotomy also require erythropoietin therapy or iron chelation treatment.

Patients with various iron overload disorders tolerate and benefit from therapeutic phlebotomy (Table 36.2). Children and adolescents with severe iron overload due to juvenile-onset hemochromatosis often need aggressive therapeutic phlebotomy. In asymptomatic persons with iron overload, therapy should not be delayed until symptoms of iron overload develop. Withholding therapeutic phlebotomy from older patients on the basis of age alone is not justifiable, although some patients are not candidates for treatment because they cannot tolerate phlebotomy or have very limited life expectancy.[2]

Iron overload may persist after successful, definitive stem cell transplantation or chemotherapy of heritable types of anemia, hematologic malignancies, or other conditions. Normal erythropoiesis is re-established after successful stem cell transplantation for beta-thalassemia major ("ex-thalassemics") (Chapter 21), permitting residual iron overload to be alleviated with therapeutic phlebotomy.[4] After remission induction of acute leukemia, transfusion iron overload can treated safely with phlebotomy.[5] Iron overload in patients with myelodysplasia, non-Hodgkin lymphoma, and autoimmune hemolytic anemia in remission after chemotherapy or transplantation can be treated similarly.

Performing therapeutic phlebotomy

Criteria for initiating phlebotomy therapy in persons without severe anemia are displayed in Table 36.3. Phlebotomy should be done by experienced persons and supervised by a physician. Ideally, it is performed in a physician's office or a blood bank, but can also be done in a medical laboratory or a patient's home. For many patients, co-operation with treatment is proportional to the skill of the phlebotomist and the confidence of the patient in the treatment staff and environment. Adequate hydration and avoidance of vigorous physical activity for 24 hours after treatment minimize the effects of hypovolemia caused by therapeutic phlebotomy. Persons with a hemoglobin concentration less than 110 g/L or a hematocrit less than 0.33 before treatment are more likely to have symptoms of hypovolemia and anemia, and phlebotomy is less efficient in removing iron. Nonetheless, many patients with chronic hemolytic anemia and iron

Table 36.3. Criteria for initiating therapeutic phlebotomy in persons without severe anemia[a]

Patient characteristics	Serum ferritin, µg/L
Persons <18 years of age[b]	≥200
Women, reproductive years, non-pregnant	≥200
Women, pregnant[c]	≥500
Women, post-reproductive	≥300
Men, all ages	≥300

Notes: [a]For control of skin lesions due to porphyria cutanea tarda, patients should undergo iron depletion therapy to reduce the serum ferritin to 10–20 µg/L. These criteria are not applicable to management of neonatal hemochromatosis.
[b]Patients with severe juvenile-onset hemochromatosis, iron overload, and cardiomyopathy or other major organ dysfunction may need combined phlebotomy and iron chelation therapy.
[c]Unless cardiac or severe hepatic dysfunction due to iron overload is present, induction of therapeutic phlebotomy should be deferred until the end of pregnancy (a normal term pregnancy removes approximately 1 g of iron from the mother).

overload tolerate phlebotomy well. The hemoglobin concentration or hematocrit and volume (or weight) of blood removed with each phlebotomy session should be documented (Chapter 4).[2]

Therapeutic phlebotomy is often performed using a large-gauge needle and a plastic bag to collect blood by gravity. This technique is typical of blood bank practice, and is necessary if the blood is to be used for subsequent transfusion. Many persons with hemochromatosis donate blood or qualify as blood donors,[6–8] and this can be used as a means of augmenting the blood supply for transfusion.[9,10] Nonetheless, many patients do not participate in such blood donation programs due to regulatory constraints, misunderstandings of blood bank personnel, or medical conditions other than iron overload that are reasons for deferring any potential donor (Chapter 38).[10]

Some patients, especially women, have insufficient venous access to permit frequent phlebotomy using a large-gauge needle. Using a small-gauge "butterfly" needle attached to an evacuated container via tubing with a roller clamp is an equally effective phlebotomy technique, and is more suitable for patients with limited venous access or in those who will require many treatments. Using the latter method, 97% of hemochromatosis probands had sufficient venous access to achieve iron depletion.[7] Sending patients to laboratories for

therapeutic phlebotomy where blood is drawn through routine diagnostic venipuncture needles and collected in evacuated glass tubes is not usually satisfactory. Informal experience suggests that implantation of indwelling central venous catheters attached to "ports" can be used for phlebotomy therapy in carefully selected patients, including children. Such patients should have peripheral venous access that is inadequate for one of the more conventional phlebotomy methods. "Ports" should only be used for phlebotomy by personnel thoroughly acquainted with them, and precautions must be taken to prevent entry of air into the great veins of the chest due to negative intrathoracic pressure. Valve-ended catheters of the Groshong type or arteriovenous shunts intended for hemodialysis are often unsuitable for therapeutic phlebotomy.

Frequency and duration of phlebotomy

Depletion of iron stores typically involves the removal of blood at regular intervals until mild hypoferritinemia occurs. Some men and persons with large body mass can sustain removal of 1.5–2.0 units of blood weekly. One-third of hemochromatosis probands diagnosed in medical care tolerated and adhered to weekly phlebotomy.[11] Some women, persons with small body mass, elderly persons, and patients with anemia, or cardiac or pulmonary disorders can sustain removal of only 0.5 units of blood weekly. Similarly, many patients with "loss-of-function" ferroportin mutations experience slow recovery of hemoglobin levels after therapeutic phlebotomy.[12] In a study of 2362 persons with *HFE* hemochromatosis, the mean rate of therapeutic phlebotomy for iron depletion was 2.6 units per month (mean duration, 13 months). Therapeutic phlebotomy rates varied by sex, age, reason for diagnosis, and severity of symptoms.[13] After a few weeks of therapeutic phlebotomy, erythroid hyperplasia permits more blood to be removed more often in many patients. Recombinant human erythropoietin also enhances erythrocyte production, but this treatment should be administered only to those patients in whom native erythropoiesis is insufficient to support phlebotomy and in whom blood levels of erythropoietin are not elevated.[14–16]

Serum ferritin and hepatic iron levels permit a relative but not absolute estimate of the amount of phlebotomy required for iron depletion.[2,17] On average, men with hemochromatosis require twice as many units of phlebotomy as women.[2,18] Persons who are homozygous for *HFE* C282Y typically have more severe iron overload than those with other *HFE* genotypes. Older persons typically have more iron overload than younger persons with the same genotype. Persons with hemochromatosis diagnosed in screening who have been regular blood donors often have less severe iron overload than do non-donors,[6,19] although this "protective" effect of previous blood donation is not apparent in most hemochromatosis probands diagnosed in medical care.[20] Some C282Y homozygotes who have common disorders that impair iron absorption such as celiac sprue or gastric bypass may require little phlebotomy to achieve iron depletion.[21,22] Hormonal factors and diet also influence the severity of iron overload in persons with hemochromatosis.

The serum ferritin level is the most reliable, readily available, and inexpensive way to monitor therapeutic phlebotomy.[2] In general, patients who have higher serum ferritin levels have more severe iron overload and need more phlebotomy than others (Chapter 4). Among patients who present with serum ferritin >1000 µg/L, it is sufficient to quantify the ferritin level every 4 to 8 weeks during the initial months of treatment. Serum ferritin should be measured more often in patients who have undergone many treatments, and in those who had mild or moderate iron overload at diagnosis. In all patients, serum ferritin should be quantified after each additional one or two phlebotomy treatments once the ferritin is 100 µg/L or less. Progress of treatment is also monitored by assessing hemoglobin concentration and hematocrit, their recovery rates, and mean corpuscular volume (MCV). Many patients with *HFE* hemochromatosis have elevated values of MCV, an inexpensive indicator of iron available for erythropoiesis.[23–25] When used in conjunction with the hemoglobin level, MCV is a clinically useful guide to the pace of phlebotomy therapy in persons with *HFE* hemochromatosis.[24] Iron depletion is complete when the serum ferritin level is 10–20 µg/L, the hemoglobin is less than 110 g/L, or the hematocrit is less than 0.33 for more than three consecutive weeks (in patients without chronic anemia).[2] These values indicate that mild iron deficiency has been induced and that potentially pathogenic iron deposits have been removed.

Typical outcomes of therapeutic phlebotomy to achieve iron depletion are summarized in Table 36.4.[2] Post-phlebotomy liver biopsy is rarely necessary to demonstrate that iron depletion has been achieved. Phlebotomy can reverse hepatic fibrosis in some patients;[26] other (but not all) associated symptoms and

disorders improve or resolve with phlebotomy. Clinicians must understand that some or all complications observed in patients with hemochromatosis, even those that are traditionally associated with iron overload, may be due to other causes. Relief of symptoms with an uncertain relation to iron overload such as fatigue and lack of endurance suggests that phlebotomy may have a placebo effect in some patients. It is also plausible that there is a iron-related molecular basis for some of these "atypical" complaints that is not presently understood (Chapter 5). Some patients who do not "respond" to iron depletion with phlebotomy are eventually discovered to have explanatory physical or psychiatric conditions unrelated to iron overload, or to have prospects of secondary gain through marital, employment, retirement, or other circumstances.

Maintenance phlebotomy

After iron depletion, the hemoglobin concentration and hematocrit are allowed to return to and remain within the normal range. Thereafter, phlebotomy may be continued to keep the serum ferritin level at ≤50 µg/L. In *HFE* homozygotes diagnosed in medical care, this requires the annual removal of 3–4 units of blood in men and 1–2 units of blood in women, on average.[2] In a large study, the mean rate of maintenance phlebotomy was 0.5 units per month.[13] Excessive phlebotomy after iron depletion has been achieved may enhance iron absorption, thus artificially increasing the need to perform maintenance phlebotomy. Many homozygotes do not require re-initiation of therapeutic phlebotomy therapy for more than 4 years.[27] Annual monitoring of body iron stores with reinstitution of weekly phlebotomy when the serum ferritin exceeds the upper reference limit is a safe alternative to long-term maintenance phlebotomy.[27]

Compliance

Approximately 97% of hemochromatosis probands diagnosed in medical care achieve iron depletion with phlebotomy.[11,28] In the first year of maintenance therapy, 84.0% of patients complied; the percentage of *HFE* C282Y homozygotes who complied was significantly greater than that of other patients. There is a constant rate of decline (~7% per year) in the percentage of *HFE* hemochromatosis patients who comply with maintenance therapy.[11]

Table 36.4. Outcomes of therapeutic phlebotomy to achieve iron depletion[a]

Abnormalities	Expected outcome(s)
None	Prevention of complications of iron overload; normal life expectancy
Weakness, fatigue, lethargy	Resolution or marked improvement
Elevated serum levels of hepatic transaminases	Resolution or marked improvement
Hepatomegaly	Often resolves
Hepatic cirrhosis	Regression in some cases
Increased risk for primary liver cancer[b]	No change[b]
Right upper quadrant pain	Resolution or marked improvement[c]
Arthropathy	Arthralgias sometimes occur; change in joint deformity rare; progression possible
Hypogonadotrophic hypogonadism	Resolution rare
Diabetes mellitus, glucose intolerance	Improves sometimes
Hyperthyroidism, hypothyroidism	Resolution rare
Cardiomyopathy	Sometimes resolves
Hyperpigmentation	Resolution
Hyperferritinemia	Resolution
Hyperferremia	Little or no change[d]
Serum non-transferrin bound iron	Reduction but not disappearance
Excess absorption, storage of non-ferrous metals	Probably little or no change
Restless legs syndrome	Symptoms may worsen
Hypogammaglobulinemia	Little or no change
Susceptibility to infections with *Vibrio vulnificus*, other bacteria	Little or no change[e]
Life expectancy	Normal in patients without iron overload complications, especially cirrhosis or diabetes mellitus; quality of life, longevity sometimes improved in others

Notes: [a]Adapted from Barton *et al.*[2]
[b]Increased risk occurs mainly in persons with cirrhosis, although primary liver cancer has been reported in *HFE* C282Y homozygotes without cirrhosis. Liver fibrosis or cirrhosis decreases or resolves in some hemochromatosis patients treated with therapeutic phlebotomy. It is unknown whether this decreases risk for primary liver cancer.
[c]Right upper quadrant pain related to hepatic iron overload usually improves or resolves. Right upper quadrant pain due to primary liver cancer, portal vein thrombosis, gall bladder disease, lesions in the hepatic flexure, or nephrolithiasis is usually unaffected by phlebotomy therapy.
[d]Serum iron levels may be normal or subnormal in persons with hemochromatosis due to severe iron deficiency, chronic inflammatory or infectious disease, vitamin C deficiency, or prolonged fasting.[2]
[e]Cirrhosis is the predominant factor that increases risk of death in patients with primary septicemia or wound infections due to *Vibrio vulnificus*.

Complications

Iron deficiency in hemochromatosis patients undergoing phlebotomy therapy should be prevented by monitoring hemoglobin levels and serum ferritin, not serum iron concentration or transferrin saturation.[29] Hemoglobin concentrations and values of MCV may be higher in iron-deficient persons with hemochromatosis than in individuals without hemochromatosis.[29] Symptomatic iron deficiency in hemochromatosis patients may be treated safely with a brief course of ferrous sulfate. Recovery is slower when iron is not given. Iron supplementation is unnecessary and not recommended for the mild, self-limited anemia, and decreased serum iron and ferritin concentrations encountered after initial iron depletion therapy for hemochromatosis.[29] Restless legs syndrome develops or is exacerbated in some hemochromatosis patients.[30] Rarely, patients report severe debilitation during therapeutic phlebotomy; the cause of this is unknown. Phlebotomy of patients who have hereditary hyperferritinemia-cataract syndrome usually results in the rapid development of iron deficiency, because most such patients do not have iron overload.[31]

Erythrocytapheresis

Erythrocytapheresis, like therapeutic phlebotomy, removes iron predominantly as hemoglobin (Table 36.1). Phlebotomy is suitable treatment for persons who have no or mild anemia, and whose rate of effective erythropoiesis is sufficient to replace phlebotomy losses rapidly. Isovolemic, large-volume erythrocytapheresis removes more blood erythrocytes per session than phlebotomy, while sparing plasma proteins, coagulation factors, and platelets. In small case series, erythrocytapheresis reduced iron measures in hemochromatosis patients with severe iron overload, intolerance of phlebotomy, or co-inheritance of beta-thalassemia;[32,33] erythropoietin administration may enhance such treatment.[33]

Erythrocytapheresis can be used as an automated method of erythrocyte exchange, especially in patients with sickle cell disease at risk for stroke. Treatment reduces hemoglobin S levels, prevents further iron accumulation, decreases body iron burdens, and eliminates the need for DFO therapy in some patients, including children.[1] Nonetheless, long-term erythrocytapheresis therapy was associated with significantly greater cardiac dysfunction than was detected in non-transfused patients, possibly due to greater pre-treatment iron overload in patients managed with erythrocytapheresis.[1,34]

Erythrocytapheresis appears to be safe and rapid; compliance with treatment has been excellent. This technique requires venipuncture with large-bore needles to accommodate the flow and pressure requirements of apheresis machines, the special apheresis apparatus itself, a skilled apheresis technician, and careful patient selection. Altogether, availability of and clinical experience with erythrocytapheresis for management of iron overload are limited, and concerns about its possible adverse effects on cardiac function in sickle cell disease are unresolved.

Iron chelation therapy

Iron chelation is the treatment of choice to alleviate severe iron overload in persons in whom iron mobilization from stores, efficacy of erythropoiesis, or severity of anemia preclude therapeutic phlebotomy (Table 36.1).[1,35–37] Accordingly, chelation therapy is the only practical means by which iron overload can be reduced in persons with either severe beta-thalassemia, other types of chronic anemia associated with ineffective erythropoiesis, or chronic erythroid hypoplasia unresponsive to erythropoietin therapy (e.g. Blackfan-Diamond syndrome, pure red cell aplasia, Fanconi anemia, severe aplastic anemia, or refractory anemia due to myelodysplasia). Iron chelation therapy can also reverse life-threatening cardiomyopathy due to siderosis of cardiac myocytes. Thus, combined therapy with iron chelation and phlebotomy therapy should be considered for immediate application in newly diagnosed patients with iron-induced cardiomyopathy. The typical underlying disorders in such patients are severe beta-thalassemia or *HJV* hemochromatosis.

The rationale, potential benefits and adverse effects, and costs of iron chelation for the management of iron overload due to *HFE* hemochromatosis and other iron overload disorders routinely treated with phlebotomy therapy are largely unproven. In *HFE* hemochromatosis and other adult-onset iron overload disorders unassociated with severe anemia, clinical trials must first determine the safety and efficacy of oral chelation drugs, and then compare long-term outcomes, costs, and acceptability of oral chelation therapy with those of phlebotomy in patients at risk to develop complications of iron overload. The pharmacology of iron chelation drugs and their clinical role in the treatment of diverse types of iron overload are reviewed in this section.

Iron stores available for chelation

Most iron in normal subjects is unavailable for chelation. Hemoglobin iron, more than two-thirds of all iron, is resistant to chelation. Likewise, transferrin-bound iron is a poor target for in vivo chelation, even though the stability constant of deferoxamine with Fe^{3+} exceeds that of transferrin. By exclusion, the iron most available for chelation is that stored in tissues as ferritin or hemosiderin, or a labile iron compartment in dynamic equilibrium with the former.[35]

Excess iron may be deposited in almost all tissues, but most is found in two types of cells: macrophages in the spleen, liver, and bone marrow; and in parenchymal cells, predominantly hepatocytes. Whereas iron accumulation in macrophages may be relatively harmless, parenchymal siderosis may cause significant organ damage. Altogether, optimal selection of an iron chelating drug requires: (a) consideration of the principal target cells or organs of excessive iron deposition based on knowledge of the underlying disorder; (b) an examination of liver, heart, or other organs by biopsy or non-invasive methods to determine the extent of overload; and (c) review of the preferential iron chelating action of the drug for iron deposits in either macrophages or parenchymal cells.[35]

In health, much of the iron in macrophages is derived from the catabolism of hemoglobin in non-viable erythrocytes; most of this iron is re-cycled within a few hours via ferroportin under the control of hepcidin (Chapter 2).[35] Hepatocytes, a major storage site for iron, take up greater quantities of iron when transferrin saturation is high and release greater quantities via transferrin when transferrin saturation is low. In contrast to macrophages, the turnover of parenchymal iron stores is very low (Chapter 2). In *HFE* hemochromatosis and other iron overload disorders in which transferrin saturation is typically elevated, there is a predominance of iron deposition in hepatocytes and other parenchymal loci (Chapters 3, 5). In transfusion iron overload unassociated with ineffective erythropoiesis or in "loss-of-function" ferroportin (*SLC40A1*) hemochromatosis, the primary site of iron deposition is macrophages (Chapter 12). In patients in whom both increased iron absorption and chronic erythrocyte transfusion occur, e.g. severe beta-thalassemia, a mixed pattern of parenchymal and macrophage iron deposition may occur (Chapter 21). Much redistribution of excessive iron may occur through diverse mechanisms.

Non-transferrin-bound iron (NTBI)

NTBI, found only after complete saturation of circulating transferrin, promotes the formation of free hydroxyl radicals and accelerates the peroxidation of membrane lipids in vitro.[35] Measurement of NTBI is not commercially available in many areas. Research studies of patients with severe thalassemia demonstrate that long-term treatment with deferoxamine or deferiprone markedly decreases their NTBI levels. Plasma NTBI is removed by intravenous deferoxamine therapy in a biphasic manner. After cessation of deferoxamine infusion, NTBI reappears rapidly, lending support to the continuous, rather than intermittent, use of chelation in high-risk patients with iron overload.[38] Recognition of NTBI as a potentially toxic component of plasma iron in hemochromatosis is useful in designing better strategies for the administration of deferoxamine and other iron-chelating drugs.[35]

Ascorbic acid and chelation therapy

Ascorbate deficiency decreases release of iron from macrophage stores, is associated with a shift of storage iron from ferritin to hemosiderin, and decreases serum iron concentrations.[39–41] Conversely, ascorbate treatment in scorbutic patients increases serum iron concentrations two to threefold within 6 hours after ascorbic acid dosing,[39] after which there is an increase in serum ferritin concentrations.[42,43] In a series of pioneering studies of iron-overloaded Bantu patients, Bothwell and colleagues showed that ascorbate deficiency is very common;[39] that it is caused by increased catabolism of ascorbate and its oxidative conversion into oxalate;[44] that deferoxamine-induced urinary iron excretion is impaired in ascorbate deficiency, but improves after ascorbate treatment in direct proportion to the severity of iron overload;[45] and that ascorbate treatment has no effect on deferoxamine-induced iron excretion in normal subjects.[45] Thalassemia patients with transfusion iron overload often have low leukocyte ascorbic acid concentrations.[42,46] In such patients, ascorbate supplementation markedly improves deferoxamine-induced iron excretion.[46] Consequently, ascorbate supplementation has been adopted by some physicians as a useful adjunct to chelation therapy.

Ascorbate supplementation is also associated with an increased availability of toxic, low-molecular-weight iron which, in combination with ascorbate, could enhance free radical formation and lead to increased organ damage.[35] In several reports, thalassemia patients treated with iron chelation therapy and oral ascorbate supplementation (500 mg/d) had striking and sometimes irreversible deterioration in left ventricular function.[47,48] Other reports describe paradoxical, rapid aggravation of cardiomyopathy in patients receiving iron chelation therapy with high-dose ascorbate supplementation.[49,50] A patient with pyruvate kinase deficiency and iron overload had rapid progression of congestive cardiomyopathy after self-administration of ascorbic acid, 500–1000 mg daily.[49] Accordingly, it has been recommended that ascorbate supplementation should not be started prior to the implementation of effective chelation therapy, and that the daily dose of ascorbate should not exceed 200 mg. It is doubtful, however, whether reducing the dose of ascorbate completely abolishes toxicity, because studies of lipid peroxidation in iron-overloaded spleens showed maximal malonyldialdehyde formation at the lower range of ascorbate concentrations; very high concentrations had an anti-oxidant effect.[35] Prospective controlled studies for establishing the role, if any, of ascorbate supplementation in iron-chelating therapy are needed.

Iron chelation drugs

Deferoxamine

Deferoxamine (DFO) is a hexadentate siderophore (M.W. 560) derived from *Streptomyces pilosus* (deferoxamine mesylate; Desferal®) (Fig. 36.1). DFO was introduced as parenteral therapy for iron overload associated with β-thalassemia major in 1976. The half-life of DFO is short (~20 minutes). Therefore, standard treatment involves the subcutaneous infusion of 40 mg DFO/kg for 8–12 hours nightly for 5–7 nights weekly using a battery-operated infusion pump.

Oral vitamin C, 200 mg, enhances urine iron excretion, but should be administered only during days of DFO infusion.[51] A stringent infusion routine is necessary for optimal iron chelation and excretion.[52] There are alternative routes of administration.[53–55] Although DFO mobilizes iron deposited in parenchymal cells and macrophages, iron mobilization from the heart occurs less rapidly than that from the liver and other sites.[56] Urinary iron excretion often wanes after several consecutive days of infusion, but usually returns to higher rates after several days off therapy.

Some adverse effects of DFO therapy are dose-dependent, although their mechanism(s) is poorly understood. The growth rate is decreased in some children with severe thalassemia whose serum ferritin levels were not greatly elevated. Abnormal skeletal growth has also been described, especially in the radius, distal ulna, and tibia. Growth rates may increase after DFO dosage is decreased. Similarly, some children treated with DFO develop high-frequency sensorineural hearing loss; some of them have relatively mild hyperferritinemia. Reducing DFO dosage may permit recovery in those whose hearing deficits are mild, but not in those with severe auditory impairment. Retinal, pulmonary, and renal toxicities have occurred in patients treated with DFO at very high dosages. None of these complications precludes continued chelation therapy. They are preventable if proper monitoring is practiced to detect early signs of toxicity. Because these adverse effects are dose-dependent and inversely related to the degree of iron

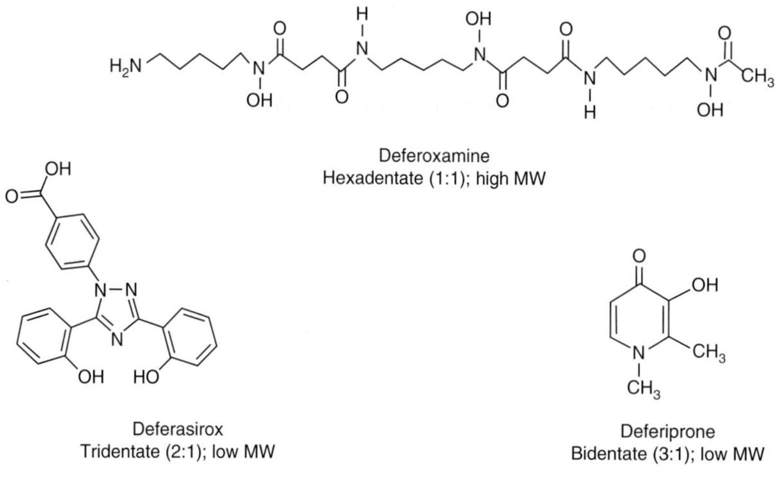

Fig. 36.1. The structure of three iron chelators. From Nick et al.[132]

Deferoxamine
Hexadentate (1:1); high MW

Deferasirox
Tridentate (2:1); low MW

Deferiprone
Bidentate (3:1); low MW

overload, their risk can be minimized by proper dose adjustment. Susceptibility to infection with *Yersinia* and perhaps other Gram-negative bacilli is increased in thalassemia patients who receive DFO therapy (Chapter 7).

Lack of compliance, cost, and physician dissatisfaction are major impediments to successful DFO therapy. Painful local reactions at the infusion site are the major reason for non-compliance, but severe allergic reactions are uncommon. Zinc deficiency can occur.

Deferiprone

Deferiprone (DFP) is an orally administered bidentate iron chelator (1, 2 dimethyl-3-hydroxypyrid-4-one (M.W. 139); L1, CP20; Kelfer®, Ferriprox®) (Fig. 36.1).[57] DFP is indicated for treatment of iron overload in beta-thalassemia major patients in whom DFO is contraindicated or inadequate. DFP traverses cell membranes more readily than DFO; this possibly accounts for the greater capacity of DFP to reduce myocardial siderosis and its ability to remove iron from other cells and from transferrin, ferritin, and hemosiderin. During therapy, daily urinary iron excretion remains constant over long periods. A "standard" dose of DFP 75 mg/kg per day (maximum 100 mg/kg per day) in three divided doses is approximately equivalent to a "standard" dose of DFO, measured by urinary iron excretion. The typical dosage of deferiprone is 75 mg/kg per day (up to 100 mg/kg daily) in three divided doses.[58,59] In beta-thalassemia major patients treated more than 3 years with DFP therapy, the prevalence of hepatic cirrhosis did not increase.

Retrospective epidemiologic data reported by Piga et al.[60] and by Borgna-Pignatti and colleagues[61] suggest that dramatic reductions in cardiac events and mortality occurred in Italian thalassemia patients given DFP instead of DFO. A randomized trial based on cardiac T2* magnetic resonance imaging suggests further that DFP can unload myocardial iron faster than DFO. Pennell et al.[58] compared oral DFP to subcutaneous DFO in 61 patients with thalassemia major who did not have symptomatic heart failure. The entry criteria required T2* to be abnormal (<20 ms) but not "severe" (<8 ms); it was required that study participants have left ventricular ejection fraction >56%. The primary outcome measure was change in myocardial T2* after 6 and 12 months. The rate of rise in T2* was significantly higher in participants treated with DFP (mean dose 92 mg/kg/d) than

in participants treated with DFO (mean dose 43 mg/kg, 5–7 d/wk). The increase in left ventricular ejection fraction in the DFP group was greater than that in the DFO group, but all values were within the "normal" range. Mean hepatic iron concentration measured by SQUID decreased slightly in each treatment group. Taken together with the epidemiologic data of Piga et al.[60] and Borgna-Pignatti and colleagues,[61] this trial provides important further evidence that DFP may be superior to DFO in decreasing myocardial iron (under the criteria specified in the studies).

Gastrointestinal symptoms occur in about one-third of patients and are usually mild. Joint symptoms may be severe enough to require interruption of therapy; their occurrence varies in different studies, possibly due to differences in degree of iron overload. Transient elevations in serum transaminase levels can occur, and are between usually reversible and not associated with other evidence of liver dysfunction. Zinc deficiency can sometimes occur and some physicians routinely provide oral zinc supplements to patients who take DFP. Agranulocytosis is a major complication of DFP therapy that occurs in about 1% of patients. Neutropenia (absolute neutrophil count 500–1500/μL) is more common (approximately 8% of patients). In some cases, patients who had recovered from DFP-associated neutropenia were retreated with DFP and did not develop recurrent neutropenia. Idiosyncratic adverse effects include erosive arthritis (common in patients in South Asian countries, from 5% to >20%).[37]

Deferasirox

Deferasirox (DFX) (4-[3,5-*bis*(2-hydroxyphenyl)-1,2,4-triazol-1-y1] benzoic acid; ICL670; Exjade®) is an orally administered tridentate iron chelator (M.W. 373) that is indicated for the treatment of transfusion iron overload in persons more than 2 years of age. DFX enters a variety of cells, especially cardiac myocytes. Iron excretion occurs primarily in the stool. Net iron excretion after 6 days of exposure is linearly related to the drug dose. Iron excretion at "standard" dose is within "therapeutic" range (7.7–28.5 mg Fe/d) for patients with beta-thalassemia major. At present, the US Food and Drug Administration approves a recommended daily dose of 20 mg/kg body weight, taken on an empty stomach at least 30 minutes before food. Doses may be escalated to 30–40 mg/kg daily after 3–6 months if there is no evidence of toxicity and sufficient follow-up and monitoring indicate that the initial daily dose is not sufficiently effective. In general, DFX is at least as effective as DFO in reducing liver iron deposits and serum ferritin levels, and DFX has a tolerability and safety profile suitable for chronic, once-daily administration in children and adults. Cappellini *et al.* demonstrated that DFX (20–30 mg/kg per day) can keep most but not all patients with severe thalassemia in neutral or negative iron balance in rough equivalence with moderate doses of DFO.[62] Some patients with high transfusion burdens will probably have rising ferritin levels and hepatic iron concentrations if treated with the approved DFX doses of 20–30 mg/kg per day.[37] The effectiveness of DFX in reducing cardiac iron overload in a manner that is superior to the action of DFO remains largely unproven.[63] Thus, DFX monotherapy is not suitable for patients with iron-induced cardiomyopathy, although it is possible that doublet chelation therapy that includes DFX may be acceptable, based on presently available reports.

The most frequent adverse reactions are diarrhea, vomiting, nausea, abdominal pain, skin rashes, and increases in serum creatinine levels. In the pivotal phase II trial of DFX in patients with thalassemia and iron overload, gastrointestinal symptoms were reported in 15% and skin rash in 11% of patients. Most patients can continue therapy with symptomatic management. A 33% elevation over baseline in serum creatinine level occurred in 38% of patients. Most patients had mild reversible elevations and treatment could be restarted safely at a lower dose. Elevation of alanine aminotransferase levels can occur and is usually mild and non-dose limiting. Auditory changes (high frequency hearing loss) and ocular abnormalities (lens opacities, cataracts, elevated intraocular pressure, and retinal effects) are rare.

Post-marketing reports include descriptions of acute renal failure (some fatal), acute hepatic failure (some fatal), severe hemocytopenias (some fatal), serious hypersensitivity reactions, and gastrointestinal ulceration and bleeding. Patient monitoring should include baseline and monthly assessments of serum creatinine level and urine protein; serum transaminase and bilirubin measurements (initiation of treatment, every 2 weeks during the first month, monthly thereafter), regular complete blood counts; and auditory and ophthalmic testing before starting treatment and yearly thereafter. DFX should be administered with caution in patients with ulcerogenic or hemorrhagic potential, such as those who take non-steroidal inflammatory drugs, corticosteroids, oral *bis*phosphonates, or anticoagulants. Nonetheless, the overall adverse effect profile of DFX is more acceptable than that of DFP if patients for chelation therapy are selected with prudence.

Investigational iron chelators

Three unlicensed chelation drugs for which some animal and limited clinical trials data have been reported include parenterally administered starch deferoxamine polymers; the orally administered compound deferitrin (GT56–252; 4,5-dihydro-2- (2,4-dihydroxyphenyl)-4-methylthiazole-4 (S)-carboxylic acid);[64] and L1NAll (1-allyl-2-methyl-3-hydroxypyrid-4-one), also an oral agent. There are unconfirmed reports that the juice of wheat grass has beneficial iron-chelation properties in patients with thalassemia intermedia and myelodysplasia.[65,66] In mice, curcumin and calcium-channel blockers have been reported to have iron chelation properties.[67,68]

Iron overload disorders treated with chelation

Chelation therapy is most beneficial for patients with iron overload caused by repeated red cell transfusions. The role of chelation in treating disorders of iron overload that can be managed satisfactorily with phlebotomy is more limited and controversial.

Severe beta-thalassemia

Severe anemia, ineffective erythropoiesis, and increased iron absorption appear in early infancy in patients with homozygous beta-thalassemia and in some patients with thalassemia intermedia genotypes. Periodic erythrocyte transfusion is necessary to sustain life, decreases cardiomegaly, hepatomegaly, splenomegaly, and bone and orthodontic abnormalities, promotes growth until adolescence, and improves well-being. All patients who receive chronic erythrocyte transfusion develop positive iron balance at the rate of 20–40 mg Fe/d (0.3–0.7 mg Fe/kg per day). Cardiac iron overload is a major cause of morbidity and mortality. Hepatic cirrhosis and primary liver cancer are also common, especially in patients with hepatitis C (Chapter 5). Guidelines of the Italian Society of Hematology for the initiation of DFO therapy in patients with severe thalassemia are displayed in Chapter 21. DFO removes liver iron more readily than cardiac iron. DFO does not reverse iron-induced cardiomyopathy in all patients, but significantly improves life expectancy.[52,69] Nonetheless, cardiac failure, the predominant cause of death after DFO therapy is initiated, is often associated with lack of compliance with DFO therapy.[70]

DFP treatment was associated with lower cardiac iron levels, less cardiac dysfunction, and fewer deaths due to cardiac disease than was DFO therapy in two retrospective studies.[56,60] Nonetheless, a significant decline in mean hepatic iron concentrations was reported in only one of six studies in which serial liver iron determinations were made in DFP-treated patients.[71] In a study of 54 children and young adults during more than 3 years, median liver iron concentration measured by biomagnetic liver susceptometry increased despite DFP treatment.[72] In another retrospective study, significantly greater liver iron concentrations were observed in patients treated with DFP than in those treated with DFO.[56] Serum ferritin concentrations often fall with DFP therapy. In a short-term study, raising the dose of DFP to 100 mg/kg per day led to reduction of serum ferritin levels in patients whose treatment at 75 mg/kg per day seemed inadequate.[73] A retrospective, multicenter study of patients with beta-thalassemia major confirms that cardiomyopathy, poor compliance with DFO chelation therapy, and high ferritin levels are significant risk factors for death. The results also suggest that including DFP in the therapeutic plan may protect against mortality.[74]

An expert group has recommended a chelation combination protocol of DFP during the day (80–110 mg/kg per day) and subcutaneous DFO (40–60 mg/kg) for a minimum of 3 nights per week.[75] After clearance of excess cardiac and liver iron, DFP monotherapy at doses >80 mg/kg per day has been recommended to prevent iron re-accumulation.[75] DFX may also be used in combinations with DFP and DFO, especially in patients intolerant of the DFP/DFO combination.[75]

DFX therapy was non-inferior to DFO therapy after 1 year in a phase III trial.[62] Patients with liver iron concentrations ≥7 mg Fe/g dry weight treated with either DFO or DFX (40 mg/kg per day) had significant and similar dose-dependent reductions in serum ferritin levels, liver iron concentration, and net body iron balance.[62]

Sickle cell disease

This group of disorders is usually associated with Hb SS, or with co-inheritance of Hb S and either Hb C or beta-thalassemia alleles (Chapter 22). Clinical syndromes are characterized by chronic anemia of variable severity, diverse complications caused mainly by intravascular sickling of erythrocytes, and increased susceptibility to infection. Iron overload, an important cause of morbidity and mortality,[76] is caused primarily by transfusion. Hepcidin levels are also down-regulated;[77] unusual patients have mutations in iron regulatory genes.[78] Stroke, a major complication, affects ~11% of patients by age 20 years; at-risk patients can be identified by transcranial Doppler examinations. Regular transfusions significantly reduce the incidence of stroke in at-risk children, but risk increases after transfusions are discontinued.[79] Some patients receive transfusions to alleviate other complications. Treatment for iron overload should be initiated as described for beta-thalassemia major.

Iron chelation with DFO has been used for many years, but compliance with therapy is suboptimal.[80] During short-term treatment, DFP can maintain negative iron balance in patients who require transfusion. In addition, DFP can remove pathologic iron deposits from sickle cells in vitro and in vivo. At "standard" doses, DFP significantly reduced serum ferritin levels and measures of hepatic iron content.[81] Nonetheless, there was no significant correlation of serum ferritin levels, liver and heart iron measures, and left ventricular ejection fraction. Compliance with DFP therapy was good, and there were no significant adverse effects.[81] It has been proposed that DFX could eventually replace DFO as the "standard" therapy for iron overload associated with sickle cell disease.[82]

Hereditary sideroblastic anemia

Meo et al. reported the results of a combined phlebotomy program and chelation therapy of iron overload in a patient with pyridoxine-refractory hereditary sideroblastic anemia that persisted after successful bone marrow transplantation. A regular phlebotomy program was started after which combination chelation therapy with DFO and DFP was administered. A 10-year follow-up showed a marked decrease in the concentration of serum ferritin, NTBI, liver iron content, normal hemoglobin level, and a good quality of life.[83] The overall rationale for using chelation therapy in this unusual class of patients who tolerate phlebotomy therapy seems similar to that for *HFE* hemochromatosis (Fig. 36.1). Further, the ideal use of chelation drugs first requires demonstrations that the drugs do not cause stem cell injury, exacerbate immunosuppression, or worsen graft vs. host disease.[36]

Other types of anemia associated with severe iron overload

Some patients with aplastic anemia or inherited bone marrow failure syndromes such as Blackfan–Diamond syndrome and Fanconi anemia are transfusion dependent. In pyruvate kinase deficiency, congenital dyserythropoietic anemia, and X-linked sideroblastic anemia due to *ALAS2* mutations, iron absorption is increased due to ineffective erythropoiesis; some patients also require transfusion (Chapters 23–25). Serious complications of iron overload have been reported in patients with these disorders. Patients with Diamond–Blackfan syndrome and other rare anemias have been treated with DFX in clinical trials,[3] In a large, 1-year, prospective, phase II study, DFX reduced iron burdens with a defined, clinically manageable safety profile in patients with various transfusion-dependent anemias, although many were excluded from further trial participation due to disease-related complications.[84]

Myelodysplastic syndromes (MDS)

This is a common, heterogeneous group of disorders characterized by hemocytopenias, dysmorphic, and genetically abnormal marrow and blood cells of myeloid lineage, and increased risk to develop acute leukemia. A majority of patients are 60–80 years old (Chapter 27). Approximately 80% of patients have anemia at presentation, more than one-half become transfusion dependent, and some develop iron overload.[85] Patients at greatest risk to develop iron overload and associated complications have refractory anemia (with or without ringed sideroblasts); 5q syndrome; a good prognosis (low or lower intermediate International Prognostic Scoring System (IPSS) score); >100 units of transfusion; or age <70 years.[86] Overall survival in many patients is limited due to age at diagnosis and common complications of MDS (e.g. infections, bleeding, acute leukemia).

Major uncertainties about the clinical importance of iron overload and the necessity for iron chelation therapy in patients with MDS who require chronic erythrocyte transfusion are unresolved.[90–92] The prevalence of impaired liver function, cardiomyopathy, diabetes mellitus, and other endocrinopathy has not been reported in large cohorts of patients with MDS. Similarly, there are few observations on whether such co-morbid conditions in MDS are due to iron overload or to other causes. The relationship, if any, of increased iron absorption in some MDS patients to inheritance of common *HFE* polymorphisms is unclear. There is a significant inverse correlation of transfusion and survival in MDS,[87] and transfusion burden and serum ferritin levels are independent negative prognostic factors.[88,89]

DFO therapy can induce negative iron balance in some MDS patients. Improvement of hemocytopenias sometimes observed after therapy may be related to effects of DFO on hematopoietic stem cells. Reports of DFP treatment include relatively few MDS patients, but suggest that rates of iron excretion may be less than those typical of beta-thalassemia major. DFP may act in synergy with defective granulopoiesis inherent to MDS to increase risks for neutropenia or agranulocytosis in some cases. Data from a phase II study of 47 MDS patients indicate that DFX therapy was effective and well tolerated.[93] Further, the US Food and Drug Administration has approved DFX for all situations in which iron overload could be a problem, but there are no specific studies showing that DFX therapy reduces complications in MDS patients.[94] In one report, it was recommended that chelation therapy be initiated in MDS patients after 20–30 units of erythrocyte tranfusion, or when serum ferritin exceeds 2500 µg/L.[95] It is probably reasonable to use DFX at a starting dose of 20 mg/kg per day in chronically transfused patients who, by virtue of low IPSS scores, are expected to live for many years.[96] Given the lack of prospective data demonstrating a benefit of DFX therapy, it should be discontinued for financial or adverse effect concerns.[94]

HFE hemochromatosis

Phlebotomy therapy is not suitable for or preferred by all patients with hemochromatosis.[1,36] Reasons patients offer for non-compliance include physiologic intolerance, anxiety, religious beliefs, time expenditure, inadequate insurance, and disinterest. Approximately 3% of *HFE* hemochromatosis probands cannot undergo routine phlebotomy therapy because they have insufficient venous access or anemia due to co-morbid conditions that is unresponsive to erythropoietin therapy.[7] Some patients with hemochromatosis live in remote areas such that compliance with routine phlebotomy therapy schedules is not feasible. Some patients who are compliant with phlebotomy indicate that they would prefer to take an oral medication if it were available. Altogether, the prevalence of hemochromatosis and the proportion of patients who cannot be treated adequately with phlebotomy or who prefer other therapy suggest that it is reasonable to conduct carefully designed trials of oral chelation therapy for hemochromatosis and related disorders.[1,36]

Chelation therapy with DFO-induced iron depletion in patients with hemochromatosis who were unable to undergo phlebotomy therapy.[97] In short-term studies, DFO treatment was as effective as phlebotomy of 500 mL weekly in removing iron from the liver.[97] Regardless, much experience with the poor compliance and acceptability of DFO therapy in non-hemochromatosis iron overload suggests that DFO treatment would not be generally satisfactory for persons with hemochromatosis. DFP and DFX also remove iron from hepatocytes, the primary site of excess iron deposition in *HFE* hemochromatosis. Because gastrointestinal and renal function are typically normal in hemochromatosis, the primary paths of absorption of oral chelators and the excretion of chelated iron are probably intact. Studies in rats suggest that DFP might also decrease the absorption of orally administered iron.[98] In *HFE* hemochromatosis, there are fewer concerns about long-term effects of chelation therapy on growth and development than in beta-thalassemia major or intermedia or sickle cell disease, because C282Y homozygotes rarely develop severe iron overload before age 40 years.[99,100] Zinc deficiency occurs in some transfusion-dependent patients who receive long-term DFO or DFP treatment. In hemochromatosis, zinc absorption is increased through divalent metal transporter-1 (DMTI) (Chapters 2, 8), and hepatic zinc concentrations are markedly increased.[101] In addition, DFX chelated iron with much greater specificity than zinc or copper in an iron-loaded marmoset model.[63] Thus, it is plausible that zinc deficiency will occur less frequently in hemochromatosis patients treated with oral iron chelation drugs than in persons with transfusion iron overload, although this is unproven.[36]

Selecting hemochromatosis patients for oral chelation therapy and determining treatment outcomes would presumably employ guidelines widely used for therapeutic phlebotomy. Typically, these include initiation of treatment when serum ferritin levels exceed 300 µg/L in men and 200 µg/L in women,[2] and monitoring progress with serum ferritin or mean corpuscular volume.[2,24] At present, there is an on-going phase I/II clinical trial of the safety and efficacy of DFX therapy

of iron overload in *HFE* C282Y homozygotes. Study participants with serum ferritin values of 300–1500 µg/L are being treated with DFX 5–20 mg/kg per day. No final results of this study have been reported. Treatment schedules of DFP or DFX applicable to the management of iron overload in previously untreated hemochromatosis patients need to be ascertained in phase II trials that also measure rates of net iron excretion and organ iron content, especially that of the liver. Treatment schedules for maintaining low body iron stores after iron depletion has been achieved must also be determined.[36]

Various measures of excess iron are greater in men than women with hemochromatosis, on the average,[2] but the incidence of agranulocytosis associated with DFP therapy may be greater in women than in men.[3] Thus, different schedules for oral chelation therapy should be considered for men and women. Phase III trials comparing phlebotomy with oral chelation therapy should be conducted, but may need to await a means to detect C282Y homozygotes who will develop progressive, injurious iron overload and therefore potentially benefit from treatment. It is also important to estimate the percentage of patients who comply with oral iron chelation treatment.[36]

Liver-related abnormalities due to iron overload, co-morbid hepatic conditions, and elevated serum concentrations of hepatic transaminases are common in persons with hemochromatosis.[2] A significant decline in mean hepatic iron concentrations occurred infrequently in persons with transfusion-dependent anemia whose iron overload was treated with DFP;[71] there are no reports of DFX therapy in persons with hepatic functional impairment. DFP and DFX cause elevated serum transaminase concentrations.[3,57,63] Altogether, clinical trials must be designed to determine if oral chelation therapy can eliminate hepatic iron deposits without causing additional liver injury, and if hepatic fibrosis and cirrhosis caused by iron overload can be reversed.[36]

Non-*HFE* hemochromatosis

Some adult age-of-onset hemochromatosis or iron overload phenotypes are caused by mutations of genes encoding ferroportin (*SLC40A1*), hemojuvelin (*HJV*), hepcidin (*HAMP*), alternate transferrin receptor (*TFR2*), H-ferritin (*FTH1*), DMT1 (*SLC11A2*), and ceruloplasmin (*CP*) (Chapters 12–16, 20, 28). Iron overload in many patients can be treated with phlebotomy or DFO; some patients may benefit from ancillary erythropoietin treatment, especially those with *SLC40A1* or *SLC11A2* mutations.

Early age-of-onset hemochromatosis phenotypes are typically associated with particular *SLC40A1*, *TFR2*, *HJV*, or *HAMP* mutations. Myocardial siderosis with consequent cardiomyopathy or arrhythmia can cause death within days after iron overload is diagnosed. Some patients appear to benefit from a combination of aggressive phlebotomy therapy and DFO infusions, or with DFO and DFP therapy.[2,102] Clinical trials of phlebotomy and chelation therapy to improve treatment of life-threatening cardiac siderosis and to alleviate non-cardiac iron overload will be difficult due to the rarity and genetic diversity of these cases.

African iron overload

This disorder, common in sub-Saharan African natives, is characterized by multi-organ iron deposition that occurs predominantly in macrophages. Contributing factors include a putative genetic factor and consumption of traditional beer that contains much iron (and sometimes other adulterants) (Chapter 18).[103] Associated disorders include hepatic cirrhosis, cardiomyopathy, osteoporosis, scurvy, primary liver cancer, and carcinoma of the esophagus. The relative importance of iron, alcohol, nutritional deficiencies, hepatitis B, and other factors implicated in the causation of these disorders is incompletely understood. Primary iron overload in African-American patients is phenotypically and genotypically heterogeneous; some patients have common *HFE* mutations.[104] Non-transfusion iron overload in African and in African-American patients with primary iron overload can be treated with phlebotomy,[104,105] but at present there are no reports of case series or clinical trials that have evaluated chelation therapy.[36]

Iron overload due to supplements

Patients who chronically ingest iron supplements and develop iron overload are rare. Some have hemochromatosis-associated mutations and mild or no anemia; phlebotomy therapy is feasible and effective, and would prevent complications of iron overload.[106] For patients with anemia that precludes phlebotomy, it is reasonable to use chelation therapy in a manner similar to that presently recommended for beta-thalassemia or sickle cell disease.[36]

Evidence-based clinical decisions

Much evidence supports the use of chelation therapy, especially oral drugs, to manage iron overload in patients with beta-thalassemia major, beta-thalassemia intermedia, or sickle cell disease. In comparison with chelation monotherapy, chelation drug doublets may enhance iron excretion and possibly decrease cardiac deaths, but may increase the overall incidence of adverse treatment-related events. There is good evidence that patients with rare forms of anemia and iron overload can be treated with DFO or oral chelation drugs, although results of long-term follow-up of large groups of patients have not been reported. Long-term studies of large cohorts of patients with MDS with iron overload have not been performed to determine if chelation therapy will reduce morbidity or mortality significantly. Therefore, chelation therapy should be used only in patients who have both high risk to develop iron overload and good prognosis. There is fair evidence to support chelation treatment of patients with hemochromatosis and severe iron overload who are unable to undergo phlebotomy, or as an adjunct for managing early age-of-onset hemochromatosis, especially in patients with cardiomyopathy. At present, there is insufficient evidence to support the routine use of chelation therapy in patients with either *HFE* or other types of adult-onset hemochromatosis, African iron overload, or African-American iron overload. It seems prudent to treat iron overload in patients with normal erythropoiesis post-transplantation or post-chemotherapy with phlebotomy, not chelation.

Methods to decrease iron absorption

Some patients may benefit from measures to reduce iron intake and absorption. All patients should avoid ingesting supplemental iron or eating excessive quantities of red meat. Ceasing consumption of traditional beer is important in the management of iron overload in native Africans. Tea consumption can decrease iron absorption in patients with beta-thalassemia major or *HFE* hemochromatosis; this effect is attributed to the binding of inorganic iron by tannate.[107,108] Other foods rich in tannates, phosphates, phytates, oxalate, or ionized calcium may also decrease the absorption of test doses of inorganic iron, but their routine use to manage iron overload is unproven. Regardless, reducing absorption of dietary iron is not expected to affect burdens of iron that have already been absorbed. Some patients treated with iron chelation drug may benefit by taking oral zinc supplements.

Other dietary topics

Patients should not ingest supplements of minerals absorbed in parallel with iron unless specific deficiencies have been demonstrated. (Chapter 8)[2,109] Susceptibility to lead or cadmium toxicity from avocational or occupational exposure and subsequent increased gastrointestinal absorption may be increased in persons whose iron absorption is also increased (Chapter 5, 8).[110–112] Patients with iron overload who have open wounds should avoid contact with water from warm seas during outdoor activities or when handling fresh finfish or shellfish. Patients with iron overload disorders should not ingest uncooked shellfish or cooked foods contaminated with seawater drippings (Chapter 7).[2,113] Ascorbic acid (vitamin C) can enhance the absorption of inorganic iron, and mobilize excessive quantities of iron from storage sites. Persons with hemochromatosis should limit consumption of supplemental ascorbic acid to 500 mg daily,[2] and those with thalassemia should limit consumption to 200 mg daily.[35]

References

1. Barton JC. Optimal management strategies for chronic iron overload. *Drugs* 2007; **67**: 685–700.

2. Barton JC, McDonnell SM, Adams PC, *et al.* Management of hemochromatosis. Hemochromatosis Management Working Group. *Ann Intern Med* 1998; **129**: 932–9.

3. Beutler E, Hoffbrand AV, Cook JD. Iron deficiency and overload. *Hematology (Am Soc Hematol Educ Program)* 2003; 40–61.

4. Angelucci E, Muretto P, Lucarelli G, *et al.* Phlebotomy to reduce iron overload in patients cured of thalassemia by bone marrow transplantation. Italian Cooperative Group for Phlebotomy Treatment of Transplanted Thalassemia Patients. *Blood* 1997; **90**: 994–8.

5. Barton JC, Bertoli LF. Transfusion iron overload in adults with acute leukemia: manifestations and therapy. *Am J Med Sci* 2000; **319**: 73–8.

6. Edwards CQ, Griffen LM, Goldgar D, Drummond C, Skolnick MH, Kushner JP. Prevalence of hemochromatosis among 11 065 presumably healthy blood donors. *N Engl J Med* 1988; **318**: 1355–62.

7. Barton JC, Grindon AJ, Barton NH, Bertoli LF. Hemochromatosis probands as blood donors. *Transfusion* 1999; **39**: 578–85.

8. Levstik M, Adams PC. Eligibility and exclusion of hemochromatosis patients as voluntary blood donors. *Can J Gastroenterol* 1998; **12**: 61–3.

9. Leitman SF, Browning JN, Yau YY, *et al.* Hemochromatosis subjects as allogeneic blood donors: a prospective study. *Transfusion* 2003; **43**: 1538–44.

10. Power TE, Adams PC. Hemochromatosis patients as voluntary blood donors. *Can J Gastroenterol* 2004; **18**: 393–6.

11. Hicken BL, Tucker DC, Barton JC. Patient compliance with phlebotomy therapy for iron overload associated with hemochromatosis. *Am J Gastroenterol* 2003; **98**: 2072–7.

12. Lim FL, Dooley JS, Roques AW, Grellier L, Dhillon AP, Walker AP. Hepatic iron concentration, fibrosis and response to venesection associated with the A77D and V162del "loss-of-function" mutations in ferroportin disease. *Blood Cells Mol Dis* 2008; **40**: 328–33.

13. McDonnell SM, Grindon AJ, Preston BL, Barton JC, Edwards CQ, Adams PC. A survey of phlebotomy among persons with hemochromatosis. *Transfusion* 1999; **39**: 651–6.

14. Bilgrami S, Bartolomeo A, Synnott V, Rickles FR. Management of hemosiderosis complicated by co-existent anemia with recombinant human erythropoietin and phlebotomy. *Acta Haematol* 1993; **89**: 141–3.

15. De Gobbi M, Pasquero P, Brunello F, Paccotti P, Mazza U, Camaschella C. Juvenile hemochromatosis associated with β-thalassemia treated by phlebotomy and recombinant human erythropoietin. *Haematologica* 2000; **85**: 865–7.

16. Mariani R, Pelucchi S, Perseghin P, Corengia C, Piperno A. Erythrocytapheresis plus erythropoietin: an alternative therapy for selected patients with hemochromatosis and severe organ damage. *Haematologica* 2005; **90**: 717–18.

17. St. Pierre TG, Jeffrey GP, Rossi E, *et al.* A new model for predicting venesection therapy requirements in hereditary hemochromatosis using non-invasive liver iron concentration measurement [abstract]. *Blood* 2005; **106**: Abstract 3596.

18. Moirand R, Adams PC, Bicheler V, Brissot P, Deugnier Y. Clinical features of genetic hemochromatosis in women compared with men. *Ann Intern Med* 1997; **127**: 105–10.

19. Witte DL, Crosby WH, Edwards CQ, Fairbanks VF, Mitros FA. Practice guideline development task force of the College of American Pathologists. Hereditary hemochromatosis. *Clin Chim Acta* 1996; **245**: 139–200.

20. Barton JC, Preston BL, McDonnell SM, Rothenberg BE. Severity of iron overload in hemochromatosis: effect of volunteer blood donation before diagnosis. *Transfusion* 2001; **41**: 123–9.

21. Barisani D, Ceroni S, Del Bianco S, Meneveri R, Bardella MT. Hemochromatosis gene mutations and

iron metabolism in celiac disease. *Haematologica* 2004; **89**: 1299–305.

22. Barton JC. Hemochromatosis, *HFE* C282Y homozygosity, and bariatric surgery: report of three cases. *Obes Surg* 2004; **14**: 1409–14.

23. Barton JC, Bertoli LF, Rothenberg BE. Peripheral blood erythrocyte parameters in hemochromatosis: evidence for increased erythrocyte hemoglobin content. *J Lab Clin Med* 2000; **135**: 96–104.

24. Bolan CD, Conry-Cantilena C, Mason G, Rouault TA, Leitman SF. MCV as a guide to phlebotomy therapy for hemochromatosis. *Transfusion* 2001; **41**: 819–27.

25. McLaren CE, Barton JC, Gordeuk VR, *et al.* Determinants and characteristics of mean corpuscular volume and hemoglobin concentration in white *HFE* C282Y homozygotes in the hemochromatosis and iron overload screening study. *Am J Hematol* 2007; **82**: 898–905.

26. Adams PC, Barton JC. Haemochromatosis. *Lancet* 2007; **370**: 1855–60.

27. Adams PC, Kertesz AE, Valberg LS. Rate of iron reaccumulation following iron depletion in hereditary hemochromatosis. Implications for venesection therapy. *J Clin Gastroenterol* 1993; **16**: 207–10.

28. Adams PC. Factors affecting the rate of iron mobilization during venesection therapy for genetic hemochromatosis. *Am J Hematol* 1998; **58**: 16–19.

29. Barton JC, Bottomley SS. Iron deficiency due to excessive therapeutic phlebotomy in hemochromatosis. *Am J Hematol* 2000; **65**: 223–6.

30. Barton JC, Wooten VD, Acton RT. Hemochromatosis and iron therapy of restless legs syndrome. *Sleep Med* 2001; **2**: 249–51.

31. Barton JC, Beutler E, Gelbart T. Coinheritance of alleles associated with hemochromatosis and hereditary hyperferritinemia-cataract syndrome. *Blood* 1998; **92**: 4480.

32. Fraquelli M, Mandelli C, Cesarini L, Barisani D, Bianchi PA, Conte D. [Survival and development of neoplasms in 56 patients with idiopathic hemochromatosis.] *Ann Ital Med Int* 1992; **7**: 26–9.

33. Kohan A, Niborski R, Daruich J, *et al.* Erythrocytapheresis with recombinant human erythropoietin in hereditary hemochromatosis therapy: a new alternative. *Vox Sang* 2000; **79**: 40–5.

34. Raj AB, Condurache T, Bertolone S, Williams D, Lorenz D, Sobczyk W. Quantitative assessment of ventricular function in sickle cell disease: effect of long-term erythrocytapheresis. *Pediatr Blood Cancer* 2005; **45**: 976–81.

35. Hershko C, Link G, Konijn AM. Chelation therapy in iron overload. In: Barton JC, Edwards CQ, eds.

Hemochromatosis. Genetics, Pathophysiology, Diagnosis and Treatment. Cambridge, Cambridge University Press. 2000; 339–54.

36. Barton JC. Chelation therapy for iron overload. *Curr Gastroenterol Rep* 2007; **9**: 74–82.

37. Neufeld EJ. Oral chelators deferasirox and deferiprone for transfusional iron overload in thalassemia major: new data, new questions. *Blood* 2006; **107**: 3436–41.

38. Porter JB, Abeysinghe RD, Marshall L, Hider RC, Singh S. Kinetics of removal and reappearance of non-transferrin-bound plasma iron with deferoxamine therapy. *Blood* 1996; **88**: 705–13.

39. Bothwell TH, Bradlow BA, Jacobs P, *et al.* Iron metabolism in scurvy with special reference to erythropoiesis. *Br J Haematol* 1964; **10**: 50–8.

40. Lipschitz DA, Bothwell TH, Seftel HC, Wapnick AA, Charlton RW. The role of ascorbic acid in the metabolism of storage iron. *Br J Haematol* 1971; **20**: 155–63.

41. Banerjee S, Chakrabarty AS. Utilization of iron by scorbutic guinea pigs. *Blood* 1965; **25**: 839–44.

42. Chapman RW, Hussain MA, Gorman A, *et al.* Effect of ascorbic acid deficiency on serum ferritin concentration in patients with beta-thalassaemia major and iron overload. *J Clin Pathol* 1982; **35**: 487–91.

43. Cohen A, Cohen IJ, Schwartz E. Scurvy and altered iron stores in thalassemia major. *N Engl J Med* 1981; **304**: 158–60.

44. Lynch SR, Seftel HC, Torrance JD, Charlton RW, Bothwell TH. Accelerated oxidative catabolism of ascorbic acid in sideriotic Bantu. *Am J Clin Nutr* 1967; **20**: 641–7.

45. Wapnick AA, Lynch SR, Charlton RW, Seftel HC, Bothwell TH. The effect of ascorbic acid deficiency on desferrioxamine-induced urinary iron excretion. *Br J Haematol* 1969; **17**: 563–8.

46. O'Brien RT. Ascorbic acid enhancement of desferrioxamine-induced urinary iron excretion in thalassemia major. *Ann NY Acad Sci* 1974; **232**: 221–5.

47. Nienhuis AW. Vitamin C and iron. *N Engl J Med* 1981; **304**: 170–1.

48. Thalassemia major: molecular and clinical aspects. NIH Conference. *Ann Intern Med* 1979; **91**: 883–97.

49. Rowbotham B, Roeser HP. Iron overload associated with congenital pyruvate kinase deficiency and high-dose ascorbic acid ingestion. *Aust NZ J Med* 1984; **14**: 667–9.

50. McLaran CJ, Bett JH, Nye JA, Halliday JW. Congestive cardiomyopathy and haemochromatosis-rapid progression possibly accelerated by excessive ingestion of ascorbic acid. *Aust NZ J Med* 1982; **12**: 187–8.

51. Porter JB. Practical management of iron overload. *Br J Haematol* 2001; **115**: 239–52.

52. Gabutti V, Piga A. Results of long-term iron-chelating therapy. *Acta Haematol* 1996; **95**: 26–36.

53. Araujo A, Kosaryan M, MacDowell A, *et al*. A novel delivery system for continuous desferrioxamine infusion in transfusional iron overload. *Br J Haematol* 1996; **93**: 835–7.

54. Borgna-Pignatti C, Cohen A. Evaluation of a new method of administration of the iron chelating agent deferoxamine. *J Pediatr* 1997; **130**: 86–8.

55. Davis BA, Porter JB. Results of long-term iron chelation treatment with deferoxamine. *Adv Exp Med Biol* 2002; **509**: 91–125.

56. Anderson LJ, Wonke B, Prescott E, Holden S, Walker JM, Pennell DJ. Comparison of effects of oral deferiprone and subcutaneous desferrioxamine on myocardial iron concentrations and ventricular function in beta-thalassaemia. *Lancet* 2002; **360**: 516–20.

57. Liu DY, Liu ZD, Hider RC. Oral iron chelators-development and application. *Best Pract Res Clin Haematol* 2002; **15**: 369–84.

58. Pennell DJ, Berdoukas V, Karagiorga M, *et al*. Randomized controlled trial of deferiprone or deferoxamine in beta-thalassemia major patients with asymptomatic myocardial siderosis. *Blood* 2006; **107**: 3738–44.

59. Taher A, Sheikh-Taha M, Koussa S, Inati A, Neeman R, Mourad F. Comparison between deferoxamine and deferiprone (L1) in iron-loaded thalassemia patients. *Eur J Haematol* 2001; **67**: 30–4.

60. Piga A, Gaglioti C, Fogliacco E, Tricta F. Comparative effects of deferiprone and deferoxamine on survival and cardiac disease in patients with thalassemia major: a retrospective analysis. *Haematologica* 2003; **88**: 489–96.

61. Borgna-Pignatti C, Cappellini MD, De Stefano P, *et al*. Cardiac morbidity and mortality in deferoxamine- or deferiprone-treated patients with thalassemia major. *Blood* 2006; **107**: 3733–7.

62. Cappellini MD, Cohen A, Piga A, *et al*. A phase III study of deferasirox (ICL670), a once-daily oral iron chelator, in patients with beta-thalassemia. *Blood* 2006; **107**: 3455–62.

63. Barton JC. Deferasirox Novartis. *Curr Opin Investig Drugs* 2005; **6**: 327–35.

64. Barton JC. Drug evaluation: Deferitrin for iron overload disorders. *IDrugs* 2007; **10**: 480–90.

65. Mukhopadhyay S, Mukhopadhyay A, Gupta PR, Kar M, Ghosh A. The role of iron chelation activity of wheat grass juice in blood transfusion requirement of intermediate thalassemia [abstract]. *ASH Annual Meeting Abstracts* 2007; **110**: 3289.

66. Mukhopadhyay S, Basak J, Kar M, Mandal S, Mukhopadhyay A. The role of iron chelation activity of wheat grass juice in patients with myelodysplastic syndrome [abstract]. *ASCO Meeting Abstracts* 2009; **27**: 7012.

67. Jiao Y, Wilkinson J, Christine PE, *et al*. Iron chelation in the biological activity of curcumin. *Free Radic Biol Med* 2006; **40**: 1152–60.

68. Ludwiczek S, Theurl I, Muckenthaler MU, *et al*. Ca^{2+} channel blockers reverse iron overload by a new mechanism via divalent metal transporter-1. *Nat Med* 2007; **13**: 448–54.

69. Olivieri NF, Nathan DG, MacMillan JH, *et al*. Survival in medically treated patients with homozygous beta-thalassemia. *N Engl J Med* 1994; **331**: 574–8.

70. Brittenham GM, Griffith PM, Nienhuis AW, *et al*. Efficacy of deferoxamine in preventing complications of iron overload in patients with thalassemia major. *N Engl J Med* 1994; **331**: 567–73.

71. Hoffbrand AV, Cohen A, Hershko C. Role of deferiprone in chelation therapy for transfusional iron overload. *Blood* 2003; **102**: 17–24.

72. Fischer R, Longo F, Nielsen P, Engelhardt R, Hider RC, Piga A. Monitoring long-term efficacy of iron chelation therapy by deferiprone and desferrioxamine in patients with beta-thalassaemia major: application of SQUID biomagnetic liver susceptometry. *Br J Haematol* 2003; **121**: 938–48.

73. Wonke B, Wright C, Hoffbrand AV. Combined therapy with deferiprone and desferrioxamine. *Br J Haematol* 1998; **103**: 361–4.

74. Ceci A, Baiardi P, Catuprano M, *et al*. Risk factors for death in patients with β-thalassemia major: results of a case-control study. *Haematologica* 2006; **91**: 1420–1.

75. Kontoghiorghes GJ, Kolnagou A. Effective new treatments of iron overload in thalassaemia using the ICOC combination therapy protocol of deferiprone (L1) and deferoxamine and of new chelating drugs. *Haematologica* 2006; **91**: ELT04.

76. Darbari DS, Kple-Faget P, Kwagyan J, Rana S, Gordeuk VR, Castro O. Circumstances of death in adult sickle cell disease patients. *Am J Hematol* 2006; **81**: 858–63.

77. Kearney SL, Nemeth E, Neufeld EJ, *et al*. Urinary hepcidin in congenital chronic anemias. *Pediatr Blood Cancer* 2007; **48**: 57–63.

78. Barton JC, Lee PL, Bertoli LF, Beutler E. Iron overload in an African-American woman with SS hemoglobinopathy and a promoter mutation in the X-linked erythroid-specific 5-aminolevulinate synthase (*ALAS2*) gene. *Blood Cells Mol Dis* 2005; **34**: 226–8.

79. Lee MT, Piomelli S, Granger S, *et al.* Stroke Prevention Trial in Sickle Cell Anemia (STOP): extended follow-up and final results. *Blood* 2006; **108**: 847–52.

80. Treadwell MJ, Law AW, Sung J, *et al.* Barriers to adherence of deferoxamine usage in sickle cell disease. *Pediatr Blood Cancer* 2005; **44**: 500–7.

81. Voskaridou E, Douskou M, Terpos E, *et al.* Deferiprone as an oral iron chelator in sickle cell disease. *Ann Hematol* 2005; **84**: 434–40.

82. Okpala I. Investigational agents for sickle cell disease. *Expert Opin Investig Drugs* 2006; **15**: 833–42.

83. Meo A, Ruggeri A, La Rosa MA, Zanghi L, Morabito N, Duca L. Iron burden and liver fibrosis decrease during a long-term phlebotomy program and iron chelating treatment after bone marrow transplantation. *Hemoglobin* 2006; **30**: 131–7.

84. Porter J, Ealanello R, Saglio E, *et al.* Relative response of patients with myelodysplastic syndromes and other transfusion-dependent anemias to deferasirox (ICL670): a 1-year prospective study. *Eur J Hematol* 2008; **80**: 168–76.

85. Gattermann N. Clinical consequences of iron overload in myelodysplastic syndromes and treatment with chelators. *Hematol/Oncol Clin* 2006; 13–17.

86. Rose C, Cambier N, Mahieu M, Ernst O, Fenaux P. [Iron overload and myelodysplastic syndromes.] *Transfus Clin Biol* 2001; **8**: 422–32.

87. Malcovati L, Porta MG, Pascutto C, *et al.* Prognostic factors and life expectancy in myelodysplastic syndromes classified according to WHO criteria: a basis for clinical decision making. *J Clin Oncol* 2005; **23**: 7594–603.

88. Takatoku M, Uchiyama T, Okamoto S, *et al.* Retrospective nationwide survey of Japanese patients with transfusion-dependent MDS and aplastic anemia highlights the negative impact of iron overload on morbidity/mortality. *Eur J Haematol* 2007; **78**: 487–94.

89. Armand P, Kim HT, Cutler CS, *et al.* Prognostic impact of elevated pretransplantation serum ferritin in patients undergoing myeloablative stem cell transplantation. *Blood* 2007; **109**: 4586–8.

90. Maggio A. Light and shadows in the iron chelation treatment of haematological diseases. *Br J Haematol* 2007; **138**: 407–21.

91. Steensma DP. Myelodysplasia paranoia: iron as the new radon. *Leuk Res* 2009; **33**: 1158–63.

92. DeLoughery TG. Iron: The fifth horseman of the apocalypse? *Am J Hematol* 2009; **84**: 263–4.

93. Gattermann N, Cazzola M, Greenberg P, Maertens J, Soulieres D, Rose C. The efficacy and tolerability of ICL670, a once-daily oral iron chelator, in patients with myelodysplastic syndromes (MDS) and iron overload. *Leuk Res* 2005; **29** (suppl 1): S76.

94. Stone RM. How I treat patients with myelodysplastic syndromes. *Blood* 2009; **113**: 6296–303.

95. Greenberg PL, Baer MR, Bennett JM, *et al.* Myelodysplastic syndromes clinical practice guidelines in oncology. *J Natl Compr Canc Netw* 2006; **4**: 58–77.

96. Greenberg PL. Myelodysplastic syndromes: iron overload consequences and current chelating therapies. *J Natl Compr Canc Netw* 2006; **4**: 91–6.

97. Nielsen P, Fischer R, Buggisch P, Janka-Schaub G. Effective treatment of hereditary haemochromatosis with desferrioxamine in selected cases. *Br J Haematol* 2003; **123**: 952–3.

98. Barr J, Berkovitch M, Tavori I, Kariv N, Schejter A, Eshel G. Acute iron intoxication: the efficacy of deferiprone and sodium biocarbonate in the prevention of iron absorption from the digestive tract. *Vet Hum Toxicol* 1999; **41**: 308–11.

99. Bacon BR, Farahvash MJ, Janney CG, Neuschwander-Tetri BA. Non-alcoholic steatohepatitis: an expanded clinical entity. *Gastroenterology* 1994; **107**: 1103–9.

100. Barton JC, Felitti VJ, Lee P, Beutler E. Characteristics of *HFE* C282Y homozygotes younger than age 30 years. *Acta Haematol* 2004; **112**: 219–21.

101. Adams PC, Bradley C, Frei JV. Hepatic zinc in hemochromatosis. *Clin Invest Med* 1991; **14**: 16–20.

102. Fabio G, Minonzio F, Delbini P, Bianchi A, Cappellini MD. Reversal of cardiac complications by deferiprone and deferoxamine combination therapy in a patient affected by a severe type of juvenile hemochromatosis (JH). *Blood* 2007; **109**: 362–4.

103. Gordeuk V, Mukiibi J, Hasstedt SJ, *et al.* Iron overload in Africa. Interaction between a gene and dietary iron content. *N Engl J Med* 1992; **326**: 95–100.

104. Barton JC, Acton RT, Rivers CA, *et al.* Genotypic and phenotypic heterogeneity of African-Americans with primary iron overload. *Blood Cells Mol Dis* 2003; **31**: 310–19.

105. Speight AN, Cliff J. Iron storage disease of the liver in Dar es Salaam: a preliminary report on venesection therapy. *East Afr Med J* 1974; **51**: 895–902.

106. Barton JC, Lee PL, West C, Bottomley SS. Iron overload and prolonged ingestion of iron supplements: Clinical features and mutation analysis of hemochromatosis-associated genes in four cases. *Am J Hematol* 2006; **81**: 760–7.

107. de Alarcon PA, Donovan ME, Forbes GB, Landaw SA, Stockman JA, III. Iron absorption in the thalassemia syndromes and its inhibition by tea. *N Engl J Med* 1979; **300**: 5–8.

108. Kaltwasser JP, Werner E, Schalk K, Hansen C, Gottschalk R, Seidl C. Clinical trial on the effect of regular tea drinking on iron accumulation in genetic haemochromatosis. *Gut* 1998; **43**: 699–704.

109. Barton JC, Bertoli LF. Zinc gluconate lozenges for treating the common cold. *Ann Intern Med* 1997; **126**: 738–9.

110. Barton JC, Patton MA, Edwards CQ, *et al*. Blood lead concentrations in hereditary hemochromatosis. *J Lab Clin Med* 1994; **124**: 193–8.

111. Tallkvist J, Bowlus CL, Lonnerdal B. *DMT1* gene expression and cadmium absorption in human absorptive enterocytes. *Toxicol Lett* 2001; **122**: 171–7.

112. Akesson A, Stal P, Vahter M. Phlebotomy increases cadmium uptake in hemochromatosis. *Environ Health Perspect* 2000; **108**: 289–91.

113. Barton JC, Acton RT. Hemochromatosis and *Vibrio vulnificus* wound Infections. *J Clin Gastroenterol* 2009; **43**: 890–3.

114. Walshe JM, Cox DW. Effect of treatment of Wilson's disease on natural history of haemochromatosis. *Lancet* 1998; **352**: 112–13.

115. Shiono Y, Wakusawa S, Hayashi H, *et al*. Iron accumulation in the liver of male patients with Wilson's disease. *Am J Gastroenterol* 2001; **96**: 3147–51.

116. Camaschella C. Understanding iron homeostasis through genetic analysis of hemochromatosis and related disorders. *Blood* 2005; **106**: 3710–17.

117. Speight AN, Cliff J. Iron storage disease of the liver in Dar es Salaam: a preliminary report on venesection therapy. *East Afr Med J* 1974; **51**: 895–902.

118. Barton JC, Edwards CQ, Bertoli LF, Shroyer TW, Hudson SL. Iron overload in African-Americans. *Am J Med* 1995; **99**: 616–23.

119. Wurapa RK, Gordeuk VR, Brittenham GM, Khiyami A, Schechter GP, Edwards CQ. Primary iron overload in African-Americans. *Am J Med* 1996; **101**: 9–18.

120. Barton JC, Acton RT. Inheritance of two *HFE* mutations in African-Americans: cases with hemochromatosis phenotypes and estimates of hemochromatosis phenotype frequency. *Genet Med* 2001; **3**: 294–300.

121. Lundvall O. Phlebotomy treatment of porphyria cutanea tarda. *Acta Derm Venereol Suppl (Stockh)* 1982; **100**: 107–18.

122. Chrobak L. Successful treatment of iron overload with phlebotomies in two siblings with congenital dyserythropoietic anemia-type II (CDA-II). *Acta Medica (Hradec Kralove)* 2006; **49**: 193–5.

123. Hofmann WK, Kaltwasser JP, Hoelzer D, Nielsen P, Gabbe EE. Successful treatment of iron overload by phlebotomies in a patient with severe congenital dyserythropoietic anemia type II. *Blood* 1997; **89**: 3068–9.

124. Lee PL, Barton JC, Rao SV, Acton RT, Adler BK, Beutler E. Three kinships with *ALAS2* P520L (c.1559 C→T) mutation, two in association with severe iron overload, and one with sideroblastic anemia and severe iron overload. *Blood Cells Mol Dis* 2006; **36**: 292–7.

125. Zimelman AP, Miller A. Primary hemochromatosis with hereditary spherocytosis. *Arch Intern Med* 1980; **140**: 983–4.

126. Valenti L, Fracanzani AL, Dongiovanni P, *et al*. Iron depletion by phlebotomy improves insulin resistance in patients with nonalcoholic fatty liver disease and hyperferritinemia: evidence from a case-control study. *Am J Gastroenterol* 2007; **102**: 1251–8.

127. Hayashi H, Takikawa T, Nishimura N, Yano M, Isomura T, Sakamoto N. Improvement of serum aminotransferase levels after phlebotomy in patients with chronic active hepatitis C and excess hepatic iron. *Am J Gastroenterol* 1994; **89**: 986–8.

128. Piperno A, Sampietro M, D'Alba R, *et al*. Iron stores, response to alpha-interferon therapy, and effects of iron depletion in chronic hepatitis C. *Liver* 1996; **16**: 248–54.

129. Guillygomarc'h A, Mendler MH, Moirand R, *et al*. Venesection therapy of insulin resistance-associated hepatic iron overload. *J Hepatol* 2001; **35**: 344–9.

130. Hramiak IM, Finegood DT, Adams PC. Factors affecting glucose tolerance in hereditary hemochromatosis. *Clin Invest Med* 1997; **20**: 110–18.

131. Piperno A, Vergani A, Salvioni A, *et al*. Effects of venesections and restricted diet in patients with the insulin-resistance hepatic iron overload syndrome. *Liver Int* 2004; **24**: 471–6.

132. Nick H, Acklin P, Lattmann R, *et al*. Development of tridentate iron chelators: from desferrithiocin to ICL670. *Curr Med Chem* 2003; **10**: 1065–76.

Chapter 37

Population screening for hemochromatosis

Before the 1980s, hemochromatosis was thought to be an uncommon disorder, but severe iron overload was common in case series of white patients diagnosed to have "classical" hemochromatosis in medical care. A high proportion of 2851 hemochromatosis patients located using patient advocacy groups, physicians, blood centers, newsletters, and the internet reported on a questionnaire that they had symptoms or other problems that were interpreted as complications of iron overload.[1] Thus, it was generally presumed for many years that most whites with hemochromatosis would eventually develop injurious iron overload. Accordingly, large-scale population screening using iron phenotyping of white populations was promoted to achieve early diagnosis and permit timely treatment to alleviate iron overload.

A pioneering screening study of 11 065 presumably healthy Utah blood donors revealed a high prevalence of hemochromatosis homozygotes defined by a persistently high serum transferrin saturation level and post-initial screening evaluations of iron stores.[2] Since the description of the *HFE* gene in 1996, it has been possible to screen for the genotype *HFE* C282Y homozygosity (and serum iron measures) associated with "classical" hemochromatosis. Additional large-scale genetic screening studies have been performed in southern California,[3,4] Norway,[5] North America,[6–8] and Australia.[9,10] Outcomes of large-scale screening programs to detect *HFE* hemochromatosis and iron overload are summarized herein (Table 37.1). The potential value of targeted screening is also described.

Large-scale screening programs
Utah blood donors

In a landmark study of the 1980s, 11 065 presumably healthy volunteer blood donors in Utah were screened using an elevated transferrin saturation criterion.[2]

Study participants who had transferrin saturation levels ≥62% after an overnight fast were offered liver biopsy with quantitative iron measurement. The prevalence of transferrin saturation ≥62% was 0.008 in men and 0.003 in women. Thirty-five participants underwent liver biopsy to assess liver histology and to measure hepatic iron levels by grading and atomic absorption spectrometry. Liver iron detected in these participants ranged from normal to markedly increased, but the proportion of subjects with hepatic fibrosis or cirrhosis was not presented in the primary report.[2] Edwards and colleagues observed that their transferrin saturation criterion identified only half as many female homozygotes as expected.[2]

Rochester, New York primary care patients

In the mid-1990s, 16 031 ambulatory patients recruited through 22 primary care practices in Rochester were screened using an elevated transferrin saturation criterion.[11] Patients with persistently high transferrin saturation levels (≥45% at initial screening and ≥55% after subsequent fasting) were offered liver biopsy testing for measurement of hepatic iron content. Twenty-five subjects had ≥50 μmol Fe/g liver dry weight (normal <25 μmol Fe/g liver dry weight). Three participants had previously occult cirrhosis. Subsequent testing for *HFE* mutations was performed on a subset of 4865 individuals;[12] 12 of them were homozygous for *HFE* C282Y. Eighty-three percent of C282Y homozygotes had transferrin saturation levels ≥55% and 42% had serum ferritin ≥300 μg/L. None had cirrhosis. No African-Americans were diagnosed to have hemochromatosis or iron overload.

Busselton, Australia population

Olynyk and colleagues obtained serum samples for transferrin saturation and ferritin testing and *HFE* mutation analysis in 3011 white adults.[9] Persons with

Table 37.1. Summary of large-scale hemochromatosis and iron overload screening studies[a]

Study (persons screened)	Utah blood donors (11 039)[2]	Rochester, New York primary care patients (16 031)[11]	Busselton, Australia population (3011)[9]	Kaiser Permanante, California health appraisal clinic (41 038)[3,4]	Nord-Trøndelag County, Norway health survey program (65 238)[5]	HEIRS Study, north American primary care clinics (99 711)[6]	Melbourne, Australia Collaborative Cohort Study (31 192)[10]
Year of primary report	1988	1998	1999	2000	2001	2005	2008
Subjects	Whites	Whites, blacks	Whites	Multiracial/ ethnic	Whites	Multiracial/ ethnic	Whites
Screening tests	TS	TS (repeated if elevated), then SF[b]	TS, SF, HFE genotyping	TS, SF, HFE genotyping	TS, then HFE genotyping	TS, SF, HFE genotyping	TS, SF, HFE genotyping
Prevalence of HFE C282Y homozygotes	(0.0045)[b]	(0.0045)[c]	0.0053	0.0037	0.0068	0.0030	0.0068
Homozygotes with elevated serum ferritin	[d]	42%	43.8%	76% (men); 54% (women)	100%[e]	88% (men); 57% (women)	28.4% (men); 1.2% (women)[f]
Percent screen-positive subjects with biopsy-proven cirrhosis or hepatic fibrosis	—	6.4	25.0	0.7	1.5	0.7	5.9[g]

Notes: [a]TS = transferrin saturation; SF = serum ferritin.
[b]These estimates were made before discovery of HFE in 1996, and therefore reflect subjects ascertained to be hemochromatosis homozygotes by iron phenotyping or family analyses.
[c]HFE genotyping was subsequently performed in a subgroup of 4865 study participants.
[d]The highest ferritin value detected in this study was 549 µg/L, but many of the homozygotes detected were young (mean age of 37.5 years for men and 34.7 years for women) and had donated blood multiple times.
[e]100% of 11 men and 1 woman who underwent liver biopsy.
[f]These estimates reflect "documented iron overload-related disease."
[g]Two of these subjects had or developed hepatocellular carcinoma.

persistently high serum transferrin saturation ($\geq$45%) or HFE C282Y homozygosity were evaluated further. Liver biopsy was recommended for those with serum ferritin $\geq$300 µg/L. Study participants were followed for 4 years after initial screening and additional data were collected. In 1999, these investigators reported that 16 study participants (0.5%) were C282Y homozygotes. Fifteen of the 16 had transferrin saturation values $\geq$45%; the other participant had transferrin saturation of 43%. Serum ferritin levels were increased in seven participants.[9] Serum ferritin increased during the 4 years of longitudinal observation in six subjects and decreased in the seventh. Eleven of 16 C282Y homozygotes underwent liver biopsy; three had hepatic fibrosis and one (who had a history of excessive alcohol consumption) had cirrhosis and microvesicular steatosis. Eight of the 16 participants had arthropathy, hepatomegaly, or increased skin pigmentation that was interpreted to be a manifestation of iron overload.[9]

Kaiser Permanante, California health appraisal clinic

Beutler and colleagues performed a large primary care-based screening study at Kaiser Permanente health appraisal clinics in southern California.[3,4] 41 038 individuals of diverse racial and ethnic backgrounds were screened using *HFE* genotyping; serum iron measures were also quantified. The screening detected 152 C282Y homozygotes; most were white. A transferrin saturation of 50% had a sensitivity of only 0.52 and a specificity of 0.908 for detection of *HFE* C282Y homozygosity. This confirmed previous observations in the Utah blood study that transferrin saturation was an imperfect screening test.[2]

In men with C282Y homozygosity, 75% had transferrin saturation >50% and 76% had serum ferritin >250 μg/L. In women with C282Y homozygosity, 40% had transferrin saturation >50% and 54% had serum ferritin values >200 μg/L. Symptoms among homozygotes were compared with those of a group of matched controls. Although many homozygotes reported symptoms such as fatigue and arthropathy sometimes attributed to iron overload, there was no significant difference between cases and controls in any of the parameters tested, except that elevated serum transaminase levels were more prevalent in C282Y homozygotes than in control subjects. Of the 152 C282Y homozygotes, only one had hepatic cirrhosis, although many did not undergo liver biopsy. The authors concluded that penetrance of *HFE* C282Y in the US is low. This study also confirmed that C282Y and C282Y homozygosity are much less prevalent in blacks, Hispanics, and Asians than in whites. Beutler and colleagues demonstrated the necessity of using adequate control groups when assessing the prevalence of relatively non-specific symptoms such as fatigue and arthropathy.[3,4]

Nord-Trøndelag County, Norway health survey program

Åsberg and colleagues invited all residents of Nord-Trøndelag county to participate in a population-based health survey program; hemochromatosis screening was one of several subprojects.[5] Initial screening was performed using transferrin saturation and serum ferritin measurements in 65 238 residents. Those with two transferrin saturation levels >50% and serum ferritin above the upper reference limit were offered a liver biopsy to assess iron stores. Testing for *HFE* mutations became available during the course of the study and was offered to all program participants who had two elevated transferrin saturation levels. The investigators diagnosed hemochromatosis in 92 women (prevalence 0.0034) and 177 men (prevalence 0.0068). Only four participants had cirrhosis on liver biopsy. When corrected for age and gender, the morbidity in persons with screening-detected hemochromatosis was not very different from the morbidity in the control group, indicating that population-based screening in Norway may not be as beneficial as anticipated.[13]

HEIRS Study, North American primary care clinics

In 2000, the National Heart, Lung, and Blood Institute and the National Human Genome Research Institute launched a large multi-center, primary care-based screening study of persons of various races and ethnicities recruited from five field centers in the US and Ontario, Canada.[6–8] This was designated as the HEmochromatosis and IRon Overload Screening (HEIRS) Study. African Americans, Hispanics, and Asians were "oversampled" to permit a greater understanding of the serum iron measures typical of these non-white sub-populations and to estimate their prevalences of common *HFE* mutations. Initial screening included measurement of serum iron, transferrin saturation, and ferritin levels. Of 99 711 individuals screened, 299 were *HFE* C282Y homozygotes. The within-person biological variability of transferrin saturation (and unsaturated iron-binding capacity) limited its usefulness as an initial screening test to detect C282Y homozygosity.[14]

Biochemical abnormalities were detected in the majority of C282Y homozygotes, most of whom reported their race as white or Caucasian. In male C282Y homozygotes, 84% had transferrin saturation ≥50% and 88% had serum ferritin ≥300 μg/L. In female C282Y homozygotes, 73% had serum transferrin saturation values greater than ≥45% and 57% had serum ferritin ≥200 μg/L. Serum ferritin levels were ≥1000 μg/L in 13% of C282Y homozygotes, suggesting that they could have advanced iron overload. Serum ferritin was as likely to decrease as increase in untreated C282Y homozygotes over a relatively brief observation period. This indicates that increments in serum ferritin are not inevitable in untreated C282Y homozygotes.[15]

Performing liver biopsies or providing phlebotomy therapy was not part of the HEIRS Study. Collection of data generated on study participants by their respective physicians indicated that screening for iron overload with ferritin and transferrin saturation detects persons with viral hepatitis and other types of liver disease. A minimum of 0.66% of C282Y homozygotes had biopsy-proven liver fibrosis.[16] Data collection on participants with iron overload phenotypes or C282Y homozygosity treated outside the study is continuing.

The HEIRS Study demonstrated that the prevalence of *HFE* C282Y is low in Hispanics, African Americans, and Native Americans, and that *HFE* C282Y is rare in Asians and Pacific Islanders.[6–8,17] African-Americans, Asians, and Pacific Islanders had significantly lower mean transferrin saturation values and greater mean serum ferritin levels than whites, even when study participants were compared for age and sex.[6–8,17] The HEIRS Study found little evidence of non-*HFE*, non-transfusion iron overload in any race/ethnicity subgroup.[6–8,17,18]

After the discovery of *HFE* in 1996, there was heightened concern about the potentially negative social implications of phenotype or genotype diagnoses of heritable disorders, especially one as common as hemochromatosis. The HEIRS Study included evaluations of such ethical, legal, and social issues. There were only minor negative emotional responses to the genetic testing.[19,20] The risk of insurance or employment problems 1 year after phenotype and genotype screening for hemochromatosis and iron overload was also very low in HEIRS Study participants.[21]

Melbourne, Australia Collaborative Cohort Study

In 2008, Allen and colleagues reported results from a large Australian study that evaluated persons of northern European descent; the participants were followed for an average of 12 years after initial screening.[10] *HFE* mutation analysis was performed in 29 676 individuals; 203 participants were *HFE* C282Y homozygotes. Clinical and biochemical data were obtained on these C282Y homozygotes and on a random sample of control subjects without C282Y homozygosity. Among the C282Y homozygotes, 21 of 74 men (28.4%) and

1 of 84 women (1.2%) satisfied study criteria for iron overload-related disease. The definition of iron overload disease included criteria such as "diagnosis by a physician owing to symptoms associated with hereditary hemochromatosis." Twelve participants had hepatic fibrosis or cirrhosis defined by liver biopsy. Allen and colleagues concluded that the likelihood of advanced iron overload in white Australians was greater than that reported in the screening studies performed in the US.[10]

Population screening vs. targeted screening

Early diagnosis and institution of appropriate treatment of hemochromatosis and iron overload can prevent organ damage and reduce disease-related morbidity and mortality. Evidence is nonetheless substantial that penetrance of disease clearly attributable to iron overload and *HFE* hemochromatosis is low, thus arguing against general population screening. In 2006, the US Preventive Services Task Force concluded that "Research addressing genetic screening for hereditary hemochromatosis remains insufficient to confidently project the impact of, or estimate the benefit from, widespread or high-risk genetic screening for hereditary hemochromatosis."[22,23] At present, there is no rationale for population screening for various types of non-*HFE* hemochromatosis and other iron overload disorders.

There is substantial and rational support for hemochromatosis screening in certain sub-populations of whites, including selected family adult members of probands,[24–26] white men,[2,27,28] persons with undiagnosed liver disease,[29] and persons with serum ferritin >1000 μg/L.[30] Unexplained chronic fatigue, diabetes mellitus, premature osteoarthritis, or porphyria cutanea tarda in persons of any race/ethnicity group should trigger assessment of serum iron levels and *HFE* genotypes by physicians after they have discussed risks and benefits of *HFE* mutation analysis with their patients.

References

1. McDonnell SM, Preston BL, Jewell SA, *et al.* A survey of 2851 patients with hemochromatosis: symptoms and response to treatment. *Am J Med* 1999; **106**: 619–24.

2. Edwards CQ, Griffen LM, Goldgar D, Drummond C, Skolnick MH, Kushner JP. Prevalence of hemochromatosis among 11 065 presumably healthy blood donors. *N Engl J Med* 1988; **318**: 1355–62.

3. Beutler E, Felitti VJ, Koziol JA, Ho NJ, Gelbart T. Penetrance of 845G→A (C282Y) *HFE* hereditary haemochromatosis in the USA. *Lancet* 2002; **359**: 211–18.

4. Beutler E, Felitti V, Gelbart T, Ho N. The effect of *HFE* genotypes on measurements of iron overload in patients attending a health appraisal clinic. *Ann Intern Med* 2000; **133**: 329–37.

5. Asberg A, Hveem K, Thorstensen K, *et al.* Screening for hemochromatosis: high prevalence and low morbidity in an unselected population of 65 238 persons. *Scand J Gastroenterol* 2001; **36**: 1108–15.

6. Adams PC, Reboussin DM, Barton JC, *et al.* Hemochromatosis and iron-overload screening in a racially diverse population. *N Engl J Med* 2005; **352**: 1769–78.

7. Barton JC, Acton RT, Dawkins FW, *et al.* Initial screening transferrin saturation values, serum ferritin concentrations, and *HFE* genotypes in whites and blacks in the Hemochromatosis and Iron Overload Screening Study. *Genet Test* 2005; **9**: 231–41.

8. Barton JC, Acton RT, Lovato L, *et al.* Initial screening transferrin saturation values, serum ferritin concentrations, and *HFE* genotypes in Native Americans and whites in the Hemochromatosis and Iron Overload Screening Study. *Clin Genet* 2006; **69**: 48–57.

9. Olynyk JK, Cullen DJ, Aquilia S, Rossi E, Summerville L, Powell LW. A population-based study of the clinical expression of the hemochromatosis gene. *N Engl J Med* 1999; **341**: 718–24.

10. Allen KJ, Gurrin LC, Constantine CC, *et al.* Iron-overload-related disease in *HFE* hereditary hemochromatosis. *N Engl J Med* 2008; **358**: 221–30.

11. Phatak PD, Sham RL, Raubertas RF, *et al.* Prevalence of hereditary hemochromatosis in 16 031 primary care patients. *Ann Intern Med* 1998; **129**: 954–61.

12. Phatak PD, Ryan DH, Cappuccio J, *et al.* Prevalence and penetrance of *HFE* mutations in 4865 unselected primary care patients. *Blood Cells Mol Dis* 2002; **29**: 41–7.

13. Åsberg A, Hveem K, Kruger O, Bjerve KS. Persons with screening-detected haemochromatosis: as healthy as the general population? *Scand J Gastroenterol* 2002; **37**: 719–24.

14. Adams PC, Reboussin DM, Press RD, *et al.* Biological variability of transferrin saturation and unsaturated iron-binding capacity. *Am J Med* 2007; **120**: 999–1007.

15. Adams PC, Reboussin DM, Barton JC, *et al.* Serial serum ferritin measurements in untreated *HFE* C282Y homozygotes in the Hemochromatosis and Iron Overload Screening Study. *Int J Lab Hematol* 2008; **30**: 300–5.

16. Adams PC, Passmore L, Chakrabarti S, *et al.* Liver diseases in the hemochromatosis and iron overload screening study. *Clin Gastroenterol Hepatol* 2006; **4**: 918–23.

17. Harris EL, McLaren CE, Reboussin DM, *et al.* Serum ferritin and transferrin saturation in Asians and Pacific Islanders. *Arch Intern Med* 2007; **167**: 722–6.

18. Barton JC, Acton RT, Leiendecker-Foster C, *et al.* Characteristics of participants with self-reported hemochromatosis or iron overload at HEIRS Study initial screening. *Am J Hematol* 2008; **83**: 126–32.

19. Hicken BL, Calhoun DA, Barton JC, Tucker DC. Attitudes about and psychosocial outcomes of *HFE* genotyping for hemochromatosis. *Genet Test* 2004; **8**: 90–7.

20. Power TE, Adams PC, Barton JC, *et al.* Psychosocial impact of genetic testing for hemochromatosis in the HEIRS Study: a comparison of participants recruited in Canada and in the United States. *Genet Test* 2007; **11**: 55–64.

21. Hall MA, Barton JC, Adams PC, *et al.* Genetic screening for iron overload: No evidence of discrimination at 1 year. *J Fam Pract* 2007; **56**: 829–34.

22. Whitlock EP, Garlitz BA, Harris EL, Beil TL, Smith PR. Screening for hereditary hemochromatosis: a systematic review for the US Preventive Services Task Force. *Ann Intern Med* 2006; **145**: 209–23.

23. US Preventive Services Task Force. Screening for hemochromatosis: recommendation statement. *Ann Intern Med* 2006; **145**: 204–8.

24. Edwards CQ, Carroll M, Bray P, Cartwright GE. Hereditary hemochromatosis. Diagnosis in siblings and children. *N Engl J Med* 1977; **297**: 7–13.

25. Barton JC, Rothenberg BE, Bertoli LF, Acton RT. Diagnosis of hemochromatosis in family members of probands: a comparison of phenotyping and *HFE* genotyping. *Genet Med* 1999; **1**: 89–93.

26. Acton RT, Barton JC, Passmore LV, *et al.* Accuracy of family history of hemochromatosis or iron overload: The Hemochromatosis and Iron Overload Screening Study. *Clin Gastroenterol Hepatol* 2008; **6**: 934–8.

27. Barton JC, Acton RT. Population screening for hemochromatosis: has the time finally come? *Curr Gastroenterol Rep* 2000; **2**: 18–26.

28. Asberg A, Tretli S, Hveem K, Bjerve KS. Benefit of population-based screening for phenotypic hemochromatosis in young men. *Scand J Gastroenterol* 2002; **37**: 1212–19.

29. Bacon BR, Olynyk JK, Brunt EM, Britton RS, Wolff RK. *HFE* genotype in patients with hemochromatosis and other liver diseases. *Ann Intern Med* 1999; **130**: 953–62.

30. Waalen J, Felitti VJ, Gelbart T, Beutler E. Screening for hemochromatosis by measuring ferritin levels: a more effective approach. *Blood* 2008; **111**: 3373–6.

Chapter 38

Ethical, legal, and social implications

Prevention or amelioration of disease is possible if risk or susceptibility factors can be identified and effective interventions are available. For example, phenotype testing of neonates for rare disorders such as phenylketonuria, other heritable amino acid metabolism defects, galactosemia, and congenital hypothyroidism is universal or mandatory because timely diagnosis and management avert disease manifestations. In diverse, typically adult-onset disorders, it is feasible to detect pathogenic germline or acquired mutations in individuals, family members, or population cohorts. Some clinicians rely on DNA analyses to assess the risk of single-mutation disorders such as familial breast and colon cancer, hemochromatosis, and Huntington disease. Among these examples, the risk of symptoms is great in Huntington disease, but the potential to prevent symptoms and consequent death is low. In *HFE* hemochromatosis, the capability to prevent disease due to iron overload is great, but the risk that subjects with a "positive" genetic test will develop severe iron overload is relatively low. Many physicians and non-medical members of the public have difficulty understanding the indications for, and interpreting results and consequences of, genetic information for risk assessment or diagnosis.

Across certain disorders, some studies and many anecdotes suggest that the potential for misuse and misunderstanding is greater for DNA-based tests than for phenotype tests, even one like hemoglobin electrophoresis that has diagnostic and predictive value equivalent to that of corresponding DNA-based testing. In the 1990s, controversy about the privacy, confidentiality, and fairness of use of genetic information increased. There were concerns that DNA-based testing would lead to employment and insurance discrimination, decreased utilization of indicated medical care, stigmatization, and emotional harm. These bioethics concerns surrounding genetic testing became known collectively in the US as ethical, legal, and social implications ("ELSI"). For hemochromatosis, additional specific quandaries developed regarding population screening, genetic counseling, use of hemochromatosis blood for transfusion, and government-mandated iron fortification of foods. This chapter reviews the current status of these "ELSI" issues (Table 38.1).

Employment and insurance discrimination

The stigma associated with being "labeled" as having a genetic disorder is a real or perceived concern that has discouraged some persons from participating in screening for genetic disorders. Insurance companies and employers may use this type of information to deny coverage for health insurance or to increase premiums.[1] Hemochromatosis is no exception to this general concern, although the real risk versus benefit can be argued in this case. This section discusses the real and perceived risks of employment and insurance discrimination associated with a diagnosis of hemochromatosis or with finding a genetic profile that may be associated with increased risk of hemochromatosis.

Basis of concern

A person with severe iron overload and associated organ dysfunction may incur testing and treatments that are very expensive. On the other hand, therapeutic phlebotomy can reduce iron stores and reduce or eliminate the risk of organ damage due to iron overload if iron overload is diagnosed before it becomes severe. The diagnostic costs associated with the diagnosis of iron overload in this latter circumstance include those of measuring serum transferrin saturation and ferritin levels, genetic testing, and liver biopsy. The costs of phlebotomy treatments vary depending on the degree of iron overload and the need for maintenance phlebotomy. In such cases, life

Table 38.1. Ethical, legal, and social issues pertinent to hemochromatosis

Employment and insurance discrimination

Acceptability of genetic testing

Population screening

Genetic counseling

Use of hemochromatosis blood for transfusion

Government-mandated food fortification with iron

expectancy is not decreased and thus it is logical that life insurance premiums should not be increased. Nonetheless, insurers make their own determinations in this regard, and some persons with hemochromatosis have reported that they were denied life insurance coverage for this reason. Because normalization of life expectancy depends on compliance with therapy, insurers, and others argue that there remains some risk of non-compliance and consequent risk of organ dysfunction.

Once organ dysfunction due to iron overload becomes irreversible, there is an on-going cost to treat complications. Diabetes mellitus, hepatic cirrhosis, and cardiac failure are associated with major treatment costs. Thus, higher health insurance premiums may be justifiable in patients with these complications. In addition, these conditions may reduce life expectancy. Higher life insurance premiums may be justifiable in such cases.

The most contentious circumstance from the standpoint of potential discrimination occurs when genetic testing detects a genotype that is associated with hemochromatosis. This scenario is common when family members of an affected patient are screened by genetic testing. The clinical penetrance associated with the common *HFE* mutations is described in Chapters 8 and 37. The occurrence of a genotype associated with no phenotypic manifestations should not cause significant morbidity or mortality. Nonetheless, such information is sometimes used by both health and life insurance carriers to exclude individuals from coverage or to increase their insurance premiums based on the theoretical increased risk of disease-related complications. Although it can be argued that this type of "labeling" and discrimination is unjustified, only appropriate follow-up and institution of treatment, if needed, can assure that no organ dysfunction will occur as a

consequence of iron overload. Because compliance with follow-up is not perfect in all cases, insurance carriers may argue that there is an actuarial risk of lack of compliance that could lead to subsequent iron-related organ dysfunction.

Impact on screening and early diagnosis

Concerns about genetic "labeling" and discrimination have led some physicians and scientists to be reluctant to recommend or implement screening programs for hemochromatosis. By their nature, insurance carriers are corporations that need to limit risk and maximize profits. Their tendency to deny insurance or increase premiums based on genetic information is in some ways predictable.

From a societal standpoint, the early diagnosis of hemochromatosis and implementation of appropriate therapy is an effective preventive health measure. Early diagnosis may result in a meaningful prolongation of productive life. If blood removed by therapeutic phlebotomy to achieve iron depletion could be used for transfusion, some argue that the benefit to society is further increased.

As a society, we tend to make decisions that favor common benefit and not individual corporate interests. Thus, legislation to protect individuals against "labeling" and genetic discrimination has been advocated by many.[2] The need for such legislation is predicated on the perceived discrimination associated with early diagnosis. Some have argued that studies that have examined this issue do not show any substantial unjustifiable discrimination by employers or insurance companies. Others report anecdotes in which persons who were denied insurance or assigned to high-premium groups were subsequently sold insurance or given premium reductions.

Impact on acceptability of genetic testing

Cases of genetic discrimination by employers and insurance companies are often publicized by the media, sometimes leading to a public perception of harm. In the context of genetic discrimination, the deterrent effect on clinically justifiable genetic screening may be due as much to public perception of genetic discrimination as it is to the actual discrimination that occurs by employers and insurance carriers. In adults, potential for genetic discrimination can be discussed when testing is contemplated. In the

US, some states require written informed consent before any type of genetic testing can be performed.

Issues related to consent are more complicated when the individual being tested is a minor. Legally, consent can be obtained from a parent or guardian, but the potential for harm later in life, particularly during early employment years, is more substantial than it is in adults undergoing testing. In the case of *HFE* hemochromatosis, the risk of significant iron overload early in life is low.[3] Accordingly, some clinicians have therefore argued in favor of serum iron tests early in life to exclude iron overload, and to withhold genetic testing until the persons undergoing testing have reached an age of majority.

Acceptability of genetic testing

The potential for "genetic labeling" and discrimination has led to public debate regarding the advisability of genetic testing.[2] On one hand, the detection of a genetic profile that may be associated with increased disease risk may be useful information if the expected disease entity can be prevented or ameliorated by appropriate measures. On the other hand, the prediction of a high-risk genetic profile may be lead to psychological distress surrounding the potential for disease and to discrimination by employers and insurance carriers. The latter is discussed in detail elsewhere in this chapter. The present discussion centers on acceptability of genetic testing from the standpoint of the individual being tested.

Basis of concern

The decoding of the human genome has led to unprecedented advances in the ability to discover the genetic basis of disease. Genetic tests for many disorders are now widely available. In many cases, the genetic information predicts the probability of disease occurrence, but little can be done to prevent the occurrence of the disease or change its natural history.[2] An example is Huntington's disease. In this case, identification of the genetic mutation leads to a high degree of certainty that disease manifestations will develop in the predictable future. Regardless, no therapy is currently available to prevent this disorder. Individuals with positive genetic tests have the psychological impact of disease inevitability and the potential for discrimination by employers and insurance carriers.[1] This may mitigate any potential benefit from knowing their genetic risk. Examples of this type have led

to media assertion and public perception that genetic testing is in some way different and always carries this type of negative potential. Many states therefore have requirements for signed informed consent before DNA-based testing can be performed. Whether the same concern applies to situations wherein knowledge of genetic predisposition may allow appropriate preventive measures to be instituted is unclear.

Perception versus reality

DNA-based testing requires special consent forms and carries the concerns associated with "genetic testing." In reality, the diagnosis of an inherited disorder is sometimes made by the clinician using tests that are not DNA based. For example, the diagnosis of hemochromatosis was often made in the past using serum iron studies before *HFE* mutation analysis became widely available. Because testing for mutations in other genes may not be commercially available, diagnosis of non-*HFE* hemochromatosis is currently often made based on phenotypic testing. Phenotypic tests may diagnose iron overload disorders before the onset of organ dysfunction. Further, every individual with elevated serum iron measures will not develop significant iron overload. Thus a "label" of hemochromatosis may be placed on a patient in the absence of DNA-based testing. Public perception regarding the harm of genetic testing does not seem to extend to this relatively common circumstance.

The approach to DNA testing should differ based on the nature of the disease being diagnosed. In testing for mutations that increase susceptibility to familial breast and other cancers using *BRCA1* and *BRCA2* mutation analyses, it has been argued that knowledge of such pathogenic mutations would lead to vigilant screening, early diagnosis, and possible prolongation of life. This should clearly counterbalance any harm related to "labeling" and discrimination,[4] although long-term advantages and risks of *BRCA1* and *BRCA2* testing are not clearly delineated.

Identification of a hemochromatosis-associated genotype can allow close monitoring of iron stores and institution of therapy to reduce body iron before organ dysfunction occurs. Genetic testing in the course of evaluation for suspected hemochromatosis can be a useful adjunct to confirm the diagnosis, often abrogating the need for invasive testing such as liver biopsy (Chapter 4).

Genetic testing for common *HFE* mutations among asymptomatic individuals results in the identification of persons who have "at-risk" genotypes but who do not have deleterious iron overload. The risk that such individuals will develop harmful iron overload may be relatively low, thus raising the concern of "labeling" these individuals with a diagnosis of hemochromatosis. This may risk psychological harm and employer and insurance discrimination. The question of true psychological harm was addressed in the HEIRS Study. There was no significant overall physical or mental effect measured by the SF-36 score, although it was reported that there was at least one negative emotional impact in individuals undergoing genetic testing.[5] Thus, the true psychological impact of such testing may be much lower than is perceived by many.

Effect of testing venue

The acceptability of genetic testing is likely to vary depending on the venue and context in which the test is performed. Few would argue against the value of performing a test for *HFE* mutations in the context of evaluating a patient with suspected hemochromatosis based on symptoms and abnormal iron studies. It is acceptable for a physician to offer genetic testing to first-degree adult family members of hemochromatosis probands after an adequate explanation of potential benefits, risks, and outcomes. Survey data suggest that patients are more likely to trust their physician with their personal genetic information than their employer or health insurance carrier. Testing outside physician offices or general population screening may be more problematic, particularly if screening is not accompanied by an informed and adequate discussion of benefits and risks.

Testing minors

It is generally recommended that minors not be tested for adult-onset heritable disorders. In *HFE* hemochromatosis, disease manifestations rarely occur before the age of 30 years in subjects identified in medical care or in population screening,[3,6] and the rate of penetrance of severe iron overload is low in adults of middle age. Testing minors for iron-related mutations is not justified unless phenotyping reveals substantive abnormalities that need further understanding or management. Even so, testing minors with genotyping requires special consideration because consent is given by a parent or guardian who may inadequately consider potential risks of psychological distress and genetic discrimination. In most cases, testing can be postponed until the individual is an adult and can make his/her informed decision.

Testing of cord blood or neonates

Anonymous screening of banked or prospectively obtained cord blood samples has provided some information regarding *HFE* mutation frequency in different geographic regions.[7–10] In routine care delivery, however, the concerns of testing of cord blood samples or neonates to detect subjects at risk for hemochromatosis and iron overload phenotypes are similar to those described above for testing minors.

A non-iron condition related to childhood-onset disease associated with *HFE* mutations is higher blood levels and increased risk of lead toxicity in infants and children exposed to environmental lead. Lead and iron are absorbed by at least one common pathway in humans and animals,[11,12] namely that involving divalent metal transporter-1 (Chapters 2, 8). Adults with hemochromatosis heterozygosity had significantly higher blood lead concentrations than control subjects.[12] Blood lead levels were significantly higher in Mexican children who had common *HFE* mutations than in those who did not.[13] Because lead intoxication in children is a major public health problem for children,[14,15] it is possible that *HFE* mutation analysis to identify children with increased risk for plumbism may become advisable.

Population screening

Principles for defining diseases that are good candidates for general population screening have been formulated by epidemiologists and public health officials.[16] The disease must have a significant impact on the quality or length of life, and be sufficiently prevalent to justify the cost of screening. The disease should have an asymptomatic phase during which detection and treatment lead to reductions in morbidity and mortality. Treatment in the asymptomatic phase must yield better outcomes than treatment delayed until the onset of symptoms. Treatment and testing strategies must be acceptable and available to the population. The tests used for screening must be sensitive enough to detect asymptomatic disease and specific enough to avoid initiating evaluations of patients without actual disease. These criteria are met by some genetic disorders, such as phenylketonuria and sickle cell anemia, both of which are less common than *HFE* hemochromatosis. Routine screening for these disorders among populations at risk is commonplace.

Hemochromatosis was initially believed to be a candidate disorder for routine screening. It is prevalent, and the early detection of disease improves outcomes by preventing irreversible end-organ damage and thereby prolongs life expectancy. Transferrin saturation and serum ferritin testing and phlebotomy treatments are easily tolerated and widely available. The need for hepatic biopsy is a major source of concern, but is generally well tolerated and safe, and indicated for a minority of patients. In many cases, the presence of typical *HFE* hemochromatosis-associated genotypes may confirm the diagnosis without the need for invasive testing. The morbidity and mortality caused by hemochromatosis with severe iron overload impose a high degree of disability on affected individuals. Several recent studies have demonstrated a relatively low disease penetrance defined as iron-related organ dysfunction (especially that of the liver), although the degree of penetrance varies moderately across populations (Chapter 8). Altogether, this reality has reduced the enthusiasm for general population screening in many regions.

Clinical practice guidelines of the American College of Physicians[17] and the US Preventive Services Task Force[18] indicated that there is inadequate evidence to support routine genetic screening for hemochromatosis or iron overload in the asymptomatic members of the general population. Although both guidelines recognize the value of early diagnosis before the onset of organ dysfunction, only aggressive testing will identify such cases before irreparable tissue injury due to severe iron overload has occurred.

Historical perspective

In the late 1990s, hemochromatosis appeared to be a strong candidate for routine population screening, based on commonly accepted criteria that have been used to justify population screening for other conditions. The phenotype tests currently used for screening (serum transferrin saturation level or unsaturated iron-binding capacity) are sensitive, and the addition of genetic testing with *HFE* mutation analysis reduces the need for invasive procedures. Although large-scale screening studies had not been

done to directly assess disease penetrance, substantial morbidity and mortality could be attributed to hemochromatosis. Because the potential risks of screening are low, it appeared reasonable to design a screening strategy for hemochromatosis.

The results of a large population-based genetic screening study performed in San Diego, California showed that the prevalence of *HFE* C282Y homozygosity was relatively great, and that disease penetrance, especially for serious organ damage such as hepatic cirrhosis, was low.[19] The study investigators did not perform clinical examinations or liver biopsies on newly found C282Y homozygotes, and some homozygotes with previously diagnosed hemochromatosis were excluded. Thus, the true penetrance of iron overload disease may have been underestimated. Nevertheless, these results and a concern regarding the potential for genetic discrimination and psychological harm that could result from identification of a genetic abnormality steered many experts away from recommending a population-based genetic screening strategy.[17,18,20]

Studies from other countries have demonstrated a more substantial risk of organ damage that can be attributed to hemochromatosis than that reported from the San Diego study. A Dutch group reported that first-degree family members of C282Y homozygous probands had a 45.7% risk of hemochromatosis-related disorders (compared with 19.4% of controls).[21] A large, multi-center study in north America reported that 13% of C282Y homozygotes had serum ferritin levels >1000 µg/L.[22] A group from Melbourne, Australia recently reported their experience using a large population sample in which participants were followed for an average of 12 years. The proportion of C282Y homozygotes with documented iron-overload disease was 28.4% for men and 1.2% for women.[23]

Psychosocial effects and genetic discrimination

If the disease penetrance of hemochromatosis is low, the vast majority of *HFE* C282Y homozygotes identified by genetic screening would remain relatively unaffected by iron overload for a lifetime. The identification of a "genetic disorder" may lead to undue anxiety and could be associated with societal discrimination.

Despite these theoretical fears, screening studies such as the HEIRS Study that have examined the

"ELSI" issues have been unable to demonstrate any significant psychological harm based on quality-of-life scores.[5,24] This suggests that fears of psychological harm and genetic discrimination may have been over-estimated and based largely on anecdotal "evidence." The advantage of early detection of iron overload is obvious and may be substantial, even if the risk of significant organ dysfunction such as hepatic cirrhosis is low. A phenotypic screening approach has the additional advantages of being less likely to detect individuals without significant disease expression than genotype testing, and detecting all types of iron overload and iron deficiency.

Genotypic vs. phenotypic screening

Genotypic screening should probably involve screening for *HFE* C282Y homozygosity. Some also recommend detecting the *HFE* H63D and S65C mutations among C282Y heterozygotes, because some compound heterozygotes develop iron overload. Genetic testing is highly specific. In countries where C282Y homozygosity accounts for the great majority of cases, such as those of ultramontane northern Europe, Australia, and the US, the sensitivity of *HFE* mutation analysis is also high.[25,26] The variable findings of disease penetrance across geographic regions suggest that penetrance in some countries such as Australia may be higher due to environmental and dietary factors. Moreover, non-*HFE*-related hemochromatosis accounts for a substantial proportion of hemochromatosis cases in some regions such as Italy. Rare mutations, such as those of the transferrin receptor 2 gene *TFR2*, have been found in some hemochromatosis cases in Italy. Sole reliance on genotypic screening for *HFE* mutations would miss such cases. Genotypic screening can identify persons with deleterious genotypes whose body iron levels are not severely elevated. Because the natural history of iron accumulation in hemochromatosis is poorly understood and thus unpredictable, the value of detecting such individuals with genotyping is uncertain. Genetic testing associated with genotyping may be needed but is not widely available, and increases costs of screening. In an office setting, however, genetic screening of first-degree family members of known hemochromatosis patients should be considered to be the standard of care.

Phenotypic screening usually involves measuring serum transferrin saturation or unsaturated iron-binding capacity. Some "non-expressing" C282Y homozygotes will be missed by such a strategy, but the likelihood that adults who have or will develop severe iron overload will be missed is low. Phenotypic screening will detect some persons with non-*HFE* hemochromatosis or iron overload. The cost of phenotype screening is low, and "genetic labeling" and discrimination are lesser issues than with genotyping. Nonetheless, the specificity of phenotyping is low. Therefore, some screening program participants must undergo further testing to evaluate initial positive screening results.

The value of screening is likely to be greatest among young adult men of northern European ancestry. The presence of a family history of hemochromatosis should lead to a high index of suspicion. Individuals with clinical features that suggest early iron overload such as elevated serum levels of hepatic aminotransferases, premature osteoarthritis, or porphyria cutanea tarda should be evaluated for hemochromatosis. In the absence of data that specifically identifies a population subgroup that clearly benefits from screening, the decision to screen should be made in the course of routine evaluation by primary care physicians who take these factors into account and discuss them, as appropriate, with individual patients.

Genetic counseling

Hemochromatosis and related disorders comprise a group of heritable disorders for which diagnostic criteria, patterns of inheritance, and most causative genes and pathogenic mutations are well understood. The risk that first-degree family members of hemochromatosis index patients also have hemochromatosis is greater than the risk of hemochromatosis in members of the general population, regardless of the type of hemochromatosis. Family members of index cases with *HFE* hemochromatosis often have hemochromatosis and morbid complications similar to those observed in index cases.[27,28] Family studies of rarer types of hemochromatosis demonstrate the same principles. It is appropriate to be directive when counseling a person at risk for hemochromatosis, because early detection of hemochromatosis in family members and treatment by phlebotomy is effective in preventing complications of iron overload and premature death.[29] Many patients with hemochromatosis rely on their physicians for genetic counseling, described as "the process by which patients or relatives at risk of a disorder that may be hereditary are advised of the consequences of the disorder, the probability of developing or transmitting it and of the ways in which this may be prevented, avoided or ameliorated".[29]

Identifying persons at risk

Collecting detailed family history of disease information is necessary to identify persons at risk and to assess family members in whom the diagnosis of hemochromatosis is not clear, e.g. persons with elevated serum ferritin levels that may be due to common liver disorders or other conditions.[30] In a study of Canadian patients, a family history of hemochromatosis was present in 3.6% of hemochromatosis patients and none of the control patients. The combination of cirrhosis, diabetes mellitus, and arthritis predicted the diagnosis of hemochromatosis in only 48% of cases.[31] In 150 family members of 61 Alabama probands with *HFE* C282Y homozygosity, 25 family members were C282Y homozygotes; 23 of these (92%) had an abnormal iron phenotype.[32] In addition, iron phenotyping using routine serum iron measures and *HFE* genotyping are complementary in diagnosing hemochromatosis among family members of probands.[32] As more genetic tests become available to identify persons at risk for hemochromatosis and iron overload disorders, it is increasingly necessary to obtain complete family history of disease information to identify those who would benefit from genetic testing.

Collecting family history of disease

The quality and completeness of a family history is increased if the information is obtained either by interview or with self-administered forms in which disorders that occurred in each relative over four generations are checked by the patient at home.[29] The latter method requires less time of the health care provider, and the amount and quality of the information obtained is greater than that acquired by interview. An accurate diagnosis is needed for all subjects reported to have a disorder. If possible, the physician should review of medical records or autopsy reports of, or interview and examine, family members reported to have hemochromatosis or iron overload.[29] Family members reported to have cirrhosis, arthritis, diabetes mellitus, primary liver cancer, or cardiomyopathy are especially important. Other associated disorders include alcoholism, porphyria cutanea tarda, and sideroblastic anemia.

The age and gender of all persons in the pedigree should be recorded. The prevalence of many complications of iron overload in *HFE* hemochromatosis increases with age. Therefore, it is important to record the date of birth for all family members.[29] The penetrance and expressivity of *HFE* hemochromatosis is greater in men than women, although iron overload and its complications are fully expressed in some women.[33] In contrast, males and females in the same kinship with early age-of-onset hemochromatosis such as that associated with *HJV* mutations are affected in approximately the same proportions, and the severity of iron overload in family members of similar age is typically similar.

Obtaining information about the racial and ethnic origin of the patient and family is helpful. *HFE* hemochromatosis is most prevalent in Caucasians of northern or western European descent, and a corresponding family history of ancestry is helpful in white patients who reside outside Europe, especially in derivative countries such as the US, Canada, Australia, or New Zealand.[34] The frequency of the *HFE* C282Y mutation among various racial and ethnic groups is consistent with the prevalence of *HFE* hemochromatosis in these groups.[22] The C282Y mutation occurs with decreasing frequency in Hispanics, Ashkenazi Jews, African-Americans, Native Americans, and Asians and Pacific Islanders, respectively.[22,35] Hemochromatosis associated with pathogenic mutations in *HJV*, *TFR2*, or *SLC40A1* has also been described predominantly but not exclusively in persons who reside in Europe or derivative countries. Primary iron overload in sub-Saharan African natives sometimes occurs in two or more members of the same family, although no causative genetic abnormality of African iron overload has been identified. In African-American patients with primary iron overload, mutations in *HFE*, *HJV*, *TFR2*, *ALAS2*, or *SLC40A1* or types of thalassemia or hemoglobinopathy have been identified in some kinships.

It is important to determine the genetic relationships of the married couples in a family. Consanguinity increases the risk that certain heritable disorders will occur, especially those transmitted as autosomal recessive traits. For example, the carrier frequency of *HFE* C282Y is ~0.1 in European white populations. Accordingly, a known carrier has a one in ten chance of marrying another carrier from the general population. If the spouse is a first cousin, the chance increased to one in eight, thus increasing the risk that their offspring will be a C282Y homozygote.[29] Many patients reported to have forms of autosomal recessive hemochromatosis associated with mutations in *HJV* or *TFR2* arise in consanguineous marriages, and the causative mutations in such kinships are often "private" and not detected in the general population.

Counseling patients and relatives

The pedigree should be constructed using standardized nomenclature, and drawn by hand or by using one of several computer programs.[29] The pedigree should be edited by the family member who provided the information, and a corrected copy should be included in the medical record. The physician or counselor should formulate a risk assessment and schedule a session for genetic counseling.[29] The American College of Medical Genetics Laboratory Practice Committee recommends that a molecular genetics laboratory report include a copy of a pedigree if a family study were conducted using DNA-based testing.[29] For newly diagnosed patients, the physician or counselor should explain the nature of the iron overload disorder, associated complications, the mode of inheritance, and the rationale of reducing body iron stores to prevent further organ injury. Discussion of expectations of treatment to achieve iron depletion must reflect the presence or absence of iron overload complications and their typical response to therapy. Using a checklist of the items to be discussed in an education and genetic counseling session assures that nothing will be omitted, and promotes uniformity of the process. The checklist should be signed and placed in the medical record.[29]

Family members at risk are identified based on the type of hemochromatosis in the index patient and in the pedigree. In autosomal recessive forms of hemochromatosis, each sibling of a proband has a 25% chance of being homozygous for the hemochromatosis gene(s) in the proband. Accordingly, siblings of newly diagnosed patients, regardless of age, should tested with serum iron measures and DNA-based testing. In *HFE* hemochromatosis in whites, it is not unusual to detect different *HFE*-associated genotypes (and phenotypes) in siblings (or parents) due to the high prevalence of *HFE* C282Y and H63D in western white populations.[36] Some family members also need counseling before (and after) testing, although most understand the rationale of a family-based risk assessment.

The probability of inheriting *HFE* mutations and developing iron overload can be estimated in family members of a proband with a *HFE* hemochromatosis genotype[37] or in other autosomal recessive forms of hemochromatosis. Each child of a parent with hemochromatosis is an obligate heterozygote, and may inherit a second hemochromatosis-associated allele from the second parent. Because approximately one in ten white Americans are *HFE* C282Y heterozygotes, the probability that a child will inherit a second hemochromatosis-associated mutation from a parent without hemochromatosis is approximately 1 in 20. This risk to develop hemochromatosis is much greater than in members of the general population (approximately 1 in 200). The risk for iron overload due to *HFE* hemochromatosis is highest in men and their C282Y homozygous brothers, and significantly lower in homozygous women. Some persons with C282Y homozygosity, especially women, never develop iron overload. Although uncommon, severe iron overload occurs in some C282Y/H63D compound heterozygotes and in some H63D homozygotes, many of whom have hepatic steatosis, alcoholism, or viral hepatitis.

In *HFE* C282Y homozygotes, significant iron overload rarely occurs before the age of 30 years.[3] Accordingly, it is recommended that children of probands not be tested for *HFE* genotypes until after the age of consent.[38,39] In kinships with juvenile or early age-of-onset hemochromatosis (usually due to *HJV* or *TFR2* mutations), all siblings of a proband should be tested as soon as possible due to the rapidly progressive nature of iron overload and its complications. Parents or siblings who are heterozygous for a *HJV* or *TFR2* mutation usually have no evidence of iron overload. In autosomal dominant hemochromatosis typical of that due to ferroportin gene (*SLC40A1*) mutations, each sibling of a proband has a 50% chance of having hemochromatosis. *SLC40A1* "gain-of-function" mutations sometimes result in a juvenile or early age-of-onset clinical picture like that typically due to *HJV* or *TFR2* mutations.

Insurance and discrimination

Insurance denial and increased premium rates are reported commonly among individuals with *HFE* hemochromatosis without end-organ damage, although all of these occurrences were not related to hemochromatosis.[40] During counseling, the patient should be informed that discrimination with respect to obtaining health, life, and disability income insurance, and employment is possible.[29] Nonetheless, the overall proportion of those with active insurance, their quality of life, and their psychological well-being were similar to those of siblings without hemochromatosis.[40]

Health care costs for persons with hemochromatosis are increased, even those diagnosed before the development of iron overload. Accordingly, costs of health care insurance are sometimes increased in the US, especially when insurance is obtained through individual or small group policies. This is not discrimination, but a reality of medical and insurance economics. Persons with severe complications of iron overload, especially those with hepatic cirrhosis, primary hepatic cancer, diabetes mellitus, or disabling arthropathy, may be unable to obtain health care, disability, or life income insurance, or only at markedly increased rates. Likewise, this is not discrimination, because such patients have increased risks for health care expenditures, disability, or death, and problems obtaining similar insurance coverage is encountered by persons with similar disorder(s) caused by factors other than iron overload.

Life and disability insurance can usually be purchased at competitive rates by persons who have completed iron depletion therapy, whose health is otherwise good, and who do not have hepatic cirrhosis or diabetes mellitus, the two complications of hemochromatosis associated with a statistically decreased length of survival.[41] Patients who appear to have no complication of iron overload, who have achieved iron depletion, and who are compliant with therapy should present an explanatory letter from a physician knowledgeable about their case to insurance underwriters at the time an application for insurance is made. This usually avoids misunderstandings regarding suitability for life or disability income insurance, and often avoids deferrals for insurability that may remain part of the patient's permanent computerized insurance record available to all insurance companies. In the US, the risk of insurance or employment problems 1 year after detection of HFE hemochromatosis and iron overload by phenotype and genotype screening is very low.[24]

Concern about genetic discrimination varies substantially by race/ethnicity, nationality, and other demographic factors.[1] Americans 65 years of age or older and adult Canadians report relatively little concern about genetic discrimination associated with HFE genotyping, probably because they are covered by nationalized health care insurance. Some states in the US have statutes to limit discrimination against obtaining health insurance and employment based on genetic risk of disease,[29] and similar statutes are expected to increase in number and specificity. Regardless, US citizens in states with some legal protections against genetic discrimination had more, not less, concern than either Canadians or US residents in states with no legal protections.[1] In the US, the Genetic Information Nondiscrimination Act ("GINA") of 2008 expanded protections for Americans from being treated unfairly by insurers or employers due to differences in their DNA.

Some patients need help in coping with the psychological burdens associated with learning that they have a heritable disorder, although the proportion of patients with HFE hemochromatosis who report such burdens is small. Often, patients and their family members remember little that was discussed in the initial counseling session. Questions that arise later can usually be discussed and resolved by telephone. A genetic counselor should be available to provide support, re-enforce the physician's recommendations, and, if necessary, refer the patient to an appropriate support service.[29]

Genetic counseling and education are strongly recommended as integral components of screening and genetic testing programs.[38,42] Unresolved issues surrounding population screening for hemochromatosis should not diminish efforts to identify individuals with a positive family history of hemochromatosis who could benefit from genetic counseling and indicated medical testing.

Use of hemochromatosis blood for transfusion

A unit of blood that is donated by a healthy person can be transfused into another person without fractionation. This is referred to as whole blood, which includes red blood cells, white blood cells, platelets, and plasma. Before transfusion, almost all whole blood is separated into different components including packed red blood cells, platelets concentrates, and plasma. These components can be transfused into different people according to therapeutic needs. All donors of blood intended for transfusion undergo careful identification and evaluation. Likewise, all blood units collected for the purpose of transfusion into another person undergo careful identification, labeling, and much evaluation and testing. Blood that is withdrawn in a setting other than a blood bank cannot be handled properly or subjected to the extensive testing that is required to determine safety for transfusion.

Basic principles of blood transfusion

Some of the important principles of collection of blood for the purpose of transfusion into others include the accuracy of the health information provided by the donors, the motivation of the donors, and the safety of the donated blood. Published data indicate that a higher percentage of units of blood that was collected from individuals who were paid to donate tested positive for infectious agents than blood that was collected from donors who did not receive compensation.[43] It is possible that some blood donors could have a reimbursement motive instead of a purely altruistic motivation, including considerations of blood safety.

Another important principle of blood transfusion is that no individual has the right to insist that his/her blood must be used for transfusion. Some hemochromatosis patients insist that their blood cannot possibly test positive for a transmissible infection, that their blood is as good as anyone else's blood, and that their blood must be used for transfusion, rather than be discarded. An obvious example of blood that cannot be used for transfusion is blood that tests positive for viral hepatitis B, viral hepatitis C, or infection by the human immunodeficiency virus. Units of blood that test positive for transmissible infections must be discarded and cannot be used for transfusion. The presence of drugs and some antibodies to erythrocyte antigens could also make the blood of some donors unusable for transfusion into others.

Charges for blood donation

Blood banks do not charge for withdrawing blood from individuals whose only motivation for donating is purely altruistic. A reasonable explanation for this is that very few healthy people would be willing to pay to donate their blood for transfusion into others. Hemochromatosis patients in several areas of the US have told the authors of this book the amounts they were charged by their local hospital or blood bank for therapeutic phlebotomy. These amounts varied

widely, from no charge up to $250 per unit of blood. Some patients were annoyed that their blood was discarded and never tested for safety. The published results of a survey of hemochromatosis patients indicated that the amount charged for therapeutic phlebotomy in different settings averaged about $90 in hospitals, $69 in a physician's office, $52 in a blood center, and $48 when performed in a home. The overall average of reported charges for therapeutic phlebotomy was $74.[44] In the same survey of hemochromatosis patients in the US, 76% of individuals indicated that their insurance paid for all or a part of the charges for phlebotomy therapy.

Altruistic vs. other motivation to donate blood

Individuals with hemochromatosis and iron overload have a medical reason to have blood withdrawn: to deplete their iron stores. If the local blood bank charges for phlebotomy therapy, hemochromatosis patients could have both a medical reason and a financial incentive not to disclose that they have a history of behavior that increased their risk to acquire a transmissible infection, or a medical reason that requires blood removal. Patients with hemochromatosis and iron overload and commercial blood donors do not satisfy the principle of altruism because they expect to achieve a health or a financial benefit from blood donation. If an individual donates blood because his/her employer provides paid time off work, or the donor wants to find out if he/she has acquired infection from hepatitis viruses or human immunodeficiency virus infection, these are self-serving motivations and do not qualify as purely altruistic reasons for donating blood.[45] A differing point of view was published by an ethicist at the Centre for Environmental Philosophy and Bioethics of the University of Ghent, Belgium. The author concluded that hemochromatosis patients can be free, voluntary, altruistic blood donors if they do not request any benefit other than blood removal.[46]

Transfusion of blood from healthy hemochromatosis patients
Experience in Canada

Blood from hemochromatosis patients whose blood meets other safety criteria has been used for transfusion in Canada since 1991.[47] Subsidies from the

Canadian government for blood banking centers may have eliminated a non-altruistic financial motivation for blood donation.

Experience in Wales and Sweden

Hemochromatosis patients whose blood meet safety standards is used for transfusion. Because these individuals had iron overload, they are allowed to donate blood more frequently than other volunteer donors.[48,49]

Experience in New Zealand

In 2000, there was no national blood banking standard about transfusing the blood from hemochromatosis patients. Investigators in Auckland reported that, in Christchurch, blood donated by healthy hemochromatosis patients was used for transfusion. Blood from hemochromatosis patients in Auckland was not used for transfusion. Investigators studying the number of units of blood removed each year from known hemochromatosis patients recommended that a national blood banking policy be developed to allow transfusion of the blood that is donated by healthy hemochromatosis patients if the blood meets all safety standards.[50]

Experience in France

Before 2001, blood from known hemochromatosis homozygotes or heterozygotes was not used for transfusion. On January 31, 2001 a multidisciplinary working group of investigators met to consider changes in this policy. The members of the working group recommended that people with one or more hemochromatosis genes be allowed to donate blood if they had a normal serum ferritin concentration and did not have liver disease, cardiomyopathy, diabetes, infection by hepatitis viruses, *Yersinia* infection, or other signs of illness. These healthy people were referred to as having hemochromatosis stage 0 or stage 1. The members of the working group recommended continuation of the policy not to allow blood donation by hemochromatosis patients who had an elevated serum ferritin concentration or evidence of iron-associated organ injury or illness. These patients were classified as have hemochromatosis stage 2 or stage 3.[51]

Experience in the US

Before 1980, local blood banks in some states used the blood from healthy hemochromatosis patients for transfusion if the blood tested negative for known transmissible infections. Later, the Food and Drug Administration required blood banks to label such units of blood, indicating that the blood was donated by an individual who had hemochromatosis or some other non-transmissible disorder (Title 21, Code of Federal Regulations, Part 640.3d). This labeling required the physician who prescribed blood transfusion to discuss the meaning of hemochromatosis with a potential recipient, and that there was no identified transmissible risk to the recipient. This added a requirement of time and a measure of complexity that was confusing or worrisome to sick potential recipients of the labeled hemochromatosis blood. Some patients asked, "If the blood is so safe, why does the label say it was donated by someone who has a disease that I have never heard about?" The net effect for some physicians was that the requirement of extra time and the complexity of the discussion were unacceptable. Accordingly, some physicians refused to use the labeled blood for his/her patients, even when the physicians believed that the blood was safe.

In April 1999, the US Public Health Service Advisory Committee on Blood Safety and Availability recommended that the Department of Health and Human Services develop policies that would eliminate any incentives for hemochromatosis patients to donate blood, and to develop policies that allowed transfusion of this blood if it met all safety standards. In August 2001, the US Food and Drug Administration (in a publication that included the US Department of Health and Human Services and the Center for Biologics Evaluation and Research) issued a policy of variances for collecting blood from hemochromatosis donors that accomplished at least four major aims: (1) the policy allowed the transfusion of blood from individuals with hemochromatosis if the blood met all known safety standards; (2) the policy eliminated financial incentives for hemochromatosis patients to falsify responses to blood bank questions about health status and about possible behaviors that increased the risk of transmissible infections; (3) the policy indicated blood banks that accepted the blood for transfusion from any hemochromatosis patient were required to provide phlebotomy therapy without charge to all hemochromatosis patients who came to the blood bank; and (4) the policy authorized a blood bank to perform phlebotomy therapy according to the prescribing physician's written orders about frequency and hematocrit/hemoglobin limits (Title 21, Code of Federal Regulations, Section 640.120 (21 CFR 640.120).

Effect of blood donation on iron stores before hemochromatosis diagnosis

In 2001, a study was published about the effect on iron overload of blood donation prior to the diagnosis of hemochromatosis. The data were obtained during a questionnaire survey of 1089 hemochromatosis patients and from 124 homozygotes who were discovered during routine medical care. Overall, less than half of the patients had donated any blood before they were found to have hemochromatosis. Only 5% of patients had donated 20 or more units of blood prior to their diagnosis of hemochromatosis. The authors concluded that the number of units of blood donated before diagnosis of hemochromatosis did not have a major effect on the amount of iron overload in these groups of patients.[52] Any individual who has donated many units of blood before the diagnosis of hemochromatosis may not require many phlebotomies to deplete his/her mobilizable iron stores, although this is not invariably the case.

Safety of blood from hemochromatosis donors

A 2001 study reported data about transfusion-transmissible viral infections in hemochromatosis blood donors and other donors. Questionnaires were mailed to 92 981 blood donors from eight blood centers in the US. Of the 52 650 donors who returned a questionnaire, 197 (0.4%) indicated that they had hemochromatosis. The hemochromatosis patients donated an average of about 3 units of blood per year; other respondents reported donating about 2 units per year. The authors of the study reported that the prevalence of transfusion-transmissible viral infections was not significantly higher among hemochromatosis donors (1.3%) than other donors (1.6%).[53]

Experts in the Department of Transfusion Medicine at the National Institutes of Health in Bethesda studied hemochromatosis patients as blood donors. They evaluated 1402 units of blood from hemochromatosis donors and concluded that, if these individuals do not have serologic results necessitating deferral, they did not pose a health risk for recipients. The authors indicated that healthy hemochromatosis donors could augment the blood supply significantly.[54] After 27 months of study, blood from hemochromatosis donors represented 14% of all blood donations at the study institution. In another report,

an ethicist at the Centre for Environmental Philosophy and Bioethics of the University of Ghent, Belgium concluded that hemochromatosis patients can be free, voluntary, altruistic blood donors if they do not request any benefit other than blood removal.[46]

Proportion of blood donations contributed by hemochromatosis patients

In a prospective intramural study at the US National Institutes of Health, hemochromatosis patients were encouraged to enter their donor pool as repeat donors. The hemochromatosis subjects kept 89% of their donor appointments compared with 75% for other donors. The investigators determined that, after 27 months, hemochromatosis subjects were contributing 14% of the center's blood donations. They also concluded that blood from hemochromatosis donors that met all known safety standards did not pose increased risk to recipients.[54] These authors demonstrated that it is possible to recruit and retain hemochromatosis donors. This high percentage could apply to other blood centers whose staff develop a sustained interest and effort to recruit hemochromatosis patients to join and remain in the center's donor pool.

In centers that do not recruit hemochromatosis patients to donate blood, the number of blood donations from hemochromatosis patients represents a very small proportion of the total number of blood collections. In a report of the data compiled from 16 blood centers in different areas of the US, hemochromatosis patients donated only 0.4% of the total 1.67 million units of red blood cells. The percentage of usable units of red blood cells ranged from 0.18% to 0.8% in the 16 blood centers.[55] In a questionnaire survey of donors from eight US blood centers, 0.8% of the 52 650 donors who responded reported that they had hemochromatosis.[53]

Government-mandated food fortification with iron
Rationale for iron fortification of foods

It is estimated that more than one billion people worldwide have anemia; its predominant cause is iron deficiency.[56–58] The prevalence of anemia varies greatly within a population and is much higher with the increased physiological iron requirements associated with growth, menstruation, and childbearing.[56]

Iron-deficiency anemia has significant health effects, especially impairment in cognitive performance in infants and toddlers.[56–58] The major strategy to control iron deficiency in a population has been to increase iron intake either by providing medicinal iron (supplementation) or by increasing the iron content of the diet (fortification).[56–59] Iron supplementation has had little success due to distribution problems and poor compliance in the targeted population.[56,57] Consequently, most authorities in the field of iron nutrition advocate iron fortification as the optimal long-term approach for controlling iron deficiency. There are two broad categories of iron fortification: universal fortification, in which iron is added to a staple food with the goal of reaching all segments of the population; and targeted fortification, in which iron is added to food items that are consumed predominantly by individuals at greatest risk of iron deficiency.[56–59] Universal fortification of wheat flour with iron began in the US in the early 1940s.[56,57] In the 1970s, widespread targeted iron fortification of infant formula and weaning foods was implemented in the US.[56]

Food iron bioavailability

The two types of dietary iron, heme iron and non-heme iron, differ markedly in their bioavailability for absorption and thus their impact on body iron status.[56] Heme iron is more bioavailable than non-heme iron, and it represents 40%–50% of the iron in beef and somewhat less in poultry and fish.[56] Heme iron is absorbed as an intact porphyrin complex and is therefore unaffected by foods consumed in the same meal. Because its absorption is approximately threefold greater than non-heme iron, it can contribute as much as 30% of the iron absorbed from the diet in industrialized countries, even though it usually represents only 10%–15% of dietary iron.[56]

Absorption of the large remaining fraction of non-heme food iron is highly variable and therefore most studies of food iron bioavailability have focused on this component. Although many factors have been reported to influence non-heme iron absorption,[60,61] only a few are important. The major facilitators are ascorbic acid and tissue foods such as meat, fish, and poultry.[56] The main inhibitors are phytic acid in cereals and grains, and phenolic compounds in tea, coffee, legumes, and some vegetables.[56]

Fortification iron

Ideally, fortification iron should be fully soluble and therefore absorbed to the same extent as the native non-heme iron in the diet.[56] Ferrous sulfate is the most available iron source in widespread use and is consequently used as the reference compound by which the absorption of other forms of fortification iron is judged.[56]

There are two main categories of iron compounds currently used for fortification. The first category is elemental iron: reduced iron; electrolytic iron; and carbonyl iron.[56] These are ground into powders of varying particle size that is a key determinant of bioavailability. The second major category of commercially-available iron compounds is iron salts. The more soluble forms are ferrous sulfate, ferrous gluconate, ferrous fumarate, and ferric ammonium citrate, all of which are absorbed to the same extent as dietary non-heme iron.[56] The less soluble iron salts contain phosphate and include ferric orthophosphate, sodium iron pyrophosphate, and ferric pyrophosphate. These relatively inert forms of iron are often used to fortify breakfast cereals and infant foods.[56]

Another compound used for fortification is sodium iron (III) ethylenediaminetetraacetic acid (EDTA) which is both soluble and highly stable.[62] Therefore, EDTA is particularly useful for fortifying foods that require prolonged storage or are prepared at high temperature. An important aspect of iron-EDTA is its unique absorption property when given with food. With a meal that strongly inhibits non-heme iron absorption, iron–EDTA is absorbed two-three times more efficiently than iron as ferrous sulfate.[62]

Food vehicles for iron fortification

Universal fortification with iron is designed to reach all segments of the population, irrespective of iron status. By adding iron to a staple food (e.g. wheat, maize, rice), delivery of the iron is roughly proportional to caloric intake.[56] The addition of iron to wheat flour that was introduced in the US, Canada, and the UK in the early 1940s is sometimes referred to as enrichment, rather than fortification.[56] Enrichment indicates that sufficient iron is added to compensate for that lost in the milling of wheat, rather than to increase substantially the native iron content of unmilled wheat. During the milling process of wheat flour in industrialized countries, the native iron content of whole wheat is decreased from about 36 ppm to 12 ppm of iron for unenriched wheat flour.[56] After fortification with a mandatory 44 ppm of iron, wheat flour in the US contains about 56 ppm of iron. Ferrous sulfate is the preferred iron source when iron is added at bakeries, and allows storage of the product for up to 3 months. Elemental iron powders are used when storage requirements are longer.[56] Other staple foods have been used for universal iron fortification, including common salt in India, sugar in Guatemala, and condiments such as soy sauce in China, curry powder in South Africa, and fish sauce in Thailand and Vietnam.[56–59]

Targeted fortification is an effective means of delivering iron to groups at high risk of developing iron deficiency. In most industrialized countries, infant formula and weaning foods are routinely fortified with iron.[56,57] Although not strictly targeted fortification, breakfast cereals are usually fortified with iron and other minerals and vitamins. Several breakfast cereals contain 100% of the recommended dietary allowance (RDA) for iron in a single serving.[56]

Criteria for iron deficiency and iron-deficiency anemia

The prevalence of iron deficiency depends on the criteria used to define it. It is common practice to define two levels of severity depending on the presence or absence of anemia.[56] The milder form, often called iron deficiency without anemia, will be referred to simply as iron deficiency. The earliest laboratory evidence of iron deficiency is a serum ferritin concentration of less than $12 \mu g/L$, which reflects the depletion of iron stores.[56] Most investigators require additional laboratory criteria to identify iron deficiency such as low serum iron concentration, low transferrin saturation, elevated red cell distribution width, low mean corpuscular volume, or elevated free erythrocyte protoporphyrin (FEP).[56] For example, in the National Health and Nutrition Examination Survey (NHANES) III (1988–1994), the definition of iron deficiency was based on three laboratory tests of iron status: transferrin saturation; FEP; and serum ferritin concentration.[63] An individual was considered to be iron-deficient if two or more of these measurements were abnormal.

In assessing the impact of iron fortification, it is preferable to use the prevalence of iron-deficiency anemia, because adverse effects due to iron deficiency have rarely been detected in the absence of anemia.[56]

Most studies use the WHO criteria of anemia: a hemoglobin concentration of less than $130 g/L$ in men, less than $120 g/dL$ in women, and less than $110 g/L$ during pregnancy.[56] In the NHANES III survey, iron-deficiency anemia was defined as anemia combined with at least two abnormal iron measurements indicating deficiency (as listed above).

The level of serum transferrin receptor (sTfR) is also useful in assessing the prevalence of iron-deficiency anemia.[56,64,65] The concentration of sTfR is proportional to the total body mass of tissue TfR and is therefore elevated with either enhanced erythropoiesis or tissue iron deficiency.[64,65] An important additional advantage of using sTfR is that it is not affected by chronic inflammation and can therefore distinguish iron-deficiency anemia from the anemia of chronic disease.[56,64,65]

Efficacy of targeted iron fortification

One of the important advances in iron nutrition in most industrialized countries has been the virtual elimination of iron deficiency in infants and preschool children by using targeted fortification.[56] This occurred in the US in response to recommendations by the Committee on Nutrition of the American Academy of Pediatrics first published in 1969.[66] It is currently recommended that all formula-fed infants should receive an iron-fortified formula until 12 months of age, and that breast-fed infants should be given an iron-fortified formula if weaned before 12 months.[67] Iron-fortified infant cereal is recommended when infants begin solid foods. These recommendations have been widely implemented and have resulted in a marked reduction in the prevalence of iron-deficiency anemia in this highly susceptible age group.[56] For example, anemia in middle-class American children surveyed between 1982 and 1987 was almost eliminated during the prior decade. These findings testify to the effectiveness of delivering adequate amounts of fortification iron to a population in need.

Efficacy of universal fortification

Universal iron fortification of wheat flour and bakery products in the US is thought to have contributed to a current low prevalence of iron deficiency anemia.[56,57] It is difficult to quantify precisely its contribution because the program began in the 1940s before iron measures were determined in the population.

The results of the NHANES III survey indicate that iron-deficiency anemia has been almost eliminated in the US, except in toddlers (3%) and women of childbearing age (5%).[56] National fortification programs that have begun more recently in developing countries demonstrate that universal iron fortification can have a substantial impact on the prevalence of iron deficiency and iron-deficiency anemia.[56–59] In contrast, the withdrawal of iron fortification of flour in Sweden in 1994 is thought to be responsible for an increase in iron deficiency in adolescent girls from 39% to 50%.[68]

Effect of iron fortification in hemochromatosis

The fundamental disturbance in iron metabolism in hemochromatosis is excessive absorption of dietary iron (Chapters 2, 8). Studies in patients with *HFE* hemochromatosis suggest that the rate of iron accumulation in persons with hemochromatosis may be faster with iron fortification, and that clinical manifestations may occur at a younger age.[69–71] These reports suggest that accelerated evolution of clinical disease may be directly proportional to the amount of fortification iron added. If dietary iron intake is increased by 20% with fortification, the time required to develop clinical manifestations in hemochromatosis subjects is predicted to be shortened by about 20%.[56] Consistent with these findings, the interval between phlebotomies was lengthened in hemochromatosis patients after iron fortification of flour was stopped in Sweden.[72] It is widely recognized from population studies that *HFE* C282Y homozygosity has incomplete phenotypic and clinical penetrance, even with iron fortification programs in place (Chapters 8, 37).

The purpose of iron fortification is to reduce the prevalence of iron-deficiency anemia. NHANES III results indicate that this goal has been largely achieved in the US, except in 5% of women of childbearing ape and 3% of toddlers.[56] Universal iron fortification is thought to be mainly responsible for this success, but other factors such as the widespread use of iron supplements and improved bioavailability of dietary iron also have played an important role. It is unlikely that any further increase in the level of iron fortification will influence the prevalence of iron-deficiency anemia in segments of the population where it persists.[56] Further reduction in iron-deficiency anemia in toddlers is probably better

achieved by modifying or enhancing the fortification of infant foods. The residual iron-deficiency anemia in menstruating women is primarily due to excessive menstrual blood loss and could be controlled more effectively by iron supplementation or targeting fortified foods to susceptible individuals.

References

1. Hall MA, McEwen JE, Barton JC, *et al.* Concerns in a primary care population about genetic discrimination by insurers. *Genet Med* 2005; **7**: 311–16.

2. Hudson KL. Prohibiting genetic discrimination. *N Engl J Med* 2007; **356**: 2021–3.

3. Barton JC, Felitti VJ, Lee P, Beutler E. Characteristics of *HFE* C282Y homozygotes younger than age 30 years. *Acta Haematol* 2004; **112**: 219–21.

4. Matloff ET, Shappell H, Brierley K, Bernhardt BA, McKinnon W, Peshkin BN. What would you do? Specialists' perspectives on cancer genetic testing, prophylactic surgery, and insurance discrimination. *J Clin Oncol* 2000; **18**: 2484–92.

5. Power TE, Adams PC, Barton JC, *et al.* Psychosocial impact of genetic testing for hemochromatosis in the HEIRS Study: a comparison of participants recruited in Canada and in the United States. *Genet Test* 2007; **11**: 55–64.

6. Barton JC, Acton RT, Leiendecker-Foster C, *et al.* *HFE* C282Y homozygotes aged 25–29 years at HEIRS Study initial screening. *Genet Test* 2007; **11**: 269–75.

7. Raszeja-Wyszomirska J, Kurzawski G, Suchy J, Zawada I, Lubinski J, Milkiewicz P. Frequency of mutations related to hereditary haemochromatosis in northwestern Poland. *J Appl Genet* 2008; **49**: 105–7.

8. Zorai A, Harteveld CL, Rachdi R, *et al.* Frequency and spectrum of hemochromatosis mutations in Tunisia. *Hematol J* 2003; **4**: 433–5.

9. Girouard J, Giguere Y, Delage R, Rousseau F. Prevalence of *HFE* gene C282Y and H63D mutations in a French-Canadian population of neonates and in referred patients. *Hum Mol Genet* 2002; **11**: 185–9.

10. Merryweather-Clarke AT, Simonsen H, Shearman JD, Pointon JJ, Norgaard-Pedersen B, Robson KJ. A retrospective anonymous pilot study in screening newborns for *HFE* mutations in Scandinavian populations. *Hum Mutat* 1999; **13**: 154–9.

11. Barton JC, Conrad ME, Nuby S, Harrison L. Effects of iron on the absorption and retention of lead. *J Lab Clin Med* 1978; **92**: 536–47.

12. Barton JC, Patton MA, Edwards CQ, *et al.* Blood lead concentrations in hereditary hemochromatosis. *J Lab Clin Med* 1994; **124**: 193–8.

13. Hopkins MR, Ettinger AS, Hernandez-Avila M, *et al.* Variants in iron metabolism genes predict higher blood lead levels in young children. *Environ Health Perspect* 2008; **116**: 1261–6.

14. Jones RL, Homa DM, Meyer PA, et al. Trends in blood lead levels and blood lead testing among US children aged 1 to 5 years, 1988–2004. *Pediatrics* 2009; **123**: e376–85.

15. Wengrovitz AM, Brown MJ. Recommendations for blood lead screening of Medicaid-eligible children aged 1–5 years: an updated approach to targeting a group at high risk. *MMWR Recomm Rep* 2009; **58**: 1–11.

16. Cadman D, Chambers L, Feldman W, Sackett D. Assessing the effectiveness of community screening programs. *JAMA* 1984; **251**: 1580–5.

17. Qaseem A, Aronson M, Fitterman N, Snow V, Weiss KB, Owens D K. Screening for hereditary hemochromatosis: a clinical practice guideline from the American College of Physicians. *Ann Intern Med* 2005; **143**: 517–21.

18. Whitlock EP, Garlitz BA, Harris EL, Beil TL, Smith PR. Screening for hereditary hemochromatosis: a systematic review for the US Preventive Services Task Force. *Ann Intern Med* 2006; **145**: 209–23.

19. Beutler E, Felitti VJ, Koziol JA, Ho NJ, Gelbart T. Penetrance of 845G→A (C282Y) *HFE* hereditary haemochromatosis mutation in the USA. *Lancet* 2002; **359**: 211–18.

20. Adams PC. Population screening for hemochromatosis—are we finding people with a disease or a biochemical curiosity? *Semin Gastrointest Dis* 2002; **13**: 89–94.

21. Jacobs EM, Hendriks JC, Marx JJ, *et al.* Morbidity and mortality in first-degree relatives of C282Y homozygous probands with clinically detected haemochromatosis compared with the general population: the HEmochromatosis FAmily Study (HEFAS). *Neth J Med* 2007; **65**: 425–33.

22. Adams PC, Reboussin DM, Barton JC, *et al.* Hemochromatosis and iron-overload screening in a racially diverse population. *N Engl J Med* 2005; **352**: 1769–78.

23. Allen KJ, Gurrin LC, Constantine CC, *et al.* Iron-overload-related disease in *HFE* hereditary hemochromatosis. *N Engl J Med* 2008; **358**: 221–30.

24. Hall MA, Barton JC, Adams PC, *et al.* Genetic screening for iron overload: No evidence of discrimination at 1 year. *J Fam Pract* 2007; **56**: 829–34.

25. Jazwinska EC, Cullen LM, Busfield F, *et al.* Haemochromatosis and *HLA-H*. *Nat Genet* 1996; **14**: 249–51.

26. Jouanolle AM, Fergelot P, Gandon G, Yaouanq J, Le Gall JY, David V. A candidate gene for hemochromatosis: frequency of the C282Y and H63D mutations. *Hum Genet* 1997; **100**: 544–7.

27. Adams PC. Intrafamilial variation in hereditary hemochromatosis. *Dig Dis Sci* 1992; **37**: 361–3.

28. Bulaj ZJ, Ajioka RS, Phillips JD, *et al.* Disease-related conditions in relatives of patients with hemochromatosis. *N Engl J Med* 2000; **343**: 1529–35.

29. Acton RT, Harman L. Genetic counseling for hemochromatosis. In: Barton JC, Edwards CQ, eds. *Hemochromatosis: Genetics, Pathophysiology, Diagnosis and Treatment.* Cambridge, Cambridge University Press. 2000; 574–82.

30. Bacon BR. Diagnosis and management of hemochromatosis. *Gastroenterology* 1997; **113**: 995–9.

31. Assy N, Adams PC. Predictive value of family history in diagnosis of hereditary hemochromatosis. *Dig Dis Sci* 1997; **42**: 1312–15.

32. Barton JC, Rothenberg BE, Bertoli LF, Acton RT. Diagnosis of hemochromatosis in family members of probands: a comparison of phenotyping and *HFE* genotyping. *Genet Med* 1999; **1**: 89–93.

33. Moirand R, Adams PC, Bicheler V, Brissot P, Deugnier Y. Clinical features of genetic hemochromatosis in women compared with men. *Ann Intern Med* 1997; **127**: 105–10.

34. Barton EH, Barton JC, Hollowell WW, Acton RT. Countries of ancestry reported by hemochromatosis probands and control subjects in central Alabama. *Ethn Dis* 2004; **14**: 73–81.

35. Beutler E, Gelbart T. HLA-H mutations in the Ashkenazi Jewish population. *Blood Cells Mol Dis* 1997; **23**: 95–8.

36. Barton JC, Rothenberg BE, Bertoli LF, Acton RT. Diagnosis of hemochromatosis in family members of probands: a comparison of phenotyping and *HFE* genotyping. *Genet Med* 1999; **1**: 89–93.

37. Adams PC, Walker AP, Acton RT. A primer for predicting risk of disease in *HFE*-linked hemochromatosis. *Genet Test* 2001; **5**: 311–16.

38. Andrews LB, Fullarton JE, Holtzman NA, Motulsky AG. *Assessing Genetic risks. Implications for Health and Social Policy.* Washington, National Academy Press, 1994.

39. Holtzman NA, Watson MS. Promoting safe and effective genetic testing in the United States. Final report of the Task Force on Genetic Testing. *J Child Fam Nurs* 1999; **2**: 388–90.

40. Shaheen NJ, Lawrence LB, Bacon BR, *et al.* Insurance, employment, and psychosocial consequences of a diagnosis of hereditary hemochromatosis in subjects without end-organ damage. *Am J Gastroenterol* 2003; **98**: 1175–80.

41. Niederau C, Fischer R, Purschel A, Stremmel W, Haussinger D, Strohmeyer G. Long-term survival in patients with hereditary hemochromatosis. *Gastroenterology* 1996; **110**: 1107–19.

42. Witte DL, Crosby WH, Edwards CQ, Fairbanks VF, Mitros FA. Practice guideline development task force of the College of American Pathologists. Hereditary hemochromatosis. *Clin Chim Acta* 1996; **245**: 139–200.

43. Alter HJ, Holland PV, Purcell RH, *et al.* Post-transfusion hepatitis after exclusion of commercial and hepatitis-B antigen-positive donors. *Ann Intern Med* 1972; **77**: 691–9.

44. McDonnell SM, Grindon AJ, Preston BL, Barton JC, Edwards CQ, Adams PC. A survey of phlebotomy among persons with hemochromatosis. *Transfusion* 1999; **39**: 651–6.

45. Pennings G. Demanding pure motives for donation: the moral acceptability of blood donations by haemochromatosis patients. *J Med Ethics* 2005; **31**: 69–72.

46. Munsterman KA, Grindon AJ, Sullivan MT, *et al.* Assessment of motivations for return donation among deferred blood donors. American Red Cross ARCNET Study Group. *Transfusion* 1998; **38**: 45–50.

47. Levstik M, Adams PC. Eligibility and exclusion of hemochromatosis patients as voluntary blood donors. *Can J Gastroenterol* 1998; **12**: 61–3.

48. Friedrich C. Blood donation by patients with hemochromatosis. *JAMA* 1993; **270**: 2928–9.

49. Worwood M, Darke C. Serum ferritin, blood donation, iron stores and haemochromatosis. *Transfus Med* 1993; **3**: 21–8.

50. Blacklock HA, Dewse M, Bollard C, Hudson P, Barnhill D, Jackson S. Blood donation by healthy individuals with haemochromatosis. *N Z Med J* 2000; **113**: 77–8.

51. Courtois F, Danic B. [Genetic hemochromatosis and blood donation.] *Ann Med Interne (Paris)* 2001; **152**: 452–4.

52. Barton JC, Preston BL, McDonnell SM, Rothenberg BE. Severity of iron overload in hemochromatosis: effect of volunteer blood donation before diagnosis. *Transfusion* 2001; **41**: 123–9.

53. Sanchez AM, Schreiber GB, Bethel J, *et al.* Prevalence, donation practices, and risk assessment of blood donors with hemochromatosis. *JAMA* 2001; **286**: 1475–81.

54. Leitman SF, Browning JN, Yau YY, *et al.* Hemochromatosis subjects as allogeneic blood donors: a prospective study. *Transfusion* 2003; **43**: 1538–44.

55. Newman B. Hemochromatosis blood donor programs: marginal for the red blood cell supply but potentially good for patient care. *Transfusion* 2004; **44**: 1535–7.

56. Cook JD. Effect of iron fortification of foods. In: Barton JC, Edwards CQ, eds. *Hemochromatosis: Genetics, Pathophysiology, Diagnosis and Treatment.* Cambridge, Cambridge University Press. 2000; 535–43.

57. Lynch SR. The impact of iron fortification on nutritional anaemia. *Best Pract Res Clin Haematol* 2005; **18**: 333–46.

58. Zimmermann MB, Hurrell RF. Nutritional iron deficiency. *Lancet* 2007; **370**: 511–20.

59. Huma N, Salim UR, Anjum FM, Murtaza MA, Sheikh MA. Food fortification strategy—preventing iron deficiency anemia: a review. *Crit Rev Food Sci Nutr* 2007; **47**: 259–65.

60. Hallberg L. Bioavailability of dietary iron in man. *Annu Rev Nutr* 1981; **1**: 123–47.

61. Charlton RW, Bothwell TH. Iron absorption. *Annu Rev Med* 1983; **34**: 55–68.

62. MacPhail AP, Patel RC, Bothwell TH, Lamparelli RD. EDTA and the absorption of iron from food. *Am J Clin Nutr* 1994; **59**: 644–8.

63. Looker AC, Dallman PR, Carroll MD, Gunter EW, Johnson CL. Prevalence of iron deficiency in the United States. *JAMA* 1997; **277**: 973–6.

64. Cook JD, Skikne BS, Baynes RD. Serum transferrin receptor. *Annu Rev Med* 1993; **44**: 63–74.

65. Skikne BS, Flowers CH, Cook JD. Serum transferrin receptor: a quantitative measure of tissue iron deficiency. *Blood* 1990; **75**: 1870–6.

66. Iron balance and requirements in infancy. American Academy of Pediatrics. Committee on Nutrition. *Pediatrics* 1969; **43**: 142.

67. Iron fortification of infant formulas. American Academy of Pediatrics. Committee on Nutrition. *Pediatrics* 1999; **104**: 119–23.

68. Hallberg L, Hulthen L. Perspectives on iron absorption. *Blood Cells Mol Dis* 2002; **29**: 562–73.

69. Bothwell TH, Derman D, Bezwoda WR, Torrance JD, Charlton RW. Can iron fortification of flour cause damage to genetic susceptibles (idiopathic haemochromatosis and beta-thalassaemia major)? *Hum Genet Suppl* 1978; 131–7.

70. Bezwoda WR, Bothwell TH, Derman DP, MacPhail AP, Torrance JD, Charlton RW. Effect of diet on the rate of iron accumulation in idiopathic haemochromatosis. *S Afr Med J* 1981; **59**: 219–22.

71. Lynch SR, Skikne BS, Cook JD. Food iron absorption in idiopathic hemochromatosis. *Blood* 1989; **74**: 2187–93.

72. Olsson KS, Vaisanen M, Konar J, Bruce A. The effect of withdrawal of food iron fortification in Sweden as studied with phlebotomy in subjects with genetic hemochromatosis. *Eur J Clin Nutr* 1997; **51**: 782–6.

Chapter 39

Directions for future research

Scientific and clinical questions are usually answered partially and in increments. Most of the questions posed by Joseph Sheldon in 1935 and at the First International Conference on Hemochromatosis in 1987 have been answered. Since the discovery of *HFE* in 1996, there has been an explosion of research interest and reports related to iron biology and diseases of iron homeostasis. Some important "unknowns" presented in the conclusion of a major 2000 text devoted to hemochromatosis have been resolved. This section presents some of the important old and new questions for which answers are needed and changes in medical care delivery are predicted. These topics of interest include the biology and genetics of iron homeostasis and iron overload, hemochromatosis and iron overload screening, advances in diagnosis, complications of iron overload, and improvements in management.

Biology and genetics of iron homeostasis and iron overload

It is assumed that the common *HFE* mutations C282Y and H63D conferred some evolutionary advantage, but the mechanism(s) by which such a putative advantage(s) was mediated is not known. C282Y, found predominantly in western European Caucasians, is the most common known mutation that has a profound effect on iron homeostasis and phenotype. Many have inferred that this polymorphism fostered an iron procurement advantage for women during their reproductive years, although this is unproven. Related possibilities include the conjecture that C282Y either increases fertility of women (or men), or promotes greater survival of fetuses *in utero* or of newborns. Iron handling is important in defense against infection, and therefore C282Y could increase infection resistance. *HFE* is a major histocompatibility complex gene, some of which influence mate selection in mice and humans. Are persons with

C282Y more attractive mates than others? Is C282Y only a surrogate marker for a tightly linked but as yet unknown gene that confers a reproductive or survival advantage? Less attention has been paid to H63D than to C282Y, perhaps because H63D is unlikely to cause severe iron overload in any genotype configuration. Nonetheless, H63D is a cosmopolitan polymorphism, and therefore over centuries it may have exerted a subtle but nonetheless profound effect on iron, reproduction, or infection defense. Seeking explanations for the possible advantages of these *HFE* polymorphisms in human populations is likely to reveal answers that have clinical implications.

There is great variability in the expression of iron abnormalities among *HFE* C282Y homozygotes diagnosed in medical care or in screening programs, regardless of the phenotype criterion selected for evaluation. This phenomenon is readily apparent in kinships affected by diverse hemochromatosis or iron disorders, wherein siblings matched for pathogenic alleles of iron-related genes have disparate phenotypes. More than a decade of research has shown that mutations in other known genes that directly control iron absorption and metabolism account for little of the variability observed in the iron phenotype of C282Y homozygotes. Accordingly, most of the genetic basis for this phenotypic heterogeneity remains occult.

Phenotype variability in C282Y homozygotes is related in part to genetic causes for which better definitions are needed. Men with *HFE* hemochromatosis develop more severe iron overload, on average, than women. The array of human leukocyte antigen (HLA) haplotypes differs between men and women with C282Y homozygosity, and gender disparity of HLA alleles or haplotypes occurs in other chromosome 6p-linked disorders. Expression of some iron-related genes differs between male and female mice. It is predicted that research to identify "new" genes that affect iron homeostasis and animal experiments that analyze sex-related control of iron metabolism will explain much about clinical observations in humans with hemochromatosis.

A recent genome scan study detected several chromosome loci other than *HFE* that have a significant influence on serum iron measures. Further analyses to identify these putative iron-related genes are needed. There are significant heritability components of serum iron phenotype that are independent of sex, age, race, and *HFE* genotype. In addition, the rate of iron loss and food choices probably include heritable components, although little research has been devoted to these possibilities. Several studies report evidence that African iron overload has a heritable component, although the putative gene(s) or mutation(s) remains unknown.

Greater understanding of the mechanisms by which mutations in *HFE*, *TFR2*, and *HJV* alter hepcidin production in the liver is needed. The roles of Smad and bone morphogenetic protein (BMP) signaling need more study in humans with iron overload phenotypes. The gene that encodes human BMP6 occurs on chromosome 6p, and mutations in *BMP6* may cause hemochromatosis in humans (as they do in mice) or "modify" penetrance of *HFE* C282Y homozygosity. Recent observations concerning erythrocyte morphology and production rates in persons with *HFE* homozygosity indicate that ineffective erythropoiesis may stimulate iron absorption. Careful erythrokinetic evaluations of C282Y homozygotes hemochromatosis are needed to increase understanding of this phenomenon. Further study of growth/differentiation factor 15 and twisted gastrulation (TWSG1), possible "erythroid stores" stimulators of iron absorption and inhibitors of hepcidin, is indicated not only in *HFE* hemochromatosis but in diverse heritable anemias associated with enhanced iron absorption and iron overload.

Phenotype variability in C282Y homozygotes is related in part to acquired conditions or environmental circumstances. Some factors are reasonably well understood. Examples include the iron cost of pregnancy and lactation, blood donation, pathologic blood loss, iron content of and iron absorbability from individual foods, beverages, or meals, the effects of chronic ingestion of medicinal iron supplements, and iron malabsorption due to diverse conditions. Other factors are not well understood. Why is the proportion of Australian C282Y homozygotes with severe iron overload greater than that of Americans, Canadians, or Norwegians with the same genotype? What are the significant non-heritable components of serum iron phenotypes that are independent of sex, age, race, and *HFE* genotype? Investigations to identify such components are needed. Answers from such inquiries are likely to inform investigators and clinicians about the development of iron overload and iron deficiency.

Screening for hemochromatosis and iron overload

Targeted screening is indicated for high-risk individuals and family members of hemochromatosis and iron overload probands. European populations or derivative countries in which the prevalence of *HFE* C282Y is relatively high are broadly suitable for targeted screening. C282Y frequency is also relatively great in some Hispanic populations. A population subgroup that represents an ideal target for screening is men from these respective countries or subpopulations. What is the ideal age at which screening should occur? Few C282Y homozygotes develop injurious iron overload before the age of 30 years, but iron overload is common in clinically unselected homozygotes aged 40 years or more. Is it better to use phenotype or genotype testing? Should we routinely test entering college freshmen or military recruits? Should primary care physicians perform the screening? The design and performance characteristics of targeted screening strategies should be investigated and reported. Ethical, legal, and social implications should also be evaluated in targeted screening, including greater understanding of the reasons why relatively few American blood banks accept persons with hemochromatosis as donors.

Diagnosis of hemochromatosis and iron overload

New knowledge about hemochromatosis and iron overload gained during the last decade must be translated into practical improvements in diagnosis. Continuing, up-to-date education of physicians about hemochromatosis and iron overload will help them meet their obligations to understand basic diagnostic and treatment criteria for iron overload disorders, interpret results of DNA-based tests, and provide genetic counseling for patients and family members.

Once clinically available, measurements of plasma hepcidin could enhance the diagnosis of anemia of chronic disease, hyperferritinemia (a common clinical presentation of iron overload), and liver disorders. Multi-mutation "chip" analyses or gene scanning to identify deleterious mutations in genes such as *HJV*, *TFR2*, *SLC40A1*, *HAMP*, and *FTL1* were feasible in exploratory studies. Availability of such testing from reference laboratories on a routine clinical consultation basis would increase understanding of non-*HFE* iron overload proven by phenotype studies that are widely available. Discovering new iron-related genes could permit more specific testing to identify susceptibility alleles related to prognosis. Greater accessibility of calibrated magnetic resonance imaging devices and knowledgeable radiologists and technicians familiar with quantification of tissue iron levels would improve care of patients with transfusion iron overload associated with hemoglobinopathy, thalassemia, myelodysplasia, or other causes.

The results of multiethnic, multiracial screening programs in north America demonstrate that mean serum iron levels are significantly lower and that mean serum ferritin levels are significantly greater in blacks and Asians than in whites matched for age and sex. Research is needed to identify the genetic and acquired components of these phenotype differences. A relatively high proportion of American blacks have increased liver iron content. It is important to determine if this is due to transferrin or ferritin alleles, increased iron absorption, common deleterious alleles in genes that encode for mediators of inflammation, or to common liver disorders such as chronic viral hepatitis, alcoholism, or non-alcoholic fatty liver disease.

Complications of iron overload

The role of excess body iron as a co-factor and modulator of disease states other than "traditional" iron overload needs additional investigation. What is the "optimal" amount of body iron to provide enough reserve against deficiency but reduce the risks of disorders that may be augmented by the presence of iron? Further investigation of the impact of iron in contributing to hepatic injury in common liver disorders, e.g., non-alcoholic fatty liver disease, chronic viral hepatitis, and alcohol-induced liver disease is needed. Some patients with insulin resistance associated with diabetes mellitus have

hyperferritinemia. A few units of phlebotomy typically decreases their insulin resistance. It is essential to delineate the physiologic and molecular components of this effect.

A distinctive form of arthropathy occurs in some persons with *HFE*-related hemochromatosis; this complication is more prevalent among women than men. Arthropathy causes much morbidity and disability, but is not correlated with the severity of iron overload in many patients. Will some homozygotes identified at a young age and treated to prevent iron loading eventually develop arthropathy characteristic of hemochromatosis? Should studies of genetic markers of heritable forms of premature osteoarthritis and other forms of arthropathy with genetic components (e.g. rheumatoid arthritis) be undertaken in patients with hemochromatosis? Additional investigation is necessary to identify predisposing genetic or environmental factors. In non-*HFE* hemochromatosis, especially early age-of-onset iron overload syndromes, the molecular basis of arthropathy must also be defined. Mouse models of human iron overload disorders may be valuable in investigating the development of distinctive patterns and pathophysiology of joint disease due to iron overload.

Cirrhosis is the major target organ complication sustained by persons with severe primary iron overload syndromes. The risk of primary liver cancer is increased in persons with cirrhosis. Further development of non-invasive indicators of cirrhosis and protocols to monitor regression of fibrosis after therapy to achieve iron depletion would be valuable to patients and clinicians. Randomized studies are needed to determine if surveillance of patients with cirrhosis associated with iron overload using liver ultrasonography, alpha-fetoprotein levels, or other markers can improve early diagnosis and thereby decrease morbidity and mortality from primary liver cancer. The underlying oncogenic events in persons with iron overload disorders remain largely undefined, although it is generally acknowledged that chronic viral hepatitis or alcoholism poses additional risk for primary liver cancer. Molecular genetics and proteomic evaluations of primary liver cancers could lead to improvements in medical treatment and perhaps prevention measures. Clinical trials of new drugs such as multi-kinase inhibitors should compare outcomes of treating patients with primary liver cancer stratified by the presence or absence of iron overload disorders.

Treatment of iron overload

During the first 40 years after the description of phlebotomy therapy for iron overload, it was believed that most patients diagnosed to have hemochromatosis should be treated with phlebotomy to achieve iron depletion and prolong life. It is now understood that iron overload is not progressive in many persons with *HFE* hemochromatosis, although more longitudinal studies of untreated C282Y homozygotes would reveal valuable information. Which C282Y homozygotes need to undergo phlebotomy treatment and who not? Is maintenance phlebotomy always necessary? If not, in whom is it likely to be beneficial?

Randomized trials are needed to determine if phlebotomy treatment to maintain low iron burdens of patients with non-alcoholic fatty liver disease or chronic viral hepatitis will decrease risks of cirrhosis, liver failure, and hepatocellular cancer. Other studies are needed to determine characteristics of patients whose cirrhosis will or will not regress after phlebotomy to achieve iron depletion. Randomized clinical trials are also needed to determine if phlebotomy treatment of patients with diabetes mellitus and insulin resistance with iron overload can improve glucose control and forestall or prevent vascular, neurologic, or hepatic complications.

New oral iron chelation drugs could improve the management of transfusion iron overload, if the oral agents are less toxic and generally more acceptable to patients than deferoxamine. Such drugs must have substantial capability to remove cardiac iron in patients with severe thalassemia. At present, it appears likely that combination iron chelation therapy holds greater promise to decrease morbidity and mortality due to cardiomyopathy and liver damage due to iron overload than single-agent chelator management. If oral iron chelation therapy were sufficiently safe and effective, it could become an alternative to phlebotomy therapy in selected patients with *HFE* hemochromatosis or other forms of primary iron overload in whom phlebotomy was not feasible.

Modulation of divalent metal transporter-1 function by L-type calcium channel blockers such as nifedipine has emerged as a potential treatment of iron overload. In mice, these drugs appear to act by mobilizing iron from liver and other storage sites and enhancing its excretion but there are no reports of effects of calcium channel blockers on iron metabolism in humans. Recombinant hepcidin or a polypeptide analog could be used to inhibit iron absorption. It may be possible to design small molecules that will alter the expression or function of ferroportin, hemojuvelin, bone morphogenetic protein, hepcidin, or GDF-15. Such agents could be used to decrease iron absorption or mobilize iron from parenchymal cells.

Conclusions

Some revelations provoke the formulation of new questions and provide the basis for perfecting scientific understanding and patient management. It is probable that many of the foregoing questions will be answered within the next decade. This will increase understanding of the molecular basis of iron homeostasis and meet the needs of improving prevention, diagnosis, and treatment of iron overload.

Index

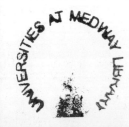